THE PROFESSIONAL PRACTICE OF NURSING ADMINISTRATION

THIRD EDITION

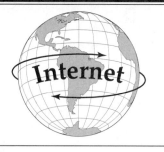

THE PROFESSIONAL PRACTICE OF NURSING ADMINISTRATION

THIRD EDITION

Lillian M. Simms, Ph.D., R.N., F.A.A.N.
Associate Professor Emeritus
School of Nursing
The University of Michigan
Ann Arbor, MI

Sylvia A. Price, Ph.D., R.N.
Professor (Retired)
College of Nursing
University of Tennessee
Memphis, TN

Naomi E. Ervin, Ph.D., R.N., C.S., F.A.A.N.
Associate Professor
Decker Chair in Community Health Nursing
Decker School of Nursing
Binghamton University
Binghamton, NY

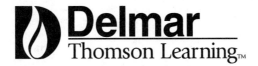

Africa • Australia • Canada • Denmark • Japan • Mexico • New Zealand • Philippines
Puerto Rico • Singapore • Spain • United Kingdom • United States

NOTICE TO THE READER

Delmar Staff:
Health Care Publishing Director: William Brottmiller
Acquisitions Editor: Cathy L. Esperti
Development Editor: Darcy M. Scelsi
Executive Marketing Manager: Dawn F. Gerrain
Project Editor: Christopher C. Leonard
Production Coordinator: James Zayicek
Art/Design Coordinator: Jay Purcell

COPYRIGHT © 2000
Delmar is a division of Thomson Learning. The Thomson Learning logo is a registered trademark used herein under license.

Printed in the United States of America
2 3 4 5 6 7 8 9 10 XXX 05 04 03 02 01 00

For more information, contact Delmar, 3 Columbia Circle, P.O. Box 15015, Albany, NY 12212-0515; or find us on the World Wide Web at http://www.delmar.com

Asia:
Thomson Learning
60 Albert Street, #15-01
Albert Complex
Singapore 189969
Tel: 65-336-6411
Fax: 65-336-7411
Japan:
Thomson Learning
Palaceside Building 5F
1-1-1 Hitotsubashi, Chiyoda-ku
Tokyo 100 0003 Japan
Tel: 813-5218-6544
Fax 813-5218-6551
Australia/New Zealand:
Nelson/Thomson Learning
102 Dodds Street
South Melbourne, Victoria 3205
Australia
Tel: 61-39-685-4111
Fax: 61-39-685-4199
UK/Europe/Middle East:
Thomson Learning
Berkshire House
168-173 High Holborn

London
WC1V 7AA United Kingdom
Tel: 44-171-497-1422
Fax: 44-171-497-1426
Thomas Nelson & Sons LTD
Nelson House
Mayfield Road
Walton-on-Thames
KT 12 5PL United Kingdom
Tel: 44-1932-252211
Fax: 44-1932-246574
Latin America:
Thomson Learning
Seneca, 53
Colonia Polanco
11560 Mexico D.F. Mexico
Tel: 525-281-2906
Fax: 525-281-2656
South Africa:
Thomson Learning
Zonnebloem Building
Constantia Square
526 Sixteenth Road
P.O. Box 2459
Halfway House, 1685

South Africa
Tel: 27-11-805-4819
Fax: 27-11-805-3648
Canada:
Nelson/Thomson Learning
1120 Birchmount Road
Scarborough, Ontario
Canada M1K 5G4
Tel: 416-752-9100
Fax: 416-752-8102
Spain:
Thomson Learning
Calle Magallanes, 25
28015-MADRID
ESPANA
Tel: 34-91-446-33-50
Fax: 34-91-445-62-18
International Headquarters:
Thomson Learning
International Division
290 Harbor Drive, 2nd Floor
Stamford, CT 06902-7477
Tel: 203-969-8700
Fax: 203-969-8751

Library of Congress Cataloging-in-Publication Data

Simms, Lillian M. (Lillian Margaret)
  The professional practice of nursing administration / Lillian M. Simms, Sylvia A. Price, Naomi E. Ervin. — 3rd ed.
    p. cm.
  Includes bibliographical references and index.
  ISBN 0-7668-0790-8
  1. Nursing—Administration. 2. Nursing services—Administration. 3. Nurse administrators. I. Price, Sylvia Anderson. II. Ervin, Naomi E. III. Title.
  [DNLM: 1. Nurse Administrators. 2. Administrative Personnel. WY 105 S592p 2000]
RT89.S58 2000
362.1'73'068—dc21   99-042118

CONTENTS

*To all professional nurses around the world who seek
to understand how to integrate their clinical and
management knowledge and skills wherever they practice*

CONTRIBUTORS

Yvonne Marie Abdoo, Ph.D., R.N.
Assistant Professor
Division of Nursing and Health Systems
The University of Michigan
School of Nursing
Ann Arbor, MI

Marcia D. Andersen, Ph.D., R.N., F.A.A.N., C.S.
President and Founder
Personalized Nursing Corporation and
    Well-Being Institute
Ann Arbor, MI

Eunice A. Bell, Ph.D., R.N., C.N.A.A.
President
Educational Consultation Services
Savannah, GA

Judith A. Bernhardt, M.S., R.N.
Medical Malpractice Consultant
Hospital Services of Louisiana, Inc.
Baton Rouge, LA

Catherine Buchanan, Ph.D., R.N.
Clinical Nurse Specialist
University of Michigan Medical Center
Ann Arbor, MI

Peter I. Buerhaus, Ph.D., R.N.
Director, Harvard Nursing Research Institute
Assistant Professor, Health Policy and Manage-
    ment
Harvard University
School of Public Health
Boston, MA

Sandra R. Byers, Ph.D., R.N., C.N.A.A.
Parish Nurse and Health & Wellness Director
Worthington Presbyterian Church
Worthington, OH

Harriet Van Ess Coeling, Ph.D., R.N.
Associate Professor
Kent State University
School of Nursing
Kent, OH

Anne F. Darga, R.N., M.S., C.S.-F.N.P.
President, Pursuit Health Formulas
Harbor Springs, MI

Ingrid A. Deininger, M.S., R.N.
Administrator and Founder
Individualized Home Nursing Care & Hospice
Ann Arbor, MI

Erica Dutton, R.N., M.S., C.S.
Director, Wellspring Counseling
Ann Arbor, MI

Paula R. Jaco, M.S.N., R.N.
Vice President of Nursing Services
Marshall Regional Medical Center
Marshall, TX

Katherine R. Jones, Ph.D., R.N., F.A.A.N.
Professor of Nursing
University of Colorado Health Sciences Center
School of Nursing
Denver, CO

Debra Keene, M.S.N., R.N.
Blue Cross Blue Shield of Tennessee
Memphis, TN

Marylane Wade Koch, M.S.N., R.N., C.N.A.A., C.P.H.Q.
Director, Community Health Outreach
Methodist Health Systems/University of
    Tennessee
Memphis, TN

Robert Koch, M.S.N., R.N., C.N.A.
Assistant Professor
Loewenburg School of Nursing
University of Memphis
Memphis, TN

Arlene Lowenstein, Ph.D., R.N.
Director, Nursing Program
MGH Institute of Health Professions
Boston, MA

Charlotte McDaniel, Ph.D., M.Ed., B.S.N., B.A., R.N., S.T.M.
Director, Contextual Education
Candler School of Theology
Faculty, Emory University
Atlanta, GA

Mary L. McHugh, Ph.D., R.N.
Associate Professor of Nursing
University of Colorado Health Sciences Center
School of Nursing
Denver, CO

Mary G. Nash, Ph.D., R.N., F.A.A.N.
Associate Executive Director and Chief Nursing
   Officer
The University of Alabama Hospital
Birmingham, AL

Phyllisis M. Ngin, Ph.D.
Lecturer
Melbourne Business School
Melbourne, Victoria
Australia

Karin Polifko-Harris, Ph.D., R.N.
Associate Professor
Christopher Newport University
Newport News, VA

Richard W. Redman, Ph.D., R.N.
Professor and Associate Dean, Academic Affairs
University of Colorado Health Sciences Center
School of Nursing
Denver, CO

Linda Roussel, D.S.N., R.N., C.N.A.
Louisiana State University Medical Center
School of Nursing
New Orleans, LA

Christine M. Smith, M.S., R.N.
Nurse Consultant for Education and Redesign
Home Business
Fitzroy Victoria
Australia

Annie J. Starr, Ph.D., R.N.
Assistant Professor
University of Western Ontario
London, Ontario
Canada

Judith Lloyd Storfjell, Ph.D., R.N.
President, Storfjell Associates & Asst. Prof.,
   U of Illinois-Chicago
Berrien Springs, MI

Ilene Warner, R.N.C., C.W.C.N., M.A., M.L.S.P., N.H.A.
Vice-President, Clinical Applications
Insight Telehealth Systems, Inc.
Valley Forge, PA

Ke-Ping Agnes Yang, Ph.D., R.N.
Nursing Supervisor and Associate Professor
Veteran's General Hospital—Taichung VACRS
Chung-Shan Medical College in Taiwan
Taichung, Taiwan
Republic of China

FOREWORD

The nursing profession is grappling with profound changes in health care delivery. The pace of change is rapid and accelerating. Technology is blossoming, new global, social and economic issues emerge, and health care research creates new opportunities and therapies to improve health status. There has been a rapid increase in integrated health care networks that rely on new economic models to deliver services.

Nursing care is an integral part of the health care delivery system. System changes profoundly affect how we as nurses use our expertise in practice today and what we will be able to do in the future. As the world moves into the new millennium, nurses have an exceptional opportunity to actively participate in determining the future direction of health care services. However, to make our presence known and to be effective in implementing our ideas, individual nurses have much to learn about working with health care administrators, other health care disciplines, consumers, and members of our own profession.

Simms, Price, and Ervin have been at the forefront of educating nurses to understand the dynamics of change in the health care system and to recognize opportunities for innovation and creativity in response to those dynamics. Improved delivery of health care services for patients, their families, communities, and society requires nurses to be proactive in designing and providing services. The effectiveness of implementing those services will also depend on establishing collaborative relationships with patients, other providers, and health care administrators in a variety of settings.

This book is a major contribution to the nursing literature that should be read by students and practicing nurses as well as nursing administrators. Through the Integrated Professional Nursing Administration Model, the authors provide an important framework that addresses the many issues facing nursing executives and practicing nurses in all settings where care is delivered. Their model is presented as a model of leadership, and nursing leadership is critical to enable us to make a difference in the evolving health care system.

As we move into the 21st century, new models of nursing leadership are emerging. Creativity and flexibility are required. Nursing leaders need the skill to evaluate outcomes so that the needs of society can be heard and addressed. Nursing leaders need to develop and improve nursing technologies. Nursing leaders need to understand cultures of their populations and their organizations. They need to be both intrapreneurial and entrepreneurial, working with and outside of health care organizations. The authors have addressed these issues in interesting and novel ways. They encourage changing the paradigms to embrace new ways of thinking and doing. These are skills that will be invaluable in years to come.

Arlene Lowenstein, R.N., Ph.D.
Professor and Director
Graduate Program in Nursing
MGH Institute of Health Professions

PREFACE

If nursing is to survive in the 21st century, the discipline must prepare flexible clinical experts who in the tradition of Nightingale and Wald are able to transform environments using leadership and management skills in addition to excellent clinical skills. This third edition firmly links community nursing with nursing in other settings of practice and addresses the need for learning new behaviors in creative learning environments that maximize human potential of nurses and consumers. The second edition was ahead of the times and now we hope the nursing world is ready for the third edition. This edition continues to blend emerging ideas from the organizational, behavioral, and management sciences with clinical nursing as it should be practiced.

This book has not been written as a traditional nursing text but rather as a book for students in professional development, leadership, or management courses in undergraduate and graduate nursing programs. Nurses in all clinical settings who wish to understand the principles of leadership, management, and personal empowerment will also find this text useful. A seminal work for nursing, this book offers a completely new look at nursing administration, which is rapidly becoming recognized as the professional level of nursing. The title of nurse executive can no longer be reserved for corporate level nurses who manage health care systems. Every professional nurse needs executive skills regardless of where they practice on this earth. As no other nursing text does, this book provides a clinical and management theoretical framework for professional nursing practice focusing on essential personal and group skills as paramount in the 21st century.

The computer has changed the way we think about our work, our organizations, and the way we practice our profession. New organizational structures are like cobwebs that can be built anywhere. To function in the new age, nurse executives must have an understanding of the knowledge and skills necessary to function in ever-changing organizations. Nursing administration is practiced everywhere and globalization of health care will soon be transformed to interplanetary health care.

Practicing in the global community demands that individual professionals take personal responsibility for lifelong learning.

If the computer has changed the way we think about working and communicating with each other, the realization that people can learn over the life span has changed the way we look at human resources and the development of effective work skills. Major emphasis has been placed, therefore, on human development and personal responsibility for quality care delivery. The work of nursing is cast in a new light, moving past the industrial models of the past. Work can be exciting, and nowhere is work more exciting than nursing care that is delivered in a wide variety of settings. The authors break loose from the traditional vision of past specialties of community health, medical-surgical, parent-child nursing and others to recognize that modern nursing administration must be practiced anywhere care is delivered: in the home, in the neighborhood, in the military, in acute care hospitals, long-term care facilities, walk-in centers, in the bush country of Africa, in rural areas, in sports arenas, and anywhere else imaginable. Our practice is not defined by the traditional divisions but rather by a vision of community that encompasses wherever humans live.

ORGANIZATION

This book provides a clinical and management theoretical framework for professional nursing administration. Chapters are organized in groups according to major themes that could pertain to any organizational structure. We want this book to be interesting and readable, to be read in its entirety or to be relished in chapters, or even pages, that have particular individual relevance. We want readers to gain new ideas about themselves and how they can view the changing world of work.

In essence, the book is delivered in sections that are relevant anywhere on earth or in space. In Part 1, the reader will move through a trajectory of a new vision of integrated practice, relevant clinical and management theories, a new look at organizations, and a soul-searching discussion of the nurse executive as a person in professional practice models. Part 2 presents a view of the context of nursing administrative practice with emphasis on community and rural settings. The importance of organizational and unit culture as important to the business of operationalizing nursing and creating learning environments responsive to innovation makes this part vital. Part 3 presents essential competencies in practice settings.

Part 4 addresses the facilitation of professional nursing administration practice in any setting. Ethical decision-making, mentoring, quality management, and nursing research are all portrayed as essential knowledge areas for the practicing nurse executive. Part 5 places major emphasis on building and managing resources in any setting. Resources include people, fiscal, and productivity abilities not usually addressed in administrative texts. Maximizing the creativity of workers in a non-zero sum-based power environment is encouraged through continual learning and functioning in flexible work groups. The chapters in Part 6 include the impact of changing demographics and managed care. Collective action and labor relations in this text extends the discussion of effective work groups to a total organizational environment.

The last section, Part 7, is truly unique. Building on the concept of quality in any environment, the section covers marketing nursing services through entrepreneurship and nursing economics and politics in a global economy. A new chapter on cultural diversity is considered essential content for any nurse executive and part of the development of executive skills. Clinical practice, teaching/ learning, research, and management must be integrated in the nurse executive role. For too long we have created great divisions in our profession by preparing special elites, the most recent being the nurse researcher. The authors believe we must bring these components together in one new revolutionary role, the nurse executive. Nursing research sits on shelves of numerous places, unused in practice because it is not seen as being relevant to practice. The clinical nurse manager must be one and the same with the researcher and teacher/learner if we are to bring wholeness to our work. The changing face of practice in the year 2000 is a fresh new chapter entitled Beyond Integrating Practices, Education and Research: The Next Steps.

NEW TO THIS EDITION

In addition to providing a superb understanding of leadership and management theories, this book includes new material on nursing as a business and provides examples of nursing businesses as described by the nurses who started them. Reality-based descriptions are provided by new age nurse executives who have started their own successful businesses. The theoretical frameworks for practice will assist the beginning student and skilled practitioner to more easily transfer across settings of practice. Coping is emphasized as an essential leadership attribute and is further developed in the chapter on humor, adding strength to the personal empowerment content introduced in the earlier editions. Frequently unrecognized in nursing texts, the impact of global aging on nursing practice patterns receives emphasis in a full chapter.

Assistive technology is addressed from the viewpoint of the practitioner and consumer with examples of application for personal living and nursing practice. Self-care is linked with cybermedicine and the importance of self-care management is introduced as a new and important concept. Managing a culturally diverse workforce is a new feature that strengthens the focus on building effective work groups.

This book is bold and not to be read by the faint hearted. We are proposing a totally new direction in nursing administration but one we believe will become the hallmark of professional nursing schools around the world. If we truly want to take our place in the "Health for All" agenda of the World Health Organization, we must take drastic steps in preparing our professionals so that we give them the tools they need to practice anywhere and develop nursing administration curricula that will appeal to diverse students with various backgrounds that could enrich our work.

The authors wish to give special acknowledgment to Richard J. Simms, Sr., who provided extensive assistance with the creation of illustrations throughout the text.

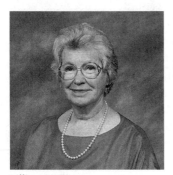

Lillian M. Simms

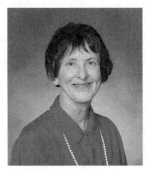

Sylvia A. Price

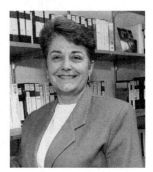

Naomi E. Ervin

PART
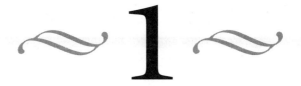
1

A Framework for the Practice of Nursing Administration

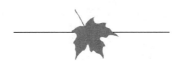

CHAPTER

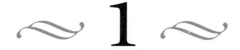

1

Integrated Professional Nursing Administration in Diverse Settings

Lillian M. Simms · Sylvia A. Price · Naomi E. Ervin

Much of what now seems basic in modern health care can be traced to pitched battles fought by Nightingale in the 19th century. *(Cohen, 1984, p. 128)*

Chapter Highlights

- Emergence of the nurse executive
- Professions and professionalism
- Professional practice disciplines
- Integrated professional nursing administration
- Operationalizing professional nursing administration

The purpose of this chapter is to present a conceptual framework for integrated professional nursing practice. Since the 1985 edition of this book, nursing administration has advanced rapidly. Modern professional nursing has become **nursing administration** and deliberations on the fit of administration with clinical nursing are beginning to cease. Professional nursing practice combines care provision and care coordination in the mature integrated discipline of nursing administration and the title of nurse administrator has changed to nurse executive in most progressive settings.

Leadership is no longer the bailiwick of a single person but is an essential skill for all professional nurses. In a paper presented at the Leadership Conference in Ann Arbor, Michigan, Dumas (1986) stated:

> We will fail in the preparation of leaders if the focus of our attention is limited to the roles of those whom we designate leaders. For we cannot fully comprehend the nature of leadership by focusing only on a single individual whom we would give the title of leader. This provides only half of the picture. The behavior and success of leaders is influenced as much by the needs, demands, and actions of followers as by the leader's own knowledge and skills, character and personality traits, needs and leadership style. Thus, preparation for leadership necessarily includes serious attention to the inextricable linkage between those whom we label leaders and those whom we label followers. (p. 4)

We have gone full circle in nursing education: from emphasizing clinical training, to integrating practice and education roles, to separating practice and education roles, to discovering management in other disciplines, to the preparation of elites in administration. We are at a crossroads and must pull it all together in schools of nursing administration or stand by and watch other health services administration programs take over (Simms, 1991).

The title of nurse executive can no longer be reserved for corporate-level nurses who manage health service systems and other health-related enterprises. Every professional nurse needs executive skills (Simms, 1991; Sovie, 1987). All professional nurses must be able to work with multiple groups. All professional nurses must develop team-building skills and knowledge essential to engage in participative management. Executive roles include head nurses, supervisors, coordinators, directors, chiefs, clinicians, managers, faculty members who manage courses, principal investigators and students, deans, vice presidents, presidents, and chief nurse executives under whatever title yet to be introduced. This does not mean there will not be senior nurse executives. These roles will change dramatically, however, and we can expect to see more visionary Nightingales and Walds who are unafraid to put theory and action together and who are unafraid to explore the development of new theories to nurture quality patient care.

EVOLUTION OF PROFESSIONAL NURSING ADMINISTRATION

Florence Nightingale (Figure 1.1) was an extraordinary person and the first nurse executive to appreciate the importance of linking care provision and care management (Simms, 1991). Modern nursing and hospital administration emerged from her work and she was never content to provide only nursing care without tackling the physicians and the environment to improve patient care. In addition to advancing the cause of medical reform, she helped to pioneer the revolutionary notion that phenomena could be objectively measured and subjected to

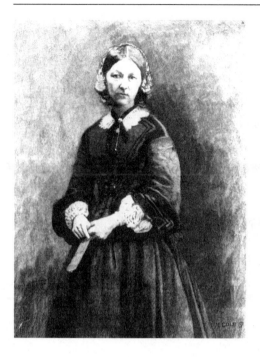

Figure 1.1 Florence Nightingale 1820–1910. Graphic by T. Cole se. Courtesy of National Library of Medicine, Bethesda, MD.

mathematical analysis. Although unaware of modern research methods, she fully understood the importance of collecting and analyzing data.

According to Cohen (1984), Nightingale not only instituted sanitary reforms in the hospitals at Scutari in 1854, she recognized the importance of medical statistics as a tool for improving medical care in military and civilian hospitals. She systematized the chaotic record-keeping practices and developed graphical representations of statistics. She invented polar-area charts, in which the statistic being represented is proportional to the area of a wedge in a circular diagram. These charts, called "coxcombs" in her writings, were used to dramatize the number of preventable deaths in the Crimean campaign (Figure 1.2). Her statistical charts and diagrams became an important part of the Royal Commission Report, a document that was widely distributed in Parliament, the government, and the army and had an important effect on the improvement of environmental conditions in hospitals.

Nightingale (Cohen, 1984) had little interest in the germ theory of disease and its implications for the treatment of contagious diseases. However, she was ahead of the times in her clinical efforts to improve ventilation, heating, sewage disposal, water supply, and kitchens. It is interesting to note that in modern times, we are again emphasizing environmental factors in disease prevention. And the major cause of death, as Nightingale noted, is still "diarrhea," which is related to poor sewage disposal, inadequate water supply, and malnutrition (Michigan League for Nursing, 1990). It is important to note that Nightingale managed patient care

DIAGRAM OF THE CAUSES OF MORTALITY
IN THE ARMY IN THE EAST

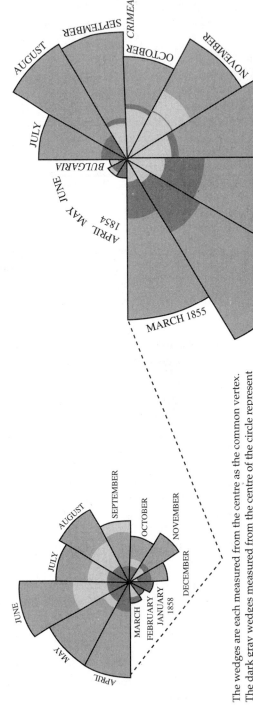

The wedges are each measured from the centre as the common vertex.
The dark gray wedges measured from the centre of the circle represent
area for area the deaths from Preventible or Mitigable Zymotic
diseases; the light gray wedges measured from the centre the deaths
from wounds, & the black wedges measured from the centre the
deaths from all other causes.

The black line across the light gray triangle in Nov. 1854 marks the
boundary of the deaths from all other causes during the month.

In October 1854, & April 1855, the black area coincides with the light gray;
in January & February 1855, the dark gray coincides with the black.

The entire areas may be compared by following the dark gray, the light
gray & the black lines enclosing them.

Figure 1.2 Florence Nightingales' coxcomb diagram. Reprinted with permission of the Houghton Library, Harvard University.

and the environment while at the same time she paid close attention to physicians and government policy makers, recognizing their influence on her freedom to practice.

Lillian Wald (Figure 1.3) also was a superb nurse executive (Kalisch & Kalisch, 1986; Wald, 1915). Wald was a public health nurse who graduated from New York Hospital School of Nursing in 1891. Unhappy with her scant nursing knowledge, she enrolled in Medical School at Woman's Medical College in New York. She used her nursing and entrepreneurial business skills to establish a nurses' settlement house in one of the slum sections of the Lower East Side. By 1909, the East Side Settlement moved to Henry Street and became the Henry Street Settlement. This very creative business included first-aid homes in densely populated sections of the city, small surgical offices for dressings, and a small obstetric service. The Henry Street Settlement grew in size from two nurses living on the top floor of a tenement house to a highly organized social enterprise with many departments. Wald and her staff provided care for inner city people and much of the care focused on that of immigrant women and children who could neither read nor write the English language. The world has the same needy populations today, and the need for nurse executives who can combine clinical and management skills is greater than ever.

In 1977, the World Health Organization (WHO) set a global objective "the attainment of Health for All citizens of the world by the year 2000" and in 1978, primary health care was introduced in Alma-Ata as the primary strategy to achieving this goal (Kiereini, 1989). Although progress has been made, many barriers

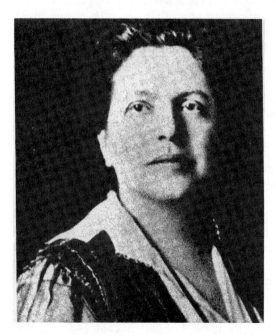

Figure 1.3 Lillian Wald. Photo Courtesy of the American Nurses Association.

still exist—perhaps the most important being the disease orientation of most health professionals, including nurses, and the relative incompetence among all health professionals to effectively develop and manage new health care systems that can meet current and emerging needs.

Maglacas (1988) forcefully states that nursing's choice for the 21st century is simple. We can participate in "health care for a few" or "health for all." This demands an integrated managerial process for national health development, stressing the concept of broad-based planning for health and development rather than for health services alone. It also places great emphasis on policy formulation, on the political and social processes in planning, and on strong links among clinical knowledge, planning, and management. Furthermore, says Maglacas, this implicitly requires reorientation of national health systems so that each system develops an appropriate structure for primary care. This has tremendous implications for the nursing profession wherein the struggle is still underway to keep at least 150 specialties alive and well despite tremendous overlap of services and competition for students. The artificial barriers that exist between nursing administration, community health, and medical-surgical nursing need to be removed. The Berlin Wall came down, why not the walls within nursing?

In many countries of the world, there is an oversupply, underuse, and unemployment of various categories of health personnel, physicians and dentists in particular. There is a tremendous shortage of nurses offering care. Health promotion as nursing's focus must go beyond responsibility for merely delivering medical care services. Nurses should be running nursing and health services around the world, not participating only in illness services. Holleran (1988) supports the need for appropriate nursing care in institutions as well. In any case, nurses must be better prepared to influence the quality of care provided in home, community, or institutional settings. Influence on health care must take place in the home, the workplace, and wherever humans abide. To accelerate the delivery of essential health services to the people of the world, particularly underserved populations, the transformation of the nursing profession is critical, and professional nurses must assume roles as leaders and active participants in these changes. All professional nurses must master the skills of visionary and strategic thinking to have an impact on the institutional and political forces that control health development.

Nursing services constitute a core function of health care delivery systems, and nurse executives conduct and control clinical nursing practice. As health care delivery systems change and as professional roles are redefined, effective nursing leadership is essential. Nurses participate in policy and decision-making, assume responsibility for managing nursing service and related activities, and work cooperatively with professionals from other health disciplines to ensure that quality client-centered care is administered. The acquisition and allocation of human and physical resources required to meet the goals of clinical care are facilitated by the nurse executive. For example, nurse executives generally influence the largest proportion of the budgets of hospitals and other health care institutions and make major decisions affecting the quality of patient care.

Because the health care industry is a human services endeavor, nurse executives must have a theoretical grounding in the behavioral sciences. It is also essential that they acquire both knowledge of administrative theory and awareness of changing concepts in the field. This knowledge will enable nurse executives to develop a conceptual framework for their nursing administrative practice in regional, national, and global environments.

DEFINITION OF A PROFESSION AND PROFESSIONALISM

Nursing is both a *profession* and a *professional practice discipline.* One must have comprehensive understanding of both terms to promote the highest level of nursing administrative practice. Many writers have discussed the history, development, definition, and application of the concept of a profession (Etzioni, 1969; Schein, 1972; Simms, 1991). Although these writers exhibit considerable diversity, there is consensus on the basic premise that *professionalism* involves autonomy, mastery of a body of knowledge, and a community of colleagues. The following are essential criteria of a *profession:*

1. Provides practical services that are vital to human and social welfare
2. Possesses a specialized body of knowledge and skills
3. Educates its practitioners in institutions of higher education
4. Attracts people who emphasize service over personal gain or self-interest and recognize their occupation as a long-term commitment
5. Formulates and controls its own policies and activities and has practitioners who function relatively autonomously in the performance of functions and activities
6. Has a code of ethics that is usually enforced by colleagues or through licensure examinations
7. Has a professional association that promotes and ensures quality of practice

It should be noted that profession is a social concept. The authority for nursing is based on a social contract that is derived from a complex social base. Donabedian (1976) states:

> There is a "social contract" between society and the professions. Under its terms, society grants the professions authority over functions vital to itself and permits them considerable autonomy in the conduct of their own affairs. In return, the professions are expected to act responsibly, always mindful of the public trust. Self-regulation to assure quality in performance is at the heart of this relationship. It is the authentic hallmark of a mature profession. (p. xiii)

Although there is some agreement as to what constitutes a professional nurse, much variation in opinion remains. One area of diversity involves the length and type of educational preparation necessary to qualify for the status of professional nurse. Another issue is whether nursing is really an occupation, rather than a profession, such as medicine, theology, and law. Writers who present this issue acknowledge that some nurses now perform expanded roles and functions, whereas others lack the educational basis for such a practice. Therefore, it is often difficult to distinguish among associate-degree, diploma, and baccalaureate-prepared nurses.

Nurses provide services in a variety of settings and assume more responsibility and accountability for the consequences of their decisions than in the past. This extension of nursing practice also involves increased collaboration with physicians and other health practitioners in the performance of their respective roles in the provision of health services. In collaborative practice, nurses emphasize psychosocial aspects of health care, coordination of patient care services, and advocacy of patient rights (Simms, Dalston, & Roberts, 1984).

As a profession, nursing has recognized the need to formulate a theoretical base for its practice and to articulate that base to others. Research is conducted in clinical areas to test nursing theories and related theories on which the practice of nursing is based. Similarly, research in the practice of nursing administration provides an empirical knowledge base for the various functions and responsibilities associated with nursing administration. Nursing must promote research to support the organizational restructuring of the delivery of nursing services, to define nurses' roles and responsibilities in interdisciplinary endeavors, and to provide a database for a systematic evaluation of the effectiveness of nursing.

Professional roles and functions of nursing are being reexamined and redesigned. The professional role of the practitioner of nursing has been expanded, leading to a repatterning of nursing education and emphasis on lifelong learning and career commitment to nursing. This trend has further emphasized the need for nurses who are creative and possess competencies to function in collegial relationships with other health care professionals.

NURSING PRACTICE

Nursing is concerned with human health and well-being. It involves the delivery of humanistic care to people to promote and maintain health, prevent illness, cure illness and restore health, and coordinate health care services to improve continuity of care.

Discussing the nature of nursing, Virginia Henderson (1961) states:

> The unique function of the nurse is to assist the individual, sick or well, in the performance of those activities contributing to health or his recovery (or to peaceful death) that he would perform unaided if he had the necessary strength, will, or knowledge. And to do this in such a way as to help him gain independence as rapidly as possible. This aspect of her work, this part of her function, she initiates and controls; of this she is master. In addition she helps the patient carry out the therapeutic plan as initiated by the physician. She also, as a member of a medical team, helps other members, as they in turn help her, to plan and carry out the total program whether it be for the improvement of health, or the recovery from illness, or support in death. (p. 42)

Nursing's Social Policy Statement (1995), first adopted by the American Nurses Association (ANA) in 1980, further specifies the social context, nature, and scope of nursing and the specializations in nursing.

Schlotfeldt (1981) emphasizes that nurses should search for a conceptual focus and definition of their profession that permit inclusion of phenomena related to human beings' seeking optimal health. She believes that a definition is needed that will help to establish nursing as a profession whose practitioners are responsible for the general health of human beings. Thus, her definition is, "Nursing is assessing and enhancing the general health status, health assets, and health potentials of human beings" (p. 298). This definition is unambiguous; focuses on nursing practice, education, and research; and conveys nurses' knowledge, practice, and scope of accountability. Because it does not encroach on the responsibilities of other helping professionals, it is conceptually appropriate and politically acceptable. Schlotfeldt emphasizes that nursing will become a recognized, learned profession and that nurses will provide essential services that will enhance the health and well-being of our society.

The nursing profession makes significant contributions to the evolution of a health-oriented system of care. Nursing practice has been health-oriented for over half of a century because of its focus on individuals as persons and on the family as the necessary unit of service (ANA, 1995).

Professional Practice Disciplines

Both the legal responsibility and the scope of nursing practice are regulated by the nursing practice acts of each state. For example, according to the State of Michigan Public Health Code (1997), the practice of nursing is "the systematic application of substantial specialized knowledge and skill derived from the biological, physical, and behavioral sciences to the care, treatment, counsel, and health teaching of individuals who are experiencing changes in the normal health processes or who require assistance in the maintenance of health and the prevention or management of illness, injury, or disability." This definition is appropriate for a professional practice discipline such as nursing. It conveys that nursing emphasizes human health and well-being, which are the concerns of nurses and determine the essential nature of nursing.

In 1981 Lysaught proposed an interactive model that included episodic (acute) care and distributive (nonacute) care. This conceptual scheme argued for variation in the educational patterning of preparatory and advanced studies to ensure the education of the variety as well as the number of nurses needed to implement a full range of client services. It provided for a commitment and career perspective that includes mobility and increments in responsibility, authority, and recognition. Furthermore, it provided for the integration of management skills that are so essential for the care coordination and action responsibilities of the modern nurse executive.

Although episodic and distributive terminology did not achieve common usage, the Lysaught interactive model laid the groundwork for nursing's later move toward integrated models with multidisciplinary linkages in diverse hospital and community settings. The Pew Health Professions Commission (1995) stresses that in many situations nursing has isolated its educational enterprise from the practice arena as it pursued a more professional basis in education and research. They state that this lack of linkage to the care delivery system is both a weakness and a strength. The weakness implies that nursing has been isolated somewhat from the clinical setting of teaching hospitals; whereas the advantage is that teaching hospitals are precarious places to reside these days. The Commission emphasizes that to correct this, nursing educators must forge new alliances with the emerging integrated health care systems. These alliances must address education, research, and patient care. Nursing faculty must understand the delivery of care in managed care settings, or they will not adequately exploit the great opportunity that now presents itself.

The Pew Commission recommends that new models of integration between education and the highly managed and integrated systems of care be developed to provide nurses with an appropriate educational and clinical practice opportunity and that model flexible work rules to encourage continual improvement, innovation, and health care work redesign.

Donaldson and Crowley (1978) distinguish between academic and professional disciplines. The purpose of academic disciplines is to know (and, for some, to apply that knowledge); therefore, they develop descriptive theories. Because the professional disciplines have an added component of service to people, their theories are both descriptive and prescriptive in nature. Whereas academic disciplines involve basic and applied research, professional disciplines also involve clinical research. Donaldson and Crowley (1978) caution that:

> The discipline, which is a body of knowledge, must not be confused with its associated practice realm, which embodies the processes of conducting research, giving service, and educating. Furthermore, some members of the profession must engage in enquiry that is not immediately applicable to current clinical practice. As a branch of knowledge, the discipline embodies more than the science of nursing and requires researchers who employ a variety of approaches from nursing's perspective. (p. 119)

Nurse researchers, clinicians, and educators use information from many disciplines and must understand or conduct research in these fields outside nursing.

Professional practice disciplines such as nursing, medicine, and dentistry are defined by the application of knowledge in relation to the health of clients. Although clinical practice is a major thrust of nursing, other components of professional practice must be considered, including research, education, and management. The four components, therefore, of integrated professional nursing administration are *(1)* clinical practice (application of knowledge), *(2)* research (development of knowledge), *(3)* education (learning and transmission of knowledge), and *(4)* management (care coordination and utilization of knowledge), as shown in Figure 1.4. These components need to be articulated and coordinated toward the full attainment of a professional practice discipline. The education component influences policy formation by administration, which in turn nurtures research-based clinical practice. Nurse executives are responsible for nursing practice, research, and education as they relate to professional nursing within an institution.

NEED FOR INTEGRATION OF SERVICE AND EDUCATION

Professional nursing practice emphasizes interdependence and collegial relationships between schools of nursing and clinical practice settings. The distinction between faculty and nursing service personnel in this relationship becomes diminished because all are participating in multiple aspects of practice. Practitioners in educational and clinical practice settings must be active participants at all

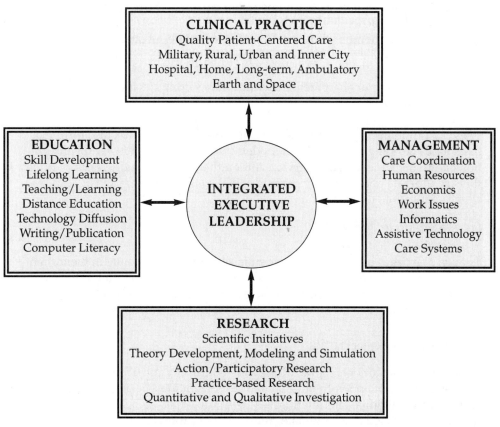

Figure 1.4 Integrated professional nursing administration.

levels of policy formulation and implementation in both the educational and clinical settings. Such professional accountability for all aspects of practice by all participants is essential.

In addition to professional accountability, mature professional practice requires the acceptance of the following assumptions:

- Clinical nursing is central to all other aspects of the profession of nursing, thus forming the unifying base for administration, education, research, and practice.
- Professional nursing is practiced in all settings, including acute, long-term, ambulatory, and home care settings.
- In these various settings, nursing care is based on the most advanced nursing knowledge.
- Nursing is responsible for nursing administration, education, practice, and research.
- The relationship between a school of nursing and a practice setting fosters a mutually productive environment that enhances the tripartite missions: education, practice, and research.
- The organizational and decision-making structures of practice settings have direct effects on the extent to which educational missions can be achieved.
- Excellence in nursing practice in health care settings facilitates nursing education.

These assumptions, although necessary for professional practice, also form the basis for developing organizational models that allow for and foster the integration of nursing education and service. Although a variety of models can provide this, the ultimate goal is quality nursing care through an integration of administration, education, research, and clinical practice.

Criteria for Integrated Models

Though marriages of service and academia are coming into vogue in the form of born-again models (20 to 30 years ago, deans were directors of nursing), the criteria are similar. The following criteria were adapted from Christman's work on centers of excellence in nursing (Christman, 1979a; Christman, 1979b).

Complete Opportunity for Practice

Educators are practitioners, practitioners are educators, and a variety of opportunities exist for joint appointments. Shared responsibilities are assumed, and research, both individual and interdisciplinary, is an expected behavior. Administration is recognized as a legitimate component of professional nursing.

Appropriateness for Size of Institution and School of Nursing

In some settings, the dean of the school of nursing may be the director of nursing. In other settings, it may be appropriate to have an associate dean for clinical practice. Top-level administrative responsibilities in practice and education are assumed by the best and most appropriately prepared nurses.

Open Communication Between Nursing Service and Education

Open communication is maintained through joint appointments and shared committee or task force responsibilities. Joint positions are crucial to maintaining open communication, and nurses in these positions are the viable linkage. For example, curriculum and research review committees, formerly considered the total prerogative of schools of nursing, have nursing service and faculty members, for they are one and the same in an integrated model.

Ability to Be Realized in a Variety of Health Care Settings

Because of the close involvement with the delivery of patient care, faculties with joint appointments can be more realistic in assignment of patients for student experience. All models portray the teacher as a participant in care rather than as a visitor to a patient care setting.

Participation in Policy-Making at the Executive Level

The size and type of institution dictate the nature of governance; however, successful implementation of any model requires the participation of the dean or director at the executive level. This includes but is not limited to voting membership on the institution and school of nursing executive boards. In academic centers, nursing bylaws are shared across education and service.

Comparable Rewards for Education, Practice, and Research

Because of the tripartite mission of most teaching hospitals, some nursing homes, and community health nursing agencies, the successful integrated model allows for comparable rewards for education, practice, and research activities. These include promotion, merit increases, and public recognition.

Promotion of Interdisciplinary Collaboration

The success of any integrated model depends heavily on the acceptance and support of other health professionals. Nurses, physicians, and hospital administrators must collaboratively define and implement an integrated model appropriate for each particular institution.

MODELS OF INTEGRATION

The mid-1970s signaled the beginning of a time of revolutionary change in the organization and operations of departments of nursing and their relationships with schools of nursing. To grasp the magnitude and scope of these changes, one has only to recognize two concurrent yet contrasting trends. At one extreme is the organizational model, characterized by the absorption of autonomous schools of nursing and departments of nursing into the medically dominated systems. An opposite trend is characterized by the integration of schools of nursing and nursing services into a unified structure for the provision of nursing care and nursing education. Between these two extremes are multiple other organizational structures in which nursing provides clinical care, education, and management of services. Whatever organizational context prevails, nursing contends with multiple authority systems and issues related to the direction and scope of practice.

Variations for models of integration exist in the real world and on the drawing board. Case Western Reserve University, Rush-Presbyterian-St. Luke's Medical Center, and the University of Rochester are well established unification models. Grace (1980) presented a taxonomy for integrated models at the Fall Conference of the Midwest Alliance for Nursing in September 1980. This taxonomy represents a progression of development:

1. Nightingale model: historical hospital training model with no organized external education
2. Medical model: current state of the art; structures in nursing match the medical organization
3. Collaborative model: characterized by consultative arrangements in selected roles and at selected levels of institutions; institution specific
4. Affiliative model: based on the "associated with" concept; found in shared services and multihospital systems
5. Independent faculty practice model: a specific mutant of the field on the edge of the movement with realignment of roles and current fiscal issues
6. Transition model: undefined conceptually and operationally; the conversational model of integration without firm commitment by any of the involved members; goal clear, but process for achievement unclear

Other model variations could potentially be established around:

1. Contract for nursing services by clinically expert faculty (e.g., gerontologic or pediatric specialists)
2. Unreimbursed adjunct appointments in the practice setting
3. Research facilitation by nurse executives
4. Collaborative research involving participants from practice and education
5. Collaborative scholarly efforts among researchers, clinicians, and educators
6. Shared teaching by faculty and clinical practitioners
7. Integration of hospital nursing services with nursing home and home care services

8. Alternating appointments by term in nursing practice and education
9. Shared nursing consultation within and across multihospital systems
10. Combination of the above in a newly designed transformation model

The extent to which integration occurs depends primarily on the creativity, flexibility, and autonomy of nurse executives in both education and service. Sharing common mission, philosophy, and goal statements is the first step in collaboration within nursing and the development of a nursing community within a geographic area. Differentiating nursing practice can then provide a transitional step to achievement of a dynamic integrated practice/education model.

Administrative support provides the environment and structure in which nursing practice can occur. The majority of nurses are employed by health care institutions, and their clinical practice must interface with administrative philosophy and policy. The amount of control that nurses have over their own practice is related to many factors in the employer-employee relationship. The following chapters cover innovative administrative approaches and factors that influence nursing practice on both conceptual and pragmatic levels. A nurse executive must consider both conceptual and pragmatic levels to construct a supportive and growth-producing environment for professional nursing administrative practice.

MODEL FOR OPERATIONALIZING PROFESSIONAL NURSING ADMINISTRATION

Because models assist one in gaining understanding of complex relationships, it is advantageous to have a model for the complex process of operationalizing professional nursing administration. The traditional steps for the development of any model are *(1)* facts are observed; *(2)* the facts are looked at as if they were the outcome of some unknown process (the model), and speculation is made about what processes might have produced these outcomes; *(3)* other implications or predictions are deduced from the model; and *(4)* whether these implications are true is questioned, and new models are produced if necessary.

For the nurse executive, the facts observed are those that, taken together, define professional nursing. The process that might result in professional nursing in a particular institution or agency is not known precisely. Although nurse executives have operationalized professional nursing based on some research findings, much has been based primarily on assumptions and the executives' individual experiences. Because the research base from nursing and other fields is inadequate as a basis for operationalizing professional nursing, any model is necessarily speculative and based on assumptions, that is, circumstances and situations that the executive supposes to be true. Given that any model will be imperfect at this point in the development of professional nursing, the following model is presented for use and revision as new information becomes available.

The model depicted in Figure 1.5 presents a basic relationship framework among the three elements for operationalizing professional nursing administration:

foundations, derived components, and operationalized results. Foundations are those theories, conceptual frameworks, and research findings that are used as the bases for developing the elements in the environment for nursing, for example, theories of nursing, management theories, organizational theory, research findings about nurse performance, leadership theories, and values. Many nurse executives assume their positions with an understanding of and leanings toward various foundation components. In such instances, it is important for the nurse executive to be aware of bias before developing a plan for implementing professional nursing.

The derived components are aspects of clinical practice and the environment most related to professional nursing. For example, if the foundation of a decentralized organizational structure is chosen, primary nursing may be one derived component related to decentralization. Operationalized results are those outcomes, from the derived components, that can be observed in terms of behavior. All results will not, of course, be those that were anticipated or desired, but with an imperfect model and incomplete data, revisions in the components are expected to be necessary. Perhaps a different foundation is required or a component needs to be operationalized in an effective manner. All results require continuous evaluation and adjustments of the components when results are not adequate.

Use of the Model

Use of the model for operationalizing professional nursing administration presumes knowledge of theories and willingness to intellectually struggle with some ideas that are in various stages of development. The major bases for professional nursing in a service agency are those used to develop the management and clinical practice components. One task of the nurse executive is to facilitate the incorporation of theoretical knowledge and research findings into the practice environment.

Some of the categories of theories and conceptual frameworks useful to the nurse executive in developing the organizational structure are organizational theory,

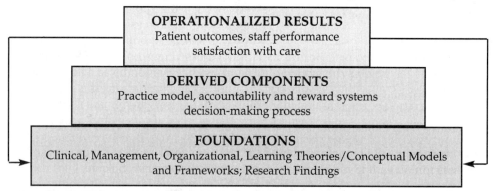

Figure 1.5 Model for operationalizing professional nursing administration.

management theory, leadership styles, communications, team building, and bureaucratic characteristics. These concepts are based on theory from psychology, sociology, and other fields. To understand these concepts, the nurse executive need not return to the study of the basic sciences, but at times, a review of a concept may be useful in attempting to operationalize some aspect of professional nursing.

Before developing or changing the organizational structure of a nursing service, the nurse executive must assess the structure of the total institution. Knowledge of theory and conceptual frameworks is also important for this assessment.

Another area in which the model for operationalizing professional nursing may be useful is in determining nursing practice patterns. Some common types of nursing assignment patterns are functional, team, and primary. In recent years, research has been completed comparing the effectiveness and efficiency of some nursing assignment patterns. Primary nursing may be more cost effective than team nursing when the nursing support system requires very little time of the registered nurse and the patients require highly skilled nursing care. Based on conclusions from study results, probably a short-term acute care community hospital would not financially benefit from primary nursing. However, from other perspectives, for example, job satisfaction, quality of care, and patient satisfaction, primary nursing may still be desirable. Knowledge of theories and concepts can be used in the model as a basis for discussion in choosing a nursing practice pattern.

Many decisions are made based on preference or subjective data. Although the use of the model for operationalizing professional nursing will not eliminate the use of subjective data by any means, it gives nurse executives an alternative approach for making changes in the nursing division. The strategies of change presented in Chapter 12 are foundations that could be used in the model as the basis of implementing a change within the division of nursing. The same change strategy may be used for several changes, or a different one may be more successful with different changes. The model for operationalizing professional nursing administration can be used to phase in various components or changes in the practice environment and to assist the development of professional practice models in diverse settings. Although planning and the use of the model to operationalize professional nursing will not prevent costly errors, a more studied approach can lead to better organizational outcomes. If cost estimates are made for each change or concept to be introduced, the nurse executive also has more concrete data on which to make decisions. Managing fiscal resources is discussed in Chapter 23.

SUMMARY

Nursing administration, as a recognized professional practice discipline, must do more than formulate a theoretical basis for its practice. Nursing theories and models provide conceptual frameworks for the implementation of nursing practice. Management theories and models provide a framework for putting action into nursing practice. This chapter has provided a conceptual framework and supporting rationale for integrated professional nursing administration. It concludes with an application to practice by presenting a basic model for operationalizing nursing in any setting. The major prerequisites for operationalizing professional nursing are administrative support, budgetary control, and authority to approve nursing practice components. These factors provide the foundation on which the operationalizing process can occur. The major components of a model for operationalizing professional nursing are foundations, derived components, and operationalized results. These components must be individualized to diverse practice settings and compatible with the overall health care organization.

STUDY QUESTIONS

1. Formulate a definition of professional nursing administration.
2. What are the distinguishing characteristics that differentiate professional and vocational nursing?
3. According to the National Commissions for the Study of Nursing and Nursing Education's interactive model, there is no single focus for nursing practice. Explain.
4. Why is the field of nursing administration considered a professional practice discipline rather than an academic one? Explain.
5. Describe the four components of professional nursing administrative practice.
6. Compare Nightingale and Wald with modern nurse entrepreneurs.
7. What are the two most important prerequisites for operationalizing professional nursing administration?
8. Discuss one way in which a model for operationalizing professional nursing could be used.
9. Write a brief paper on the lives of Nightingale and Wald and their approaches to integrating theory and practice.
10. Create a model of your practice setting identifying the four components of professional practices as they currently exist. Identify areas that need development.
11. What is meant by a professional practice discipline?

REFERENCES

American Nurses Association. (1995). *Nursing's social policy statement.* Washington, DC: American Nurses Publishing.

Christman, L. (1979a, October). *The center of excellence in nursing: The conceptual model.* Paper presented at the Third Annual Nurse Educator Conference, Detroit, MI.

Christman, L. (1979b). On the scene: Uniting service and education at Rush-Presbyterian-St. Luke's Medical Center. *Nursing Administration Quarterly, 3*(3), 7–40.

Cohen, I. B. (1984). Florence Nightingale. *Scientific American, 250*(3), 128–137.

Donabedian, A. (1976). Foreword. In M. Phaneuf, *The nursing audit and self-regulation in nursing practice* (2nd ed.). New York: Appleton-Century-Crofts.

Donaldson, S., & Crowley, D. (1978). The discipline of nursing. *Nursing Outlook, 26*(2), 113–120.

Dumas, R. G. (1986). *Preparing adults for leadership roles in the 1980's and 1990's.* Presented at the University of Michigan National Nursing conference on Leadership, Ann Arbor, September 17, 1986.

Etzioni, A. (Ed.). (1969). *The semi-professions and their organization.* New York: The Free Press.

Grace, H. (1980, September). *Taxonomy of unification models.* Paper presented at the Fall Conference of the Midwest Alliance for Nursing on Designs for Collaboration: Nursing Service and Nursing Education. Rapid City, SD.

Henderson, V. (1961). *Basic principles of nursing care.* London: International Council of Nurses.

Holleran, C. (1988). Nursing beyond national boundaries: The 21st century, *Nursing Outlook, 36*(2), 72–75.

Kalisch, P. A., & Kalisch, B. J. (1986). *The advance of American nursing* (2nd ed.). Boston: Little, Brown.

Kiereini, E. M. (1989, May 26–27). *Health policy: Barriers and means of achieving health for all by the year 2000.* Paper presented at the conference on Nursing Leadership: Using Research for Policy Making in Primary Health Care. Yonsei University: Seoul, Korea.

Lysaught, J. P. (1981). *Action in affirmation: Toward an unambiguous profession of nursing.* New York: McGraw-Hill.

Maglacas, A. M. (1988). Health for all: Nursing's role, *Nursing Outlook, 36*(2), 66–71.

Michigan League for Nursing. (1990). Nurses desperately needed in the developing world, *Nursing Focus, 7*(3), 5, 9.

Pew Health Professions Commission. (1995). *Critical challenges: Revitalizing the health professions for the twenty-first century.* San Francisco: UCSF Center for the Health Professions.

Robbins, S. P. (1991). *Management* (3rd ed.). Englewood Cliffs, NJ: Prentice-Hall.

Schein, E. H. (1972). *Professional education.* New York: McGraw-Hill.

Schlodtfeldt, R. (1981). Nursing in the future, *Nursing Outlook, 29*(5), 295–301.

Simms, L. M. (1991). The professional practice of nursing administration: Integrated nursing practice, *Journal of Nursing Administration, 21*(5), 37–46.

Simms, L. M., Dalston, J. W., & Roberts, P. W. (1984). Collaborative practice: Myth or reality, *Hospital and Health Services Administration, 29*(6), 36–48.

Sovie, M. D. (1987). Exceptional executive leadership shapes nursing's future, *Nursing Economic$, 5*(1), 13–20.

State of Michigan, Act 368 of 1978 as amended (1997). *Michigan Public Health Code:* Occupational Regulation Sections.

Wald, L. D. (1915). *The house on Henry St.* New York: Henry Holt & Company.

CHAPTER

2

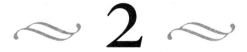

Nursing Theories
and Conceptual Models

Robert Koch • Linda Roussel

There is nothing more difficult to take in hand, more perilous to conduct, or more uncertain in its success than to take the lead in the introduction of the new order of things. (Niccolo Machiavelli)

Chapter Highlights

- Theories
- Orem's self-care theory
- Roy adaptation model
- King's general systems theory
- Levine's conceptual model for nursing
- Leininger's transcultural care model
- Implications for nursing administrative practice

The purpose of this chapter is to introduce the concept of theory and its relationship to nursing administrative practice. Nursing theories and models provide the conceptual framework for patient-centered nursing practice. In a practice discipline such as nursing, conceptual frameworks are necessary in directing the thinking of scholars, in the development of theories, and in guiding the observation of practitioners as the processes of assessment and intervention are implemented.

This chapter focuses on nursing theories that are patient centered with patients considered to be biopsychosocial beings and partners in the care delivery process.

THEORIES

A theory consists of a set of interconnected propositions designed to describe, explain, and predict an event or phenomenon. Chinn and Kramer (1991) envision a theory as a systematic abstraction of reality intended to serve some purpose. A systematic abstraction is defined as an organization pattern underlying the creation and design of theory as well as the notion that theory is not reality itself. Chinn and Kramer imply that what is systematized is also abstract; that is, it is a representation of reality, not reality itself. Approaches to theory development are themselves organized and patterned or systematic. The systematization of abstractions requires rigorous thought and action. The words and symbols that comprise a theory are labels associated with an object, property, or event in the real world. For example, the word "computer" represents an abstraction that denotes a real object. A theory consists of words (such as the label "computer") that represent abstractions, such as the mental image of a computer, that denote reality, such as the object "computer." Words and other symbols enable theories to be communicated and understood.

In general, theories are constructed either deductively or inductively. In deductive theory construction, the concepts under study proceed from general to specific. Thus, deductive theory construction begins with general axioms and propositions. Deductive theories are developed through a logical process that relates concepts in general statements so that increasingly specific statements can be deducted from them.

The process of inductive theory construction proceeds from the specifics of empirical situations to generalizations about the data. This approach is best illustrated in the grounded theory of Glaser and Strauss (1967). This process involves sequential formulation, testing, and redevelopment of propositions until a theory is generated that is integrated, consistent with the data, and in a clear form, operationalized for later testing in quantitative research.

Theory formulation in the discipline of nursing provides a guide for professional nursing practice. Some nurse theoreticians use the deductive process with selected concepts from fields such as sociology, psychology, and physiology. They begin with general concepts and use these as parameters for analyzing specific nursing situations. Other theoreticians use the inductive approach to theory building in nursing; Wald and Leonard (1964) speculate that theorists begin with practical nursing experience and develop concepts that they feel will fit.

In their classic work, Dickoff, James, and Weidenbach (1968) describe the relationship of inductive theory to practice. They emphasize that a theory is neither a useless fairy tale nor a picture of the real. As such, the various kinds of theories can be grouped into four levels: *(1)* factor-isolating theory; *(2)* factor-relating, or situation-depicting theory; *(3)* situation-relating, or predictive, theory; relationships; and *(4)* situation-producing, or perspective, theory. In this classification, each higher level presupposes the existence of theories at the lower level. Dickoff et al. (1968) state that a "situation is depicted in terms of actors already isolated; predictive or promoting theories conceive relationships between depictable situations; and situation-producing theories prescribe in terms of available predictive and promoting theories, and use depicting theories in the characterization of goal-content" (p. 420).

The *factor-isolating* theory, or naming, must be considered first because all scientific theory begins with the naming of factors. The essential function of naming is to facilitate reference to and communication about the factor associated with the name. This theoretical activity is called classifying or the introduction of technical terminology. To neglect factor-isolating theory is particularly detrimental when a theory is self-consciously being developed for the first time, as in nursing.

After factors are identified, they should be observed in relationships. This level of theory is *situation-depicting* in that it relates the factors that have been identified. Theories that depict or provide conceptions of interrelations among factors, as opposed to among situations, are correlations: the presence or absence or range of variation between two factors. Correlations do not imply causation or reference to time sequence; the two factors simply coexist.

Theories classified in the third level are *situation-relating*. Factors are related in such a way that predictions can be made, because predictive theory can state relationships only between such situations as are depictable, which is dependent on what factors have been identified. Causal relationships must show the qualities of priority and direction among variables. For example, if A causes B, one must show that A precedes B, that when A occurs, so does B; that when A increases, B increases; and that when A decreases, B decreases. Therefore, situations may be connected causally.

The highest level of theory is *situation-producing* theory. This level exceeds predictive theory by stating not only that A causes B but also how to bring about A or how to facilitate A's production of B (Figure 2.1).

Dickoff et al. (1968) contend that to have an impact on practice, nursing theory must be at the highest level: situation-producing theory. Nurses confronted with a variety of complex situations must have a prescription for action. This prescription is made as a result of situation-producing theory.

Newman (1979) emphasizes that for a theory to have direct application, it must meet the following criteria:

1. The focus is on human beings.
2. The purpose is understanding the patterns of the life process that relate to health.

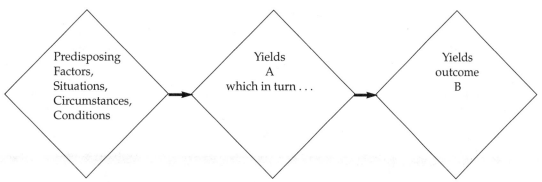

Figure 2.1 Situation-producing theory

3. A total elaboration of the theory contains an action component that facilitates health.

These criteria are consistent with the current conceptual models of nursing that include prescriptive-level theory.

Recently, additional categorizations of theories have emerged. Fitzpatrick and Whall (1996) categorize theories in three divisions: practice theory, mid-range theory, and grand theory. *Practice theory* examines phenomenon at the micro level. This type of theory produces specific direction for practice. Research related to tube feedings, intramuscular injection methods, and therapeutic massage are examples of practice theory. Practice theory is designed specifically for application into clinical practice.

Mid-range theory is an area of theory development that is presently receiving the most attention from nursing scholars. This type of theory is not as abstract as the grand theories, yet less circumscribed as practice theories. Examples of mid-range theory include family stress theories, health promotion theories, and maternal-bonding theories. Unfortunately, there has been little development of mid-range theory specific to nursing administration. Closely analyzing the practice of nursing administration and developing theoretical models for utilization and testing are mandates for nurse leaders. However, until such mid-range theory is developed, nursing administrators will have little nursing theory to guide administrative practices or adopt theories categorized as grand theories.

Grand theory is the most abstract of all theory. It contains concepts (or constructs) that refer to an entire complex entity. This type of theory suggests the relationships between society, person, and environment. Grand theory plays an important role within each discipline. This type of theory establishes the disciplinary beliefs and domains important to that specific discipline.

During the 1990s, additional developments emerged concerning theory. In nursing administration, multiple phenomena must be considered. The use of one theory exclusively may not comprehensively explain the process of nursing in health care organizations today. Pedhazur and Schmelkin (1991, p. 182) said the following about theory: "(Theory is) a way of seeing, a theory is also a way of not seeing . . . even blinding." These authors suggest that one theory only provides one viewpoint and in itself may cause us to ignore simultaneously other phenomenon.

Theory triangulation, new to nursing, is a process of selectively combining various theories. This process may allow the nursing administrator to more fully define the scope of nursing practice. When theories are triangulated or combined they are done so "carefully and purposefully" (Bennett, 1997). Triangulation is not for the purpose of creating a hybrid or eclectic approach to nursing practice. However, it is a mechanism to develop a more complete description of all the phenomena occurring. This approach may prove beneficial in allowing the nurse administrator to use nursing theory in all practice areas.

One example that illustrates theory triangulation is to examine two theories related to adaptation. Two models that embrace the concepts of "systems theory" are Roy's Adaptation Model (Roy, 1976) and Senge's Learning Organization Model (Senge, 1994). The traditional nursing model described by Roy examines nursing care in context to the patient or client, whereas Senge examines how individuals operate within an organization or system.

Using both theories, it is important that nursing administrators consider how patients and staff members learn. Both theories address this process. Adaptive learning (a concept in Roy's theory) is about coping and adjusting to a changing world. Senge introduces the concept of generative learning; this type of learning refers to creating and seeing how the overall system controls events and circumstances.

The use of only one theory exclusively blocks the perception of the nursing leader and in this case can inhibit other possibilities. Blending theories gives a clearer picture, is more inclusive of various circumstances, and allows greater flexibility in defining and working with the phenomenon.

However, theory triangulation is not without its critics. Nursing administrators must be mindful that some theorists think that theory triangulation is nothing more than a "piecemeal" approach to theory application. The mechanics of this process have yet to be defined by nursing scientists. It is interesting to note that nursing theory is not dead, but simply reaching a new level of debate and inquiry.

CONCEPTUAL MODELS AND THEORIES OF NURSING PRACTICE

The relationship between variables may be depicted by a model. Hardy (1974) states that an investigator may formalize a theory, identify its postulates, identify or derive its propositions, and then decide that the problem of relationships is best represented by a model. A model is a simplified representation of a theory, certain complex events, structures, or systems. It is a conceptual representation of a reality situation.

Conceptual models provide a framework that directs the work of scholars in the formulation of theories. Differences among the various conceptual models of nursing are apparent in terms of emphasis, underlying assumptions, definition of health and illness, and designation of the goal of nursing.

The following nursing theories and conceptual models illustrate these differences. The objective of this discussion is to familiarize the nurse executive with selected nursing models and theories that are currently being implemented in nursing practice. It is important that nurse executives be knowledgeable about differences in emphasis so that they may adapt these models to interface with the philosophy of nursing practice within the context of their organizational (practice) setting. These models offer guidelines for nursing practice.

Theories and conceptual models are categorized in different ways depending on use, purpose, concepts, and discipline. Selected models presented in this chapter are used to demonstrate integration of theory into nursing administration practice.

Orem's Self-Care Theory

Dorothea Orem's (1991) general theory of nursing is a descriptive explanation of the human foundations of nursing and of nursing actions. She emphasizes that nursing is a response of human groups to one recurring type of incapacity for action to which human beings are subject, that is, the incapacity to care for oneself or one's dependents is limited because of the health or health care needs of the care recipient.

From the nursing perspective, human beings are viewed as needing continuous self-maintenance and self-regulation through a type of action termed "self-care." Self-care is care that is performed by oneself for oneself when this individual has reached a state of maturity that enables one to take consistent, controlled, effective, and purposeful action. Self-care involves the practice of activities that people initiate and perform on their own behalf in maintaining life, health, and well-being.

Her major concepts include *(1)* self-care; *(2)* self-care agent or provider of self-care; *(3)* dependent-care agent or provider of infant care, child care, or dependent adult care; *(4)* the agent who is the person taking action; *(5)* the nursing agency refers to the provision of nursing to individuals and families requiring that nurses have specialized abilities that enable them to provide care; and *(6)* the nursing system refers in a general way to all the actions and interactions of nurses and patients in nursing practice situations.

Orem's general theory of nursing is referred to as the self-care deficit theory of nursing because it explains the relationship between the action capabilities of individuals and their demands for self-care or the care demands of children or adults who are their dependents. Deficit is the relationship between the action that individuals take (action demanded) and the action capabilities of individuals for self-care or dependent care. It is important to note that deficit should be interpreted as a relationship, not a human disorder. However, these self-care deficits may be associated with the presence or human functional or structural disorders.

The essence of Orem's model is on the individuals' self-care needs and their capabilities for meeting these needs. She stresses that self-care has purpose. It is action that has pattern and sequence when it is effectively performed, contributes to human structural integrity, human functioning, and human development.

Orem stresses that self-care related to the need for normalcy may be directed toward the promotion of integrated human functioning or the protection and care of the body. It is important to note that when individuals perform sets of actions for meeting these needs, they are enhancing their health and well-being.

Health-deviation self-care requisites exist for persons who are ill or injured; who have specific forms of pathology, including defects and disabilities; and who are under medical diagnosis and treatment. Obvious changes in (1) human structure, such as edematous extremities or tumors, (2) physical functioning, such as dyspnea or joint immobility, and (3) habits of daily living (e.g., sudden mood changes, loss of interest in life) focus a person's attention on him- or herself. When a change in health status results in total or almost total dependence on others for the needs to sustain life or well-being, the person moves from the position of self-care agent to that of patient, or receiver of care. The role of nursing focuses on assisting the individual, family, or significant others to meet universal self-care demands or develop new methods of providing self-care.

In implementing Orem's model in nursing practice, the major emphases of the nursing assessment are the individual's self-care requisites, self-care agency or capabilities, and the influencing components related to the self-care agency. On the principle that nurses, patients, or both can act to meet patients' care requisites, three variations of basic nursing systems are recognized. These are (1) wholly compensatory, (2) partly compensatory, and (3) supportive-educative (Figure 2.2). The nursing system is formed by the nurse's selection and use of methods of assisting patients and prescribes particular roles for the nurse and the patient.

The criterion measure for determining the need for a wholly compensatory nursing system exists when the patient is unable to engage in those self-care actions requiring self-directed and controlled ambulation and manipulative movement. These patients cannot or should not engage in any form of deliberate action. In the partly compensatory, the nurse and the patient perform care measures or other actions involving manipulative tasks or ambulation. It is intended for situations in which the patient can perform some, but not all of, the care measures required. In the supportive-educative system a patient can or should learn to perform the required self-care measure but cannot do so without assistance.

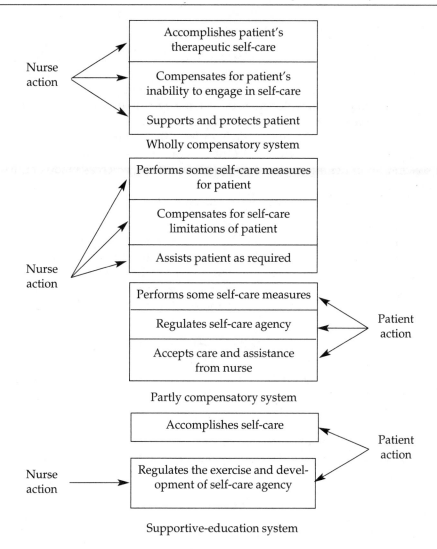

Figure 2.2 Basic nursing systems. From Orem, D. E. (1991). *Nursing: Concepts of Practice* (4th ed.). St. Louis: Mosby-Year Book. Copyright 1991 by Mosby-Yearbook. Reprinted with permission.

The family, community, and environment are important components considered in self-care actions, but the primary focus is on the patient. The outcome measures for evaluating nursing care are used to determine whether the patient's self-care requisites are met, and if the patient can achieve self-care management and does perform therapeutic self-care measures on an ongoing basis. The goal of nursing action is to involve the patient in his or her own self-care activities whenever possible.

Roy's Adaptation Model

Sister Callista Roy's (1976, 1989) adaptation model of nursing practice can be viewed primarily as a system model even though it also contains interactionist levels of analysis. The person is a biopsychosocial being who, to be understood, has parts or elements linked together in such a way that force on the linkages can be increased or decreased. Roy emphasizes that increased force, or tension, occurs because of strains within the system or from the environment that impinges on the system. The units of analysis of the nursing system are the system of the person and his or her interaction with the environment, whereas mode of nursing intervention involves the manipulation of parts of the system or the environment. See Chapter 27 for an example of person-centered care.

Roy has identified that the person has four subsystems: *(1)* physiologic needs, *(2)* self-concept, *(3)* role function, and *(4)* interdependence (Roy, 1976, p. 14). The self-concept and role function systems are envisioned as developing in an interactionist framework. This interaction process is one of the elements to be assessed with the system. Roy stresses that one of the nurse's primary tools in manipulating elements of the system or the environment is one's interaction with the patient.

In Roy's model, an assumption is a statement accepted as true without proof. These assumptions may be explicitly stated or implied with the discussion of the model and are based on the model's approach to the concept of person and to the process of adaptation. The following are the basic assumptions of the Roy adaptation model:

1. The person is a biopsychosocial being.
   The nature of the person includes a biologic component (such as anatomy and physiology) along with psychological and social components. The behavior of the individual is related to the behavior of others on a group level. Methods of analysis of the person must come from the biologic, psychological, and sciences, and the person must be viewed from those perspectives as a unified whole.
2. The person is in constant interaction with a changing environment. Daily experience with such things as vicissitudes of the weather or traffic conditions supports this assumption. The person confronts physical, social, and psychological changes in the environment and is continually interacting with these.
3. To cope with a changing world, the person uses both innate and acquired mechanisms (biologic, psychological, and social in origin). These acquired mechanisms are used to cope with the world (an example of this is dressing to suit the weather). Other mechanisms are innate (natural reaction of thirst in response to water loss through perspiration).
4. Health and illness are one inevitable dimension of a person's life. Each person is subject to the laws of health and illness. This dimension is one aspect of the total life experience.

5. To respond positively to environmental changes, the person must adapt. A changing environment demands a positive response, which is hopefully adaptive.
6. Adaptation is a function of the stimulus a person is exposed to and his or her adaptation level. The person's adaptation level is determined by three classes of stimuli: *(1)* focal stimuli, which are stimuli immediately confronting the person; *(2)* contextual stimuli (all other stimuli present); and *(3)* residual stimuli (such as beliefs, attitudes, or traits, which have an indeterminate effect on the present situation).
7. The person's adaptation level is such that it comprises a zone indicating the range of stimulation that will lead to positive response. If the stimulus is within the zone the person responds positively; whereas, if the stimulus is outside the zone, the person cannot make a positive response.
8. The person is conceptualized as having four modes of adaptation:
   a. Person adapts according to his or her *physiologic needs* (adaptation to temperature).
   b. Person's *self-concept* is determined by interactions with others (outside stimuli cause the person to adapt according to his or her self-concept).
   c. *Role function* is the performance of duties based on given positions within society (the way one performs these duties is constantly responsive to outside stimulation).
   d. *Interdependence relations.* In relations with others, the person adapts according to a system of interdependence, which involves ways of seeking help, attention, and affection. (Roy, 1989, pp. 106–108)

Roy emphasizes that the elements of a practice-oriented model imply values and include goal patency, source of difficulty, and intervention. The model implies values that, taken together, point to the desirability of the model's goal content. The basic values behind the goal can be summarized as follows:

1. Nursing's concern with the person as a total being in the areas of health and illness is a socially significant activity.
2. The nursing goal of supporting and promoting patient adaptation is important for patient welfare.
3. Promoting the process of adaptation is assumed to conserve patient energy; thus, nursing makes an important contribution to the overall goal of the health team by making energy available for the healing process.
4. Nursing is unique because it focuses on the patient as a person adapting to those stimuli present as a result of his or her position on the health-illness continuum. (Roy, 1989, p. 109)

The Roy adaptation model states that the goal of nursing is the person's adaptation in the four adaptive models previously described. Roy emphasizes that all nursing activity will be aimed at promoting the person's adaptation in physiologic needs, self-concept, role function, and relations of interdependence during health and illness. The criterion used for judging when the goal has been reached is generally any positive response made by the recipient to the stimuli present that frees energy for responses to other stimuli. This is applied to each specific nursing intervention for which a specific goal of adaptation has been set.

Roy envisions the person as an adaptive system receiving stimuli from the environment inside and outside of its zone adaptation. The recipient of nursing is the person in the dimension of his or her life related to health and illness. For example, the patient may be ill, or at risk of illness and in need of preventive services. The person may be adapting positively or not. It is important to emphasize that if the patient is adapting, the nursing goal is to maintain that response.

The newest element of this model is the source of difficulty that is described as the originating point of deviations from the desired state or condition. A need is described as a requirement in the individual that stimulates a response to maintain integrity. Roy implies that as internal and external environments change, the level of satiety for any need changes, and when this satiety changes, a deficit or excess is created. This deficit or excess then triggers the appropriate adaptive mode. Coping mechanisms whose activity is aimed at integrity are with each of the adaptive modes. The manifestations of this activity are the adaptive or ineffective behaviors. The source of difficulty is the coping activity that is inadequate to maintain integrity in the event of a need deficit or excess.

Intervention includes both focus and mode. This intervention focus involves the kind of problems found when deviations from the desired state occur that describe the kinds of disturbances that are to be prevented or treated. Each adaptive mode is related to underlying needs. For example, the physiologic adaptive mode is related to the need for physiologic integrity (such as exercise and rest, nutrition and elimination, fluid and electrolytes). The intervention mode is the means of preventing or treating the problems identified in the intervention focus; that is, it is the action that can be used to change the course of events toward the desired end product. It is what the nurse can do to promote patient adaptation. According to Roy's model, the nurse acts as an external regulatory force to modify stimuli affecting adaptation either by increasing, decreasing, or maintaining stimulation. This occurs within the nursing process, a problem-solving approach to diagnosing patient problems and to planning, performance, and evaluating patient care.

Roy's theory development is explanatory and an example of situation producing because it explains how the nurse can encourage adaptation through the manipulation of stimuli. The nurse must be able to consider each client as an individual, assess his or her needs, and act, accordingly. The model encourages the nurse to become more proficient in the total assessment of the patient through observation, interviews, and the performance of a variety of nursing care activities. An understanding of Roy's four adaptive modes for responding to change enables the nurse to bring a broad perspective to the planning and evaluating of nursing care based on individual client needs.

King's General Systems Theory

Imogene King's (1981) theory of nursing is based on the concept that patients and nurses are personal systems that coexist with other personal and group systems, as well as society as a whole. It is based on general systems theory as introduced by von Bertalanffy (1968) as a "complex of elements standing in interaction." He noted that general systems theory is a general science of "wholeness . . . in itself purely formal but applicable to the various empirical sciences" (p. 37). The distinguishing characteristics of systems include goals, structure, functions, resources, and decision-making. Individuals are influenced by their interactions with both the internal and external environment and they, in turn, influence the environment. Three dynamic interacting systems comprise King's theory. These are *(1)* personal systems (individuals); *(2)* interpersonal systems (dyads, triads, and small and large groups); and *(3)* social systems (family, school, industry, social organizations, and health care delivery systems) (King, 1981).

King stresses that the goal of her conceptual system of nursing is health. Nurses help individuals attain and maintain their health, and if some disturbance occurs such as an illness or disability, nurses' actions are goal directed to assist the individual in regaining health or to help the individual live with a chronic disease or disability. Therefore, health is a dynamic state of an individual in which change is constant and an ongoing process.

King states that perception is a comprehensive concept in personal systems. This varies from one individual to another because each human being has different backgrounds of such things as knowledge, skills, abilities, needs, values, and goals. These perceptions of nurses and patients influence their interactions. Perception along with communication provide a channel for relaying information from one person to another. Self, growth and development, learning, body image, time, and space are concepts that also relate to individuals as personal systems.

A comprehensive concept in interpersonal systems is interaction. King emphasizes that knowledge of interaction is essential for nurses to understand a fundamental process for gathering information about human beings, and that purposeful interactions lead to transactions. Communication, transactions, role, and stress are related concepts. King notes that knowledge of the concepts identified in personal systems is also used to understand interactions.

Organization is a comprehensive concept in social systems because knowledge of organization is essential for nurses to understand the variety of social systems with which individuals grow and develop. Related concepts are power, authority, status, decision-making, and control. King further states that all the concepts from personal and interpersonal systems provide knowledge for use within the social system.

In King's theory, concepts of the general systems framework are applied in nursing through the interaction-transaction process model. This model is defined as a "dynamic interpersonal process in which nurse and patient are viewed as a system with each affecting the behavior of the other and both being influenced by the factors within the situation" (Daubenemire & King, 1973, p. 513).

King's conceptual framework is a system of processes, which includes those of perception, communication, purposeful interactions, information, and decision-making. She defined nursing as a "process of action, reaction, and interaction whereby nurse and client share information about their perceptions in a nursing situation. Through purposeful communication they identify specific goals, problems or concerns. They explore means to achieve a goal and agree to means to the goal" (King, 1981, p. 2).

Nursing is described as a process of human interactions between nurse and patient in which each perceives the other and the situation. By means of communication, they mutually explore and set goals and agree on means to achieve those goals. The consequences or outcomes of the attained goal is also proposed. The basic premise of the theory is the interrelationship that exists between the nurse and the patient through action, interaction, and transaction for the purpose of achieving mutual goal attainment.

Levine's Conceptual Model for Nursing: The Four Conservation Principles

Myra Levine's theory (1973, 1989) of nursing is based on the concept of "wholeness" of the individual and the need to provide total patient care, from which she derives four conservation principles that serve as the basis for her nursing model. She emphasizes that the unity, integrity, the oneness, and the wholeness of human experience are universal.

Levine's theory (1973) reflects her definition of nursing in which she makes the assumptions that nursing is a human interaction, a discipline rooted in the dependency of people and their relationship with other people, and is based on intervention that supports or promotes the person's adjustment (pp. 1–3). She envisions nursing as holistic, individualized to meet each person's needs, and supporting adaptation. Therefore, the components of her theory are:

1. The patient is in the predicament of illness.
2. The nurse must recognize the patient's holistic response, which indicates the nature of the adaptation to illness.
3. The nurse who participates actively in every patient's environment must recognize the organismic response of the patient, make an intervention in the patient's environment, and evaluate the intervention as therapeutic or supportive. (Levine, 1973, p. 13)

Levine makes the assumptions that the nurse-patient interaction is determined by *(1)* the conditions in which the patient enters the health care setting, *(2)* the functions of the nurse in the situation, and *(3)* the responsibilities of the nurse in the situation. The theory implies that the nurse is able to make judgments that will promote or support the patient's adaptation to the situation based on knowledge. The nurse also is expected to possess the skills necessary to implement these interventions. Levine refers to the environmental setting of the nurse-patient interaction as the hospital.

Supporting her holistic beliefs, Levine views a person holistically as requiring four elements to be in a state of health. These are *(1)* structural integrity, *(2)* personal integrity, *(3)* social integrity, and *(4)* energy to be in state of health. If any one of these elements is disrupted or changed, the person is in a state of altered health. Health and disease are patterns of adaptive change and they are never static entities. Nursing interventions are based on the conservation of these four elements. Levine defines conservation as the "keeping-together" function that should be the major guideline of all nursing interventions where it occurs. The purpose of conservation is to maintain the unity and integrity of the patient. The four conservation principles are:

1. Conservation of energy of the individual.
   Energy is eminently identifiable, measurable, and manageable. For example, changes in the energy of heat production in the individual provide signals as to how effectively his or her body is functioning. Pulse rate, respiratory rate, measurement of blood gases are energy measures. Energy conservation is an empirical activity of nursing care.
2. Conservation of structural integrity of the individual.
   This conservation principle is concerned with healing. Individuals are taught to have confidence in the ability of bodies to heal, that is, to restore wholeness and continuity after injury or illness, and to return to their pristine state. Healing is the defense of wholeness and is also a consequence of an effective immune system. Nurses have empirical awareness of the necessity to defend the structural integrity of individuals (such as proper positioning to prevent subluxations and other skeletal deformities or preventing pressure areas where decubiti might occur).
3. Conservation of personal integrity of the individual.
   The conservation of personal integrity implies that the sense of "self" is much more than a physical experience of the whole body, although it is a part of that awareness. The defense of self is reaching into the person. Everyone seeks to defend his or her identity as self. Even in those instances where the relationship with others is intimate and close—between parent and child, husband and wife—only by analogy it is known that our experience of selfhood is somehow an expression of personal identity. Nothing threatens that pride of self more than vulnerability of dependence. It is impossible for one individual to surrender his or her privacy to another, no matter how much the individual must depend on the good offices of the caregiver. It is much more difficult to articulate the anxiety created by a threat to self—to share it with another individual. The emphasis over the years on extracting psychosocial information about patients neglects the inevitable guarding of the privacy that cherishes self. It is possible that the use of private information as a component of the nursing care plan may be more damaging to the personal integrity of the individual than respecting a desire to withhold information. It may be that the most generous psychosocial approach would

be to limit the recording of confidences to only those generalizations that actually make a difference in the choice of treatment plans. Individuals must participate freely in decisions that affect them.

4. The conservation of social integrity of the individual.
   This concept refers to the acknowledgement of the individual within the context of his or her social environment. Selfhood needs definition beyond the individual and this is the message of the conservation of social integrity. Individuals define themselves by their relationships (an identity places one in a family, a community, a cultural heritage, a religious belief, a socioeconomic slot, an educational background, a vocational choice). Coping refers to the way in which the individual responds to given social instant. Coping patterns are judged by the social acceptance of the behavior that is manifested. For example, coping patterns are categorized as everyday responses that have proved to be adequate and acceptable for the individual in the past. (Levine, 1989, pp. 331–336)

Levine emphasizes that the conservation principles do not operate singly and in isolation from each other. "They are joined within the individual as a cascade of life events, churning and changing as the environmental challenge is confronted and resolved in each individual's unique way" (p. 336). The nurse as caregiver becomes part of the environment bringing his or her own cascading repertoire of skill, knowledge, and compassion. She believes it is a shared enterprise and each participant is rewarded.

Similar to Orem's conceptual framework, Levine's nursing theory focuses on the individual (patient). The nurse is concerned with the patient's family and significant others as they influence the patient's progress. Levine's theory depicts nursing as an independent practice profession. Because her focus is on the hospital-based practice arena, Levine does not consider the collaborative relationship of nursing within the total health care setting. However, nurses in acute care settings could use this model. For example, the theory emphasizes the patient's dependency (illness) states with limited participation in planning his or her care. In such settings, the nurse has the major responsibility for assessing the patient's ability to participate in his or her own care, which is in contrast to Orem's self-care deficit theory model.

Leininger's Transcultural Care Model

Cultural diversity is present in every aspect of nursing. Not only are clients more diverse in their cultural orientation, but nursing personnel are more culturally diverse than ever before. Leininger's culture care theory provides the nursing executive with an excellent framework for administrative practice. (See Chapter 31 for related discussion.)

"Culture is defined as the learned, shared, and transmitted values, beliefs, norms, and lifeways of a particular group that guides their thinking, decisions, and actions in patterned ways" (Leininger, 1997, p. 47). Leininger's theory suggests that care diversities and commonalities exist in all cultures. Leininger postulates that there are generic and professional care meaning, symbols, patterns, processes, and practices transculturally, but they might not be the same everywhere. It is essential that nurses, educators, practitioners, as well as nursing administrators consider worldviews, social and cultural structures, languages, and ethnic histories.

Additionally, Leininger suggests that for nurses to assist people of diverse or similar cultures, three dominant actions and decision modes are essential. These three modes include culture preservation and maintenance, culture care accommodation, and culture care restructuring (Leininger, 1997).

Culture preservation and maintenance refers to those assistive, supportive, and facilitative activities that enable professions to help people to retain and preserve cultural values. Such preservation will assist in the maintenance of optimal well-being. Cultural care accommodation refers to the professional actions and decisions that help individuals of a designated culture adapt to others for a beneficial outcome, whereas "cultural repatterning" refers to those activities that assist in reordering, changing, or greatly modifying patterns, cultural beliefs, and cultural values to improve health status.

Just as individual nurses consider the cultural factors of the individual client, the nurse administrator considers the culture of the organization in planning, developing, and implementing nursing services. The nurse administrator takes into account the cultural background and values of the nursing personnel individually and collectively. Efforts to foster positive, productive mores are emphasized. Because Leininger predicts that providing culturally, congruent, meaningful care would have positive health benefits to recipients of care, it is critical that nursing administrators examine cultural influences on all aspects of the nursing organization and services (Leininger, 1996).

Many of the concepts of organizational culture have roots in the anthropological views as described by Leininger. Organizational cultures add yet another dimension to cultural care as posited by this theorist.

Table 2.1 depicts the central theme and concepts of Orem's self-care model, Roy's adaptation model, King's open systems framework and theory of goal attainment, Levine's theory of nursing, and Leininger's transcultural care model.

IMPLICATIONS FOR NURSING ADMINISTRATION PRACTICE

Nursing administrators have been functioning for years without formalized theory. Today's changing environment requires that leaders influence the direction of nursing's contribution to an evolving health care system. This commission can only be achieved and successfully measured if nursing's efforts are compared to established models of practice. The nurse administrator's mission is to project a well-defined view of nursing and its contribution within an interdisciplinary health care field. Such a view will only be developed and articulated within the framework of nursing models and nursing theory.

Table 2.1 Selected Nursing Theories

Theorist	Central Theme & Concepts
Orem's Self Care Model	➢ Nursing is directed towards self-care activities—Meeting self care needs through learned behavior. ➢ Illness results in the person's inability to maintain self-care.
Roy's Adaptation Model	➢ The person in constant interaction with a changing environment. ➢ All conditions and circumstances ultimately influence the organism.
King's Open Systems Framework and Theory of Goal Attainment	➢ Theorizes concepts related to the process of human interaction. ➢ Nursing is directed toward communication, mutual goal setting, exploration of means, and agreement on achieving desired outcomes.
Leininger's Transcultural Care Model	➢ Emphasizes cultural specific care. ➢ Nursing care is directed towards personalized care behaviors of the client and promoting health behaviors that have physical, psycho-cultural and social significance.
Levine's Theory of Nursing	➢ Conservation—The holistic person. ➢ Defines nursing as a discipline that focuses on human and the complexity of relationships with the environment.

If nursing leaders are to clearly articulate the value of the nursing profession, they must move past the question "Do nursing models work?". Instead nursing administrators must create environments and practice settings that support the development and utilization of conceptual models and theories in nursing practice. The nurse executive can serve as a catalyst for instituting the use of nursing theoretical models as well as inspire, challenge, and influence clinical nursing practice within a health care organization.

BENEFITS OF THEORY-BASED NURSING SERVICE ORGANIZATIONS

There are multiple reasons why nursing theories are beneficial to nursing administrators. Through understanding these benefits, theory utilization can become a reality to the profession.

When specific nursing theories are used to govern the practice of nursing in a health care organization, the model provides a means for the nurse to view the recipient of care in a particular and unified manner. Furthermore, the model can provide a framework within which assessments and observations can be made. Nurses practicing under one common conceptual model use one language in categorizing and diagnosing patient problems. Language is essential to "passing on" cultural values, standards, and ways of doing business.

Using one central nursing theory also helps establish the guidelines for intervention, conditions for implementation, and evaluation. Moreover, the integration of a conceptual model in nursing administration defines the unique purpose of nursing services and the focus of nursing care in the clinical agency.

Theory-based nursing practice is perceived by some nursing administrators as aiding nurse recruitment and retention. Many nursing service organizations recognize their role in the career development of nurses as a way to enhance the quality of care. Therefore, theory-based practice is considered a means to clarify the role of the nurse. It establishes the focus and domains of nursing whereby the nurse can function responsibly and autonomously. Additionally, theory-based nursing practice stimulates learning and promotes innovation and creativity. Another perceived benefit of the theory-based nursing organization is that it may help in costing out nursing by delineating nursing responsibilities.

Consider the following example. Historically, nursing has vacillated between taking on various functions (such as housekeeping, clerical duties, and material management) and abdicating other functions (such as ambulating patients, pulmonary care, and venipucture). When these tasks are examined with a specific nursing theory in mind, it becomes evident what the true role of nursing is meant to be. This is not to say that nurses should not become willing and responsive team members in a health care organization. However, in these days of tight budgetary constraints, nursing administrators must possess a clear understanding of the role and responsibilities of the professional nurse.

OBSTACLES AND CHALLENGES TO BUILDING A THEORY-BASED NURSING ORGANIZATION

Unfortunately, the use of nursing theory to guide nursing administration is far from a reality. Although there are several benefits to adopting a central governing nursing theory for a nursing service division, such an endeavor is not easily accomplished. Significant barriers to implementation are present. Decisions to embrace one theory over another should be done cautiously because total integration will affect all areas of nursing practice.

Congruence between the institution's mission, the philosophy of nursing, and the selected theory must exist. A division of nursing should not choose a nursing theory that is contradictory to one's philosophy, because it is both nursing theory and nursing philosophy that are integrated into each component of service within the nursing department.

Furthermore, the service lines of the organizations should also be closely scrutinized before selecting a nursing theory to guide clinical practice. Health care organizations range from acute care to chronic care, from inpatient to outpatient, from ambulatory care to long-term care. Such variations must be examined because particular theories may not be applicable to the organization's purpose.

The pragmatic issues, which surround adopting nursing theory to govern nursing operations, must also be considered. For the model to be clearly evident within the institution, nursing administration must develop policies and procedures that clearly reflect the selected conceptual model at the patient care level. Nursing documentation must be changed to make them consistent with the model chosen. Even shift reports must change so that patient problems are identified in accordance with the model.

However, nurse executives must recognize that one major problem exists. A large number of nurses have limited or no knowledge of conceptual models and theories. The nursing administrator must consider that the majority of nurses who work at the bedside in hospital and long-term care settings are graduates of associate degree nursing programs or diploma graduates. Although these nursing programs use the nursing process throughout their curriculum, typically there is heavy emphasis on the medical model as their organizing framework. Graduates of these programs, who have not had the knowledge or the experience of working with a model in conjunction with the steps of the nursing process, are less likely to know how to use nursing models in nursing practice.

Existing nursing personnel must be oriented to the selected model just as new nursing employees must have this information included in their orientation to the health care facility. Ongoing continuing in-service education must also be presented in the context of the theoretical model if the change to a governing theory is to be effective and lasting.

Another obstacle that exists is that many nursing theoretical models use complex language that adds to the confusion and uncertainty about the theory. This is often perceived as lacking a "real world view" of care delivery and not communicated pragmatically. Nursing executives who adopt theoretical models to guide administrative and practice issues must be aware that the rhetoric of the theory may be perplexing. With jargon such as physiologic mode, space-time continuum, and affiliative subsystems, it is little wonder that nurses find theory to be essentially useless in practice. Because nursing historically has lacked any formalized or unifying language, it is essential for the nurse executive to clarify terminology and to simplify meanings and definitions. Even though selection of a "nursing jargon" may be confusing initially, it can eventually become a part of the daily speech of the practicing nurse (Laschinger, 1991). Table 2.2 summarizes the advantages and disadvantages of the theory based nursing service organization.

AN EXAMPLE OF THEORY-BASED NURSING ORGANIZATIONS

The following is an example of how nursing theory can be integrated into nursing administration practices. The number of possible nursing theories as well as

Table 2.2 The Theory-Based Nursing Service Organization

Advantages	Disadvantages
• Clearly establishes goals and objectives for nursing practice.	• Confusing to nurses uneducated in theory and requires extensive orientation and ongoing education.
• Distinctly identifies beneficiary of nursing interventions.	• Must be compatible with existing mission and philosophy of institution.
• Defines nursing domains and independent nursing interventions.	• Difficulty in operationalizing abstract concepts and propositions.
• Establishes nursing outcome measures.	
• Clarifies taxonomy and communication efforts among nursing personnel.	

organizational theories that can be used in practice are too numerous to discuss in this text. However, the true excitement is derived from "trying on" a nursing theory within the context of the organization and the patient care setting. The following example is to serve as a guide to the nurse executive. It is only through a method of investigation, trial and error, and inquiry that theory becomes practice and pertinent to specific nursing service organizations.

Orem's theory of self-care lends itself to such an example in a rehabilitation facility. Nursing assessments and nursing diagnoses would focus on the patient's ability to care for self. Such patients who suffer from cerebral vascular accidents or head injuries may well benefit from application of this nursing theory.

Orem's theory posits that "self-care is the practice of activities that individuals initiate on their own to maintain life and sustain health." Nursing personnel using this model would assess the patient's ability to identify what they can do (self-care) and what they cannot do (self-care deficit). The assessment data are the foundation from which all nursing care on that unit would be derived. Nurses would use this theory to prescribe, design, and plan the nursing care to meet the patient's self-care deficits.

Documentation of the patient's problems, status, and progress would focus on the self-care needs of the individual. Patient-centered conferences are directed toward identifying self-care deficits; methods of assisting the patient to optimal self-care occur on this nursing unit.

Using this model of care the patient's self-care needs determine the patient's classifications, acuity systems, and budgeted personnel demands. A patient acuity system might have several levels of care. Acuity level, hypothetically, could be assigned for those unable to engage in any form of self-care. This patient population requires intense and complex nursing care. An acuity level 2 would be for those who are aware of themselves and the environment but cannot engage in self-care secondarily to motor inability. The amount of support, guidance, and teaching, in addition to acting for and doing for the patient, would vary based on the acuity level.

Another example, Imogene King's system framework theory, is applicable to nursing administration. King suggests that a social system is an "organized boundary system of social roles, behaviors, and practices developed to maintain values and the mechanisms to regulate the practices and rules." King's thoughts on boundaries can easily be used to explain nursing accountability and scope of practice. This theory can provide valuable insight into the nursing decision-making process in an organization. Lines of authority and scope of responsibilities can be seen in the context of boundaries. Social systems, a key concept in this theory, easily relate to organization, authority, power, status, decision-making, and control. In a clinical setting, patients are viewed as living systems. Nursing assessments and interventions, using King's theory, are directed toward identifying and maintaining social roles, behaviors, values, and belief systems. In caring for a client with three small children, the nurse would consider this individual as being an integrated part of a larger system. Efforts would be directed toward ensuring optimal functioning and preservation of the overall family unit.

In conclusion, to be effective the theoretical model must be evident in every aspect of the management and administration of the nursing service organization. The selection and implementation of a selected nursing theory will, in most cases, prompt a significant culture change within the nursing organization. The nursing administrator must recognize that this type of paradigm shifting takes time and energy. Traditions, habits, and patterns of thinking are extremely resistant to change and difficult to overcome. The adoption of a nursing theoretical model entails major change for any nursing service organization. It is through the use of strategies for "planned change" that such endeavors are successful. There must be commitment on the part of all nursing administration to successfully implement a nursing conceptual model in the patient care setting. Although this process requires extensive effort, the benefits are well worth the venture.

SUMMARY

Nursing is attempting to formulate a theoretical basis for its practice. Many nurse scholars have advanced postulates, theories, and conceptual frameworks as a mechanism to achieve this goal. Orem focuses on the individuals' self-care needs and their capabilities of meeting these needs. Her belief is that self-care has a purpose because it emphasizes action that has pattern and sequence when it is effectively performed that contributes to human structural integrity, human functioning, and human development. Nursing actions are directed toward enhancing the self-care ability and therapeutic self-care ability of individuals. Roy's adaptation model of nursing practice can be perceived primarily as a systems model. The units of analysis are the person and his or her interaction with the environment, whereas mode of nursing intervention involves the manipulation of parts of the system or the environment. Roy espouses that nursing is an interpersonal process that is initiated by the individual's maladaption to change in the environment. The goal of nursing is to assess the adaptation level and intervene to promote positive adaptation and integrity. Similar to Roy, King's theory of nursing is a systems approach depicting patients and nurses as personal systems with other personal and group systems within the confines of society as a whole. King implies that through a systems approach by means of communication, nurses and patients will mutually explore and set goals and agree on means to achieve those goals, and the outcomes attained will become evident. Levine emphasizes the conservation principles of energy, structural integrity, and personal and social integrity. The goal of nursing is the wholeness of the individual that occurs by conservation in four areas when adaptive needs are manifested. She stresses an important point: that individuals (patients) must participate freely in decisions that affect them. Leininger's transcultural care theory suggests that care diversities and commonalities exist in all cultures. She postulates that symbols, patterns, processes, and practices have relevant meaning and are essential when engaging with other individuals. It is imperative that nursing executives consider alternative worldviews, social and cultural structures, languages, and ethnic histories with patients, staff, and colleagues.

Chapter 3 addresses the major concepts and theories of management that are applicable to nursing administrative practice.

STUDY QUESTIONS

1. Formulate a definition of theory.
2. What are the major differences between an inductive and a deductive theory?
3. Explain the rationale for the statement by Dickoff and James that the highest level of theory building is situation-producing theory. Why must nursing theory be at this level?
4. Formulate a definition of a model.
5. Distinguish among Orem's, Roy's, King's, Levine's and Leininger's conceptual models of nursing practice.
6. Select from among the preceding nursing conceptual models the one that would be most applicable to incorporate patient-centered nursing practice within your health care organization. What are the implications for nursing administration in the application of the model to nursing practice?

REFERENCES

Bennett, J. A. (1997). A case for theory triangulation. A case example of nurses attitudes about AIDS. *Nursing Science Quarterly, 10*(2), 97–106.

Chinn, P., & Kramer, M. K. (1991). *Theory and nursing: A systematic approach* (3rd ed.). St. Louis: Mosby-Year Book.

Daubenmire, M., & King, I. M. (1973). Nursing process models: A systems approach. *Nursing Outlook, 21*(8), 512–517.

Dickoff, J., James, P., & Weidenback, E. (1968). Theory in a practice discipline—Part I. *Nursing Research, 17*(5), 415–434.

Dickoff, J., James, P., & Weidenback, E. (1968). Theory in a practice discipline—Part II. *Nursing Research, 17*(6), 545–554.

Fitzpatrick, J. J., & Whall, A. L. (1996). *Conceptual models of nursing—Analysis and application* (3rd ed.). Stamford, CT: Appleton & Lange.

Glaser, B., & Strauss, A. (1967). *The discovery of grounded theory.* Chicago: Aldine.

Hardy, M. (1974). Theories: Components, development, evaluation. *Nursing Research, 23*(2), 100–107.

King, I. M. (1981). *A theory for nursing.* New York: Wiley.

Laschinger, H. S. (1991). Nurses' attitudes about nursing models in practice. *Journal of Nursing Administration, 21*(10), 12–18.

Leininger, M. (1996). Culture care theory, research and practice. *Nursing Science Quarterly, 9*(2), 71–78.

Leininger, M. (1997). Overview of the theory of culture care with the ethnonursing research method. *Journal of Transcultural Nursing, 8*(2), 32–52.

Levine, M. (1973). *Theory development in nursing* (2nd ed.). Philadelphia: Davis.

Levine, M. (1989). The conservation principles of nursing: Twenty years later. In J. Riehl-Sisca, *Conceptual models for nursing practice* (3rd ed., pp. 325–337). Norwalk, CT: Appleton & Lange.

Newman, M. (1979). *Theory development in nursing. Philadelphia:* Davis.

Orem, D. (1991). *Nursing: Concepts of practice* (4th ed.). St. Louis: Mosby-Year Book.

Pedhazur, E. J., & Schmelkin, L. (1991). *Measurement, design, and analysis: An integrated approach.* Hillsdale, NJ: Erlbaum.

Roy, C. (1976). *Introduction to nursing: An adaptation model.* Englewood Cliffs, NJ: Prentice-Hall.

Roy, C. (1989). The Roy adaptation model. In J. Riehl-Sisca, *Conceptual models for nursing practice* (3rd ed., pp. 105–114). Norwalk, CT: Appleton & Lange.

Senge, P. M. (1994). *The fifth discipline: The art and practice of the learning organization.* New York: Doubleday.

von Bertalanffy, L. (1968). *General systems theory.* New York: Braziller.

Wald, F., & Leonard, R. (1964). Towards theory development of nursing practice theory. *Nursing Research, 13*(4), 309–313.

CHAPTER

3

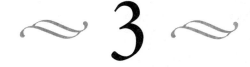

Evolving Theories of Management

Sylvia A. Price • Paula R. Jaco

The old scientific management was about ensuring control. The new will be about making sense out of chaos. (Freedman, 1992, p. 26)

Chapter Highlights

- Classical writers
- Bureaucratic model
- General systems theory
- Contingency management movement
- Chaos theory
- Contemporary organizational theorists

The purpose of this chapter is to trace the development of management and organizational theories. Because nurse executives are responsible and accountable for clinical nursing practice, education, and research in a variety of health care settings, they must be knowledgeable about classical management theories. The following discussion of the major management approaches will familiarize nurse executives with pertinent concepts and principles in the field. Selected contemporary organizational theories are also presented.

Management is a process of effectively and efficiently coordinating both human and material resources toward the accomplishment of the organization's goals.

Robbins and Coulter (1996) envision it as the process of getting activities completed efficiently and effectively with and through other people. Many believe the practice of managing is an art, whereas the organized knowledge fundamental to this practice is a science. Management and organization are not mutually exclusive and the science underlying management is still evolving and imprecise.

The management process also refers to the planning, organizing, leading, and evaluating that occur to accomplish organizational goals. Goals are an essential activity that must be directed toward some end or accomplishment. Although Nightingale sometimes described the science of administration as "the driest, most technical, and the most difficult . . ." (Cope, 1958, p. 28), she recognized that the health of each individual and a nation's well-being depended on proper management of patient care by nurses at the bedside, in communities, and in organizations (Henry, Woods, & Nagelkerk, 1990). Administrators must not only be effective, but efficient in achieving the goals within the scope of limited resources.

Administrators may be viewed negatively, especially by their subordinates. Administration often refers to powerful individuals who are in situations where conflict is frequently evident. Others see administrators as only those in corporate or top level administrative positions with luxurious offices, chauffeured limousines, private jets, and exorbitant salaries and benefits. In today's society, however, an administrator's role varies with the setting but regardless of position, title, or level, it is an extremely challenging one. This role involves critical decisions that affect such variables as production, performance, and morale, which, in turn, significantly influence corporate culture.

Early in this century, the study and formulation of theories of modern management began. Over the years, several administrative or management theories have developed, such as classical, behavioral, management science, general systems, and contingency approaches. Concepts from all of these approaches have been incorporated into the field of nursing administration.

CLASSICAL WRITERS

The classical theory of management emphasizes the functions of a manager. The classical writers focus on prescriptive management theory: on how managers should perform their functions. According to this approach, the function of management is to discover the "one best way" to perform manual tasks. This approach is based on the classical economic theory that human beings are basically motivated by a desire for economic betterment. The classical theorists identify three components of the management process: planning, organizing, and controlling. This approach consists of scientific management, or the management of work, and classical organizational theory, or the management of organization.

Taylor

One of the major contributions to the field of scientific management is Frederick W. Taylor (1911) who was a mechanical engineer at the Midvale Steel plant in

Pennsylvania. In 1911, he published *The Principles of Scientific Management.* This work, along with studies conducted before and after its publication, established Taylor as the father of scientific management. He focused on making management a science rather than an individualistic approach that was based primarily on experience. In it, he defines guidelines for improving production efficiency. At the turn of the century, business was expanding and new products were being developed, but labor was in short supply. To offset these labor shortages, two solutions were available: either substitute capital for labor or use labor more efficiently. Taylor theorized that the cause of industrial conflict was the inefficient use of scarce resources. His work concentrated on the observation of the worker's performance as he performed his task. He observed the phenomenon of "that men were," which means that men were producing far less than their capacities would permit. Taylor's principal interest was to increase production efficiency to reduce costs and increase profits and worker earnings through their higher productivity. The inducement was economic reform. The solution to increases in productivity was more efficient work performance. His premise was that workers had to be shown a better organized, more methodological way to work.

Taylor's philosophy and work techniques are still being implemented today. Industries produce products on an extensive scale within a specified time frame and base worker compensation on individual productivity. Taylor's four principles of scientific management are *(1)* develop a science for each man's work, *(2)* select and train workers scientifically, *(3)* accomplish work objectives through the cooperation of management and labor, and *(4)* divide responsibility more equitably between managers and workers.

Gantt

A colleague of Taylor's at the steel plant was a young engineer named Henry L. Gantt who was concerned with improving worker efficiency at the shop-floor level. He also recognized the human element of production work. Gantt developed a chart (called the Gantt chart) that compares the relationship between work planned and work completed on one axis and time elapsed on the other. This facilitates the administrative functions of planning, controlling, and evaluation by establishing designated outcome points.

The Gilbreths

Taylor's efforts inspired others to continue his work. Frank and Lillian Gilbreth, a husband and wife team, conducted time and motion studies. Lillian Gilbreth was an industrial psychologist who received her doctorate in that field in 1915. She raised 12 children and was depicted in the book and movie *Cheaper by the Dozen.* The Gilbreths directed their efforts toward work arrangements, eliminating unnecessary hand and body motions, and designing the proper tools for optimizing work performance. Frank Gilbreth worked as an apprentice bricklayer and observed the work of the skilled bricklayers. He was convinced that many of the body movements could be combined or eliminated so that the procedure would be simplified and production increased. He also emphasized that when applying principles of scientific management, one must consider the workers and understand their personalities and needs. The Gilbreths concluded that it is not the monotony of work that results in worker dissatisfaction but, rather, management's lack of interest in the worker.

Fayol

Contemporary with the work of Taylor is that of Henri Fayol, who worked as the managing director of a large coal-mining company in France. This experience provided Fayol with the background for his impressions about the managerial process. He sought to discover principles of management that determine the "soundness and good working order" of the firm. His ideas were first committed to writing in 1916 when Fayol contributed to the bulletin of a French industrial association. A more comprehensive statement of these ideas did not appear until 1929 with the publication of his book entitled *General and Industrial Management*. However, no English translation was widely available in the United States until 1949. Fayol was also concerned with principles of organization and the functions of an administrator. He defines administration as consisting of the functions of planning, organizing, commanding, coordinating, and controlling.

Fayol developed 14 management principles to guide the thinking of managers in resolving concrete problems and to direct the design, creation, and maintenance of an organizational structure. These principles are depicted in Table 3.1.

Over the years, Fayol's principles have been discussed and criticized in management literature, especially those principles concerning centralization, scalar chain of authority, and order. Fayol's principles do not focus on degree or specificity. He emphasizes that the balance of the 14 principles and the moral character of the manager determines the ultimate outcome of management.

BUREAUCRATIC MODEL

Max Weber (1952), a German sociologist, studied man, his work environment, and productivity. His primary concern was the bureaucratic structure and how this affected productivity. Weber described the bureaucratic organization as a highly structured, formalized, and impersonal organization.

Weber viewed this bureaucratic organizational design as the most efficient model that could be used for complex organizations. Rational-legal authority is the major management premise evident in bureaucratic structures. Rational-legal authority is defined as the "right to exercise authority based on position." Legal authority facilitates depersonalization and promotes legal obligation and obedience to the established order. In the case of legal authority, it extends to the people exercising the authority of the office under it only by virtue of the formal legality of their commands within the scope of the authority vested in that office.

Table 3.1 Fayol's 14 Management Principles

- *Division of work*
  Specialization of labor results in increased productivity through reduction of job elements expected of each worker.
- *Authority and responsibility*
  Authority is the right to give orders and the power to exact obedience, which is balanced by responsibility for performing necessary functions.
- *Discipline*
  Obedience to agreements reached between parties in the firm must be exercised. Good discipline results from effective leadership, clear understanding of the organization's rules, and prudent use of penalties for violation of these rules.
- *Unity of Command*
  Employees should receive orders from only one superior.
- *Unity of Direction*
  Each group of activities having the same purpose should operate under one head and one plan.
- *Subordination of Individual Interest to General Interest*
  The overall objectives that the group seeks to achieve take precedence over the objectives of the individual.
- *Remuneration of Personnel*
  Compensation for workers should be based on a systematic attempt to reward well-directed effort.
- *Centralization*
  The degree to which subordinates participate in decision making.
- *Scalar Chain*
  A graded chain of authority from top to bottom through which all communications flow.
- *Order*
  The material and human instruments of business must be arranged logically. The organization must provide an orderly place for all individuals.
- *Equity*
  The enforcement of established rules tempered by a sense of kindliness and justice should pervade the organization.
- *Stability and Tenure of Personnel*
  Top management should implement practices, which encourages the long-term commitment of employees, particularly of managers, to the firm.
- *Initiative*
  Employees must be encouraged to think through and implement a plan of action. The opportunity to exercise initiative is a powerful motivator.
- *Esprit de Corps*
  Unity of effort through harmony of interests. Promoting teamwork will encourage harmony within the organization.

It must be emphasized that the rational-legal authority is based on the position within the organization. When this authority evolves into an organized administrative staff, it takes the form of a bureaucratic structure. Within this organizational structure, each member of the administration occupies a position where there is *(1)* a specific delineation of power and compensation in the form of a fixed salary, *(2)* the various positions are organized in a hierarchy of authority, *(3)* fitness for office is determined by technical competence, and *(4)* the organization is governed by rules and regulations. Power is in the position or office, not in the individual, and proper respect is due because of the position. There is an assigned division of labor so that each task performed by employees is systematically established and legitimized as an official duty.

Weber's analysis tends to be descriptive (what he saw and how it should be interpreted), whereas Taylor ascribes to a prescriptive approach (how it must be done). The preceding dimensions are present in varying degrees, resulting in a highly mechanical model. Weber's discussion of bureaucracy is an example of a closed-technical system. The emphasis of this model is on the internal workings of the organization, with little attention given to environmental factors. In this highly impersonal approach, Weber views individuals as "officials" without personality or individual variations.

As a complex organization, the hospital is seen as a bureaucracy as previously described. The typical characteristics are *(1)* a hierarchical structure, with each managerial member responsible for subordinates' actions and decisions; *(2)* clear division of labor; *(3)* control by rules and regulations, so that official decisions and actions are uniform, anticipated, and stable; *(4)* impersonal relationships, so control over individuals and activities in the organization can be efficiently established; and *(5)* career mobility.

Organizations dominated by professionals often do not fit the traditional Weberian bureaucratic model. For example, nursing professionals, who are employed in a bureaucratic setting, procure a relatively standard body of knowledge on which they are examined and licensed. Their education evolves outside of the organizations, and staff nurses are hired for their basic level of skill. Their practice is regulated through an official board of nurse examiners. Nurses define an appropriate code of ethics for practice affecting both patients and nurses. Thus, professional authority is granted because of nursing's unique body of knowledge. The professional organization, the American Nurses Association (ANA), is the group that develops standards of practice. Control of the professional nursing practice in the hospital is through standards delineated by a variety of accrediting or regulatory agencies external to the organization.

HUMAN RELATIONS AND BEHAVIORAL SCIENCE APPROACHES

Behavioral scientists have challenged some established classical theories, especially the assumption that human beings are basically economically motivated. In the 1940s and early 1950s, the first branch of the behavioral school used a human relations approach and the second branch, begun in the 1950s, used a behavioral science approach.

The human relations approach modifies the premises of the classical theorists to consider differences in individual behavior and the influence of the work group on the individual. The movement began when a group of researchers headed by

Elton Mayo from Harvard University were requested to conduct studies at the Chicago Hawthorne plant of Western Electric. The purpose of the studies was to determine the relationship between employee productivity and physical working conditions. Illumination, temperature, and other working conditions were selected as representative features of the physical environment. Experiments were conducted to determine the effects of illumination changes on productivity. The conclusions were that working conditions, fatigue, and pay were secondary factors in productivity aspects. Major factors were the human aspects, such as the presence of a friendly, nonauthoritarian supervisor and increased participation in decision-making. The Hawthorne studies found that employee productivity improved when people were noticed and that when they received a lot of attention, they produced more and had a higher morale. The results of these studies indicated that social variables were more important than physical variables in affecting production.

Behavioral science theorists believed that employee satisfaction was an important variable; a satisfied worker was believed to be more productive. Douglas McGregor (1960) suggests that organizations can achieve their goals more effectively if they address the human needs of organizational members and use their potential. He believes that the vertical division of labor proposed by the classical management theorists is based on a set of negative assumptions many managers have about their employees. He formulated two sets of assumptions about human nature. What McGregor calls theory X is based on traditional autocratic assumptions about people; theory Y is founded on behaviorally based assumptions about people. Most management actions flow directly from the particular theory of human behavior that individual managers espouse.

Theory X refers to an autocratic approach to managing. It assumes that most people dislike work and will try to avoid it if at all possible. Because of this dislike of work, most people must be coerced, controlled, and threatened with punishment to get them to put forth adequate effort toward the achievement of the organization's goals. According to this theory, people have little ambition and avoid responsibility. The average human being prefers to be directed, lacks responsibility, has little ambition and wants security above all.

In contrast, theory Y implies a humanistic and supportive approach to the management of people. It assumes that people are not inherently lazy and indolent but that they may become so as a result of experience. According to this theory, the average human being learns, under proper conditions, not only to accept but also to seek responsibility. Avoidance of responsibility, lack of ambition, and emphasis on security are generally consequences of experience, not inherent human characteristics. Commitment to the organization's objectives is a function of the rewards associated with their achievement. They have potential along with imagination, ingenuity, and creativity that can be applied to their work situation.

McGregor argues that the conventional management approach ignored the facts about people because these managers adhere to theory X and follow an outmoded set of assumptions about their employees. McGregor contends that most people are close to the theory Y assumptions. The theory X manager will have a predisposition to develop autocratic or paternalistic approaches. These managers should change to a whole new theory of working with people: theory Y.

Both the human relations writers and the behavioral science workers examine the underlying determinants, types, characteristics, and roles of work groups. The behavioral science approach to the study of management is defined as "the study of observable and verifiable human behavior in organizations, using scientific procedures. It is largely inductive and problem centered, focusing on the issue of human behavior, and drawing from any relevant literature, especially in psychology, sociology and anthropology" (Filley, House, & Kerr, 1976, p. 8).

The behavioral science approach added to the earlier body of knowledge, because the behavioral scholars provided a means to test the earlier theories. Donnelly, Gibson, and Ivancevich (1975) state that advocates of the behavioral science approach were concerned that both practitioners and scholars had accepted without scientific validation so much of the management theory that preceded them. Through the work of the behavioral scientists, some aspects of the early theories have been modified, whereas others have withstood the test of scientific validations. Classical writers overemphasize the technical and structural components of management, whereas the human relationists exaggerate the psychological aspects.

MANAGEMENT SCIENCE APPROACHES

The proponents of the management science approach attempt to apply scientific knowledge to the solution of large-scale management problems in all types of organizations. Management science can be considered an extension of scientific management. The primary emphasis of this approach is on the establishment of normative models of organizational behavior for maximizing efficiency. This approach is also referred to as management science, operations research, or decision science and is related to industrial engineering and mathematic economics.

Although attempts have been made to distinguish between operations research and management science, it is very difficult to do. Several writers emphasize that the term "management science" is broader than the term "operations research" because it encompasses such fields as mathematical economics and the behavioral sciences and is also closely related to the physical sciences and engineering. Operations research is operationally oriented, whereas management science is directed toward the establishment of a broad theory. There is also a close relationship between management science and industrial engineering. Both disciplines are concerned with the same problems and often use similar techniques.

Kast and Rosenzweig (1985) emphasize that although management science and operations research represent a loose conglomeration of interests and approaches, several key concepts permeate the field:

- Emphasis on scientific method
- Systematic approach to problem-solving
- Mathematical model building
- Quantification and utilization of mathematical and statistical procedures
- Concern with economic-technical rather than psychological aspects
- Utilization of computers as tools
- Emphasis on the systems approach
- Seeking rational decisions under varying degrees of uncertainty
- Orientation toward normative rather than descriptive models (p. 90)

GENERAL SYSTEMS THEORY

The development of general systems theory has provided a basis for the understanding and integration of scientific knowledge from a variety of specialized fields. Kast and Rosenzweig (1985) define a system as "an organized, unitary whole composed of two or more interdependent parts, components, or subsystems and delineated by identifiable boundaries from its environment suprasystem" (p. 103).

When one applies the definition and key concepts of general systems theory to organizations, it is imperative also to define the structure and characteristics associated with that particular organization. The information obtained from this dissecting process provides a basic understanding of the organization in terms of its functional and operational capabilities.

The key general systems theory concepts that are common to all systems are as follows:

- A system is more than the sum of its parts; it must be viewed as a whole.
- A system has boundaries that separate it from its environment.
- Systems have subsystems and are also part of a suprasystem; they are hierarchical.

Systems can be further identified as open or closed. Open system organizations interact with their external environment, whereas closed system organizations exist within their own environment. The key concepts associated with open and closed systems are depicted in Table 3.2.

Organizations can be considered in terms of an open system model. The internal functioning of an organization must be congruent with the demands of organizational tasks, technology, external environment, and the needs of its members if the organization is effective.

The view of an organization as an open system suggests a different and more challenging role for the nurse executive than his or her role would be in a closed system. The open system interacts with its environment and moves toward a steady state while maintaining capacity for work flow and energy transforma-

Table 3.2 Comparison of Open and Closed System Models in General Systems Theory

Open System	Closed System
Exchanges information, energy, or material with its environment	Does not interact with its environment
Receives inputs from its environment	Does not receive inputs from its environment
Does not experience entropy if the inputs from the environment are as great as the energy the systems use plus the energy and materials used in the operations of the system	Subject to entropy due to lack of inputs being received from their environment; this results in the failure of the entire system
Exchanges information, energy, or material with its environment	Does not interact with its environment
Dynamic equilibrium is achieved when there is a balance or steady state; open systems have a greater potential to remain in a dynamic equilibrium through their ability to allow the inflow of materials, energy, and information	Dynamic equilibrium can be achieved in closed systems for a period of time until the lack of available resources, such as materials, energy, and information are depleted
The feedback of information required to maintain a steady state may come from inside or outside the system	The feedback of information required to maintain dynamic equilibrium may come only from inside the system
Tends toward increased elaboration, differentiation, and a higher level of organization	Tends toward entropy and disorganization
Equifinality is a process used by open systems to achieve desired results; established expected outcomes may be accomplished in a variety of ways, using assorted inputs	The cause and effect relationship is the common process associated with closed systems; regimentation and specified sequencing result in the designed or expected outcomes

Comparison of Open and Closed Systems Models in General Systems Theory, From *Organization and management: A systems and contingency approach* by F. Kast and J. Rosenzweig, 1985, New York: McGraw-Hill. Copyright 1985 by McGraw-Hill. Adapted with permission.

tion. Management must deal with external uncertainties and ambiguities and be flexible to adapt to new and changing requirements. For example, the hospital organization receives input from its external environment in the form of personnel, financial and material resources, and information. These inputs facilitate the accomplishment of outcomes expected of health care organizations. In addition, employee participation is reinforced and rewarded for achieving organizational goals.

An early systems theorist was Chester Barnard, who in 1938 wrote *The Functions of the Executive*, based on his years of experience as president of the New Jersey Bell Telephone Company. He focuses on the psychosocial aspects of organization and management. Barnard (1938) considers the organization a social system in his definition of a formal organization as "a system of consciously coordinated activities or forces of two or more persons" (p. 73). He defines the functions of the executive in a formal organization as the following: *(1)* the maintenance of organizational communication through a scheme of organization coupled with loyal, responsible, and capable people; *(2)* the securing of essential services from individuals in the organization; and *(3)* the formulation and definition of purpose.

Katz and Kahn (1978) conceptualize the role of the executive or manager as one of a number of organizational subsystems. Such subsystems operate together to meet needs and accomplish necessary tasks. They identify maintenance structures that function to maintain stability and predictability in the organization. The purpose of such structures is to preserve a steady state of equilibrium. Such structures may result in a tendency toward organizational rigidity, the preservation of the status quo in absolute terms, or they may necessitate mediation between task demands and human needs to keep the structures in operation. Such mechanisms for maintaining stability seek to formalize, or institutionalize, all aspects of organizational behavior.

The boundary structures of procurement of materials and personnel and product disposal involve transactional exchanges with the environment. These mechanisms concern acquiring control of sources of supply and creating an organizational image.

Adaptive structure concerns the survival of the organization. Both the maintenance and adaptive structures move in the direction of preserving constancy and predictability in the conditions of organizational life. Katz and Kahn (1978) emphasize that the adaptive function can focus either on attaining control over external forces, and maintaining predictability in the operations of the organization or on achieving internal modifications of organizational structures to meet the needs of a changing world.

The managerial subsystem cuts across all the operating structures of production, maintenance, environmental support, and adaptation. The managerial system is the controlling, or decision-making, aspect of the organization. The authors further state that "the complexity of organizational structures implies that the functions of management are also complex. Three basic management functions can be distinguished: *(1)* the coordination of substructures, *(2)* the resolution of conflicts between hierarchical levels, and *(3)* the coordination of external requirements with organizational resources and needs" (p. 91).

The goals, resources, and outcomes as well as technical, adaptive, psychosocial, and managerial subsystems, are all essential elements of the overall organizational structure within a general systems model framework. For example, because they were concerned with developing management principles and improving production efficiency, classical management theorists focused on the structural and managerial subsystems. The human relations and behavioral science approaches, on the other hand, emphasized the psychosocial aspects, differences in individual behavior, and the influence of the work group on the individual. The contemporary systems approach envisions the organization interacting with all of its subsystems and the external environment.

CONTINGENCY MANAGEMENT MOVEMENT

Investigators who examine the functioning of organizations in relation to the needs of their members, the internal environment, and the external forces impinging on the organization emphasize the contingency approach to management. The contingency management perspective involves understanding the interrelationships of systems and subsystems within an organization as well as the dynamics occurring between the organization and its environment.

Contingency theory originated in the late 1950s when Woodward (1958), a British researcher, attempted to determine whether the principles espoused by the scientific management theorists had any relationship to business success. She studied 100 British manufacturing firms, measuring success in relation to productivity, market standing, reputation of the firm in the community, and rate of supervisory turnover. Woodward measured the relationship between organizational structure and success, but no consistent pattern emerged. She examined the firms according to production techniques and complexity. Woodward's findings implied that different technologies imposed varying demands on individuals and organizations that had to be met through an appropriate organizational structure. This study questioned the classical theorists "one best way" approach as organizational technology was contingent on the appropriate organizational structure.

Robbins and Coulter (1996) stress that the contingency approach to management is intuitively logical. Because organizations are diverse in size, activities or tasks to be done, and individual variations, it would be unlikely to find universally applicable principles that would work in all situations. It is one thing to say, "It all depends," and another to say what it depends on. Management researchers have been attempting to identify these "what" variables. The authors describe the following four contingency variables:

- Organization size. The number of individuals in an organization is a major influence on what managers do. As size increases, so do the problems of coordination.
- Routineness of task technology. For an organization to achieve its purpose, it uses technology, that is, it engages in the process of transforming inputs into outputs. Routine technologies require organizational structures, leadership styles, and controls systems that are different from customized or nonroutine technologies.

- Environmental uncertainty. Uncertainty caused by political, sociocultural, economic, and technological change influences the management process. What works best in a stable and predictable environment would not be appropriate in a changing and unpredictable environment.
- Individual differences. Individuals differ in their desire for growth, maturity, autonomy, tolerance for change and ambiguity, desires, and expectations. These and other individual differences must be considered when managers choose motivation techniques, leadership styles, and job designs. (p. 54)

Compared with the systems approach, contingency views of organizations emphasize more specific characteristics and patterns of interrelationships among subsystems. Some theorists make no distinction between open systems and contingency theory. Others emphasize that the purpose of the contingency approach is to specify functional relationships between independent environmental and dependent management variables.

Three components of the contingency approach are the environment, management concepts, and techniques. The relationship between each of these components contributes to the functional understanding and operation of an organization using contingency theory. For example, management concepts and techniques may be classified as *(1)* process variables, including planning, organizing, directing, commanding, and evaluating; *(2)* quantitative variables such as decision-making, linear programming, and operations research models; *(3)* behavioral variables, including learning, behavior modification, motivation, and group dynamics; and *(4)* systems variables, including general systems theory, systems design, and management information systems. The contingency approach is designed to relate the environment to these various management concepts and techniques.

CHAOS THEORY

Chaos theory is a new model of how things work. Gleick (1987) explains that the chief catalyst for chaos theory was the research of Edward Lorenz, a research meteorologist at MIT, in the early 1960s. Lorenz was able to create a mathematical system of 12 equations that, although oversimplifying weather, did allow him to construct models in an attempt to predict it. He developed a computer program that simulated a weather system. It is interesting to note that science and measurement during that period gave only passing acknowledgement to measurement error, therefore, assuming that trivial errors in measuring physical systems could safely be ignored. Lorenz formulated a primitive set of graphics that would depict changes in weather patterns over time. He selected a variable such as the direction of the airstream and designated it by the letter a. The a's then marched down the role of computer paper making a series of hills and valleys that represented the way the west wind would swing north and south across a continent.

One day in the winter of 1961, Lorenz wanted to examine one sequence at greater length so he decided on a shortcut. Instead of repeating the whole run, he started midway through it. He typed the numbers from the earlier printout. Then he left the laboratory to get away from the noise to have a cup of coffee. When he returned, "he saw something unexpected, something that planted the seed for a new science" (Gleick, 1987, p. 16).

What Lorenz expected was that the run should have exactly duplicated the old one. He noticed that the weather was diverging so rapidly from the pattern of the last run that within a few months all resemblance had disappeared. The problem was due to the numbers he typed. The computer stored six decimal places: .506127. To save space he typed just three: .506. He had entered the shorter, rounded off numbers thinking that the difference—one part in a thousand—was inconsequential. This seeming inconsequential difference in a starting value had a profound and totally unpredicted effect. This sensitive dependence on initial conditions where tiny differences in input yield enormous differences in output is one of the hallmarks of chaotic systems. Robinson (1982) implies that the idea is that trajectories that begin from "arbitrarily close" initial points will, over time, diverge exponentially. Lorenz discovered that even the most minuscule of changes caused drastic alterations in weather patterns.

Scientists from other areas began experimenting with simulations of other physical systems and discovered the same phenomenon. A small change in initial conditions could have a dramatic effect on the evolution of an entire system. Freedman (1992) gives the illustration of water dripping from a faucet. If you speed up the rate of flow ever so slightly, the pattern by which drops fall changes radically. If you repeat this experiment again, the pattern will be completely different. The pattern of drip formation changes in ways that no one can model. Even a supercomputer cannot predict when the next drip will fall.

Freedman eloquently states this basic insight that minute changes can lead to radical deviations in the behavior of a natural system, which has inaugurated an equally radical shift in how scientists see the world. The 19th century emphasis on predictability and control has changed to a late 20th century appreciation for the power of randomness and chance. The behavior of relatively simple physical systems is fundamentally unpredictable.

Chaos theory's second basic insight is that patterns do lurk beneath the seemingly random behavior of these systems. These systems do not end up just anywhere; certain paths apparently make more sense or occur more frequently. Chaos theorists refer to these paths as "strange attractors." Strange attractors enable scientists to determine within broad statistical parameters what a system is likely to do, not exactly what it is going to do.

The way scientists identify predictable patterns in a system has been turned on its head. Freedman (1992) implies that instead of trying to break down a system into its component parts and analyze the behaviors of those parts independently as the reductionist tradition that so influenced Taylor, many scientists now use a more holistic approach. They focus more on the dynamics of the system rather than attempting to explain how order is designed into its parts. Scientists now emphasize how order emerges from the interaction of these parts as a whole.

To gain insight into and make use of the order that emanates from chaotic systems is the subject of Waldrop's (1992) book on the science of complexity. This is an area that is so new and wide-ranging that no one knows quite how to define it or even where the boundaries lie. Complexity research is trying to "grapple" with questions that defy conventional categories. For example:

1. How can Darwinian natural selection account for such intricate structures as the eye or the kidney?
2. What is a life, anyway?
3. What is a mind? (p. 10)

These questions all have the same answer "Nobody knows." When you examine them they actually do have a lot in common. All of the questions refer to a system that is complex with many independent agents interacting with each other. The richness of these interactions allows the system to undergo spontaneous self-organization. For example, genes in a developing embryo organize themselves in one way to make a liver cell and in another way to make a muscle cell.

These self-organizing systems are adaptive in that they do not passively respond to events; they actively try to turn whatever happens to their advantage. These systems rearrange themselves as the effects of previous actions or changes in external conditions ripple through the system. As these conditions change, the structure of the system automatically changes. Waldrop stresses that these self-organizing systems tend to change so rapidly and completely that it is meaningless to talk about agents of groups "optimizing" their behavior.

He describes research from the Santa Fe Institute, a New Mexico think tank that specializes in the analysis of "self-organizing" systems. The scientists focus on the ways that the simple actions of independent components can combine to produce extremely complex behaviors, even in the absence of central intelligence or control. An example given is how molecules organize themselves into self-reproducing proteins. Biologists determine how cells arrange themselves into immune systems.

In the process, the Santa Fe researchers developed some basic rules that Waldrop calls "complex adaptive systems," which are among the most successful in nature. Examples are ecology of tropical rain forests, colonies of ants, and the human brain. These systems have several characteristics in common, because they are "self-managed" and consist of a network of "agents" that act independently of one another and without guidance from a central control. Waldrop (1992) gives an engaging example of this phenomenon. Each of the brain's roughly 100 billion neurons is a kind of miniature chemical computer that follows its own independent pattern of behavior. Remove a neuron out of the brain, and it is still able to function. There is no master neuron or central area of the brain that is able to control what each neuron does.

These agents are capable of engaging in cooperative behavior by forming groups or communities that cooperate in producing higher order behaviors that no single agent could accomplish on its own. In the example of the brain, each neuron is connected to millions of others. Some of these communities of neurons that are clustered in certain areas of the brain specialize in functions such as language or visual recognition. These interactions among neurons produce human intelligence.

These complex adaptive systems discovered in nature contain individual agents that network to: *(1)* create self-managed highly organized behavior, *(2)* respond to feedback from the environment and fit their behavior accordingly, *(3)* learn from experience and incorporate that learning in the structure of the system, and *(4)* reap the advantages of specialization without being "stuck" in rigidity. Waldrop implies that few complexity researchers have implemented the concepts of their emerging field to organizational problems that managers face. One area of research at the Santa Fe Institute is moving in that direction. Economists are creating computer simulations of economic transactions similar to what Lorenz simulated with weather systems. They are attempting to model complex market behaviors by constructing them from a limited set of simple building blocks. Waldrop writes that "instead of viewing the economy as some kind of Newtonian machine they would see it as something organic, adaptive, surprising, and alive" (p. 252). These scientists believe that their replication of ideas is allowing them to understand the spontaneous, self-organizing dynamics of the world in a way that no one has ever done before. Their work will have potential for immense impact on the conduct of economics, business, and even politics.

CONTEMPORARY ORGANIZATIONAL THEORISTS

Senge (1990) in *The Fifth Discipline* states that the organizations that will truly excel in the future will be the organizations that discover how to tap people's commitment and capacity to learn at *all* levels in an organization. Learning organizations are possible because not only is it our nature to learn but individuals love to learn. What will distinguish learning organizations from traditional authoritarian "controlling organizations" will be mastery of the disciplines of certain basic disciplines.

His approach focuses on system thinking by contemplating the whole, not any individual part of the pattern. This is a conceptual framework, a body of knowledge and tools that attempts to make the full patterns clearer, and helps us see how to change them effectively. Senge and colleagues (1994) emphasize that the core of the learning organization is based on five "learning disciplines"—lifelong programs of study and practice.

- **Personal Mastery.** Learning to expand our personal capacity to create the results we most desire, creating an organizational environment that encourages all members of the team to develop themselves toward the goals and purposes they choose.
- **Mental Models.** Reflecting on, continually clarifying, and improving our internal pictures of the world, and seeing how they shape our actions and decisions.
- **Shared Vision.** Building a sense of commitment in a group, by developing shared images of the future we seek to create, and the principles and guiding practices by which we hope to get there.
- **Team Learning.** Transforming conversational and collective thinking skills, so those groups of people can reliably develop intelligence and ability greater than the sum of individual members' talents.
- **Systems Thinking.** A way of thinking about, and a language for describing and understanding, the forces and interrelationships that shape the behavior of systems. This discipline helps us to see how we change more effectively, and to act more in tune with the larger processes of the natural and economic world. (pp. 6–7)

In organizations, Senge and coworkers (1994) believe the individuals who contribute the most to the enterprise are the ones who are committed to the practice of these disciplines for themselves. They are expanding their own capacity to hold and seek a vision, to reflect and inquire, to build collective capabilities, and to understand systems. Senge's ideas are explored further in Chapter 22.

Gareth Morgan (1993), a modern organization theorist, explores the challenges facing modern organizations as they move from a mechanistic to an information-based world focusing on more creative, intuitive, empowered approaches to management. He emphasizes that we are departing the age of organized organizations and moving into an era where we need to facilitate and encourage processes of self-organization that allows "organized" activity to evolve and flow with change. His position attempts to reorganize the paradox that reality is simultaneously subjective and objective. Individuals engage objective realities subjectively by placing ourselves into what we "see," in such a way that actually influences what we see. This process is described as one of "engagement" and "co-production," which involves both subjective constructions and concrete interactions between real "others."

Morgan (1993) describes the process of imaginization as a mode of theorizing and an approach to social change that seeks to help people mobilize highly relativistic, open-ended, evolving interpretive frameworks for guiding understanding and action. As an approach to change, imagination seeks to mobilize the potential for understanding and transformation that is within each of us. It challenges taken-for-granted ways of thinking and opens and broadens our ability to act in new ways. He believes that individuals are *(1)* active in constructing their worlds, *(2)* can benefit from greater awareness of the process through which this occurs, and *(3)* can become simultaneously more provocative in shaping the way social reality unfolds.

He demonstrates the metaphorical basis of organizational theory and illustrates how different perspectives can generalize different insights. If individuals view organizations as cultures they begin to understand how they are held together through patterns of shared meaning, values, ideologies, rituals, and belief systems, whereas if we envision organizations as political systems, attention is on conflicting interests and power plays shaping everyday reality. If they are seen as psychic prisons we begin to realize how individuals and groups become trapped by their belief systems. In reality, organizations tend to combine all these different characteristics. Images and metaphors can be used as "mirrors" through which individuals can see themselves and their situations in fresh light, thus creating an opportunity for reflection and change. Morgan describes this process as one involving "mirrors" and "windows." If one can look in the mirror and see oneself in a new way, the mirror becomes a "window" because it allows one to see the rest of the work with a fresh perspective. It opens new "horizons," creating opportunities for new actions. Organizational windows are described in Chapter 6, offering an application of Morgan's ideas to clinical organizations.

Morgan stresses that when we see things in old ways, it is very difficult to act in new ways. This is one of the major problems with organizations and management today. For example, charts and diagrams tend to dominate our thinking about organization design. Organizational charts describe the structure of the organization. They are useful but can be extremely limiting because they convey the idea that one's organization is a structure that can be engineered and reengineered to produce appropriate results. A redesigned chart is often seen as a solution to the organization's problems. However, it can leave the basic problem unchanged. When you reshape or "downsize" a bureaucracy, you usually just end up with a smaller bureaucracy. One has to go beyond tinkering with existing organization structures. Morgan emphasizes that the challenge now is to imaginize: to infuse the process of organizing with a spirit of imagination that goes beyond bureaucratic boxes. We need to find creative ways of organizing and managing that allow individuals to "go with the flow," using new images and ideas as a means of creating shared understandings among those seeking to align their activities in an organized way.

SUMMARY

Classical management theory focuses on the structure of formal organization, the process of management, productivity, and the functions of the manager. The human relations and behavioral science approaches modify the premises of the classical theorists examining the underlying types, characteristics, and roles of the work group. The proponents of the management science approach attempted to apply scientific knowledge and mathematical modeling of systems to the solution of management problems in organizations.

Systems concepts provide the conceptual framework for understanding organizations. General systems theory includes concepts related to the understanding and integration of knowledge from a variety of disciplines. Systems theorists generally view an organization as an open system interacting with its environment. The contingency approach to management emphasizes that there should be a congruence between the organization and its environment and among its various subsystems.

The contemporary organizational approach emphasizes enterprises that will thrive in the future are the ones who respond to the needs of its members, empower individuals, and establish milieu that encourages employees' commitment. The learning organization fosters the opportunity for individuals to learn to act in the interest of the whole enterprise, and react more quickly to environmental changes because they know how to anticipate changes that are going to occur (Senge et al., 1994). The focus is on people and outcomes. Management and organizational skills are essential in professional practice.

We dream, we imagine, we create learning environments but in the final analysis works get accomplished, books are written, mountains are climbed through a complex network of management of self, time, and resources. This is why nurse executives must continually study and absorb the principles of management. Understanding good management is basic to assembling effective work groups and creating empowering environments in which vision and action lead to achievement of goals.

Drucker (1988) eloquently states that "Management is about human beings. Its task is to make people capable of joint performance, to make their strengths effective and their weaknesses irrelevant. That is what organization is all about, and it is the reason that management is the critical determining factor" (p. 75). The nurse executive should select a management theory or model that is compatible with the required work and purpose of the organization. These models provide a framework for evaluating the outcomes of both nursing administrative and clinical practice. Chapter 4 addresses the nature of organizations as people-centered workplaces.

STUDY QUESTIONS

1. What is the major premise of the classical theory of management, the human relations and behavioral science approach, and the management science approach?
2. Describe the contributions of the following individuals to their respective approaches: Taylor, Fayol, the Gilbreths, Weber, Mayo, and Barnard.
3. Which of Fayol's management principles have influenced nursing administration?
4. What assumptions do theory X managers and theory Y managers make about people?
5. Discuss the emergence of the systems approach in the study of organizations.

6. What is the difference between open and closed systems?

7. What is meant by a contingency view of an organization?

8. Explain chaos theory. How would you as a nurse executive implement this theory in your practice?

9. What distinguishes learning organizations from traditional authoritarian organizations?

10. What is the process of imaginization? How would you apply this as an approach to change?

REFERENCES

Barnard, C. (1938). *The functions of an executive.* Cambridge, MA: Harvard University Press.

Cope, Z. (1958). *Florence Nightingale and the doctors.* London: Museum Press.

Donnelly, J., Gibson, J., & Ivancevich, J. (1975). *Fundamentals of management.* Dallas: Business Publications.

Drucker, P. (1988). Management and the world's work. *Harvard Business Review, 66*(5), 65–76.

Fayol, F. W. (1949). *General and industrial management.* London: Sir Issac Pitman & Sons.

Filley, A., House, R., & Kerr, S. (1976). *Managerial process and organizational behavior.* Glenview, IL: Scott, Foresman.

Freedman, D. H. (1992). Is management still a science? *Harvard Business Review, 70*(6), 26–38.

Gleick, J. (1987). *Chaos: Making a new science.* New York: Viking.

Henry, B., Woods, S., & Nagelkerk, J. (1990). Nightingale's perspective on nursing administration. *Nursing & Health Care, 11*(4), 201–206.

Kast, F., & Rosenzweig, J. (1985). *Organization and Management: A contingency approach* (4th ed.). New York: McGraw-Hill.

Katz, D., & Kahn, R. (1978). *The social psychology of organizations.* New York: Wiley.

McGregor, D. (1960). *The human side of enterprise.* New York: McGraw-Hill.

Morgan, G. (1993). *Imaginization: The art of creative management.* Newbury Park, CA: Sage.

Robbins, S., & Coulter, M. (1996). *Management* (5th ed.). Englewood Cliffs, NJ: Prentice-Hall.

Robinson, Q. (1982). Physicists try to find order in chaos. *Science, 218*(5), 554–556.

Senge, P. M. (1990). *The fifth discipline: The art and practice of the learning organization.* New York: Doubleday.

Senge, P. M., Kleiner, A., Roberts, C., Ross, R. B., & Smith, B. J. (1994). *The fifth discipline fieldbook.* New York: Doubleday.

Taylor, F. W. (1911). *The principles of scientific management.* New York: Norton.

Waldrop, M. M. (1992). *Complexity: The emerging science at the edge of order and chaos.* New York: Simon & Schuster.

Weber, M. (1952). The essentials of bureaucratic organization: An ideal-type construction. In R. K. Merton et al. (Eds.), *A Reader in Bureaucracy* (pp. 18–27). Glencoe, IL: The Free Press.

Woodward, J. (1958). *Management and technology.* London: Her Majesty's Stationary Office.

CHAPTER

~ 4 ~

Professional Practice Models

Naomi E. Ervin • Katherine R. Jones

Any given design is necessarily an interplay of resources, possibilities, creativity, and personal judgment by the people involved. (Patton, 1990, p. 13)

CHAPTER HIGHLIGHTS

- Environments for professional practice
- Concept of environment
- Restructuring care delivery
- Collaborative practice within nursing
- Interdisciplinary collaborative practice
- Selected professional practice models

The purpose of this chapter is to discuss the concept of environments for professional nursing practice and to present examples of selected professional practice models in hospital and community environments. The term *environment* is commonly used to mean the conditions and structures outside an organization. However, both external and internal conditions of an environment influence or have an effect on professional practice models. Components or aspects of the *external environment* important for organizations are technological, legal, political, economic, demographic, ecological, and cultural including the beliefs of organized groups. The term *internal environment* refers to conditions and characteristics within an organization. The internal environment for professional nursing practice for this discussion includes all organizational elements described as tangible and intangible. Tangible elements include the physical plant, equipment, and staff; intangible elements include communication patterns, philosophy of the agency, individual values and beliefs, leadership styles, and climate.

The climate of the organization is an important aspect of the internal environment and is classified in this chapter as an intangible element of the internal environment. Climate is defined as "the psychological atmosphere that results from and surrounds the operation of the structure" (Jones, 1981, p. 160). Organizational climate is the quality of the total organizational environment that is a result of the interaction of the formal organizational policies, the personality factors, and the stress created when individual and organizational goals are integrated. The climate of an organization is considered an important factor because it serves as a link between such variables as policies and orgaizational sturcutre and such end result variables as satisfaction and turnover.

The specific aspects of an environment for professional nursing practice will vary with different settings, regional customs, and institutional history. However, the general concepts and frameworks presented herein may be adapted to fit a particular situation.

ENVIRONMENTS FOR PROFESSIONAL PRACTICE

The environment created by a nursing service in any setting serves as the foundation of the four components of professional nursing: clinical practice, administration, education, and research. Although all four components may not exist simultaneously in each practice setting, the established environment can ease the introduction of additional components at different points in time. Nurses and nursing leadership create the environment that serves as the foundation for the four components of professional nursing practice.

Unfortunately, the environment created by nurse executives does not constitute the total environment for professional nursing practice. Some aspects of the total institutional or societal environment will no doubt have more impact on the nursing staff at times than does the nursing environment. If these other aspects are negative, nursing practice may stagnate even with a well-planned basis for the nursing environment. On the other hand, the nursing-created environment may cushion the impact of some aspects of the broader environment. For example, if a nursing shortage or cost-containment initiative forces an institution to hire additional, less skilled staff, aspects of the nursing environment, such as detailed position descriptions, appropriate practice policies, and comprehensive orientations, could reduce the potential negative impact on the overall quality of nursing care (Bromley, 1997).

In addition to their accountability for quality nursing care, nurse executives have numerous reasons to provide leadership in creating the environment for professional nursing practice. Included in these reasons are their roles as members of the clinical management team, maintaining a reputation for high quality that attracts potential employees and customers, and increasing demands to report privately and publicly specific quality indicators.

THE CONCEPT OF ENVIRONMENT

Conceptual approaches to environment have been identified in the fields of business, organizational behavior, and more recently in nursing. The external environment of an organization includes the forces of society, economics, and geography as well as elements of concern to the health care organization: competitors, government regulators, accreditors, suppliers, clients and their families, the community, and general economic conditions (Decker & Sullivan, 1992). McDonagh (1993) has identified several global trends that continue to influence health care delivery: the struggle for human freedom and self-determination, ecological preservation, power shifts, shift from competition to collaboration, the changing workforce, and rapid rise in technology.

Most conceptual approaches are geared to the environment external to the organization. The health-organization environment model (Figure 4.1) represents one approach that includes both the internal and the external environment. This model provides a basis for assessing the structure, processes, and outcomes before changes are made. The health-organization environment model has values as the core. Values are reflected in the philosophy that defines the purpose for which the organization was established and the reason for its existence. The structure consists of the systems needed to carry out the goals. The climate component of the intangible internal environment is the psychological atmosphere that results from and surrounds the operation of the structure; it is both a result of and a determinant of the behavior of individuals within the structure (Jones, 1981). The outermost ring of the model depicts the many aspects of the external environment with which an organization must interact to accomplish its goals.

For purposes of analyzing and designing an internal environment for nursing practice, the health organization-environment model arbitrarily separates the internal environment into tangible and intangible aspects. Both types of aspects are viewed as having structure, process, and outcome components, which are primarily used in models for quality assessment and improvement. In a quality improvement model, the structure components are the human, physical, and financial resources needed to provide care. Structure includes the number, distribution, and qualifications of personnel, as well as the equipment, the physical facility, the care delivery system, and the organizational structure of the health care setting. The process components involve the activities of health care providers in their management of patients. Outcomes are the end results of care for the patient (Donabedian, 1980).

In the health organization-environment model (see Figure 4.1), the process and outcome improvement components are not the same as those of a quality improvement model. The process components in the environment are those activities

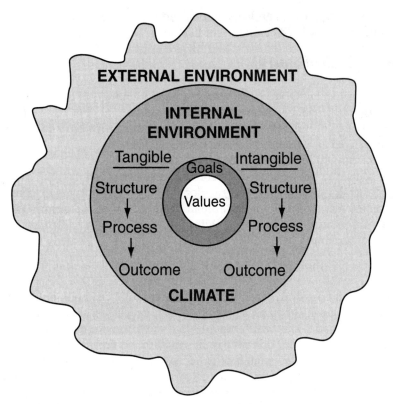

Figure 4.1 Health organization-environment model.

carried out to implement the goals and objectives of the organization, for example, patient care conferences and decision-making procedures, such as shared governance and communication strategies. The outcome components are the aspects of the environment that result from the processes and structures, for example, staff satisfaction, staff turnover, and achievement of objectives. The relationships among structure, process, and outcomes are discussed in Chapter 17.

Using the Environment Model

To use the health organization-environment model, the nurse executive must begin with an assessment of the current situation, including data collection and the identification of problems. An environmental assessment is also the first step in the strategic planning process. Because an assessment of every component of the environment is not practical, the process should begin with those aspects of the department that are considered priorities, and the other aspects should be incorporated into the long-term plan for nursing service.

How does the nurse executive know which components are priorities? Several approaches may be used to identify priorities:

- Observational studies
- Survey of the nursing staff
- Survey of key stakeholders and selected others in the organization
- Focus groups
- Combination of approaches

Interviews of key informants could be conducted by internal or external groups. External groups will be more objective and may be seen as more credible.

Attempts to study or survey broadly for all possible components results in frustration in the typical institution. However, a well-designed study of a few key areas could result in a valid basis for recommendations for creating the environment for nursing practice. A beginning point for looking at the current environment could be the assessment of the formal systems of the organizational structure: reporting relationships, communication patterns, decision-making procedures, norms, accountability system, and reward system (Jones, 1981). The area or areas that appear to be troublesome should be assessed in more depth, but a few key questions to the staff about each area could be included in a survey.

The environment model provides a systematic approach to environment development as well as to a study or series of studies of a nursing service. Table 4.1 depicts some of the structure, process, and outcome components of the internal organization environment and provides a compilation of the major items defined in this chapter as part of the environment for nursing practice. Components have been arbitrarily placed in a category, but they may be arranged differently without harming the concept.

Several of the components are explained in depth in other chapters. The reader should refer to those sources for definitions, conceptual frameworks, and discussion. For purposes of example, a component from each category is discussed briefly here.

As structure components, policies provide guidelines for the staff. Policies should free the nursing staff from the burden of making routine decisions, while not restraining the practice of professional nursing. Because policies reflect the philosophy and mission of the nursing service, they are a reflection, in turn, of the organization's goals and mission. In creating an environment conducive to nursing practice, policies should be congruent with statements such as the American Nurses Association (ANA) Code for Nurses, the ANA Standards of Nursing Practice, the state nursing practice act, the ANA Standards for Nursing Services, standards of accrediting bodies, and requirements of regulatory agencies. Precisely what policies should be developed and how they should be stated are decisions to be made by appropriate nursing staff with nursing administrative approval.

Table 4.1 Internal Environment Components

Structure Components	Process Components	Outcome Components
Organizational structure	Patient care documentation system	Staff/consumer satisfaction
Philosophy and mission statements	Nursing care plans/ therapies	Achievement of objectives
Policies and procedures	Patient care criteria and standards	Achievement of criteria and standards
Nursing practice patterns	Management objectives/ work plans	Staff morale
Staff numbers and mix	Decision-making patterns	Trust and openness
Job descriptions	Clinical judgments	Staff support
Staff qualifications	Clinical pathways	Reduced stress
Performance criteria	Disease management protocols	Reduced risk
Equitable compensation	Delegation of tasks/ responsibilities	Cost-effective care
Computerized information systems	Interdisciplinary collaboration	Positive interdisciplinary relationships

Nursing care plans using standardized nursing language are process components that provide for continuity of nursing care and constitute one mechanism of professional accountability. Care plans should be written so as to become a permanent part of patients' records. The contents should be individualized for each patient, even if standardized nursing care plans are used for some patient populations. Among other characteristics, a system for planning patients' care should aim for economical use of the nurse's time, be readily accessible to all staff, incorporate standards of care, and emphasize nursing care. In addition, the staffing of the supportive environment should be sufficient to allow enough time for care planning.

An example of an outcome component of the environment model is staff satisfaction. Although many variables affect satisfaction, several of these variables for nurses are within the nursing department and may be influenced by the nurse executive. The National Commission on Nursing (1981) cited evidence to support this: "Although they are accountable for nursing care, nurses at all levels often have insufficient decision-making authority in management of patient care and in other areas of the environment in which nurses practice (p. 9)." Furthermore, staff nurses reported that the nursing administrator's position and influence in the institution were important factors in their job satisfaction.

RESTRUCTURING CARE DELIVERY

Restructuring care delivery to produce successful professional practice models involves redesigning systems, processes, and jobs in ways that improve patient and organizational outcomes. Restructuring supports the development of high-quality work environments in which to practice. To redesign the basic flow of work in the internal environment requires integrating the thoughts and creativity of the many disciplines involved in patient care delivery (Flarey, 1995). Various reasons exist for redesigning care delivery: expense of an all-professional work force, fluctuating inpatient census, the shift to ambulatory care and shorter lengths of stay, the decline in and changing nature of reimbursement, the imposition of quality of care mandates, mergers and consolidations in the health care industry, managed care constraints and challenges, and integrated service networks (Flarey, 1995). Three major goals of work redesign have been identified: *(1)* to improve quality of the care being delivered, *(2)* to manage the cost of care more effectively, and *(3)* to improve the quality of work life of staff (Skeggs, Vestal, & Walter, 1991).

Redesign entails changes in people, work processes, culture, services and products, communication patterns, attitudes and behaviors, and rewards and requires systems thinking and integration. It cannot be viewed as only a nursing agenda or initiative—or it is doomed to failure. Work redesign must be examined within the context of the whole organization or enterprise. It must have an organization-wide perspective, integrating all departments into one system redesign. Everyone within the system and served by the system needs to be included in the planning process (Flarey, 1995; Jones, DeBaca, Tornebeni, & Yarbrough, 1995).

Strategies for identifying system problems and issues prior to redesign (Jacob, 1993) include surveys and focus groups of key constituencies—employees, patients, physicians, and managers. These target groups can be helpful in identifying inefficiencies in the care delivery process and in identifying opportunities for change. Within work redesign, the organization must define its model of care. The model must be consistent with the mission, resources, culture, values, and product lines of the enterprise. Flarey describes several models, including case management, theory-based models (Orem), patient-centered (Lathrop, 1993), work flow (Fritz, 1992), or service unit. The selected model must provide the necessary support services for the nurses to deliver high-quality care (Yancer, 1990).

McDonagh (1993) identified three work redesign models for hospitals:

1. Nurse extender models—providing less skilled employees to assist nurses to provide care. Extenders may perform clinical tasks, similar to traditional

nursing assistants or aides, or unit support functions, such as housekeeping, transport, or dietary tasks. For example, Jones, Redman, VandenBosch, Holdwick and Wolgen (1999) describe the multifunctional worker model implemented in one Midwest community hospital.

2. Patient-focused approach—restructuring operations around patient care needs. Requires cross-training at all levels (professional and nonprofessional). Many services are decentralized to patient care units, including pharmacy, routine laboratory, phlebotomy, admissions, and discharge. Patient aggregation according to diagnosis and level of need is done as well as bedside documentation by exception. This model is said to reduce compartmentalization, to make more employees accessible for direct patient care, and to reduce structural inefficiencies. One patient-focused care model has been described in detail by Jones and coworkers (1995).

3. Expanded/alternative roles—an expansion and enhancement of professional practice of nursing. The professional role of the nurse is defined, then appropriate support staff are deployed to the unit to assist the nurse. The model does not involve cross-training of personnel. Examples of integrated client care services models have been described by Flarey (1995).

McDonagh also identified several organizational enablers: case management, shared governance, documentation by exception, critical pathways, supply management systems, communication links, and scheduling systems. These enablers support the work of the professional staff and help ensure efficient and effective care delivery, regardless of the model selected.

Case management models rely heavily on the use of clinical pathways or care maps. Clinical pathways are believed to enhance quality, integrate services, reduce length of stay, and assist in resource management (Lumsdon & Hagland, 1993). Case management models vary tremendously across settings: case managers may be unit or institution based, may be clinical nurse specialists, bachelor's-prepared nurses, any RNs, or non-RN (social worker, lay person). The model may be within the walls of the institution only or include subacute care and home care. The evidence of effectiveness of these models in reducing costs and enhancing quality is mixed and sparse.

The patient-focused care model relies on the creation of new roles to support patient care delivery. Caregivers are trained to be multiskilled, blurring disciplinary boundaries. Services are decentralized to the patient care unit, reducing compartmentalization within the organization and subsequent down time. Many disciplines become unit based and report to one manager, usually the nurse manager (Sheedy, 1993). The role of the RN becomes one that emphasizes cognitive activities and highly skilled tasks. Teams of caregivers are assigned to patients rather than a single professional nurse. The structure and roles of management have also been redesigned. Administrative structures have been flattened and responsibility spheres eroded. Management is no longer solely responsible for conveying a common organizational vision for the transformation, and then providing the leadership to ensure the vision is realized (Flarey, 1995). Today's environment calls for greater levels of leadership, not management. Required skills include coaching, mentoring, self-governance, continuous quality improvement, enterprise-wide perspective, collaboration, partnerships, strategic vision, horizontal management, fiscal accountability, and innovation (Flarey, 1993).

COLLABORATIVE PRACTICE WITHIN NURSING

The development of partnerships with physicians and other health professionals is a key strategy to improving the community's health (Bolton, Georges, Hunter, Long, & Wray, 1998) and is the primary step in building professional practice models. In the final analysis, however, it is unreasonable to talk about joint or collaborative practice with physicians if there is no collaboration within nursing. Integration (internal collaboration) can and should occur in any setting where professional nursing is practiced. All nursing units in any practice setting have at a minimum, practice and quality improvement committees or councils. Is this not the first level of integration? Is this not an opportunity for faculty involvement? All schools of nursing have curriculum committees. Are these not opportunities for service involvement? The education of students should be a high priority for nurse executives, and opportunities for clinical practice and research should be available for nursing students. Figure 4.2 depicts a collaborative nursing model, freestanding from medical structure, that could optimize communication between and among educators and practitioners.

The collaborative model could be modified to meet the needs of any professional practice approach in any acute, community, or long-term care setting. The model builds on trust, mutual respect, and pride in professional nursing. Although the same person could be in the designated positions, this is not necessary. In a collaborative approach, two or more nurses can work together to achieve common goals related to excellence in practice, education, and research. This is especially important as we mount outcomes management programs and implement evidence-based practice.

Interdisciplinary Collaborative Practice

Not long ago, the relationship between physicians and nurses was clear-cut. Nurses understood their place in the world, and physicians were captains of the health care team. The team consisted of two people: the physician and the nurse. Today, the relationship has changed dramatically as care has become more complex and there is more need for multidisciplinary patient-centered care. Moreover, collaboration, as a relationship of interdependence, requires that the parties involved recognize complementary roles (Fagin, 1992).

In today's world, there seems to be a lack of opportunity for interpersonal understanding. Many more nurses are ready to do battle over real or perceived nonrecognition. Where once the alliance of medicine and nursing was strong, there is increasing evidence of a bonding between administration and medicine. This has

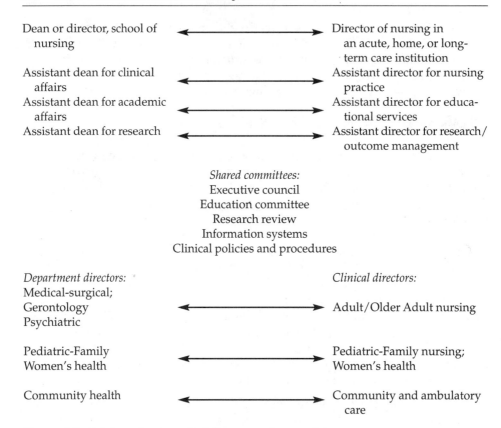

Figure 4.2 Collaborative intradisciplinary nursing model.

been driven by financial reimbursement and reforms, requiring that physician and hospital incentives be in alignment. At the same time, financial pressures have resulted in proposals to reduce the nursing budget, a large proportion of the organization's labor budget. This has led to dissatisfaction with staffing levels, concerns about quality of care, and tense contract negotiations.

In the late 20th century, the National Joint Practice Commission (1981) offered four different but typical hospitals the opportunity to demonstrate how to successfully alter the physician-nurse relationship with resulting benefits to patients, nurses, physicians, and the hospital. The commission, supported by the American Medical Association, the American Nurses Association, and the W.K. Kellogg Foundation, established guidelines for nurses and physicians to use in collaborating as colleagues in providing patient care. The work of the Joint Practice Commission has paved the way for the development of collaborative models.

The emphasis on collaborative practice can be attributed to reasons related to changing times and changing professional goals:

1. Emergence of specialty professional nursing roles
2. Increased interest in patient-centered care

3. Conflict in images of nursing projected by nursing service and nursing education
4. Gaps in communications among health professionals
5. Emergence of integrated delivery systems
6. Need to manage patients as they move across the continuum of care

Intra- and interdisciplinary collaboration is essential for the success of any professional practice model. Collaborative models reflect a flexible process of ongoing interaction, assertiveness, and creativity between individuals from two or more disciplines that influence the direction of patient care. They require communication and interdependent decision-making regarding patient care. Although developed around a particular newborn diagnosis, Lassen et al. (1997) found that implications from collaborative practice can be generalized. Results following implementation of a collaborative model yielded:

• Decrease in number of diagnoses across disciplines resulting in few complications
• Decrease in family anxiety and confusion
• Promotion of continuity and consistency of care leading to fewer gaps in care delivery
• Reduction in patient potential harm from treatments
• Reduction in consultation costs

Nurse-physician collaboration includes mutual power-control, separate and combined practice spheres, mutual concerns, and common patients' goals. Mutual power-control is present in interactions when nurses and physicians value and are aware of opportunities to participate with each other in conversations about patients. Separate practice spheres are mandated by state practice acts, but nurses and physicians have an overlap in responsibility. It is important for patient care that nurses and physicians agree on who is responsible for particular aspects of care. Some redefinition of these spheres of responsibility is occurring in some chronic care settings with the use of nurse case managers. These models also allow greater roles for patients and their caregivers.

Effective collaboration in the area of mutual concerns requires the right amounts of assertiveness (attempt to satisfy one's own concerns) and cooperativeness (attempt to satisfy the other person's concerns). Collaboration also requires that agreement be reached over goal responsibility before nurses, physicians, and other health professionals assume responsibility for care of patients. This agreement allows for working on common goals while not neglecting any discipline-specific goals (Jones, 1994). More change is occurring as health care moves from care of individuals to care of populations.

The goal of collaborative practice is to improve health care, not to protect or preserve professional prerogatives. Interdependent relationships and willingness to reformulate roles are facilitated when practitioners are mature, experienced, and comfortable in their own role. The extent to which collaboration occurs among physicians, nurses, and administrators depends on the support of professional autonomy and the sharing of care activities between and across participating disciplines.

Multidisciplinary collaborative practice can be conceptualized, planned, supported, and evaluated, taking into account the specific characteristics of the organization and the individual patient care situation. In determining either the need for or planning the evaluation of selected models, one might well raise the question: How does one know if collaborative practice exists in an institution? Its existence can be recognized by the following criteria: *(1)* effective communication patterns, verbal and written, between and among physicians, nurses, and administrators; *(2)* the rewarding of improved patient care on units in which it is practiced; *(3)* established efficient and effective support services; *(4)* patient involvement and participation, and documented clinical outcomes; and *(5)* a climate of mutual trust and respect.

SELECTED PROFESSIONAL PRACTICE MODELS

Differentiated practice is perhaps the best known professional practice model along with collaborative practice in hospital settings. American nursing has differentiated practice by roles for decades with different assignments for RNs, LPNs, and aides. Differentiated nursing practice is a phrase used to describe the sorting of roles, functions, and work of RNs according to some identified criteria, education, clinical experience, and competence (Baker et al., 1997). The goal is to provide distinct levels of nursing practice based on educational preparation. Little research has been done on the effects of differentiating practice. With cross-training of workers and self-care becoming increasingly more common, this practice model is likely to receive little attention in the 21st century. Indeed, Buerhaus (1997) has recently raised serious economic and political questions regarding staffing regulations that would lock nurses into fixed roles. The health care system is changing dramatically, almost on a daily basis, and it behooves nurse executives to look beyond nurse-centered practice models.

Patient-focused care (PFC), which first appeared as the Planetree Model (described in other chapters), is a model frequently chosen by many hospitals to compete in the marketplace (Myers, 1998). It is viewed as a means for decreasing cost of care while improving quality. Multidisciplinary teams or patient needs teams are groups of health care professionals who oversee patient care needs from admission to discharge.

Myers conducted a search of the health care literature from 1991 to 1997, covering a variety of implementation studies of PFC models in facilities of various size from all parts of the United States. All sources agreed in a general description of PFC as a model that seeks to integrate the organization's values and culture with its operational excellence, vision, and processes to achieve a customer-focused organization. Major cultural change is required to implement this model. Organizations with deeply held traditional hierarchical values will have difficulty changing from physician-centered models. The resultant reorientation of division of labor places nurses in leadership roles in multidisciplinary teams with multi-skilled workers. In these PFC models, traditional departmentalization of services is lost.

Jones, DeBaca, and Yarbrough (1997) support the need for understanding existing culture and subcultures before attempting to change to a PFC model. The authors describe PFC as a model of care delivery built around self-contained units staffed by multidisciplinary caregivers who can provide 80% of what patients need in their rooms. This reflects a substantial change from traditional structures, roles, and operations of health care organizations. Walls between disciplines are removed, which can threaten deeply held professional norms and values. However, key components of PFC are consistent with those of continuous quality improvement. Much of the work is accomplished by interdisciplinary teams and a major focus is on the process of care delivery—thus eliminating redundant steps. Hierarchical hospitals, such as academic centers and unionized environments, may not have the flexibility to introduce these models.

The PFC models are a good example of boundary-less management discussed in Chapter 6. In one model, care pairs replaced traditional categories of RNs, pharmacists, and LPNs. Research by Jones and coworkers (1997) is relevant because it measured cultural changes before and after introduction of care partners in a hospital setting using Quinn's competing values framework (Quinn, 1988). Care partners or pairs were labeled: *(1)* clinical partner (licensed health professional), *(2)* technical partner (licensed care technician or assistant, *(3)* service partner (provides support services), and *(4)* administrative partner (combined unit secretary/receptionist). Interestingly, they did not include the consumer in their model, which seems generic to patient-centered models described in other literature.

The PFC models can be found in community settings where they are beginning to flourish. Individualized home nursing care (IHNC) is described in detail in Chapter 27. A parish nursing model developed by Sandra Byers and the LIGHT model developed by Marcia Anderson are described in detail in the appendix.

SUMMARY

The internal environment of a health care organization consists of the conditions and characteristics within the organization. The health organization-environment model is one approach the nurse executive can use in assessing, planning, and implementing the environment in which nurses will practice. According to this model, the internal environment is composed of tangible and intangible elements. The categories of structure, process, and outcome can be used to classify the components of an organization. The authority to make changes and approve nursing practice components is necessary for the effective performance of a nurse executive undertaking the establishment of an environment for nursing practice. Restructuring care delivery is essential for successful implementation of professional practice models. This chapter has described several professional practice models including collaborative practice, differentiated practice, and patient-focused care. The importance of intra- and interdisciplinary collaboration is emphasized. Two community professional practice models are introduced in this chapter with more detailed descriptions provided in the appendix.

STUDY QUESTIONS

1. What do you consider the two most important structure, process, and outcome components in the nursing practice environment?
2. What are some other components that could be added to each list?
3. Develop a model other than the health organization-environment model that could be used for assessing and planning the environment for nursing practice.
4. Discuss the factors related to restructuring care delivery systems.
5. Trace the history of collaborative practice, practice partnerships, and the development of professional practice models.
6. Compare and contrast patient-focused care delivery models in the hospital and community settings.

REFERENCES

Baker, C. M., Lamm, G. M., Winter, A. R., Robbeloth, V. B., Ransom, C. A., Conly, F., Carpenter, K. C., & McCoy, L. E. (1997). Differentiated nursing practice: Assessing the state of the science. *Nursing Economic$, 15*(5), 253–264.

Bolton, L. B., Georges, C. A., Hunter, V., Long, O., & Wray, R. (1998, Spring). Community health collaboration models for the 21st century. *Nursing Administration Quarterly, 22*(3), 6–17.

Bromley, G. E. (1997). An executive nurse in action. In S. R. Byers (Ed.), *The executive nurse* (pp. 14–22). Albany: Delmar.

Buerhaus, P. I. (1997). What is the harm in imposing mandatory hospital nursing staff regulations? *Nursing Economic$, 15*(2), 66–72.

Decker, P. J., & Sullivan, E. J. (1992). *Nursing administration: A micro/macro approach for effective nurse executives.* Norwalk, CT: Appleton & Lange.

Donabedian, A. (1980). *The definition of quality and approaches to its assessment* (vol. 1). Ann Arbor, MI: Health Administration Press.

Fagin, C. M. (1992). Collaboration between nurses and physicians: No longer a choice. *Academic Medicine, 67,* 295–303.

Flarey, D. L. (1993). The changing role of the nurse manager. *Seminars for Nurse Managers, 1*(1), 41–48.

Flarey, D. L. (1995). *Redesigning nursing care delivery: Transforming our future.* Philadelphia: Lippincott.

Fritz, L. (1992). Changing the structure of daily operations: The work flow model of the future. *Healthcare Executive, 7*(4), 24–26.

Jacob, R. (1993). Beyond quality and value. *Fortune, 127*(10), 39–52.

Jones, J. E. (1981). The organizational universe. In J. E. Jones & J. W. Pfeiffer (Eds.), *The 1981 Annual handbook for group facilitators.* San Diego, CA: Pfeiffer & Company.

Jones, K. R., DeBaca, V., Tornebeni, J., & Yarbrough, M. (1995). Implementation and evaluation of patient-centered care. In K. Kelly & M. Maas (Eds.), *Health care work redesign: Vol. 7. Series on nursing administration.* Thousand Oaks, CA: Sage.

Jones, K. R., DeBaca, V., & Yarbrough, M. (1997). Organizational culture assessment before and after implementing patient-focused care. *Nursing Economic$, 15*(2), 73–80.

Jones, K. R., Redman, R. W., VandenBosch, T. M., Holdwick, C., & Wolgen, F. (1999). Evaluation of the multifunctional worker role: A stakeholder analyses. *Outcomes Management for Nursing Practice, 3*(3), 128–135.

Jones, R. A. P. (1994). Conceptual development of nurse-physician collaboration. *Holistic Nursing Practice, 8*(3), 1–11.

Lassen, A. A., Fosbinder, D. M., Minton, S., & Robins, M. M. (1997). Nurse/physician collaborative practice: Improving health care quality while decreasing cost. *Nursing Economic$, 15*(2), 87–91.

Lathrop, J. P. (1993). *Restructuring health care: The patient focused paradigm.* San Francisco: Jossey-Bass.

Lumsdon, K., & Hagland, M. (1993, October 20). Mapping care. *Hospitals & health networks,* pp. 34–40.

McDonagh, K. J. (Ed.). (1993). *Patient-centered hospital care.* Ann Arbor, MI: American College of Healthcare Executives.

Myers, S. M. (1998). Patient-focused care: What managers should know. *Nursing Economic$, 16*(4), 180–188.

National Commission on Nursing. (1981). *Initial report and preliminary recommendations.* Chicago: Hospital Research and Educational Trust.

National Joint Practice Commission. (1981). *Guidelines for establishing joint or collaborative practice in hospitals.* Chicago: Neely Printing.

Patton, M. Q. (1990). *Qualitative evaluation and research methods* (2nd ed.). Newbury Park, CA: Sage.

Quinn, R. E. (1988). *Beyond rational management.* San Francisco, CA: Jossey-Bass.

Sheedy, S. (1993). The head nurse role in redesign. *Journal of Nursing Administration, 23*(7/8), 14–15.

Skeggs, L., Vestal, K., & Wolter, R. (1991). *Redesigning care delivery.* Chicago: American Organization of Nurse Executives.

Yancer, D. (1990). Redesigning the work. *Aspen's Advisor for Nurse Executives, 5*(8), 4–5.

CHAPTER

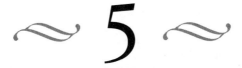

~ 5 ~

The Person in a Leadership Role

Lillian M. Simms • Annie J. Starr

The wise leader does not intervene unnecessarily. The leader's presence is felt but often the group runs itself. (Heider, 1985, p. 33)

Chapter Highlights

- The nurse executive as a leader
- Maslow, McClusky, and the development of leadership
- Leadership styles and theories
- Personal attributes of successful nurse leaders
- Personal resources and support systems
- New age leadership
- Developing leaders and followers

The purpose of this chapter is to emphasize the person in a leadership role of nurse executive by focusing on the importance of personal attributes and leadership skills. It is a myth that only those who cannot practice, teach, and those who cannot teach, administrate. Leaders who love the challenge and hard work of creating a climate in which professional nursing practice can occur are catalysts not only for their own activities but for those of others. The effective nurse executive must possess the highest level of ability and the greatest personal skills. Such leaders are not bound by thinking about what cannot be done. Rather, they see the same puzzles others see, but they envision different ways of putting them together in diverse settings and positions.

There is a leadership crisis in nursing and a critical shortage of executives with the political, psychological, and social management skills needed to cope with today's changing world (Simms, 1991). Nurses have been unprepared or unwilling to assume leadership roles. Women are not socialized to assume leadership roles, nor do existing nursing programs really address the need to prepare nursing leaders who are effective administrators. Chaska often spoke of the nursing profession as being in a "mist" of conflicting views about professionalism and professional practice. By 1990, however, Chaska confirmed that nursing is in the midst of advancing change with multiple evidence of turning points in the profession.

The hospital is no longer the primary area of employment for nurses. Nurses are employed in diverse settings in a variety of executive roles as discussed in Chapter 8.

Regardless of the setting for practice—whether hospital community health agency or long-term care setting—nurse executives must know how to compete effectively in a businesslike world.

THE NURSE EXECUTIVE AS A LEADER

Nurse executives cannot create a climate for professional practice unless they are leaders as well as clinical managers. Administration can be carried out by non-nurses, but true leadership in a professional practice setting must be manifested by a nurse with leadership skills. The work of nurse executives differs from that of other hospital administrators in that nursing involves professionals, or what Drucker (1980) calls "knowledge workers." The productivity of knowledge workers requires that people be assigned where there is potential for results and not where knowledge and skill cannot produce results. The utilization of nursing resources according to level of education, experience, and strengths is of critical importance today for all nurses in administrative posts.

There are no known ways of training great leaders, and the preparation of leaders in nursing has become the challenge of this decade for schools of nursing. Most deans and program directors will claim to be preparing leaders, but the fact remains that true leaders simply are not emerging from nursing graduate programs.

According to Zaleznik (1981), managers and leaders differ fundamentally in their world views, perceptions, and personal characteristics as portrayed in Table 5.1.

- Attitudes toward goals: managers tend to adapt impersonal attitudes toward goals; leaders adapt personal and active attitudes toward goals.
- Conception of work: managers act to limit choices as they seek the accomplishment of specific tasks through predetermined combinations of people and ideas; leaders work to develop fresh approaches to long-standing problems and to open issues for new options.
- Relation with others: managers prefer to work with people, avoid solitary activity, and relate to people according to the roles they play; leaders are

Table 5.1 *Differences between Managers and Leaders*

Characteristics	Managers	Leaders
Attitudes toward goals	Adapt impersonal attitudes toward goals	Adapt personal and active attitudes toward goals
Conception of work	Act to limit choices to specific tasks and people	Work to develop fresh approaches to problems
Relation with others	Relate to people according to their role, avoid solitary activity	Concerned with workers as people who are affected by events and decisions
Sense of self	Once-born personalities; belong to institution	Twice-born personalities and separate from their environment; never belong to organization

more empathic and are concerned with the effects that events and decisions have on participants.

- Sense of self: managers are once-born personalities and belong to the institutional environment; leaders tend to be twice-born personalities and separate from their environment; they may work in organizations but never belong to them.

Managers develop through socialization, and leaders develop through personal mastery. For a leader, self-esteem does not depend solely on positive attachments and real rewards. Leaders cannot be bought by the institution. They have visions and dreams that managers may never see. As nursing seeks to become recognized as a profession, it is increasingly important to have visionaries in leadership roles to find new answers to old, unresolved questions. Who, then, are leaders? They are people who:

- Know where they are going.
- Know how to get there.
- Have courage and persistence.
- Can be believed.
- Can be trusted not to sell their cause for personal advantage.
- Make missions important, exciting, and possible.
- Make subordinates feel that their roles in the mission are important.
- Make others feel capable of performing their roles.

Managers, says Drucker (1980), are paid to enable people to do the work for which they are paid. Nurse executives do not earn their pay if they do not create a professional practice climate in which nurses can do their work. Leaders make a difference in the lives of those who work for them and with them.

MASLOW, McCLUSKY, AND THE NURSE EXECUTIVE

The able nurse executive is not only self-motivated but is also able to create an environment in which others are motivated. To motivate others requires a strong self-concept and a high place on the ladder of Maslow's hierarchy of needs (1962). In other words, the able executive is one who has reached or is approaching the stage of self-actualization. New style organizations demand leaders who are interested in the development of others, not just their own personal success. Such leadership involves self-development and a true sense of knowing oneself intellectually, bodily, emotionally, and spiritually (Kinsman, 1998).

Maslow's Theory

Maslow's theory of motivation can be applied to almost every aspect of human life, but it has special significance for those who lead and guide others. Maslow's theory provides a basis for the higher needs of psychological growth. People are initially motivated by basic physiologic needs. As those needs are satisfied, the individual moves toward the level of higher needs and becomes motivated by them. This is the heart of Maslow's theory. Most previous studies assumed that needs could be isolated and studied separately. Maslow considered the individual as an integrated whole. The identification of needs for growth, development, and utilization of potential are an important part of self-actualization. Maslow has described this need as the "desire to become more and more what one is, to become everything that one is capable of becoming" (1962).

Figure 5.1 depicts Maslow's hierarchy of needs. Maslow's hierarchy has been applied to patient needs. It also has significant application for the nurse as a person. Nurse executives as nurse persons and leaders of other nurse persons have a special need to reach the level of self-actualization. Nurse persons were first described by Simms and Lindberg (1978) as fully functioning individuals who are comfortable with using the self as well as technical skills in professional practice. This implies the need for growth and development of the nurse as a person.

Self-actualization is the desire for self-fulfillment, to make actual all one's potentialities. Maslow related potential to the concept of growth, and by growth, he meant the constant development of talents, capacities, creativity, wisdom, and character. To play a role satisfactorily, a person must have a self-concept that fits the role.

McClusky's Conceptual Framework

Howard McClusky (1974) of the University of Michigan, delineated educational needs for older people, ranging from survival through maintenance to growth and beyond. The McClusky conceptual framework is readily adaptable to the growth and development of nurse executives and provides a companion schema to Maslow's hierarchy. Within the framework of ranges of needs, McClusky

Self-actualization	Transcendence
Influence	Growth
Esteem, love and belongingness	Contributive
Safety and security	Expressive
Physiological	Coping
Maslow	**McClusky**

Figure 5.1 A comparison of Maslow's and McClusky's hierarchies of needs.

proposed a theory of margin. According to this theory, people are constantly engaged in a struggle to maintain a margin of energy and power.

"Margin" is a function of the relationship of "load" to "power." "Load" refers to the self and the social demands a person must meet to maintain a minimal level of autonomy. "Power" is made up of the resources, abilities, possessions, positions, allies, and so on, that a person can command to cope with load. Margin can be increased by reducing load or increasing power. Margin can be decreased by increasing load or reducing power.

The crucial element in this scheme is the surplus, or margin of power in excess of load. This margin confers autonomy on individuals, gives them an opportunity to exercise a range of options, and enables them to achieve growth and development. A major force in the achievement of this outcome is education that will assist in creating margins of power for the maintenance of well-being and continuing growth toward self-fulfillment.

Figure 5.1 also demonstrates the scope of needs in McClusky's hierarchy, ranging from coping needs to transcendence. The first level "coping needs," refers to the need for basic education for survival and self-sufficiency. The second category, "expressive needs," is based on the premise that people have a need to engage in activities for the sake of the activity itself. The human personality is capable of a wide range of expression beyond habitual routines. Talents and interests flower if properly cultivated.

Category 3, "contributive needs," refers to the assumption that all people have a need to give to others and society, a desire to be of service. "Influence needs" comprises category 4. People must exert influence on the circumstances of living and the world about them. Applied to nursing, the right kind of education and utilization of experience can greatly enhance the nurse executive's power base and ability to influence others. McClusky's category 5, the need for "transcendence," matches Maslow's level of self-actualization. Although McClusky envisioned transcendence as uniquely relevant to the later years, it is also pertinent to the nurse executive who must move beyond self in motivating others. One rarely reaches this level early in life. According to McClusky, achieving the highest level of one's existence is a feature of the later years.

Figure 5.2 depicts an adaptation of the McClusky hierarchy of education in terms of the developing nurse executive. A great educator, Howard McClusky believed that education is not an option but, rather, an indispensable means of existence. For the fully functioning professional person, lifelong learning is mandatory and leadership can be learned at any point in one's worklife.

Many nurses rebel at the possibility of becoming an executive. They are bound up in the care functions and feel that unless they personally deliver hands-on care, they have somehow abandoned the profession. They fail to see that influencing others to deliver quality care can have greater impact on the quality of care than any individual effort could. As Dumas (1999) asserts, leadership development is a lifelong process and self-development is nurtured by perpetual learning.

What, then, is the able executive like? What characterizes the Ruth Freemans, the Lillian Walds, the Florence Nightingales? To begin with, they all conveyed a sense of togetherness—wholeness, confidence, wisdom. They were teachers, rational thinkers, dreamers, and independents. They did not seek to emulate others' leadership styles. They had their own. In true Maslovian fashion, they moved up the ladder to strong self-concept and self-actualization. They were the sum total of their individual lives, educations, genes, and experiences. Nurse executives should be leaders; if they are not leaders, they should not administrate.

PERSONAL ATTRIBUTES OF SUCCESSFUL NURSE LEADERS

Donna Diers (1979) aptly discussed the personal attributes of successful nurse executives as the softer aspects of leadership—those characteristics that do not fall conveniently into boxes in a diagram. They are intangible traits that are not easily researched, for example:

- Visioning
- Political skills
- Creativity
- Charisma
- Knowledge of other peoples' motivations and pressures
- Ability to read the dynamics of a situation

Heider (1985) would add the ability to listen and to let others have credit. It is not enough to be able to plan, organize, set goals, and achieve goals. One must be

SAFETY AND SECURITY
Beginning work experience
Comfortable with clinical knowledge
Little if any risk taking
Increased involvement in professional
nursing organizations

SELF-ESTEEM
Recognizes self as a fully functioning
nurse executive
Additional education and specific
interests
Personal anchors and supports in
place
Self-directed learning

HIGH SELF-ESTEEM
Regard for needs of others;
international perspective on
health for all
Able to follow others as well as
to lead
Visionary executive leadership
in a variety of roles
Not threatened by competition;
able to take risks
Active in professional nursing
and health organizations

PHYSIOLOGIC
Basic education in nursing
Beginning involvement in
professional nursing organizations
Beginning recognition of interest in professional career

LOVE AND BELONGINGNESS
Comfortable in clinical world
Middle management skills in line or
staff positions
Head nurse, clinical manager or
clinical specialist roles
Graduate education at either the
master's or doctoral level

OWN LEADERSHIP
STYLE
Builds on own unique-
ness
Established lifelong
learning pattern
Motivates self and others
Integrates management
activities in every-
day activities regard-
less of role

Figure 5.2 The developing nurse executive.

able to dream—to envision the future. Says Diers, "A vision serves as an energy source, a star to guide us, a hook on which to hang dreams of glory. Goals, on the other hand, are achievable end points, termini to measure progress. A good vision will outlive any leader; it gives one a legacy" (p. 7).

Often people in leadership roles get so involved with their work that they never step back to see if they are on target. They do not take the time to assess their personal and professional goals or their strengths and weaknesses. Professional nurse executives must pursue excellence in themselves to improve the quality of life in their institutions. This means developing and maintaining their knowledge base, keeping up to date, sharing knowledge with colleagues, and taking time to "smell the flowers" (Dumas, 1999).

Noting that the leadership literature has been more art than science, Goleman (1998) proposes a different way of looking at the components of leadership. He has studied effective performance and concludes that effective leaders all have a high degree of emotional intelligence. He defines emotional intelligence as the ability to work with others and lead change. Like Dumas (1999), Goleman cites self-awareness and growth of self as the most important components of emotional intelligence. Self-awareness, self-regulation, and motivation are all self-management skills. The ability to work with others is found in empathy and social skills according to Goleman.

The importance of Goleman's work is that it supports the softer side of leadership as described earlier by Diers (1979) and Dumas (1999). Emotional intelligence is born largely in the neurotransmitters of the brain's limbic system, which governs feelings, impulses and drives. It is not that regular intelligence (IQ) and technical skills are irrelevant says Goleman. However, emotional intelligence is the key to leadership and nurturing change.

Successful executives in nursing must have goals and dreams and ideas and a love of their work. Benjamin Mays (1980), at the White House Conference on Aging, expressed his views on professional administration in the following statement:

> It must be borne in mind that the tragedy in life doesn't lie in not reaching your goal. The tragedy lies in having no goal to reach. It isn't a calamity to die with dreams unfulfilled, but it is a calamity not to dream. It is not a disaster to be unable to capture your ideal, but it is a disaster to have no ideal to capture. It is not a disgrace not to reach the stars, but it is a disgrace to have no stars to reach for. Not failure, but low aim, is sin. (p. 7)

Personal Resources

This text has been known over the years for its emphasis on personal development and self-responsibility for lifelong learning as the most important prerequisites for executive leadership. Based on the ever-changing organizational literature and their years of experience in leadership positions, the authors have identified the following skills as essential personal resources: *Courage, Conviction, Creativity, Communication, and Coping* (Figure 5.3). One's development as an effective nurse executive depends on the nurturing of these skills. Although communication is included in Figure 5.3, it requires more extensive discussion than a sub-section here and therefore is the main theme of Chapter 13.

Coping skills are basic to the achievement of human needs according to both Maslow and McClusky. More recently Shechtman (1998) has supported the need for coping skills in personal transformation. Grieving for and discarding *old familiars* is an important part of crystallizing *new familiars* and working toward growth and development in our personal and professional lives. Thus coping becomes an essential skill for successful nurse executives as they move through and respond to multiple role and position changes during their career.

Courage

A nurse executive with courage has the mental or moral strength to venture, persevere, and withstand danger, fear, or difficulty. Courage implies a firmness of mind and will in the face of difficulty and a determination to achieve one's ends. Courage is synonymous with mettle, spirit, resolution, and tenacity.

One may not ordinarily think of the nurse executive as courageous, but he or she assuredly should be. It takes courage to make changes that need to be made, even though those changes are unpopular and little appreciated. It is very risky to move into uncharted water. For example, establishing a professional practice model between nursing service and nursing education in an environment of alienation and distrust can be very stressful. The nurse executive attempting to

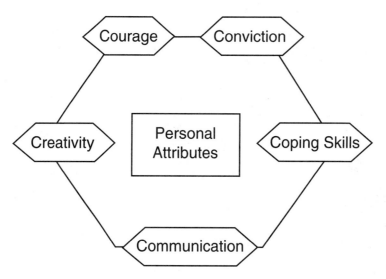

Figure 5.3 Important attributes for nurse executives.

establish such a model must be prepared to withstand personal and professional criticism. Many barriers must be broken down and many friendships established before the two groups can collaborate within a total nursing community.

Courage may also be required to establish meaningful joint practice modalities ranging from integrated charting to true collaborative care planning and implementation. Nurse executives must listen to all the arguments against joint practice and still persevere toward establishing a feasible institutional or unit model. They must be prepared to face the wrath of nurses and physicians alike who are unwilling to collaborate in a professional, meaningful way.

Nurse executives must be willing to meet one to one, in small groups or in large groups—whatever it takes to nurture discussion and identify opposition. Allowing one's ideas to be thoroughly challenged and questioned enables one to verify those ideas and to remain in one's goal without becoming known as a stubborn tyrant. Stubbornness is not to be confused with courage, for stubbornness implies a closed mind, one that is not willing to test out new ideas.

It takes courage to work in the midst of negative criticism. It takes courage to meet with opponents and try to achieve a meeting of the minds. It also takes courage to face the opposition and maintain presence of mind and dignity without becoming pompous or resorting to shallow thinking. It takes courage to swim daily with the sharks as well as the friendly dolphins. It takes courage to maintain composure and not show one's wounds, though some may be deep. Above all, it takes courage to remain dry eyed, even when angered to frustration and tears (Cousteau, 1981).

Conviction

A conviction is a strong persuasion and belief, an opinion held with complete assurance despite opposing arguments, a belief stronger than an impression and less strong than positive knowledge. One cannot have courage without convictions, and one cannot have convictions without strong inner discipline and high ideals. One who has conviction about nursing ideals is willing to attempt to convert others to the same way of thinking and to establish goals that are meaningful to nursing and the institution.

With conviction comes the ability to communicate one's opinion. Not only does one have an opinion, but one is also able to communicate that opinion orally and in writing. A lot is written about communication in the nursing literature, but little is written about having something to communicate. The nurse executive must communicate from a base of knowledge and experience that reflects understanding of the issues under discussion.

The nurse executive with conviction is a nagger, one who keeps needling away at others to move toward goals of worth: when others believe an idea has been dropped, they soon realize they are being bombarded from another quarter.

Executives with courage and conviction bring about change and desired internalization of ideas in others without force. They bring about such results by planting the seeds of a desired change and then rigorously making sure the seeds grow and multiply.

Creativity

A distinctly human quality, creativity is not any one thing, but contains the common elements of all creative thought: divergent thinking, flexibility, fluency, and originality. Creativity is the highest order of conceptualization and problem-solving. By definition, to create is to evolve something from one's own thought. True innovation must come from within. Innovating means not succumbing to the fallacy that there is not enough time to be creative. It comes from a can-do, rather than a cannot-do, philosophy.

Creativity sets the excellent executive, the true leader, apart from the minimum-level performer. Anyone can be taught the four maxims of management: planning, organizing, implementing, and evaluating. One can learn to memorize the rules of delegation and time management and still not have anything to delegate or any reason to save time.

Successful nurse executives are creative problem solvers. To be creative, they must free themselves from their own premature judgment. They must allow themselves time for theorizing and hypothesizing. Many creative people recognize that they give intermittent attention to problems of interest; that is, they are aware of incubation periods when much subconscious activity may be occurring. it is important, therefore, to develop an increased awareness of the problems to which one would like to direct attention. Functioning creatively, one can combine intuition and scientific principles to achieve superlative problem-solving. Such functioning is the highest level of professional skill. Creativity is truly the art of seeing what everyone else is seeing but thinking what no one else has thought.

The essential problem for teachers of the professions is the difficulty of providing a transition from academic experience to work experience. Many educators struggle over how to teach nurses the qualities of a leader and leadership skills. The competency-based movement in education threatens to shroud further the development of creative leaders. There is a difference between competence and the full functioning of excellence in the practice of administration.

The excellent executive is a leader who is creative. Creativity can be recognized only if it is observable by others. The outcomes of creativity are recognized in the results of one's labors, either as accomplished, recognizable feats or as changed behavior of fellow workers.

The creative leader is in fact an effective teacher, one who influences the thinking and behavior of others. The creative leader is one who can take advantage of teachable moments and seize opportunities for infiltrating the minds of others. Such a leader is also well able to take advantage of optimal "learning movements" in which vision and understanding of complex problems occur.

The highest level of creativity requires the ability to conceptualize, the ability to lift any idea or problem from the mundane to a level of abstraction so that it may be treated and studied in an innovative manner. In building a conceptual framework for nursing administration, one uses concepts from nursing, basic sciences, and behavioral sciences. Concepts can serve as powerful organizational tools for thinking, and the sorting and matching of concepts is a practical skill of creativity. Consider, for example, the conceptualization of a new organizational structure. Organizational charts are usually complex concepts developed first in one human brain, transmitted to others by a teaching-learning exercise, and completed on paper only when firmly understood by all concerned. Creativity, then, produces the paths to achievement of those dreams, visions, and goals.

Coping Skills

Throughout life, people struggle to make sense out of what happens to them and to provide themselves with a sense of order and continuity (Lazarus & DeLongis, 1983). This struggle is centered in divergent personal beliefs and commitments, shapes cognitive appraisals of stressful transactions and coping, and therefore has profound consequences. The invisible side of leadership includes the ability to cope with work and life. The cognitive phenomenological approach to coping taken by Lazarus and Folkman (1984) relates stress (environmental factors) to appraisal and coping (cognitive factors) and to outcome or change in functioning (response factors).

Cognitive appraisal is the evaluative process that determines why and to what extent a particular transaction between the person and the environment is stressful (Lazarus & Folkman, 1984) and consists of primary and secondary appraisal. In primary appraisal, one determines what is at stake. The person evaluates the significance of a specific transaction with respect to well-being. Stressful appraisals include a harm/loss that has been sustained, a threat of a harm/loss that is anticipated, or challenge for gain and growth. Secondary appraisal takes into account which coping options are available, the likelihood that a given coping option will accomplish what it is supposed to, and the likelihood that one can apply a particular strategy effectively. Coping resources, which include physical, social, psychological, and material assets, are evaluated with respect to the demands of the situation.

Lazarus and Folkman (1984) define coping as constantly changing cognitive and behavioral efforts to manage specific external and internal demands that are appraised as taxing or exceeding the resources of the person. The way a person copes is determined by resources and constraints that mitigate the use of resources. Coping refers to efforts to manage demands, regardless of the success of those efforts.

In any encounter with the environment, the key problem is to make a series of realistic judgments about its implication for one's well-being. A mismatch between primary appraisal and what is actually happening can take two basic forms: either the person will appraise harm/loss, threat, or challenge in instances and ways in which they do not apply, or the appraisal will reflect the failure to recognize harm/loss, threat, or challenge in instances where they should be recognized. This is particularly true in persons who must continually readjust appraisals of their situation.

Secondary appraisal is crucial to every encounter, because the outcome depends on what, if anything, can be done, as well as what is at stake. Secondary appraisal is the process of evaluating coping options. The resources a person believes are available are arrayed psychologically against the dangers and harms being faced. This then determines the form, amount, and appropriateness of coping behavior undertaken by that individual.

Lazarus and Folkman (1984) make a distinction between coping that is directed at managing or altering the problem causing the distress (problem-focused coping), and coping that is directed at regulating emotional response to the problem (emotion-focused coping). Emotion-focused forms of coping are likely to occur when there has been appraisal that nothing can be done to modify harmful, threatening, or challenging environmental conditions. On the other hand, problem-focused forms of coping are more probable when such conditions are appraised as amenable to change. Problem- and emotion-focused coping can both facilitate and impede each other in the coping process and almost always occur concurrently. No one strategy is considered inherently better than any other. The goodness (appropriateness and efficacy) of a strategy is determined only by its effects in a given encounter and its effects in the long term.

The relationship between coping and adaptation outcomes is subtle and complex. It involves interdependent coping strategies, and coping resources directed at a variety of interrelated outcomes such as social functioning, morale, and health (Lazarus & Folkman, 1984). Morale over the long run probably depends on a tendency to appraise encounters as challenges, to cope with negative outcomes by putting them in a positive light, and to manage effectively a wide range of demands. Quality of life and one's physical and mental health are linked with the ways people evaluate and cope with the stresses of living and working.

Active learning according to Karasek and Theorell (1990) occurs in situations that require challenge and decision-making capability. As individuals choose how to cope with stressors, new coping strategies will be learned. Successful leaders have developed the ability to appraise stressful encounters and have learned positive coping responses. Both Heider (1985) and Adams (1998) stress the importance of learning through listening and secondary appraisal in problem situations. Without the ability to cope, it is unlikely that nurse leaders will be able to stimulate learning environments for self or others.

Cognitive appraisal (primary and secondary appraisal) is perhaps the most important aspect of the stress-coping process and how an individual appraises a situation has a powerful effect on that individual's adaptive behavior (Starr, 1989). The nurse leader determines if she has control of a situation and can do something about it. Perhaps there is no choice but to accept the situation as is and sometimes more information is needed. The leader accepts responsibility for dealing with whatever happens even in uncertainty.

How a nurse executive appraises various situations is crucial to assisting team members with the demands and difficulties of everyday work. Crises in the health field are occurring continually and the handling of these problems reflects the effectiveness of the nurse leader. For example, job security and role change issues garner feelings of helplessness and powerlessness; and the nurse leader must be aware of and sensitive to these feelings. There is a continual need to reappraise harm/loss, threat, or challenge for gain and growth. Appraisal allows leaders to formulate realistic goals and expectations and use these goals and objectives to define desired outcomes.

Leaders use their coping skills to deal with external economic pressures such as diminishing resources. Over a lifetime of practice, the nurse leader builds up a repertoire of coping skills. Seeking out information from others in similar situations about their experiences, and sharing common experiences are two problem-solving coping strategies used by the leader. Other coping options of the nurse leader include planning, developing, decision-making, determining, identifying, and problem-solving. These options may involve observing, listening, recording, and making suggestions.

Problem- and emotion-focused coping almost always occur concurrently and the successful nurse leader seeks to strike a balance between the two forms of coping. Emotion-focused forms of coping directed at lessening emotional distress include strategies such as avoidance, minimization, distancing, selective attention, positive comparisons, and a positive value from negative events. Although persons experience stressors differently and cope differently, they need reassurance that their responses are "normal" (Starr, 1989). Awareness and knowledge of coping strategies provide insight into how well one adapts and insight into the coping skills of others. The utilization and exploration of a wide range of coping responses would be appropriate for anyone in a leadership role. Being open to new ideas and using creativity and curiosity allows for the building of new coping skills. Awareness of the nature of the stress appraisal and coping process and understanding the importance that appraisal plays is essential to being an effective leader.

PERSONAL SUPPORT SYSTEMS

There is more to life than work. Work time is measured in terms of work-related objectives, and personal time is measured in terms of satisfaction, emotional gain, quality of relationships, and fulfillment or service to others. Personal goals and objectives are part of the whole human picture of the nurse executive. They constitute an essential dimension of self-actualized, fully functioning leaders with the capability for mature relationships.

Other management literature suggests that personal life goals cannot be left out of performance plans. Management by objective and performance appraisal processes as typically practiced may be self-defeating if attention is not given to personal life goals and their relevance to organizational objectives. Workers whose personal and work lives are in flow are significantly happier, more creative, and more satisfied (Csikszentmihalyi, 1990).

Whatever supports are important to the individual must be identified and nurtured. Who are those individuals or groups whom one can laugh with and love? Who supports and understands one? What serves as a release for confusion and frustration? Where are the quiet and restful corners at home where comfort and solace are ensured? What hobbies and activities produce the greater sense of optimism and positive thinking? Pets, for example, can be the most significant available others an executive can have, and their value should not be underestimated.

Humor in all settings leads to greater sensibility and an appreciation of the temper of other people. It is a social lubricant and a human connection. The ability to see humor in various situations is a means of releasing the energy accompanying excessive tension. A sense of humor is both a personal attribute and a personal support system. Humor is a powerful weapon that can help establish trust and fellowship at work, at home, and in group interactions. In 1980 Jackson first proposed the use of humor as a deliberate nursing technique, "Laughing with someone enfolds him/her within a network of human love, understanding, and support" (p. 12).

The phenomenon of burnout deserves special attention and is more fully addressed later in this book. Burnout is not unique to executives, but they are prime victims of what is known to the military as battle fatigue. Burnout is a "syndrome of emotional exhaustion and cynicism that frequently occurs among people who do 'people' work—who spend considerable time in close encounters" (Simms, 1991). Nurse executives need to recognize that burnout can happen to them and that steps should be taken to mitigate its occurrence. Personal support systems become extremely important in providing channels through which individuals can tune off their work role and its demands. Female executives, especially, must see their families as support systems rather than handicaps. Too often, children of working women are perceived as interferences with productivity rather than as assets.

LEADERSHIP STYLES AND THEORIES

The leadership literature is voluminous, and yet no theorist has been able to fully describe the "perfect 10," the effective leader-administrator who is a self-actualized person who can lead common people to do uncommon things in a productive fashion. Robbins and Coulter (1996) discuss three basic approaches to explaining effective leaders:

1. Trait studies are designed to find universal personality traits that leaders have to a greater degree than nonleaders.
2. Behavioral research is undertaken to explain leadership in terms of behavior.

3. Contingency models are constructed to explain situational variables as well as leadership traits and behavior.

Personality Traits

Research efforts to isolate traits have resulted in inconsistent conclusions. Intelligence, extroversion, self-assurance, and empathy may be related to achieving and maintaining a leadership position. Although requisite traits are inconsistent, the following traditional and emerging leadership styles can be observed in practice:

1. Autocratic leader: demonstrates aggressive dominance; commands and expects others to follow.
2. Participative leader: includes followers in decision-making; assumes followers can be motivated to self-direction, self-actualization, and creative performance.
3. Laissez-faire leader: permits group members to have freedom to function and set goals independently of the leader.
4. Instrumental leader: exhibits rational rather than supportive behavior; plans, directs, organizes, controls, and coordinates the activities of followers.
5. "Great man" leader: behavior based on the belief that people can learn leadership from studying the examples of the lives of great men.
6. Teacher-learner leader: an emerging model based on the belief that leading is learning and good management is teaching. (Adams 1998)
7. Transformed leadership: belief that leadership is shared and the leader's basic tool is one's self and self knowledge. (Adams, 1998)

Behavioral Research

Two classic behavioral studies were conducted by Kerr, Schriesheim, Murphy, and Stogdill (1974) at Ohio State University and Kahn and Katz (1969) at the University of Michigan. These studies identified two dimensions of leadership behavior: *(1)* initiating structure and *(2)* consideration. Initiating structure refers to the extent to which a leader defines and structures his or her role and those of subordinates. Consideration refers to the interpersonal relationships variable. Blake, Mouton, and Tapper (1981) later addressed two concerns: *(1)* production of results and *(2)* concern for personnel as people. None of the three approaches addressed the social situations in which leaders must act.

For example, the social situation varies according to the characteristics of the group, the nature of group tasks, and the particular circumstances relevant to a given leadership position. Hershey (1984) studied the relationship of the psychological, or person, dimension to the sociological, or role, dimension in specific situations. Their work added to the leadership literature in terms of self-understanding, group tasks, the concept of group behavior, individual behavior within a group, and the importance of interpersonal relationships within a given situation.

Contingency Models

Other leadership research produced the contingency models, with *(1)* the auto-cratic-democratic continuum, *(2)* the Fiedler, and *(3)* the path-goal models be-coming the best known (Robbins & Coulter, 1996). The autocratic-democratic model depicts two extreme positions on either end of a continuum, with many positions between. The contingency approach suggests that neither the democra-tic nor the autocratic extreme is effective in all situations.

The Fiedler (1967) model suggested three contingency dimensions:

1. Leader-member relations: how well liked, respected, and trusted the leader is
2. Task structure: the procedural nature of job assignments
3. Position power: the degree to which the leader has influence over power variables

The basic premise of Fiedler's theory is that the performance of a group is contin-gent on the style of the leader and how favorable the situation is for the leader. Robert House (1971), of the University of Toronto, has proposed a contingency path-goal model of leadership that integrates the expectancy model of motiva-tion with the structure and consideration research developed by Kahn and Katz (1969). The model described the leader as being responsible for "increasing the number and kinds of personal payoffs to the subordinates for work-goal attain-ment and making paths to these payoffs easier to travel" (House & Mitchell, 1974). The path-goal model proposes that the scope of the job and the characteris-tics of the subordinates moderate the relationship between a leader's behavior and subordinates' performance and satisfaction.

In applying path-goal theory to nursing, the leader uses skills in structuring and consideration to increase worker motivation. The leader initiates structure by defining his or her own role and the roles of subordinates toward goal achieve-ment. Volunteers need a high level of direction, staff nurses less, and clinical nurse specialists very little. The leadership skill lies in knowing how to balance structure and consideration with the particular situation.

Mintzberg Model

Current beliefs about leadership are more accurately reflected by Mintzberg (1994) who notes a remarkable change in unit leadership at the head nurse level. Mintzberg describes a model of work flowing together in a natural rhythm, a blend of clinical and management responsibilities that he calls "standing up" management by nurse executives who are continuously within earshot of associ-ated people. They constantly interpret environmental signals and successfully link with the rest of the hospital and patients' relatives as well as outside agen-cies. Thus, the unit nurse executive is able to communicate, control, lead, link, and do within a blend of clinical and systems linkages.

Leadership seems to be the key to this performance and the unit nurse executive strives to develop nurses individually and into a smoothly functioning team. The unit executive must be fully informed and involved with patient care on the unit as well as be an effective interpersonal leader. Management at the unit level includes responsibility for budgets, people, and materials as well as budget cuts. In this environment management is on the run and "goes with the wind" so to speak. In this model knowledge workers respond to inspiration not supervision (Mintzberg, 1998).

Continuum-Based Leadership Model

Porter-O'Grady, Bradley, Crow, and Hendrich (1997) describe changes in transformational leadership models, addressing the option for continuum-based leadership, which eliminates the need for the single nurse executive position in integrated systems. Specific service pathways are led by a nurse pathway administrator who coordinates and integrates all necessary services and supports within the pathway. With 7 to 10 pathways, and an administrator for each, a team-based service structure with clinical leadership can be provided that is service based and a continuum-driven design. In such a system, no one group controls resources and strategies without considering the impact on other units (Figure 5.4).

The model for the year 2000 may be a truly interdisciplinary, decentralized approach, not a single individual group or profession. Past roles and behaviors of leadership no longer apply to emerging models of health service delivery. The frame of reference for thinking about organizations and relationships is greatly altered in the quantum relationship proposed by Porter-O'Grady (1997). The old perception of leader as the person at the center of decision-making does not apply in the knowledge society. The notion that leader equates with manager is not validated in quantum thinking. Leaders emerge from various places and leadership emerges where it is needed in the quantum age.

Dependence on the knowledge worker moves the locus of control in systems from the hierarchy to point of service or front-line in a truly decentralized organization. Porter-O'Grady (1997) further states that quantum theory thinking provides a broader foundation for thinking about all relationships at every level of complexity in the universe. Quantum mechanics is the understanding that all particles are waves and all waves are particles depending on the conditions and circumstances that influence how they are viewed and in what manner they are applied. As we leave the industrial command and control age for the quantum age, we need to move from linear age processes to a quantum frame of reference.

All systems work from the inside out, not from the top down or bottom up. Healthy systems live in the tension between stability and chaos in a constant state of disequilibrium that creates conditions and energy to ensure response to evolution and change. Development of leadership competencies may be the key to achieving quality patient outcomes and financial viability. Leadership skills

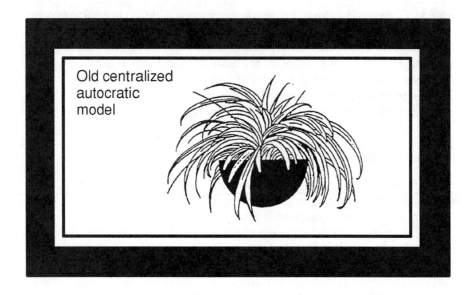

Old centralized
autocratic
model

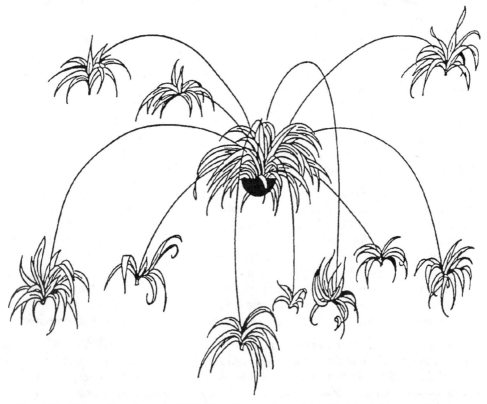

Figure 5.4 Model for the year 2000: Continuum-based leadership. Adapted with permission from Morgan, G. (1993). *Imaginization* (pp. 72–73). Newbury Park, CA: SAGE.

and knowledge can no longer be the exclusive purview of persons in traditional management positions (Krejci & Malin, 1997). Managed care has changed role expectations for all professional nurses and roles now mandate outcome management skills, team coordination, and attendance to continuity of care. Organizations on the move are now investing in leadership for all professional nurses not only those in management positions.

All nurse executives should be leaders; if they are not, they should develop the capability or be replaced. The morale and motivation of staff nurses are highly dependent on the leadership skills of the nurse executive and on the work climate.

NEW AGE LEADERSHIP

The organizational model for health care settings of various descriptions, public and private, in the 21st century will bear little resemblance to today's hierarchical structures. The new nurse executive in transformed organizations must have flexible and action-oriented personality qualities, possess executive level business management skills, have completed some graduate level work, and be an expert on clinical affairs (Smith, Parsons, Murray, Dwore, Vorderer, & Okerlund, 1994). In a survey of 5,000 nurse executives and managers, Gelinas and Manthey (1997) documented changes in nurse leader roles at all levels. Successful nurse leaders are expected to:

1. Be change masters and to lead across cultural, functional and departmental boundaries
2. Promote teamwork and build and maintain effective teams
3. Manage personal growth by objectively challenging their own behavior and beliefs
4. Promote continued development of the nursing profession in the integrated patient care environment
5. Tolerate ambiguity related to rapid perpetual change in technology and sociological forces

In 1985, and reconfirmed in 1998, John Adams and his colleagues came to the astounding conclusion that every professional person is a manager and there should be no superior/subordinate relationships, no reporting chains. Leading is learning in the new age and the successful organization is a learning community. Work becomes a developmental process and management is the art of developing people through work rather than getting work done through people. The nurse executive role in learning organizations is discussed in Chapter 6.

Developing Leaders and Followers

An important part of leadership is the ability to identify potential leaders. The willingness to nurture a potential leader at the risk of developing competition for one's own role is the mark of outstanding leadership. The nurturance of followers of institutional goals is one of the major challenges in organizations, for it is easier to set up personal friendships and loyalties. Identifying potential leaders based on personal friendships is a pitfall that nurse executives should avoid. Because friendship tends to blind one to a friend's faults, it is difficult for the nurse executive to objectively evaluate the performance of a friend.

Nurses skilled in clinical practice or education are often moved into administrative positions without the benefit of administrative preparation. Programs designed to develop administrators require integration with institutional performance improvement. To improve organizational performance, it is necessary to develop the institution or the institutional unit. The development of individual administrators is an important part of the overall schema.

The development of individual administrators and institutional development are highly interdependent tasks requiring an approach that integrates the needs of both the institution and the individual. Such an approach involves the setting of institutional goals by top management, followed by the development of participating administrators to move toward those goals. Translated to nursing, programs designed to improve the administrative capability of clinical directors and head nurses do not improve the performance of the nursing department unless they are planned to integrate with nursing department goals.

The nurse executive can encourage self-development efforts by establishing, with the employee, individual performance objectives and periodic performance evaluation. The administrator's attention to his or her own self-development further encourages such behavior in others. A positive climate for developing leadership can emerge from requiring administrators to assume the responsibility for the growth and development of their staff and assigning individuals to administrative responsibilities appropriate for their experience and interests. The active involvement of the supervisor is balanced with the encouragement of self-evaluation and personal goal setting.

The concept of supervision as a professional growth-producing process is not new, but, except in public health nursing, it is not widely practiced in the nursing field. The supervisory process requires that each staff member receive one-to-one guidance much more often than once a year for performance evaluation. The nurse executive sets the example for this process through conferencing on a regular basis with each employee who reports directly to him or her. The conferences, of course, provide the opportunity for exchange of information, but they also give the nurse executive time to review objectives, performance, strategies, and problems with each key person. This time is also used for coaching the employee so that he or she can gain new skills and develop new approaches to old problems.

The followers of today will be the leaders of tomorrow. Setting the pace for the growth and development of the staff involves presenting an image of excitement and enthusiasm for excellence in the nursing department. Technology changes daily, but the need for nurses to develop and grow within a physically exhausting environment presents a major challenge to the nurse executive. The nurse executive has the responsibility to provide leadership in creating a climate in which nurses can practice at their highest level of expertise while continuing to develop as individual professional practitioners. The nurse executive alone cannot create this climate but has the knowledge and skills to lead the nursing divisions to this end.

TIME AND CHANCE

The self-actualized, fully functioning nurse executive has mastered time management, for time management is really self-management. McCarthy (1981) emphasizes that one cannot really manage time. To be a good self-manager, one must have a positive professional self-image and enough initiative to change oneself. McCarthy stated that there are five degrees of initiative, ranging from waiting to be told what to do to acting on one's own.

To determine personal and career goals, one must conduct a formal time analysis. Most people have about 2 hours a day to do various personal things. Executives can determine how they currently spend their time in eight broad areas and then decide how they would like to spend their time. The things people value most can be divided into these eight categories: career, family, social life, financial stability, health, personal development, spiritual development, and leisure. To achieve a satisfying, fulfilling life, one must control one's life and decide how one will spend one's time in these areas. Every day, each person has a new 24 hours to unfold and to spend and a chance to write a new page of one's life.

The focus of this chapter has been the person. Within the conceptual framework, time can be seen as a personal resource that enhances one's power to cope with the demand, or load, of one's job. The surplus of power—the margin—enables individuals to be autonomous. Time is perhaps the single resource over which the individual can maintain a large degree of control. Powerless executives are "can't" people, "never have enough time" people. Lack of time is an excuse for all manner of uncompleted tasks.

The fully functioning nurse executive maintains a margin of power and energy through time management and timing. Time and chance are linked, and time is perceived as opportunity. In administration, one has seconds, minutes, days, seasons, and years to accomplish one's goals. Many conferences and books address the issue of time management. None provides a formula that works unless the individual sees time as an energy and power resource.

SUMMARY

Personal attributes and leadership skills are crucial to the role of the nurse executive. Personal attributes, personal support systems, and learned coping behaviors combine with clinical management skills to produce a competent leader. Knowing one's strengths and weaknesses, building on one's educational and work experiences, and the uniqueness of one's life experiences and leadership capabilities are essential components of a satisfying, rewarding experience in administration. The work of Maslow and McClusky in developmental psychology is a useful conceptual framework for the development of the self-actualized, transcended leader capable of creating a climate of motivation and productivity for others. In this new paradigm, leaders are followers and followers are leaders. Together, change and organizational energy are created. Leadership as continuous learning is the model for the 21st century.

STUDY QUESTIONS

1. Explore Maslow's concept of self-actualization and McClusky's concept of transcendence in terms of your own development. Where do you perceive yourself on the ladder?
2. Relate the concepts of courage, conviction, coping and creativity to a situation in your practice. To what extent does your personal leadership style influence the operationalization of these concepts?
3. Update your curriculum vitae every 6 months.
4. Examine the concept of personal support systems as it applies to you.
5. Regularly develop a personal and professional performance plan.
6. Assign yourself new learning activities based on weaknesses identified in your self-assessment and CV update.

REFERENCES

Adams, J. D. (Ed.). (1998). *Transforming leadership.* Alexandria, VA: Miles River Press.

Blake, R. R., Mouton, J. S., & Tapper, M. (1981). *Grid approaches for managerial leadership in nursing.* St. Louis: Mosby.

Chaska, N. L. (1990). *The nursing profession.* New York: McGraw-Hill.

Cousteau, V. (1981). How to swim with sharks: A primer. *American Journal of Nursing, 81*(10), 1960.

Csikszentmihalyi, M. (1990). *Flow. The psychology of optimal experience.* New York: Harper & Row.

Diers, D. (1979). Lessons on leadership. *Image, 11*(3), 3–7.

Drucker, P. F. (1980). *Managing in turbulent times.* New York: Harper & Row.

Dumas, R. (1999). President's message (about leadership). *Nursing and Health Care, 20*(1), i, 34.

Fiedler, F. E. (1967). *A theory of leadership effectiveness.* New York: McGraw-Hill.

Gelinas, L. S., & Manthey, M. (1997). The impact of organizational redesign on nurse executive leadership. *Journal of Nursing Administration, 27*(10), 35–42.

Goleman, D. (1998, November–December). What makes a leader? *Harvard Business Review, 76*(6), 93–102.

Heider, J. (1985). *The tao of leadership.* New York: Bantam Books.

Hershey, P. (1984). *The situational leader.* New York: Warner Books.

House, R. J. (1971). A path goal theory of leader effectiveness. *Administration Science Quarterly, 16*(3), 321–328.

House, R. J., & Mitchell, T. R. (1974). Path-goal theory of leadership. *Journal of Contemporary Business, 3*(4), 81–97.

Jackson, M. M. (1980). The nurse who laughs, lasts: The comic spirit in nursing. *The Michigan Nurse, 53*(4), 12–14.

Kahn, R., & Katz, D. (1969). Leadership practices in relation to productivity and morale. D. Cartwright & A. Zauder (Eds.). *Group dynamics: Research and theory* (2nd ed.). Elmsford, NY: Row Paterson.

Karasek, R., & Theorell, T. (1990). *Healthy work.* New York: Basic Books.

Kerr, S., Schriesheim, C. A., Murphy, C. J., & Stogdill, R. M. (1974). Toward a contingency theory of leadership based upon the consideration and structural literature, *Organizational Behavior and Human Performance, 12*(1), 62–82.

Kinsman, F. (1998). Leadership from alongside. In J. D. Adams (Ed.). *Transforming leadership* (pp. 19–38). Alexandria, VA: Miles River Press.

Krejci, J. W., & Malin, S. (1997). Impact of leadership development on competencies. *Nursing Economic$, 15*(5), 235–241.

Lazarus, R. S., & DeLongis, A. (1983). Psychological stress and coping in aging. *American Psychologist, 38*, 245–254.

Lazarus, R. S., & Folkman, S. (1984). *Stress, appraisal, and coping.* New York: Springer.

Maslow, A. H. (1962). *Toward a psychology of being.* New York: Van Nostrand.

Mays, B. (1980). *Report from the White House Conference on Aging, no. 2.*

McCarthy, M. J. (1981). Managing your own time: The most important management task, *Journal of Nursing of Administration, 11*(11,12), 61–65.

McClusky, H. Y. (1974). Education for aging: The scope of the field and perspectives for the future. In S. M. Grabowski & W. D. Mason (Eds.). *Education for the aging.* Syracuse, NY: ERIC Clearinghouse.

Mintzberg, H. (1994). Managing as blended care. *Journal of Nursing Administration, 24*(9), 29–36.

Mintzberg, H. (1998). Covert leadership: Notes on managing professionals. *Harvard Business Review, 76*(6), 140–147.

Morgan, G. (1993). *Imaginization* (pp. 72–73). Newbury Park, CA: Sage.

Porter-O'Grady, T. (1997). Quantum mechanics and the future of healthcare leadership. *Journal of Nursing Administration, 27*(1), 15–20.

Porter-O'Grady, T., Bradley, C., Crow, G., & Hendrich, A. (1997). After a merger: The dilemma of the best leadership approach for nursing. *Nursing Administration Quarterly, 21*(2), 8–19.

Robbins, S., & Coulter, M. (1996). *Management* (5th ed.). Englewood Cliffs, NJ: Prentice-Hall.

Schechtman, M. R. (1998). *The internal frontier.* Los Angeles: New Star Press.

Simms, L., & Lindberg, J. (1978). *The nurse person.* New York: Harper & Row.

Simms, L. M. (1991). The professional practice of nursing administration: Integrated nursing practice. *Journal of Nursing Administration, 21*(5), 39–46.

Smith, P. M., Parsons, R. J., Murray, B. P., Dwore, R. B., Vorderer, L. H., & Okerlund, V. W. (1994). The new nurse executive role. *Journal of Nursing Administration, 24*(11), 56–62.

Starr, A. J. (1989). The stress-coping process in kidney transplant recipients and their family members. Doctoral dissertation, The University of Michigan, 1989. *Dissertation Abstracts International, #9014018.*

Zaleznik, A. (1981). Managers and leaders: Are they different? *Journal of Nursing Administration, 11*(7), 25–31.

PART
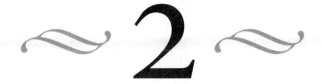
2

The Context of Nursing
Administrative Practice

CHAPTER
~ 6 ~

Through the Looking Glass: Making Sense of Organizations

Lillian M. Simms

The proliferation of complex organizations has made almost every human activity a collective one. We are born, raised and educated in organizations. We work in them and rely on them for goods and services. Many of us will grow old and die in organizations. (Bolman & Deal, 1991, p. 5)

Chapter Highlights

- Perspectives on organizations
- The human side of clinical administration
- Participatory approaches to organizational design
- The learning window
- The nurse executive role in learning organizations
- Professional associations
- Managing boundaries

There is a great need for professional nursing administration to reorganize its services, practice settings, and educational policies if nurse executives are to be able to function in current and emerging environments. Attention to the development of the "self" must be seen as a vital and integral part of continuing learning experiences, AND attention to persons in groups is equally vital. Most nursing administration texts are written about managers to describe the hierarchy of managers and the span of control of managers. Very little attention is paid to the work of the organization or workers. Organizational theorists have tended to focus on either public or private organizations, whereas all organizations have similarities. Nurse theorists have tended to focus on theories of nursing without any understanding of organizations. This chapter seeks to provide a way of looking at health care organizations as composed of autonomous, yet tightly coupled groups with various interacting networks. It assumes a different theme, that every nurse is an executive and every nurse executive is a worker in multiple organizations. It also assumes that traditional organizational theories no longer explain modern organizations, which are now viewed as networks or linkage points of distinctive competencies or areas of specialization on a global scale (Schneider, 1991).

Most traditional organizational charts are pecking orders for managers with the front-line workers perceived to be off the page somewhere. Health care organizations have been the ultimate of pecking orders with the physician always at the top in capital letters. To understand the concept of organization, let us for the moment assume that organization refers to Webster's dictionary definition: "the unification and harmonizing of the elements of work for a defined purpose." Organizations exist in nature, and may or may not have buildings as we know them. The ants have their nests, the bees their hives, and the wolves their caves for extended families. Organizations provide environments for work in which humans can struggle to provide for food, shelter, clothing, and tools for survival. In rural cultures, work seems closely tied to subsistence—less so in urban communities and especially health care organizations where work is linked with professional behavior. All in all, the understanding of work is essential to the understanding of workers in organizations. The neurosurgeon operating in a modern hospital, the nurse executive coordinating care in various settings, the potato picker in the field are all working.

The traditional organizational map describes a world that no longer exists. In the emerging boundary-less organization, the walls that separate groups from each other are knocked down and group labels such as management, professional, salaried, or hourly workers are erased or ignored. In such a world, the boundaries are more psychological than organizational and according to Schneider (1991), the old boundaries of hierarchy, function, and geography disappear in a new set of relationships among managers and workers. Knowing how to recognize and use new boundaries productively is essential in restructured organizations.

Vertical integration is a common method that aligns dissimilar but related entities such as a hospital, home care agency, rehabilitation center, and long-term care facility. An alternative proposed by Craft and Spilotro (1997) is the virtual organizational model, which brings together various entities for a limited period of time to reach a specific goal. Like the termite mound, the virtual organization is borderless, flexible, and agile and synergy of member agencies achieves more than each could do on its own. The termite mound organizational structure first proposed by Gareth Morgan (1993) may well be the most efficient organizational structure in the future. Figure 6.1 portrays such a mound in South Africa and is a beautiful example of the unstructured workplace. Morgan's theory of management in unstructured organizations can be found in Chapter 3.

Within the corporate structure, it will be necessary to create an entirely new set of organizational and structural relationships (Craft & Spilotro, 1997; Morgan, 1993). New technologies, fast changing markets and global competition are revolutionizing relationships in health care and the roles that people play and the tasks they perform have become blurred and ambiguous. Professional nursing will either rise or fall in this new era. Everyone in nursing, must figure out the roles they will need to play and what kind of relationships are essential for productive work. In addition, workers must assume responsibility for their own continuous learning rather than see career development as only an institutional goal. This will become increasingly possible as nurses work in decentralized environments with participatory management and shared governance (discussed later in this chapter).

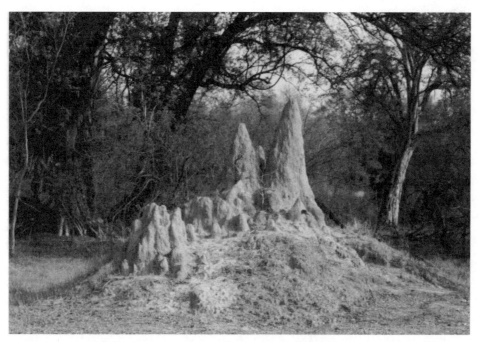

Figure 6.1 The organizational model of the future: A termite mound in South Africa. From the photo files of Simms, L. M. and Simms, R. J., 1996.

PERSPECTIVES ON ORGANIZATIONS

Bolman and Deal (1991) have consolidated the major schools of organization thought into four perspectives or frames to characterize the major vantage points. These frames are structural, human resource, political, and symbolic. They define frames as both windows on the world and lenses to bring the world into focus. Every manager, consultant, or policy maker, they say, uses a personal frame or image to make judgments and determine how to get work done. The structural frame emphasizes the importance of formal roles and relationships. Commonly depicted by organizational charts, structures are created to fit an organization's environment and technology. The human resource frame is based on the premise that organizations are inhabited by human beings with skills, needs, feelings, and prejudices. The political frame views organizations as arenas in which different interest groups compete for power and scarce resources. Conflict abounds during this competition. Bargaining, negotiation, coercion, and compromise are everyday organizational activities. In the symbolic frame, organizations are viewed as tribes, theater, or carnivals. In this view, say Bolman and Deal (1991), organizations are cultures that are propelled more by rituals, ceremonies, stories, heroes, and myths than by rules, policies, and managerial authority. This is especially true in health care delivery settings where health professionals play numerous roles in various parts of the organization many times on the same day.

In observing a day in the working life of a head nurse (unit nurse executive), Mintzberg (1994) notes the remarkable way in which the elements of clinical management flow together in a natural rhythm. He calls it "standing up" management in which the unit leader is within earshot of associated people having both clinical and systems linkages. Like a personal hub, the head nurse blends communication, control, lead, link, and do while constantly interpreting environmental signals. In a true executive role, the nurse manager links with the rest of the hospital, patients, and relatives, as well as outside agencies, and has a well-defined network of external contacts.

Our goal is to break the gap between managers and workers, to realize that managers are workers and workers are managers and that other perspectives or frames must be brought into account if nurse executives are to understand the multiple environments in which they practice. Nurse executives no longer practice in settings but rather in systems of care that now have extended boundaries in other countries and soon, on other planets. A change in position descriptions and role relations via restructuring is no longer adequate for developing optimal work environments for clinical practice and patient care delivery. We propose the following windows as essential to understanding the various ways nurse executives could look at organizations (Figure 6.2). Figure 6.3 graphically portrays the interacting systems in clinical organizations.

Successful empowered environments, discussed further in Chapter 22, will be built on the collaboration of multiple health-related disciplines. Earlier models

WINDOW	PERCEPTION OF VIEWER
Personal	Personal perception of place(s) where and how work is accomplished in organizations; innovation and resource discovery are possible; organizations viewed by some as chaos and others as places for creativity.
Structural	Organizational charts depicting formal roles and relationships; boxes and lines cloud vision of potential; rule by policies and managerial authority; some see boxes; others see only information links between boxes; others see only local and global networks.
Political	Arenas in which different groups compete for power and resources. Bargaining, negotiation, coercion and "dog eat dog" are everyday activities.
Symbolic	Public or private cultures that are orchestrated by rituals, ceremonies, stories, heroes, rumors, and myths. History, tradition, and celebrations are important. Different theater playing in different units.
Systems	Combined clinical management approaches to care delivery. Solutions are chosen from multiple alternatives. Commonly described as a tool for selection of actions based on competing resources and benefits.
Geographic	Spheres of influence with flexible boundaries that separate an organizational system from its environment; boundaries also delineate the parts and processes within the system. Maps would make a better organizational picture.
Work	Socio-technical systems with emphasis on machine and human productivity and interdependence; elements of flow and play; accomplishment of meaningful work outcomes; interactions with clients.
Play	Least recognized window. In childhood, our play is our work; adults search for ways to make work joyful and exciting; personal and work activities in synchrony; stress and monotony-breaking activities.
Clinical	Community of competent and trusted human and health care resources for the treatment of physical and mental discomforts; comfort, safety, and machine care available; a healing site; a health education center or central place either to be cured or learn how to cope with discomfort. Birth to death scenarios—daily scripts of health to illness to death phenomena and travel through diverse health care delivery settings.
Learning	Perception of organizations as learning environments with all workers sharing learning and power.
Professional	Perception of health care organizations as a stage for health professionals, professional practice considered the major role in everyday life; self-disciplined clinical professional groups.

continued

WINDOW	PERCEPTION OF VIEWER
Associations	View of organizations as professional associations; cause of major conflict in organizations where professional organizations are bargaining units also provide arenas for managers and workers to meet on common ground to discuss topics of mutual interest in a nonthreatening environment.
Laboratories	Houses of research for clinical research with animal and human research in separate sections of adjacent or separate buildings.
Knowledge	Information-based enterprises composed largely of knowledge and service specialists who direct and discipline their own performance or are managed by others; offer knowledge-based services.
Symphony	An orchestra wherein all the players (workers) are specialists and the chief executive knows how to make good music and knows something about each instrument but does not pretend to be an expert in each specialty.

Figure 6.2 Through the looking glass: windows on clinical organizations. (A synthesis of ideas by author Simms drawn from Drucker, 1988; Csikszentmihalyi, 1990; Bolman and Deal 1991; Morgan, 1993; and Schneider, 1991.)

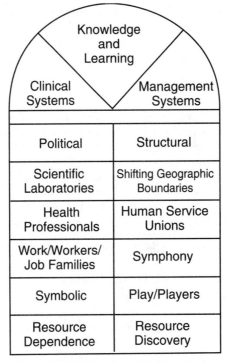

Figure 6.3 Interacting windows in the clinical organization.

focused on nursing and medicine and did not recognize the contribution of other team members or paraprofessionals and support service staff. Collaborative patient-centered practice legitimizes and sharpens the roles of each discipline. It also integrates "care" and "cure" philosophies, which are essential in seamless care. Collaborative people-centered care efficiently uses personnel in roles they are prepared to assume. Patient/family in treatment regimens should be at all points of seamless care from entry into point of service to discharge. Patient involvement has been a part of hospital-based educational programs but only in a passive role. In the future, patient involvement will be increasingly important and should be part of evaluation procedures as well. Clinical outcomes reflecting positive response to therapeutic measures will continue to have a major influence on reimbursement patterns.

Csikszentmihalyi (1990) has described positive work experiences when people are in "flow," linking psychic energy with optimal goal achievement and the work experience. He claims that people make their own optimal experiences happen and these experiences occur when people stretch their minds to the limit to accomplish something difficult and worthwhile. They become creative and self-motivated when they are in "flow." Surely, health care organizations can also be in flow, and like the amoeba, be without permanent organelles or supporting structures that restrict creativity and decision-making (Figure 6.4).

Personal and social relations not established by formal authority constitute the informal social system of work groups, with the political structure creating the environment for goal setting, distributing authority, and setting the stage for power to affect and control resources. Without organizations, there are no leaders and followers and no opportunity for followers to be leaders. Political leadership can be defined only in terms of and to the extent of realization of purposeful substantive change in the conditions of peoples' lives.

Idour (1980) described the need for health organizations to be a total community effort (Figure 6.5). The community or society is not only a unit of organization, according to Idour, it is also a unit of living, interdependent individuals. The nurse executive must be able to work with other members of society—professional and lay—to design organizational models of care delivery that meet client/customer needs and priorities. Health is no longer seen as the absence of disease but rather as a sociocultural phenomenon related to availability of numerous health professionals and services. Idour further noted that illnesses that prevail are increasingly of a chronic nature requiring community boundary changes beyond traditional health institutions. Futuristic in the 1980s, Idour's model could become a blueprint for health in the 21st century.

Patient involvement in collaborative practice is one factor rarely mentioned. With consumer interest in health care and self-care, it is important to have patient representation on various joint practice activities. Patients could be involved in discharge planning. The effectiveness of planning could therefore be measured in terms of patient compliance with health regimens as prescribed by caregivers.

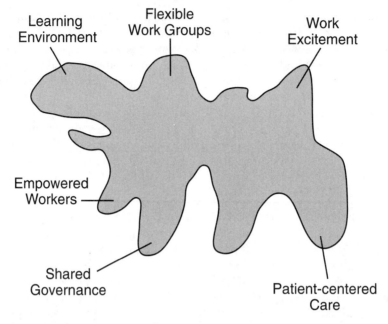

Figure 6.4 Organization in flow.

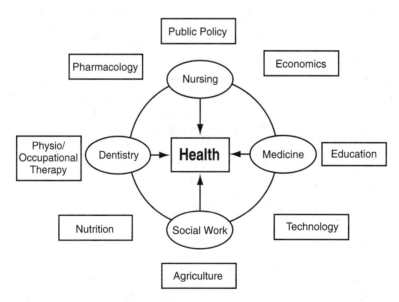

Figure 6.5 Health as a total community effort.

There are several reasons for supporting patient representation on discharge planning teams. Currently, consumers are interested in disease prevention, health promotion, and self-care. Patient involvement is a rapidly emerging part of hospital-based educational programs. Nationally, concern exists about increased health care costs and the decreased financial support. Individuals want more control of their own health; they want to assume responsibility for present and potential health care needs. More patients seek involvement in the decision-making process regarding their own care. They reject the role of passive recipients with decisions made by physicians and nurses without patient input. In the future, patient involvement will become increasingly important and should be a part of evaluation procedures.

PARTICIPATORY APPROACHES TO ORGANIZATIONAL DESIGN

Although recent attention has been focused on the introduction of shared governance in nursing, little attention has been given to participatory action research methods in redesigning clinical work groups in nursing. Shared governance, described as a philosophy, model, or structure in which nurses have explicit and legitimized control over nursing practice, has become a "buzz" word for transformation without empirical underpinnings (Perry, 1991). Furthermore, early literature on shared governance suggested governance be shared at the nursing department general policy level. Later the importance of shared governance at the nursing unit level was emphasized so that staff nurses could be actively involved in the day-to-day clinical decision-making process (Kramer, 1990; Wake, 1990). Few studies have examined the impact of nursing work redesign on patient outcomes.

Several authors have linked participatory management to the human relations theorists such as Likert, McGregor, and Argyris (Perry, 1991), but there has been no theoretical development of how participatory management relates to shared governance. Weick (1979) clarified the importance of each individual worker actively participating in the formation and maintenance of an organization. Although Weick has been influential in describing the process of organizing, a process that comes about by the active involvement of each individual worker, he has not delineated a theoretical framework for his emphasis on the worker, as contrasted with the usual organizational emphasis on the manager. This focus on interactions between rank-and-file workers is often referred to as a "bottom-up" or action approach as compared with the traditional "top-down" approach. The symphony orchestra model first proposed by Drucker (1988) could serve as one of the flexible organizational designs in the 21st century.

However, bottom-up approaches with clear pathways to redesigning clinical work and practice patterns in nursing do not exist. Quite divergent definitions of primary nursing, case management, team nursing, functional nursing, total patient care, and integrated nursing exist in the literature and in practice. Even though interest in collaborative practice in health care has increased, little attention has been given to meaningful interdisciplinary and intradisciplinary flexible work groups. Unnecessary duplication of effort exists across health care disciplines and between professional and technical nurses. With the exception of the Planetree Model for training patients to be partners in care (Martin, Hunt, Hughes-Stone, & Conrad, 1990), patient involvement in care planning efforts is frequently discussed, but inadequately implemented.

Impact on the Organizational Design of Care Delivery Systems

The Patient Intensity for Nursing Index study using Division of Nursing definitions suggests that only one-third of nursing time is spent in direct clinical care (Prescott, Phillips, Ryan, & Thompson, 1991). Other work-sampling studies reported by these authors confirmed this finding. The majority of time (over 50%) is spent in combined indirect care or unit management activities. Reducing inefficiencies in information flow and charting routines and reassigning aspects of unit management could save approximately 48 minutes per nurse per shift. Staff nurses have little creative personal time and only spend about 14% in activities such as meals, breaks, personal phone calls, or socializing with coworkers. The Prescott et al. (1991) research supports *(1)* the redesign of work and work groups through restructuring the role of the registered nurse, *(2)* developing assistive nursing personnel, and *(3)* implementing labor-saving assistive technologies.

During the past decade, revolutionary changes have involved every aspect of health care in this country. Extensive basic medical research has yielded an expanding array of diagnostic and monitoring equipment. Life support systems permit surgeons to remove, repair, or replace components of the body as never before in the history of the human race. The manned space programs have yielded a tremendous amount of knowledge related to physiology and communication systems. Major advancements in robotics and the development of assistive technology are dramatically changing patient education and rehabilitation for self-care. Because nurses are the principal caregivers in various health care delivery settings, it is essential to take a new look at the nature of the work of nursing and propose innovative models for nursing practice that take into account emerging labor-saving assistive technologies as well as rapidly changing health care needs. In essence, nurses must change the way they do their clinical work and how they spend their time in clinical practice. Nurse executives must develop new organizational models for care delivery that reflect changing thought about organizations.

THE LEARNING WINDOW

The importance of work group culture and worker learning is beginning to be recognized as important in organizational analyses and technology transfer. One aspect of culture is a group's readiness to change. Receptivity to innovation may be the critical factor in orchestrating change and learning to use technology. Schein (1984) notes that excessive stability may prevent innovation unless large numbers of people are redistributed or replaced or the organizational culture is changed and the workers become involved in decision-making.

Changing technology and work environments have created a new potential for worker learning as well as a need for better approaches to the learning process. In fact, Deutsch (1989) has proposed a new norm that it is okay to spend time learning at work. A key point stressed by various researchers is the need for effective organizations to strive consciously toward a participatory work environment to best utilize technology and human resources. Worker learning and the shaping of the work environment are important aspects of human growth and development, especially in the face of rapid technological change. Crisis conditions have accented the need for worker learning in anticipation of changed work environments. The key role of new technology cannot be overstated; it is revolutionary and "the greatest challenge for those involved in worker learning efforts will continue to be to devise ways to move from the narrow and technical to broader issues of worker knowledge, active involvement, and an ever-expanding base of learning how to learn in an on-going process" (Deutsch, 1989, p. 251). Deutsch further suggests a model for expanded learning that increasingly goes from workplace specific issues to larger matters of the work situation depicting a fluid process for everyday learning.

Senge, Kleiner, Roberts, Ross, and Smith (1994) suggest that learning is not the process of amassing data and working is not a series of unenlightening lower level routines but rather both are closely interrelated sense-making, reflective, culture-bound activities. They see human learning as the bottleneck through which innovation must pass. Conversely, innovation is becoming the learning burden of those whose working practices are constantly being changed. Senge et al. (1994) further suggest that working, learning, and innovation are related processes and if innovation can be developed out of or in relation to workplace learning, the bottleneck of human learning and burden may be avoided. The authors suggest that the activity of small groups and individuals can lead to insightful learning and this learning is potentially innovative at the organization level. Thus, the small group around the coffee pot, the drinking fountain, or the lunch room should not be assumed to be wasting time. In these small informal groups, real working knowledge about real working practices is commonly exchanged and developed. The lack of personal time at work must be viewed as detrimental to creative thinking and interaction in the workplace (Csikszentmihalyi, 1996).

Achieving goals of workplace democracy and freedom to take personal time depends on informed, growing, and self-confident individuals and groups within a supportive work group culture. Johnson and Johansson (1991) have shown how workplace participatory research can be viewed as a colearning process where researchers and workers share in some or all stages of work research. Increased learning through participative empowerment processes can make a fundamental contribution to organizational outcomes as confident workers are competent workers. Kornbluh and Greene (1989) proposed a learning consciousness in an organization model that focuses on four areas:

- Developing learning enabler roles for managers and workers
- Developing work organizations as learning milieu
- Developing meaningful participatory processes
- Developing a work climate committed to learning

The way work is organized affects the quantity and quality of worker learning; dull, repetitive, fragmented work does not produce a positive learning milieu. Workers can be deeply involved in processes of research related to their work situations and workers and researchers can be colearners.

Kornbluh, Pipan, and Schurman (1987) also related empowerment to learning and defined empowerment learning as unlimited energy in an organization. Human learning is considered an organizational asset, and in transformed organizations, human learning and problem-solving abilities are viewed as vitally important resources in empowering people—a continuous source of energy. Their thesis questions the zero-sum conception of power in command and control organizations that assumes that power is a finite commodity in which some may gain only if others lose. In turn, a radically different approach is proposed—a non-zero-sum model of power in which the total amount of power is always expanding. This situation is believed to occur in a learning environment. Learning is not a process of receiving verbal information. At the workplace, learning is the process of continually expanding coherence, collaboration, and innovation within a particular community of practice. The creation of a learning environment empowers workers to use their intellectual abilities to individual development and work-group advantage. In this model, every worker is respected and every worker exerts control over performance and quality of work and life variables. Worker participation and learning environments go hand in hand, and work redesign should be regarded as a continuous process, not a goal. Further discussion of learning environments can be found in Chapters 19 and 22.

THE NURSE EXECUTIVE ROLE IN LEARNING ORGANIZATIONS

The need for creativity in the role of the nurse executive has never been greater. Middle managers are frequently threatened by an educative, participative work environment, even though a climate of sharing information is fundamental to professional nursing practice. With the shift to consumer locus of control and demands for high quality patient-centered care, the head nurse as the front line nurse executive is extremely important in creating work environments in which integrated professional practice can occur. The classical view of the manager as the organizer, coordinator, planner, and controller becomes less important in organizations that support participatory management. Mintzberg (1990) suggests that effective management incorporates a balance of cerebral and insightful aspects. He further suggests that the effective manager's role involves interpersonal, informational, and decisional activities. The manager's effectiveness is significantly influenced by insight into the nature of the work.

The learning enabler facilitator role needs to be learned by managers (Kornbluh & Greene, 1989). A very different role compared with traditional management roles, the facilitator role involves performing the function of enabler of learning and constantly creating the conditions for learning. Learning in groups has enormous potential, as described by Hirschhorn (1988), in studying training and learning needs of workers in the new computer-based work organization. Drucker (1988) supports the notion of participatory management because the work force has changed with the introduction of the better educated knowledge worker. This suggests that the manager's primary task is to support joint performance by nurturing common goals, common values, the right structure and ongoing training, and development needed to perform and respond to change. Much of the redesign literature has focused on factors related to redesigning the work of staff nurses. Flarey (1991) asserts that first-line managerial roles must change as well. The role of the first-line manager must take on new dimensions to facilitate quality patient care and patient care provider outcomes.

Failure of unit nurse executives to use professional nurses congruent with their education and expertise is perceived by many nurse leaders to be contributing to the continuing nursing shortage. Prescott et al. (1991), however, debunk arguments of nursing shortage and make a strong case for the idea of inadequate professional nursing practice. Based on work sampling studies about how nurses spend their time, they conclude that hospitals use nurses inappropriately in two ways: nurses do the work of other departments and clinical decision-making authority of nurses is severely limited in many hospitals. Both result in too little professional nursing practice and inappropriate use of nurses' time.

In general, too much emphasis has been placed on limited organizational variables and too little emphasis has been placed on workplace and learning variables. The concept of work excitement, first introduced in a publication by Simms, Erbin-Roesemann, Darga, and Coeling (1990), has tremendous potential for affecting nursing practice. This research supports Pressler and Fitzpatrick (1988), who believe that patient behavior in response to nursing action is of considerable importance for nursing practice. If one considers behavior to be part of nursing action, then the link between work excitement and nursing practice is an important issue to explore. Behavior of health care providers is thought to significantly influence patient clinical outcomes.

The shift to consumer/customer locus of control, emphasis on clinical outcomes in health care, and the increasing availability of various personal assistive technologies mandate different approaches to nursing practice. Decisions regarding changes in staff numbers have generally been determined by management with little opportunity for staff nurse involvement or consumer input. Job redesign solutions have seldom included workers' input. In the future, worker/management/consumer participatory discussion will be essential to decision making about technological change and will be a fundamental component of organizational learning processes.

THE PROFESSIONAL ASSOCIATIONS

A basic element of any profession is the formal organization of professional associations—for example, the American Nurses Association (ANA), the National League for Nursing (NLN), the American Medical Association (AMA), and so forth. Such groups are highly visible phenomena in society and give credibility to participant members as legitimate professionals (McCloskey & Grace, 1997). Professional associations play a vital role in activities of professional life and offer a common ground for discussion and dealing with political issues of conflict among managers and workers who cannot regularly meet in fruitful conversation in the regular world of work. However, they should not be viewed as the equivalent of care delivery organizations. They have very different missions and goals. Professional associations offer wonderful opportunities to learn negotiation, bargaining, and sound management skills in a relatively friendly environment and this is one of the major reasons why nurse executives at all levels should encourage active participation in professional organizations.

MANAGING BOUNDARIES

How boundaries are managed and how that relates to levels of differentiation and integration necessary for effective functioning within organizations has become an issue of paramount importance for nurse executives at all levels. Schneider (1991) provides a meaningful perspective on the concept in her discussion of boundaries as both defined and flexible. Boundaries separate a system from its environment and delineate the various parts and processes within that system. As systems develop, they require increased differentiation and integration. As the continuum of care moves health services outside of institutional parameters, different skill sets, relationships, and behavioral patterns will be required. Entrepreneurial skills will be expected of every professional nurse (Porter-O'Grady, 1997).

In family systems, managing the boundaries between members is considered important. In organizations, the management of boundaries between and among job families is equally important. Relatedness is forced through concern for patients and quality patient care. Job-family fighting may be a symptom of threatened individuals or particular family autonomy. For example, the infighting between nurses, physicians, and social workers over responsibilities for patient care reflect the relatively low autonomy of nonmedical health workers. Descriptions of hospitals as medical care facilities rather than health care facilities further denies the existence of nonmedical health professionals.

The boundary issues present at the group level also exist between groups within organizations and between organizations and their environments (Schneider,

1991). The extent of external control greatly influences boundary management. During reorganizations and work redesign, boundaries are redrawn and redefined. The renegotiation of boundaries is frequently marked by anxiety and a scramble for power among group members. The resolution of boundaries should be dynamic and continuously changing and should restore the necessary requirements for interdependence and interaction. In other words, says Schneider (1991), organizations need appropriate levels of differentiation and integration with boundaries established within that are firm yet flexible. Firm but flexible boundaries enable interpersonal intimacy, group cooperation, and organizational interdependence. An effective nurse executive must define and redefine flexible work groups within the central organization while negotiating and planning with networking groups. Today, organizations are viewed as networks, as linkage points of distinctive competencies or specialties on a global scale that require greater and greater efforts at integration without losing differentiation (Ghoshal & Bartlett, 1990). Differences between internal and external stakeholders have become less clear; for example, organizational members such as staff nurses have become customers as well. The role of the nurse executive is to manage the boundary between what is outside to preserve the integrity of groups (nursing and nonnursing job families) and the internal coherence of the system.

Boundary problems between professional roles and tasks can create continuing problems with tensions especially pronounced between nurses and physicians. Overlapping services create blurred boundaries that require negotiation for staffing, responsibility, and accountability. Other hostilities are created by ideological boundaries of a community-oriented versus medical-model approach to care (Schneider, 1991). Competing camps vie for reimbursement of overlapping services. Professional boundaries are jealously guarded and without the National Institutes of Health (NIH) and the Joint Commission for Accreditation of Healthcare Organizations (JCAHO) mandates for attention to patient outcomes, it is likely that patients would have stayed forever at the bottom of the hierarchy with the least to say about their treatment.

SUMMARY

The way clinical organizations are viewed is extremely important and everything in this chapter is essential content for those nurse executives considering organizational innovation at any level. Basic to understanding the chapter theme, it seems important to believe that: *(1)* boundaries are necessary and need to be established for appropriate levels of differentiation and integration and *(2)* autonomy for individual workers is essential to self-development. Boundaries cannot be managed without autonomy of individuals and groups. Allowing projects to develop outside established organizational structures and policies provides the rationale for "skunkworks," which are loosely coupled with the parent structure but not strays, by any means. The nurse executive at all levels must be conscious of unit, organizational, and external boundaries. The process of managing flexible boundaries can be learned and is essential during birth, innovation, work redesign, and creation of new departments and businesses.

Reframing or changing your organization is a four-dimensional process (human, structural, political, and symbolic frames) with major investment in learning activities. New organization models will bear little resemblance to industrial models of the past. Nursing divisions with numerous levels of managers have been structured as factory models. In the coming organizations, health care delivery businesses will be knowledge-based organizations composed largely of specialists who direct their performance through organized feedback from colleagues, customers, and headquarters. Computer technology will make information, formerly considered only for managers, available to everyone who needs it. Successful information-based organizations will have no middle management at all. Senior executives will function more like orchestra conductors. Decentralization into autonomous units with flexible task forces will be essential. Physicians and nurse executives will function collaboratively with health services administrators in a variety of new practice patterns and work groups. What will you see when you look through the looking glass at your organization?

STUDY QUESTIONS

1. How does a termite mound portray a flexible organizational structure?
2. Why are the "windows" of clinical organizations different from other organizations? Explain what is meant by the learning window.
3. What is meant by the human side of clinical administration?
4. Idour uses the term total community. What does this mean in terms of nursing and health organizations?
5. How does managing in boundary-less organizations differ from managing in traditional organizations?

REFERENCES

Bolman, L. G., & Deal, T. E. (1991). *Reframing organizations.* San Francisco: Jossey-Bass.

Craft, J. S., & Spilotro, S. L. (1997). Integration for the future: Forming a virtual organization. *Journal of Nursing Administration, 27*(4), 3, 20.

Csikszentmihalyi, M. (1990). *Flow—The psychology of optimal experience.* New York: Harper & Row.

Csikszentmihalyi, M. (1996). *Creativity.* New York: HarperCollins.

Deutsch, S. (1989). Worker learning in the context of changing technology and work environment. In H. Leymann & H. Kornbluh (Eds.), *Socialization and Learning at Work* (pp. 237–255). Brookfield, VT: Gower.

Drucker, P. F. (1988). The coming of the new organization. *Harvard Business Review, 88*(1), 45–53.

Flarey, D. L. (1991). Redesigning management roles. *Journal of Nursing Administration, 21*(2), 40–45.

Ghoshal, S., & Bartlett, C. A. (1990). The multinational corporation as an interorganization network. *Academy of Management Review, 15*(4), 603–625.

Hirschhorn, L. (1988). Psychodynamics of the workplace. In *The Workplace Within* (pp. 1–15). Cambridge, MA: MIT Press.

Idour, M. G. (1980). *The social context and the relevancy of nursing curricula.* Unpublished thesis. Massey University, New Zealand.

Johnson, J. V., & Johansson, G. (eds.). (1991). *The psychosocial work environment: Work organization, democratization and health.* Amityville, NY: Baywood.

Kornbluh, H., Pipan, R., & Schurman, S. J. (1987). Empowerment learning and control in workplaces: A curricular view. *Zeitschrift Fur Sozialisationsforschung Und Erziehungssoziologie (ZSE) J. Jahrgang/Heft 7*(4), 253–268.

Kornbluh, H., & Greene, R. T. (1989). Learning, empowerment and participative processes. In H. Leymann & H. Kornbluh (Eds.), *Socialization and learning at work* (pp. 256–274). Brookfield, VT: Gower.

Kramer, M. (1990). The magnet hospitals: Excellence revisited. *Journal of Nursing Administration, 20*(9), 35–44.

Martin, D., Hunt, J. R., Hughes-Stone, M., & Conrad, D. A. (1990). The planetree model project: An example of the patient as partner. *Hospital & Health Services Administration, 35*(4), 591–601.

McCloskey, J., & Grace, H. K. (1997). *Current issues in nursing* (5th ed.). St. Louis: Mosby.

Mintzberg, H. (1990). The manager's job: Folklore and fact. *Harvard Business Review, 68*(2), 163–172.

Mintzberg, H. (1994). Managing as blended care. *Journal of Nursing Administration, 24*(9), 29–36.

Morgan, G. (1993). *Imaginization.* Newbury Park, CA: Sage.

Perry, B. (1991). *Shared governance in nursing: A review and critique of the literature.* Unpublished manuscript. University of Michigan, Ann Arbor.

Porter-O'Grady, T. (1997, Fall). The private practice of nursing: The gift of entrepreneurialism. *Nursing Administration Quarterly, 22*(1), 23–29.

Prescott, P. A., Phillips, C. Y., Ryan, J. W., & Thompson, K. O. (1991). Changing how nurses spend their time. *IMAGE: Journal of Nursing Scholarship, 23*(1), 23–28.

Pressler, J., & Fitzpatrick, J. (1988). Contribution of Rosemary Ellis to knowledge development for nursing. *IMAGE: Journal of Nursing Scholarship, 20*(1), 28–30.

Schein, E. L. (1984). Coming to a new awareness of organizational culture. *Sloan Management Review, 25*(2), 3–16.

Schneider, S. C. (1991). Managing boundaries in organizations. In M. K. deVries (Ed.). *Organizations on the couch* (pp. 169–190). San Francisco: Jossey-Bass.

Senge, P. M., Kleiner, A., Roberts, C., Ross, R. B., & Smith, B. J. (1994). *The fifth discipline fieldbook.* New York: Doubleday.

Simms, L. M., Erbin-Roesemann, M., Darga, A., & Coeling, H. (1990). Breaking the burnout barrier: Resurrecting work excitement in nursing. *Nursing Economic$, 8*(3), 177–186.

Wake, M. M. (1990). Nursing care delivery systems: Status and vision. *Journal of Nursing Administration, 20*(5), 47–51.

Weick, K. E. (1979). *The social psychology of organizing.* Reading, MA: Addison-Wesley.

CHAPTER

7

Blending Clinical Practice with Organizational Design

Sylvia A. Price

It is impossible to develop new styles of organization and management while continuing to think in old ways. (Morgan, 1993, p. 63)

Chapter Highlights

- Fit between organizational design and context for practice
- Mission, values statement and vision
- Effective team management
- Organizational work units
- Authority relationships
- Types of organizational structures
- A decentralized organizational model

Scientific and technological advances have significantly influenced the pattern of delivery of health care services. The majority of these health services are delivered within an organizational environment. Health care organizations orchestrate human and technological resources to create an environment in which care delivery can occur.

The focus of this chapter is to analyze various patterns of relationships associated with design or structure of health care organizations as they relate to the context for nursing administrative practice. It further identifies concepts that apply to analyzing, developing, or restructuring a nursing department or division. As selected designs of organizations are identified, it will become evident that, for a health care organization, a structure—the formal relationships among individuals in various positions—combines a set of variables involving technology, tasks, and human resources that will enable the organization to accomplish its purpose, mission, and goals. Nurse executives and other health care professionals must be knowledgeable about organization design. They must be able to recognize the most appropriate organizational design, the criteria for its selection, and how the organizational structure influences the behavior of individuals and groups.

FIT BETWEEN ORGANIZATIONAL DESIGN AND CONTEXT FOR PRACTICE

Organizations consist of people performing tasks within formal or informal organizational networks. Whenever individuals join in a collaborative effort, organizations should be used to obtain effective and productive results. The interrelated conditions, in which professional nursing administrative practice occurs, comprise the organization design of not only the nursing division but also other patient care areas.

The goal of organizational design is to identify the specific structures and processes that best accommodate the types of individuals and nature of the work to be performed in a given organization. Organization design is the way in which authority, responsibility, and information system networks are blended within the organization. Organization elements can be designed to include departments or divisions into sections or units, determination of the number of levels of management, locus of control of decision-making, accessibility of information, and the physical facility.

Leatt, Shortell, and Kimberly (1994) state that when a new organization is formed a new design will be created. This is an ongoing process where the design needs will change as the organization's needs change. If a hospital decides to diversify its product lines and expand to new patient programs, it may be deemed necessary to rearrange the organization's division of labor. If an extended care facility decides to close a geriatric day care program, it may be necessary to rearrange services within the organization. Another important component of organizational design is the nature and content of the information system needed by the enterprise. The design specifies who has power to make the decisions, which positions need what type of information and at what times. It should also be stressed that organization design also has implications for how performance will be evaluated and for the degree to which the reward system of the organization is congruent with achievement or performance. The knowledge gleaned from performance will indicate feedback to subsequently influence the organization's mission.

Mintzberg (1981) asserts that "a great many problems in organizational design stem from the assumption that organizations are all alike: mere collections of component parts to which elements of structure can be added and deleted at will, a sort of organizational bazaar" (p. 103). The opposite assumption is that effective organizations achieve coherence among their component parts; that is, one part cannot be changed without considering the consequences to all the others. To design effective organizations, managers need to determine the most effective structure for the set of units that constitutes the organization as a whole.

MISSION, VALUES STATEMENT, AND VISION

In designing the appropriate organizational structure one must be cognizant of the parent organization's mission, vision, and values statement. *Mission statements* are formal statements of the purpose of the organization. They reflect the nature, purpose, and setting of the organization. The mission statement of an academic health center will emphasize its commitment to training new professionals and provide for education and research activities. An example of a mission statement for a home health care organization is illustrated by the following: "Parker Homecare Agency will provide high quality health care services to the individuals of Adams and surrounding counties. We are committed to excellence and seek to constantly improve the health of people in our region."

Vision refers to what the organization desires to be. Simms and Calarco (1998) emphasize that "An inspiring vision that clarifies the direction of the organization serves as the force that assists each department, unit, and individual employee to align their missions to the organization's future direction" (p. 176). This is reflected in the following vision statement of a regional health care facility: "To be the health care provider of first choice for individuals within this region. One of the top health care systems in the United States."

Values are normative judgments held by individuals as to what is good and desirable. These values provide standards under which persons are influenced by their choice of actions. Social values indicate a system of shared beliefs concerning desired goals for conduct. Value statements describe how the organization's vision will be accomplished and must be precisely defined and reflect action-oriented behaviors. Organizations are dependent on shared values among its employees and society for their existence. These statements reflect the organization's values of compassion, personal excellence, trust, integrity, and collaboration. The driving value of the Parker Homecare Agency is "putting clients and families first ensures their active participation in all aspects of their care. This agency respects the uniqueness of all individuals and the richness of diversity in gender, ethnicity, and religious practices."

EFFECTIVE TEAM MANAGEMENT

Within the total organization and in nursing or patient care divisions there are usually formal or informal mechanisms for allocating functions. To accomplish customary functions, nursing or patient care organizations often create teams, councils, or committees. Functions are identified, and a group structure to fulfill these functions is developed. Groups are a necessary and integral part of organizational life. It is important to emphasize that these groups or teams arise out of a need and are established for a specific purpose.

A team may be classified according to the following characteristics: their purpose, mission, specified time period, membership, and structure. A team may be involved in redesigning the organization structure or formulating new projects or programs. Functional department teams, such as the finance department, are part of the formal organizational structure because members are from that department. Temporary teams are usually task forces, project, or problem-solving teams that are formed to accomplish a particular purpose such as analyzing an innovative approach to the cost effectiveness of a new procedure.

Teams may be either supervised or self-managed. A supervised team is under the direction of a manager who is responsible for guiding the team in setting goals, performing work activities, and evaluating performance. A self-managed team is explanatory as it assumes responsibilities for managing itself. The three most common types of teams are:

- Functional team
- Self-directed or self-management teams
- Cross-functional teams

Functional teams are composed of a manager and employees from a particular functional area. Issues such as authority, decision-making, leadership, and interactions are relatively understandable. These teams may be involved in efforts to improve performance or work activity or solve particular problems related to the functional area.

A popular team used in organizations is the self-directed or self-managed team. This refers to a formal group of employees who function without a manager and are responsible for a work process that delivers a product or a service to consumers. The self-directed team is accountable and responsible for getting the work accomplished and managing themselves. A cross-functional team is a hybrid group of individuals, who are specialists in various areas and who come together across department lines to work on various tasks of the organization.

Robbins and Coulter (1996) pose the question "Why use teams?" They state there is no single explanation for the recent popularity of teams. They propose the following reasons for the use of teams:

- Creates esprit de corps. Team members expect and demand a lot from each other, which facilitates cooperation and improves employee morale. Team norms tend to encourage members to excel, and at the same time, create a climate that increases job satisfaction.
- Allows management to think strategically. By using teams, especially self-directed ones, managers are able to do more strategic planning. When tasks or jobs are designed around employees, managers often spend an inordinate amount of their time supervising people and "putting out fires." They

are too busy to do much strategic planning. By using work teams these managers are able to redirect their energy and concentrate on issues such as long-range plans.

- Speeds decisions. Moving decision-making vertically down to teams allows the organization greater flexibility to make faster decisions. Team members are better informed and closer to the work-related issues than are managers. Therefore, decisions are often made more quickly when teams exist than when jobs are designed around individuals.
- Facilitates workforce diversity. The old saying that two heads are better than one is particularly applicable to work teams. Groups consisting of individuals from diverse backgrounds and experience often envision things that homogenous groups do not. The use of diverse teams may result in more innovations and better decisions than if individuals alone made the decision. (p. 509)

Because professionals need to participate in the decision-making process, health care administrators should design an organizational structure that allows such participation. An excellent example of team building is in the community health clinical practice area. Case management as a care delivery model has been practiced in the community health settings for several years. The team approach in this area may be either cross-functional or self-managed. Nurse managers coordinate the client's health care with team members such as home health aides, physicians, social workers, and physical and occupational therapists. Professional nurses in home health care are often more autonomous because they manage their own practice.

The cost of team meetings in relation to time is usually very significant. Several variables that affect group outcomes are length of meetings due to excessive deliberation, travel time required by members, and cost of personnel time in terms of salaries. It is essential that, when a decision is made to form a team or task force, consideration should be given as to whether a group decision is necessary or whether an individual decision would be as appropriate. The question arises as to whether the benefits of a team are worth its cost especially when the emphasis in many organizations is on cost containment. Often these benefits, such as increased morale and satisfaction or the experience of teamwork, are difficult to measure. Teams do function effectively when costs are justified, authority for decision-making responsibility is defined, the scope of the subject matter is considered, members are representative of the interests they serve, and sufficient resources are allocated.

ORGANIZATIONAL WORK UNITS

Work units enable the organization to achieve its purposes, goals, and objectives. Organizations have activities that must be performed. This type of structure is founded on the functional basis of departmentalization, which is a process of grouping individuals into units, divisions, or departments to facilitate the attainment of the organization's goals. For example, in the hospital setting nurses may be placed within the division of nursing and pharmacists within the pharmacy division. With the emphasis on cost containment and reductions in hospital size, integration of patient care activities across departments is becoming more evident. A major trend in the hospital setting is the shift from functional specialization to a more generalist worker who has multiple task responsibilities.

In the home health care setting the structure is usually a simple structure with a functional design. However, home care is the fastest-growing segment in health care. The organizational design will likely change to the integration of a functional and divisional structure as the home health service industry is becoming more complex and changing rapidly. For example, reimbursement for home care is moving from a fee-for-service to contract pricing and capitation. The integration of clinical, financial, and human resources and patient outcome information are factors that will influence the organizational design of the home care agency.

When one analyzes an organization, it is important to scrutinize the various systems that exist to accomplish the work of the enterprise. This includes delineating the processes or procedures that have been developed to coordinate the work to be done. To conceptualize how the organization functions, it is imperative to know the recruitment practices, the method of selecting individuals for positions, the reporting relationships, and the informational network.

Authority Relations

Concepts of line and staff authority are frequently inadequately defined, often referring to functions or authority relationships. Early classical administrative writers made a distinction between line and staff authority. They defined managers with line authority as exercising direct responsibility for accomplishing organizational objectives, whereas staff authority was envisioned as supporting the line in the achievement of those objectives.

The concept of *line authority* is clear when it is designated that a supervisor exercises direct control over a subordinate; such a structure consists of a direct vertical relationship and reflects Fayol's scalar principle. The principle is applicable to this concept in that the clearer the line of authority from the executive-level management position to the subordinate position, the responsibility for decision-making and communication will be more effective (see Chapter 3). Line refers to a position and describes managers who have direct impact on the achievement of the organization's objectives.

Staff authority is advisory and it is given to individuals who support and assist others who have line authority in implementing their managerial activities. Staff authority is depicted as an advisory relationship and does not entail the authority to enact policy decisions for the organization. An important distinction is that line and staff are differentiated by their authority relationships, not by department functions. For example, a human resource management activity such as placement of personnel at Parker Homecare Agency is considered staff, whereas at Davis Home Health Care Agency, placement of personnel is a line function. In a staff relationship, the clinical nurse specialist (CNS) or advanced practice nurse (APN) has responsibilities and functions that are advisory. This individual is not in a command position; the line manager makes decisions that are developed in consultation with the CNS or APN.

An organizational chart is a graphic representation of reporting relationships within the division of nursing and other departments. In a visual sense, the chart maps the entire operation of the organization. It is necessary to reevaluate and update these charts frequently to reflect changes in the enterprise. A futuristic decentralized organizational chart with rotating team leaders is depicted in Figure 7.1.

Span of Management

The number of subordinates who report directly and are supervised by a manager is referred to as the span of management or control. There is a limit to the number of individuals a manager can supervise that is dependent on the impact of several underlying factors. The contemporary perspective of span of management recognizes that various factors influence the number and frequency of contacts the managers have with their employees. Koontz and Weihrich (1990) identify the following factors that affect the span of management:

- The better the training of subordinates, the less of their manager's time and also less contact with them is necessary.

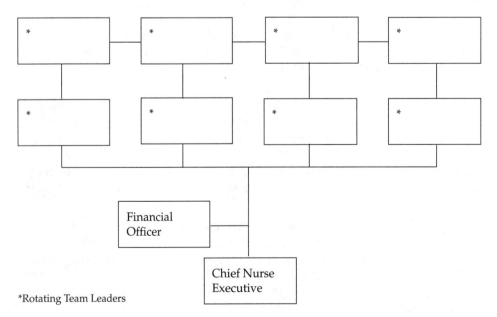

Figure 7.1 Nursing organizational chart for the year 2000 (reprinted as projects change).

- Clarity of delegation of authority—identifying the work tasks and clearly defining authority relationships enables the subordinate to perform the task with a minimum of manager's time and attention.
- Clarity of plans provides a framework of operations to guide the subordinates, which necessitates fewer contacts with managers.
- The use of objective standards enables the manager to delegate in confidence and reduce unnecessary control-centered relationships.
- Rate of change refers to stability in policies so those subordinates have guides to thinking and do not have to appeal for policy decisions and directions.
- Communication techniques—ability to communicate plans and directions clearly and concisely increase a manager's span.
- Amount of personal contact needed—allowance is given for cases where the subject matter demands personal contact.
- Variation by organization level is that the size of the most effective span varies by organizational level.

As reflected in an organizational chart, a wide span of management usually has two to four levels and is referred to as a flat, or horizontal, organizational structure. A narrow span of management has many levels and is referred to as a tall structure.

Delegation of Authority

The delegation process involves responsibility, authority, and accountability. This process is vital to an organization because it enables superiors to pass authority downward to subordinate managers, giving them certain rights as well as prescribing limits within which they must operate. Administrative personnel are authorized to make certain decisions and to direct the staff under their jurisdiction. They are also accountable for the results. When an activity is delegated to subordinates, the supervisory personnel retain responsibility for it. Subordinates are responsible to the individual who delegated the task to them. Therefore, delegation includes assigning an activity to subordinates, granting them the authority necessary for it to be fulfilled, and acceptance by subordinates of responsibility and accountability for satisfactory performance of the activity.

An interesting question arises as to whether responsibility can be delegated. Classical administrative theorists note that because the delegator is held responsible for the action of the delegatees, responsibility cannot be delegated. Robbins and Coulter (1996) recognize two forms of responsibility: operating and ultimate responsibilities. Managers give out operating responsibility but retain ultimate responsibility. Robbins and Coulter state that a manager is ultimately responsible for the actions of subordinates to whom operating responsibility has been given. It is imperative to delegate operating responsibility equal to the delegated authority. Ultimate responsibility can never be delegated.

TYPES OF ORGANIZATIONAL STRUCTURES

The concepts of centralization and decentralization are related to delegation of authority. The degree of delegation of responsibility, power, and authority to the lower levels in an organization is used to classify the organization as centralized or decentralized.

Decentralized Organizational Structure

Decentralization reflects a particular philosophy of organization and management. In a decentralized structure, decision-making, responsibility, authority, and accountability are incorporated at the operational, or practitioner, level of the organization. Decentralization fosters autonomy in practice. The concept of decentralization emphasizes the importance of human relationships within an enterprise. It requires careful selection of which decisions will be made at the operational level and which will be decided at the executive level. Decentralization entails granting subordinates authority to make decisions, determining which decisions will be made at the operational level, and enacting policies to guide decision making. Dale (1952) formulated some objective criteria that can be useful in determining the extent of decentralization. He implies that the degree of decentralization is greater when:

1. More decisions are made lower down the management hierarchy.
2. More important decisions are made lower down the management hierarchy.
3. More functions affected by decisions are made at lower levels.
4. Less checking is required on decisions. (p. 118)

In a decentralized nursing service, professional nurse practitioners participate in the management of services to their patients/clients and in decisions that affect their nursing practice. The decisions are usually made by individuals with the clinical expertise to provide quality nursing care. In this structure, managers at the first and middle levels are involved in decisions regarding the implementation of programs, because staff are more knowledgeable than upper level managers about the details of day-to-day operations and are able to implement those decisions. This expanded responsibility has encouraged the development of self-managed teams. See Figure 7.1 as an example of a decentralized structure.

At the operational level, nurse managers have greater authority than in a centralized structure and are held accountable for operations at this level. Their participation in the decision-making process provides a high degree of congruence with organizational goals and objectives.

Decentralization generally increases motivation and satisfaction of staff at the middle- and first-management levels. The advantages of decentralization are job enrichment because there is more effective utilization of managerial skills, greater potential for innovation and creativity in fulfilling the responsibilities of the position, more autonomy encouraged in decision-making, and an increase in overall satisfaction.

Limitations of decentralization are based on such contingency factors as the size of the organization. Size is a critical determinant of decentralization. An organization may not be large enough to warrant decentralization because it may not be feasible or cost effective to have autonomous units within the agency. Senior executive-level administrators may not desire decentralization, because they may not want to relinquish authority to subordinates who do not have the managerial abilities and motivations to make effective decisions. Division managers may identify with one unit to the point of developing favoritism toward it; this may result in competition among units to the extent that is detrimental to the overall objectives of the enterprise. In addition, fragmentation may occur due to problems of control and nonuniform policies.

Centralized Organizational Structure

Centralization implies a tightly controlled communication network, uniformity of policy and action in decision-making, identification of power and authority with the position, and controlling authority over financial resources, planning, and the mandating of changes of direction or programs for the organization. It is usually advantageous to centralize those activities or functions within an enterprise that interacts with the overall environment. For example, in nursing specialized functions may be centralized such as in-service education, computerized information systems, and quality management programs. See Figure 7.2 as an example of a centralized structure.

What determines whether an organization will move toward more centralization or decentralization? Daft (1994) identifies several factors that influence the amount of centralization that an organization has. For more centralization these factors include:

- Environment is more stable.
- First-level managers are not as capable or experienced at making decisions.
- Decisions are more significant.
- Organization is facing a crisis or the risk of company failure.
- Company is large.
- Effective implementation of the organization's strategies depends on managers retaining more say over what happens. (p. 298)

The disadvantages of centralization are often the result of investiture of decision-making authority at the top level, which may result in the delay of implementation at the operational, or practitioner, level. Innovative thinking and creativity tend to be stifled, and changes imposed from the top often become subverted and do not get implemented.

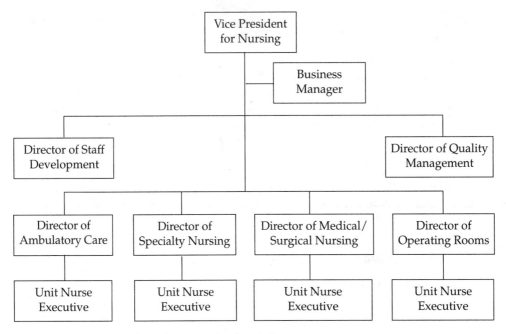

Figure 7.2 Division of nursing organizational chart.

Matrix Organization

Matrix management has become increasingly popular in recent years. Matrix organizations were initially developed in the aerospace industry, where the focus was on products and markets as well as on technology.

The matrix organization superimposes a project or program management directly over a functional, hierarchical organizational structure. This allows for maintenance of the day-to-day operations and implementation of new projects or programs within an enterprise. The single most characteristic element of the matrix organization is a dual authority, or chain of command, in that both the heads of the functional areas and the project (product-line) managers have authority over those working in the matrix unit. Within this dual authority structure, responsibilities are assigned to functional departments oriented toward specialized resources.

Three critical management roles are distinguishable in a matrix structure: the top leader; the matrix bosses, or managers, who share subordinates; and the two-boss managers. Lawrence, Kolodny, and Davis (1977) state that the matrix approach requires a strong, unified command at the top executive level to ensure a balance of power at the next level. The role of the top executive involves three unique aspects: power balancing, managing the decision, and standard setting.

First, the top executive has authority over, or controls, both of the organization's command structures: administrative and technical. The existence of dual pressures requires balanced decision-making that considers both structures to establish and sustain a reasonable balance of power between the two sectors. The second aspect of the role relates to the necessary condition for an effective matrix; that is, a very high volume of information must be processed and focused for use in making key decisions. This requires that authority and responsibility for decision-making be shared. Third, the top executive sets the standards of performance. This aspect is vital to the allocation of financial and human resources. Unless the top executive has high expectations for the organization, it is unlikely that the matrix organization will respond to the environmental pressure for resource deployment.

The matrix manager holds a middle management position and shares many of the decisions such as tasks, assignments, and performance evaluations with product-line, business, or other functional managers. In contrast to the situation in a traditional pyramidal organization, no individual manager in a matrix organization is autonomous or controls his or her own destiny. Rather, each manager has unit objectives that are partially determined by the resource demands of projects and businesses.

The most challenging aspect of the matrix organization is the often-conflicting demands of the two-boss managers. Conflicts may arise between the demands of the manager's functional position and those of the project team. Such conflicts emanate from multiple demands from above and beyond a manager's immediate command. The manager must heed the competing demands, make trade-offs, and manage the conflicts that cannot be resolved. Such situations can create anxiety and stress from above, but it is important to emphasize that two-boss managers must also be responsible for their subordinates. This role need not be shared. Any skillful politician knows that alternative sources of power increase one's flexibility, which is the key to successful performance as a two-boss manager.

Matrix organizations are a challenge to manage. Because personnel in the matrix have two bosses, conflicts within the system are inevitable. To cope with such conflicts, managers must develop a high level of interpersonal skills and a willingness to take risks. They must rely on their own personal qualities and the ability to persuade through their own knowledge and expertise.

Hospitals have been classified as matrix organizations because of their hierarchical coordination through departmentalization and their formal chain of command and horizontal coordination across departments through patient care teams. Each team has a leader and members representing technical, social, and service departments. In the nursing model, the professional nurse, a nurse manager, is responsible for coordinating patient care.

Bartlett and Ghoshal (1990) stress that most successful organizations are those whose top executives recognize the need to manage the new environmental and competitive demands by emphasizing less on the quest for an ideal structure and more on developing the abilities and performance of individual managers. One senior executive stated "The challenge is not so much to build a matrix structure as it is to create a matrix in the minds of our managers." Bartlett and Ghoshal emphasize that "developing a matrix of flexible perspectives and relationships within each manager's mind, however, achieves an entirely different result. It lets individuals make the judgments and negotiate the trade-offs that drive the organization toward a shared strategic objective" (p. 145).

Because the matrix organization focuses on a specific product line or products, it is able to generate information and mobilize resources needed to respond quickly to changes. The matrix structure should be implemented when an organization has unique problems in a market area or requires increased specialization associated with the technological requirements of the environment.

A DECENTRALIZED ORGANIZATIONAL MODEL

Shared governance is a decentralized organizational model that incorporates accountability, a sense of responsibility, autonomy, control, personal empowerment, and shared decision-making within the nursing staff. It is critical that nurses at all levels be involved in this process. Nurse practitioners must be directly responsible and accountable for decisions affecting their practice.

Porter-O'Grady (1997) depicts shared governance as a structure that ensures the nurse participates at the point of service and in the organizational structure in decisions that affect the delivery and financing of care; relationships necessary to disseminate that care; and decisions that ensure the facilitation of patient care across the continuum of services. The shared governance structure encompasses the total organization. It provides an opportunity for nurses to participate in decisions affecting their practice and changes the locus of control and authority for those decisions from the middle and top management hierarchy to the point of service (unit, or service place in the organization where the majority of nurses practice).

A degree of risk is involved in implementing a shared governance model because the organization must make commitments necessary to truly empower the staff to make the decisions they already own. Porter-O'Grady stresses that it is vital that management move its locus of control to the staff, give up much of the authority needed to control, and learn the skills of facilitating, coordinating, and integrating decision-making, which is the opposite of directing and controlling the decisions for the staff. Whole system shared governance is a model that is a framework for integrating multidisciplinary organizational systems.

The shared governance structures of an organization usually have the following characteristics:

- An overall organizational structure where nurses may participate fully in decisions about their practice.
- A council, forum, or other means where nurses participate fully in decisions affecting the strategy, direction, financing, and application of the priorities of the organization and nursing's role in relationship to it.

- A decision-making structure at the point of service is evidence that the decision-making process is ongoing, operating, and effective, and that nurses should be a part of the evaluation process of the system.
- An expectation that all nurses participate in decisions affecting their practice; rotating of authority for making decisions on councils, forums, and congresses between and among all the nursing staff; full participation is evident.
- A format linking decisions made at the system and organizational level, service and unit level of the organization; the mission, purposes, and objectives of the organization, and the principles and priorities of the profession are linked and integrated along the decision-making pathway. This seamless integration of decision-making is one of the fundamental characteristics of effective shared governance systems (p. 44).

Implementation of a Shared Governance Model

Prince (1997) describes the implementation of a unit-based shared governance model in a Mother/Baby- Gynecology 900-bed tertiary care facility in Alabama. The desired benefits for implementing shared governance were to increase staff participation, improve communication, and increase job satisfaction. A Likert-type survey tool was administered to the staff members to evaluate and benchmark staff perceptions regarding work empowerment, opportunity, teamwork, and satisfaction. The results of the preimplementation phase indicated that the respondents believed they received the information necessary to do their work, were generally satisfied, and participated in the traditional staff meetings. The response regarding staff meeting participation was incongruent as records demonstrated a monthly attendance of one-third of the staff. Based on the results of the survey, the nurse manager decided to pursue development and implementation of a shared governance model. Planning sessions were conducted and the team unit leadership identified a common vision for the future. A model for action was developed including the formation of council groups, and leadership and staff roles were defined.

A postimplementation survey was administered after more than 1 year of participation in the shared governance model. Results noted significant improvement in job participation with a high level of meeting attendance. A strong positive response regarding the importance of councils was also reported. There was confusion noted in the staff member's committee participation. Although 69.3% of the staff reported they attended council meetings 9 of 12 months, only 30.7% indicated they were active in committees. This is contradictory because both the council and committee responsibilities were fulfilled simultaneously by participation in the council meetings. Responses to communication indicated slight improvement. Even though the respondents noted they obtained information needed in a timely manner, they noted that the staff did not always receive information that affected their work. This contradictory response was a result of their interpretation of the statements. The team members felt that the manager informed them of the information they needed to do their job, but at times the manager was unsure or unaware of organizational decisions until the last moment. Job satisfaction was less than desirable and actually decreased. This was attributed to an increased workload.

Both the pre- and post-surveys indicated that the greatest satisfier was patient interaction as evidenced by a love of teaching and caring for their patients. Teamwork was a valuable asset. Prince states that "the sharing of power and opportunity yielded both the benefits and the challenges of responsibility and autonomy. The staff's commitment to quality patient care and to each other was inspirational." (p. 35)

SUMMARY

Organizational design facilitates the accomplishment of the work of nursing and structure accommodates the types of individuals and nature of the work to be performed within a given system. The organizational structure should be designed to be congruent with the institution's mission, values, and vision. To ensure such congruity, the executive must understand the types of authority relationships and the models of organizational structure that best apply to the enterprise. Nurse executives must be knowledgeable about organizational designs and their effect on human behavior.

STUDY QUESTIONS

1. Why is it important that nurse executives be knowledgeable about the organizational design process?
2. Why are mission, values, and vision necessary for a division of nursing?
3. Describe the characteristics of a functional, self-directed or self-managed, and cross-functional team. What is the importance of team leadership in the organization?
4. In the 21st century are formal organizational structures essential? What would you suggest to replace this concept?
5. Design a futuristic organizational chart. What management strategies would you recommend for this organization?
6. Describe and analyze the concept of shared governance. How would you implement this organizational model in your agency?

REFERENCES

Bartlett, C., & Ghoshal, S. (1990). Matrix management: Not a structure, a frame of mind. *Harvard Business Review, 68*(4), 138–145.

Daft, R. (1994). *Management* (3rd ed.). Fort Worth, TX: Dryden Press.

Dale, E. (1952). *Planning and developing the company organization structure.* Research Report 20, New York: American Management Association.

Koontz, H., & Weihrich, H. (1990). *Essentials of management* (5th ed.). New York: McGraw-Hill.

Lawrence, P., Kolodny, H., & Davis, S. (1977). The human side of matrix. *Organizational Dynamics, 6*(1), 43–61.

Leatt, P., Shortell, S., Kimberly, J. (1994). Organization design. In S. Shortell, A. Kaluzny, et al. (3rd ed.). *Health care management: Organization design and behavior*. Albany, NY: Delmar.

Mintzberg, H. (1981). Organization design: Fashion or fit? *Harvard Business Review, 59*(1), 103–116.

Morgan, G. (1993). *Imaginization*. New Park, CA: Sage.

Porter-O'Grady, T. (1997). Workplace advocacy, shared governance, and collective bargaining: Rights and opportunity. In C. A. Anderson (Ed.). *Nursing student to nursing leader: The critical path to leadership development*. Albany, NY: Delmar.

Prince, S. (1997). Shared governance: Sharing power and opportunity. *Journal of Nursing Administration, 27*(3), 28–35.

Robbins, S., & Coulter, M. (1996). *Management* (5th ed.). Englewood Cliffs, NJ: Prentice-Hall.

CHAPTER
8

Community and Rural Practice Settings

Naomi E. Ervin

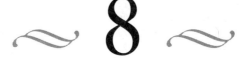

A society that spends so much on health care that it cannot or will not spend adequately on other health-enhancing activities may actually be reducing the health of its population. (Evans, Barer, & Marmor, 1994, p. 55)

Chapter Highlights

- Foci of community and rural practice
- Current and emerging community practice settings
- Practice in rural communities
- The global society and beyond
- Future roles for nurse executives

The purpose of this chapter is to discuss practice settings for nurse executives in a changing society and health care system. The professional practice of nursing administration is carried out in a variety of settings where the opportunities for leadership at all levels of administration have never been greater. Professional nursing administration is practiced wherever professional nursing is part of health care delivery.

As the knowledge base for health care has increased, health care system changes have expanded toward more high technology care and more interest in health promotion, and disease and injury prevention. In addition, community and rural areas have become important foci for innovations in the delivery of nursing services. Community-based services are seen as a way to control costs as well as to meet the needs of over 90% of the population who are not institutionalized for health care. This chapter will explore these and related areas.

FOCI OF COMMUNITY AND RURAL PRACTICE

Nursing practice in community and rural settings is often characterized by a focus on a defined population. Because of this focus, practice must consider multiple determinants of health. To some extent nursing practice in community and rural settings is also characterized by a focus on health promotion and disease and injury prevention. Continuity of care is an important factor in nursing care in community and rural settings because of the differences in the ways that services are delivered. These three foci of practice will be explored next.

Determinants of Health

Based on an ever-increasing research base supporting that health and illness are the result of multiple factors, the health care system is slowly evolving from a system that prizes high technology and tertiary medical care to one that incorporates a variety of approaches for achieving and maintaining health. For example, many studies over the years have demonstrated a correlation between life expectancy and measures of social status, for example, income, education, occupation and residence (Wilkinson, 1992).

Although recognition that multiple factors are related to health could be adequate to drive change, alas, it is not. The change because of economic issues is far greater than any change scientific knowledge could claim. This has affects on nursing administration in many ways, for example:

- Design and redesign of nursing services
- Move to community-based health care services
- Increasing continuity in the design of services
- More variety of services in health care organizations to capture a population base for support of inpatient facilities and fiscal viability

In the United States, as well as internationally, the determinants of health are rooted in political, social, and economic realities (Morrow, 1982). Poverty and lack of education are the outstanding inhibitors for health in the developing countries. One should not be surprised that the same factors exist to a lesser degree in the United States. Of interest to nurse executives is the result of a World Health Organization (WHO) analysis of the factors that were inhibiting improvement in the health status of the world's poor populations in the 1970s. This analysis shows that increasing resources for the health sector did not improve health status for the following reasons, among many:

1. Limited national resources were largely devoted to curative, urban, hospital-based services, which were inaccessible to the rural poor.
2. The greatest need for health care was for simple, preventive and promotive services that did not require highly trained personnel with sophisticated equipment.
3. The services required participation of the people.
4. Successful attainment of an integrated approach to health care required cooperation from other sectors, for example, agriculture, public works, education, and social welfare.

An analysis of factors that inhibit improvement of the health status of the poor population of the United States would reveal similar, if not the same, results. Nurse executives must be knowledgeable about the economic, social and political factors that affect health care and must work to change those factors for better health care for all.

In designing nursing services, nurse executives can incorporate aspects of the determinants of health in various, yet cost-effective, ways. For example, the research on social support demonstrates that positive relationships with care providers and others are important variables in the recovery from illness (Ornish, 1998). Providing support for patients is important in all settings where nursing is provided, but not always easy to do because of staffing constraints and the high turnover among nursing personnel often experienced in health care settings.

All job descriptions could contain aspects of providing support to patients and their families. In-service education about ways to be supportive and provide a caring approach could be mandatory in all practice settings. Even though nurses are educated about caring and individualized care, they do not always have the skills to provide what patients need in terms of social support.

The design of nursing services to incorporate other types of social support may also be cost effective. For example, group sessions for many types of patients and clients are effective for meeting the needs of newly diagnosed diabetics, new mothers, newly diagnosed cancer patients, and numerous other types of patients who receive care on the inpatient and ambulatory basis. These support groups may be led by a nurse who also sees the patients and their families on an individual basis.

Another example of where support is especially needed is in crisis situations as those encountered in emergency services. Nursing practice models and interventions for patients and families in crisis are necessary parts of a quality emergency service. Even though other disciplines, such as chaplains and social workers, may competently provide solace, the nurse is the one care provider who understands both the physical and emotional aspects of the situation. Nurse executives can be instrumental in designing nursing services that incorporate various aspects of social support for emergency services.

Health Promotion and Disease and Injury Prevention

Florence Nightingale established the importance for nursing of health promotion and disease prevention with her emphasis on the restoration and preservation of health and the prevention of disease. She identified that the basic principles inherent in nursing and health are the same (Chaska, 1990).

Today, the concepts of health promotion and disease and injury prevention are equally, if not more, important, because many diseases and conditions result from life-style or behavior in interaction with multiple factors in the environment. To continue to extend the life span, science and health care must concentrate on how to facilitate life-style and environmental changes to prevent death and disability. This rationale is part of the basis for the increased interest in these areas of health care. However, the interest is not totally altruistic, being also related to the desires of health care agencies to increase their revenue levels and sources.

Although many programs and services are directed toward health promotion and disease prevention, these terms have not been clearly defined or consistently used. In general, the concept of health promotion is health care aimed at growth and improvement in well-being. Disease prevention is a separate concept and refers to health care provided to protect from or defend against disease (Brubaker, 1983).

Until recently, health promotion and disease prevention have been a small segment of the health care industry. However, current economic factors and price competition are directly affecting the development of services based on these concepts. Community-based and ambulatory facilities and organizations provide home health care, outpatient rehabilitation and therapy, health and fitness, hospice, diagnostic, and therapeutic services. The importance of the relationship between health promotion and ambulatory care is based partially on the following:

1. New technologies that increase the possibility of giving care on an outpatient basis
2. Insurance coverage expanded to include ambulatory care
3. Reimbursement based on cost efficiency and the resultant encouragement for hospitals to use less costly alternatives
4. Private entrepreneurs opening ambulatory care facilities (Gilbert, 1983)

For the nurse executive, knowledge of the concepts of health promotion and disease prevention will become more important as increased emphasis is placed on developing new programs in these areas. Because these are areas of nursing expertise, nurses should be included in key positions in implementing the new and expanded programs of health promotion and disease and injury prevention. Although there will be competition with nursing for positions in new programs, nurse executives can be prepared to present sound rationale for why nurses are best employed in many of the positions where one-to-one counseling and group guidance are provided, for example:

1. Nurses are knowledgeable about health and illness so they can make appropriate assessments and referrals of presumably well individuals.
2. Nurses use a comprehensive view of clients and thus can be more effective.
3. Nurses are cost effective because they can function in various phases of health promotion and disease prevention.

Although health promotion and disease and injury prevention have been integral parts of nursing, practice environments have not always encouraged or allowed nurses to adequately include the concepts in their practice, except perhaps in public health nursing. Current practice settings, especially acute care settings, may not have the resources for or goal of implementing health promotion but could increase the content of disease and injury prevention in the practice of nurses through small projects. For example, discharged patients with familiar histories of specific diseases could be given literature or referrals to appropriate counseling agencies, or an injury prevention program could be developed and implemented for both patients and employees. These examples also contribute to increasing the implementation of the concept of continuity of care, which should be a part of all nursing services.

Continuity of Care

Continuity of care means that care is provided throughout time, from setting to setting and across the wellness-illness continuum. The concept of continuity of care also encompasses the goal of coordinated and uninterrupted services as well as comprehensive care, including health promotion, disease prevention, health maintenance, acute care, rehabilitation, custodial care, and terminal care. The major thrust of continuity of care is prevention, whether it is prevention of chronic disease through health promotion programs or prevention of rehospitalization (Bealty, 1980). Much of the earlier emphasis of continuity of care was on referral from the hospital to public health nursing, home care, or visiting nurses. The thrust is now included in the process of discharge planning that was mandated in 1972 Medicare and Medicaid amendments (Public Law 92-603) for hospitals, skilled nursing facilities, and home health agencies (Crittenden, 1983). Although discharge planning has been a component of quality nursing care and continuity of care, inpatient settings may still not be organized to consistently meet the patient's and family's needs on discharge. A renewed interest in continuity of care has resulted from several changes in society and the health care field.

A monumental increase in the number of older people has created what Sommers (1983) describes as the geriatric imperative. This imperative has created new health care problems that demand health care policies that recognize prevention of disease and postponing or controlling chronic conditions. Maintaining quality of life in the later years depends on the availability of ambulatory, acute, and long-term care services.

The geriatric and cost-containment imperatives of the 1980s have greatly contributed to the new emphasis in the health care industry on functional independence rather than cure. Prevention of disease is emphasized at all ages, and patient education programs and departments have become part of many hospital-based human resources departments. In addition, there is common agreement among health professionals that public financing should be impartially distributed among diverse services rather than primarily to acute care. This will involve transfer of some resources from acute care to primary and long-term care.

The goal of functional independence, rather than cure, for patients demands a change in thinking on the part of health professionals. Continuity of care and discharge planning are processes, not end points. Both processes involve the patient and a team of individuals from various disciplines working together to facilitate the transition of the patient from one environment to another. These environments are usually hospitals, nursing homes, or the patient's home.

Because patient participation is a cardinal principle of continuity of care, the concept of self-care is fitting for incorporation into a nursing practice setting. By embracing the self-care framework, nursing is able to focus attention on assisting patients in self-care practices and on increasing self-care abilities through education. Orem (1991) stresses the importance of human agency and self-care agency. Human agency is the knowledge, power, or ability of a person to act, including cognitive knowledge, affective feelings, and psychomotor development. Self-care agency is the ability of a person to initiate and perform health activities for himself or herself in maintaining life, health, and well-being.

Levin is an outspoken proponent of self-care. Health professionals, according to Levin (1981), are so rarely willing to trust people to make decisions about their own health that they have developed a negative view of people's roles in health. The health establishment has encouraged the growth of a "serviced society" in which health professionals seek to provide a service for every need and to stimulate a need for every service. Health services have emerged as an industry with values, operational styles, and plans for expansion like any other industry. A recent rise in public awareness of the limits of resources in health has added to the interest in self-care. Self-care is certainly part of continuity of care, wherein people function on their own behalf in health promotion and disease prevention in such roles as health maintenance, self-diagnosis, self-medication and self-treatment, and participation in professional care. These roles are carried out in collaboration with health professionals. Nursing services can contribute to the enhancement of self-care roles for patients as part of implementing the concept of continuity of care.

CURRENT AND EMERGING COMMUNITY PRACTICE SETTINGS

Health care services in the community offer expanding opportunities for the nurse executive in public health, nursing centers, managed care, primary care, and home health care. Entrepreneurial and intrapreneurial opportunities abound for the nurse executive who is interested in providing services for unmet needs, especially in community and rural settings, and who is willing to take risks.

Since 1988 when the *Future of Public Health* report was published by the Institute of Medicine, official public health agencies have been refocusing their efforts on three core functions: assessment, policy development, and assurance. *Assessment* is the systematic collection and analysis of information about the health of the community. *Policy development* refers to the development of comprehensive public health policies by encouraging use of the scientific knowledge base in decision-making about public health and by leading in this effort. In the 1988 report, agencies are recommended to offer *assurance* to their constituents that services are provided to meet the agreed-on goals by either encouraging their development by others, requiring the services be provided, or making the services directly available (Institute of Medicine, 1988).

The redesign of public health agencies at the federal, state, and local levels is resulting in many changes in the configuration of the workforce and the work of the workforce. Projects have been instituted to update public health workers' skills and make the necessary arrangements with community agencies to provide services once offered by the official public health sector. The managed care sector of the health care system has been one area of intersection with public health that has great opportunity for nurse executives.

Public Health and Managed Care

Managed care is a system of capitated financing arrangements for an enrolled population. Under the current evolving systems for medical care delivery and financing in the United States, managed care plans and public health have overlapping, if not identical, responsibilities. Managed care plans are given the responsibility to promote behavior that reduces risks for disease and injury to forestall costly treatment in the populations they serve. This focus requires the need for population-based information on health status and health risks. In addition, managed care systems are contracting to provide services to Medicaid and Medicare beneficiaries (Halverson, Kaluzny, & McLaughlin, 1998).

In 1996, 12.8 million Medicaid beneficiaries were enrolled in 511 managed care plans, 349 of which were health maintenance organizations (HMOs). The level of enrollment represented 38.6% of all Medicaid beneficiaries and 50% of low-income adults and children covered by Medicaid (Aday, Begley, Lairson, & Slater, 1998).

The result of this shift in care delivery systems is that both public health and managed care organizations claim responsibility for activities in disease prevention, health promotion, community assessment, and care of vulnerable populations.

Nurse executives for both public health and managed care settings share the need to have knowledge and skills in population-based management of care systems and identifying trends, problems, and wellness indicators in the populations served by agencies and health care organizations. The ability to look beyond the "usual patient" population is an asset in the current and evolving health care system.

Several examples of managed care options currently exist in the community and some are especially pertinent for nursing management. Three types of managed care entities will be briefly described: community nursing organizations, health maintenance organizations, and social health maintenance organizations.

Community Nursing Organizations

Community nursing organizations (CNOs) were developed as a Medicare demonstration project by the Health Care Financing Administration (HCFA) as a response to section 4079 of P.L. 100-203, the Omnibus Budget Reconciliation Act of 1987. This legislation was passed primarily through activities of the American Nurses Association. Four sites were funded initially for 3 years: Carle Clinic in Urbana, Illinois; Carondelet Health Services in Tucson, Arizona; the Living at Home/Block Nurse Program in St. Paul, Minnesota; and the Visiting Nurse Service of New York (VNSNY), in New York City (Daly & Mitchell, 1996).

The four sites tested a capitated reimbursement system with a bundled group of Medicare community-based services, including home health care, outpatient therapies, social work, psychology, home medical equipment and prosthetic devices, and ambulance services. Success of the project will be measured by reduction in costs and utilization of all Medicare reimbursed services, improvements in health status and well-being of enrollees, and maintenance of enrollee satisfaction (Storfjell, Mitchell, & Daly, 1997).

If CNOs were successful in the demonstration phase, they may continue into the future and expand. In the first 3 years of functioning, the CNO of the VNSNY had been able to maintain fiscal viability with the capitated system. In addition, there was a reduction in the use of home health services compared with regular VNSNY clients. The project in New York used both a case management and a community-focused approach to implement nurses' responsibilities (Storfjell et al., 1997).

Health Maintenance Organizations

Health maintenance organizations (HMOs) are the most popular model for managed care and the most familiar to nurses. Although HMOs do not usually employ large numbers of nurses, there are wonderful opportunities to provide excellent nursing care to the population served by an HMO. Medicaid beneficiaries are a part of many HMOs and require special attention to identify unmet needs for such items as transportation, adequate food and housing, and referral to community agencies. Many of these functions are the realm of nursing, especially community health or public health nursing.

Social Health Maintenance Organizations

Social health maintenance organizations (SHMOs) are programs to bridge the gap between the acute and long-term care systems to prevent premature institutionalization of aged Medicare beneficiaries. The SHMO model includes: enrolling a broad-based elderly Medicare population; prepaid capitated financing; Medicare parts A and B with a full range of providers; and expanded medical benefits such as prescription drugs, eyeglasses and hearing aids, which are integrated into a benefit called Expanded Care. Included in Expanded Care are in-home, community-based long-term care services such as personal care, homemaking, adult day care, respite care, personal emergency response systems, nonemergency medical transportation to appointments, and short-term nursing home care (Leutz, Greenlick, & Capitman, 1994).

Nursing Centers

Nursing centers, also called community nursing centers, nurse-managed centers, and nursing clinics, are organizations that provide direct access to professional nursing services. Nursing centers have existed in the United States since the late 1800s, and have recently had a revival of interest among the nursing community (American Nurses Association, 1987). Lillian Wald was the first nurse to establish a nursing center, the Henry Street Settlement, in a populated section of New York (Figure 8.1).

In a 1990 survey, 56.2% of 80 nursing centers reported being affiliated with a parent organization; 43.8% described themselves as freestanding. The centers reported serving higher proportions of racial minorities, the very young, the very old, and the poor compared with the general population (Barger & Rosenfeld, 1995).

Nursing centers play a valuable role in a community where little opportunity exists for contact with health care providers except for illness. Often opportunities for prevention and health promotion are missed in an illness-oriented service because only the presenting problem is addressed. For example, when young children are taken to a health care facility for an illness, immunization status may not be assessed. An ill child may often safely be given an immunization or an appointment given for a return visit to a primary care site. Nursing centers are concerned with the total health of the child or adult and, thus, go beyond the presenting problem.

Primary Care

Primary care has become a major focus in integrated health care systems to provide a base for the various components. Entry into the health care system and continuous care are two characteristics of primary care. In addition to continuous

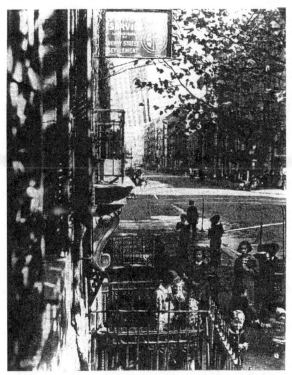

Figure 8.1 Henry Street Settlement. Courtesy of Visiting Nurses Service of New York.

care, primary care models may focus on having the same provider see the same patients over time. Advanced practice nurses, especially nurse practitioners and certified nurse-midwives, have been welcomed into primary care practices.

The incorporation of nurse providers has been a necessary component of health centers in rural and inner city locations because of a shortage of primary care physicians. HCFA administered the first federal reimbursement for nurse practitioners through Medicaid and Medicare funding in 1990. The incentive to hire nurse providers was thus put into place. Private insurance companies had been reimbursing advanced practice nurses, including clinical nurse specialists, for some time before it was mandated for entitlement programs.

Home Health Care

The services provided through home health care agencies are varied and continue to expand as changes in the health care system and payment mechanisms evolve. Home health care is generally an interdisciplinary approach to providing care to individuals in their homes after hospital discharge. Because the largest revenue source for home health care agencies is Medicare, home care patients are generally elderly and home bound. Physicians' orders are required for reimbursable care to be given under guidelines from HCFA. Reimbursement from other payers, such as private insurance and Medicaid, and self-pay comprise smaller portions of revenue for home care agencies.

In addition to nursing care, home health care agencies provide services in physical therapy, speech therapy, occupational therapy, and social work. Home health aides may provide assistance with activities of daily living. Homemaker services may be provided by a home health care agency or a separate community-based organization. These services vary a great deal by locale and are not found as frequently in rural areas of the country.

Hospice services may be provided by a separate agency or by a home health care agency. In addition to hospice services being provided in the home, the model for hospice services may be inpatient, a residential setting, or a nursing home. Because hospice services are also covered by Medicare, the availability has increased in the last several years. Chapter 27 discusses hospice services in greater detail.

PRACTICE IN RURAL COMMUNITIES

Nursing practice in rural communities is not entirely different from urban settings, but differences may be found in staffing options, resources, care options, and transportation.

Practice Settings in the Rural Community

Rural health clinics provide access for large numbers of residents but do not meet all the needs for care in rural communities. Often staffed by advanced practice nurses, rural health clinics are frequently subsidized to continue to remain open. Farmers, low-income families, and homeless people in rural areas often do not have health insurance and are not eligible for Medicaid coverage. Thus, free or subsidized care is the only option for some rural area residents.

Nursing centers also exist in rural areas. Variations in nursing center models include mobile vans, private practice by an advanced practice nurse, and group practice of advanced practice nurses. Fiscal viability is a major issue for nursing centers in all areas, but the low population density makes survival especially difficult in rural areas.

The Rural Community

Rural communities are defined as geographic areas outside cities with suburbs that total 50,000 people and population densities of fewer than 100 persons per square mile. The 1990 census showed that 8.2 million older people (which constitutes 26% of the total elderly population) lived in nonmetropolitan areas. In addition about 90% of the rural elderly are reported not to be living on farms (Bureau of the Census, 1992). Data indicate that rural elders not living on farms have the worst health status of all older people (Bull & DeCroix Bane, 1993).

Rural areas in the United States are characterized by greater poverty, less adequate housing and transportation systems, poorer health, greater incidence of chronic health conditions and a lack of a wide range of services as compared with urban areas (Krout, 1994). These facts alone demonstrate a need for more services in the rural areas of the United States, especially for the elderly population.

Changing U.S. demographics have brought great changes to the life of rural families. No longer is it common to have two or three generations of families living in close proximity as in decades past. Moreover, the elderly in rural areas often depend on informal caregivers to fill the gap in the lack of formal services (Coward & Cutler, 1989).

During the 1980s, 10% of rural hospitals closed, and this pace of closure continued into the 1990s (American Hospital Association, 1992). With the closure of hospitals often comes the loss of other health services. Primary care providers leave the area and community-based services close. Access to emergency and acute care becomes more difficult (Shreffler, 1996). Those hospitals remaining have been able to survive often because of legislation that allows different configurations of bed use. In the small rural hospital under swing bed reimbursement regulations, patient categories range from acute care to intermediate care to long-term care, depending on the needs of the community (Supplitt, 1982). Such a setting requires a nurse executive with different clinical knowledge and skills than that of the nurse executive functioning at the corporate level in a multihospital system in a large urban area.

Role of the Nurse Executive in the Rural Community

The role of the nurse executive in the rural community is not different from that in other settings, but some skills require more development if the nurse executive is to be a contributing member to the efforts of the small agency, which is often one of a few or the only one in a large geographic area.

The challenges of the nurse executive in rural areas relate to the demands and cost of delivering services to individuals and families spread over great distances, lower rates of reimbursement than for urban areas, staffing problems, and lack of transportation, among many others (Parker et al., 1992). Because of the difficulty recruiting qualified staff, often the nurse executive is required to fill several roles. Maintaining skills for delivering direct care as well as to provide orientation and skill training for staff is more important for nurse executives in rural areas than in settings where a greater supply of qualified staff is available.

Knowledge and experience in finance of health services are critical for the nurse executive who guides the largest department in most health care settings, but especially important for the survival of rural health services. Because reimbursement alone may be inadequate to meet expenses, the nurse executive in rural settings may be asked to develop grant proposals for funding operations as well as special projects (Berry & Seavey, 1994).

In small health agencies, such as those found in rural areas, the nurse executive is often responsible for several departments or staff of several disciplines. These responsibilities call for a wide base of knowledge not always acquired in formal educational programs. The nurse executive in rural areas may be in need of additional course work or continuing education to meet the challenges of the rural health care setting.

THE GLOBAL SOCIETY AND BEYOND

The shift to a global society has led to a massive change in thinking about "who does what" in health care. The old barriers between nurses and physicians are crumbling as the world moves toward the goal of "Health for All by the Year 2000." There is increasing interest by the public and by many health care providers to enact a universal access patient-centered health plan for millions of Americans who are without insurance benefits. Grasping the concept of uninsured in America has led to a better understanding of the world populations who are without basic subsistence health care.

The "Health for All" agenda emerged in 1977 at the World Health Assembly of WHO. It was decided at that meeting that the main social target of governments and of WHO should be the attainment by all people of the world by the year 2000 a level of health that permits them to live socially and economically productive lives (Little, 1992). In 1978, the WHO and UNICEF adopted and published the now famous Declaration of Alma-Ata and further stated "An acceptable level for all the people of the world by the year 2000 can be attained through a fuller and better use of the world's resources, a considerable part of which is now spent on armaments and military conflicts" (Little, 1992). In 1981, the World Health Assembly unanimously adopted a "Global Strategy for All by the Year 2000."

The major strategy used for achieving "Health for All" was primary health care. "Primary health care is essential health care based on practical, scientifically sound and socially acceptable methods and technology made universally accessible to individuals and families in the community through their full participation and at a cost that the community and country can afford to maintain at every stage of their development in the spirit of self-reliance and self-determination" (WHO, 1978, p. 3).

The primary health care approach contains at least these eight elements:

- Education about prevailing health problems and the methods of preventing and controlling them
- Promotion of a food supply and proper nutrition
- An adequate supply of safe water and basic sanitation
- Maternal and child health care, including family planning
- Immunization against major infectious diseases
- Prevention and control of endemic diseases
- Appropriate treatment of common diseases and injuries
- Provision of essential drugs (WHO, 1978)

Every country differs in how primary health care is carried out depending on available resources and the priorities of the country.

Physicians in America responded to the challenge. Medical schools changed curricula to emphasize preparation of the general practitioner who can serve in primary care and family practice. Nursing responded to the challenge by restructuring educational programs in nursing schools by increasing primary care and community content. Although the goal of "Health for All" was not achieved by 2000, progress has been made in restructuring education and organizations to meet the needs of a larger segment of the U.S. population.

Computerized information systems will allow nurses and physicians to collaborate in newly designed centers of care that can reach human beings from all walks of life and social levels. These are exciting times in nursing. National Nursing organizations are working closely together and the relationship with the International Council of Nurses (ICN) is excellent. In the new age, however, nurses must work closely with physicians and other health care providers in flexible work groups with transdisciplinary patient-centered goals. The need for executive and primary care skills for nurses and physicians has never been greater.

Health of the population is an important factor for all countries. It is widely recognized that health depends on social and economic development and, in turn, contributes to the development of a country. Chapter 34 provides more discussion about the globalization of nursing and related issues.

FUTURE ROLES FOR NURSE EXECUTIVES

As indicated in the discussion about the rural community, the nurse executive often must demonstrate a variety of skills that may range from the staff nurse to the chief financial officer. It is, of course, almost impossible to maintain such a wide range of skills with equal competence in each. However, the nurse executive in small community-based and rural agencies may be required to carry out many such divergent, yet critical, responsibilities. Examples of combined roles will next be explored.

The development and implementation of many community-based services require that the expertise of nursing be involved from the initial vision to the operation of such an entity. For example, nursing centers are often envisioned by nurse leaders who not only identify the need, but also coalesce with others to write the proposal, obtain funding, and attend to all the detail to open for business (Ervin & Young, 1996). Often nursing centers are planned by nurses who serve as both the executive and the primary care provider. Such combinations of skills require that the nurse have both administrative and nurse practitioner preparation.

Another example of skill combination is in the area of home health care. Nurses who have advanced practice preparation as a nurse practitioner or a clinical nurse specialist and a nurse executive may be much in demand in small home care agencies. Dual preparation will meet needs such as assessment of patients in their homes when hospitalization is considered. For example, in rural areas transport to a hospital is a costly process not to be undertaken without good reason.

The assessment of a patient in the home by an advanced practice nurse would be a good investment of time for a home care agency.

Dual preparation as mental health clinical nurse specialist and nurse executive would meet a very large unmet need for mental health services in rural areas. These kinds of roles would be valuable in nursing centers, home health care agencies, and other community-based service agencies such as alcohol and drug treatment programs. Prevention and education in mental health are rare services provided anywhere, but are especially uncommon in rural areas (Aday, 1993).

Nurses are often reluctant to give up their direct care provider roles to become nurse executives. The potential for future roles in community-based and rural areas could resolve this dilemma for many nurses. The rewards of administration are multiplied as nurse executives see how their efforts have a broader impact on improving access to and quality of care for a larger group of people.

SUMMARY

Opportunities for nurse executives in community and rural practice settings are increasing as society and the health care system change (Figure 8.2). Multiple determinants of health are important factors to address in the development of nurs-

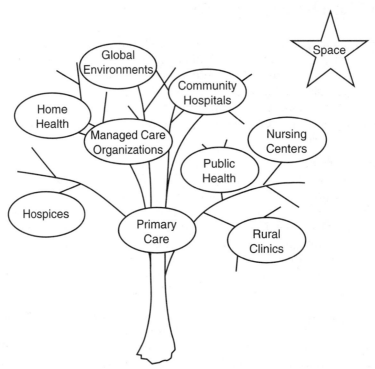

Figure 8.2 Opportunities for nursing practice in community settings.

ing services for the community and rural areas. Health promotion, prevention of disease and injury, and continuity of care will play increasingly important parts in health care services in a variety of settings.

Future roles for nurse executives in community and rural settings call for formal preparation in dual and complimentary areas. Often small agencies cannot afford to employ highly educated nurses who serve only in an administrative role. The ability to fulfill both clinical and administrative responsibilities enhances the nurse's employability and the agency's ability to serve more clients.

STUDY QUESTIONS

1. Describe some entrepreneurial settings in which nursing administration is and will be practiced.
2. Discuss the impact, actual or potential, on nursing of one economic, one social, and one political issue.
3. How do health promotion and disease prevention differ?
4. Define continuity of care.

REFERENCES

Aday, L. A. (1993). *At risk in America.* San Francisco, CA: Jossey-Bass.

Aday, L. A., Begley, C. E., Lairson, D. R., & Slater, C. H. (1998). *Evaluating the healthcare system* (2nd ed.). Chicago: Health Administration Press.

American Hospital Association. (1992). *Hospital closures 1980 through 1991: A statistical profile.* Chicago: Hospital Data Center.

American Nurses Association. (1987). *The nursing center: Concept and design.* Kansas City, MO: Author.

Barger, S., & Rosenfeld, P. (1995). Models in community health care: Findings from a national study of community nursing centers. *Nursing and Health Care, 14,* 426–431.

Bealty, S. R. (Ed.). (1980). *Continuity of care: The hospital and the community.* New York: Grune & Stratton.

Berry, D. E., & Seavey, J. W. (1994). Health care management challenges in rural environments. In J. E. Beaulieu & D. E. Berry (Eds.), *Rural health services: A management perspective* (pp. 143–161). Ann Arbor, MI: AUPHA Press/Health Administration Press.

Brubaker, B. H. (1983). Health promotion: A linguistic analysis. *Advances in Nursing Science, 5*(3), 1–14.

Bull, C. N., & DeCroix Bane, S. (1993). Growing old in rural America: New approach is needed in rural America. *Aging Magazine, 365,* 18–25.

Bureau of the Census. (1992). *Statistical abstracts of the United States: 1990, national general population characteristics.* Hyattsville, MD: Author.

Chaska, N. L. (1990). *The nursing profession: A time to speak.* New York: McGraw-Hill.

Coward, R. T., & Cutler, S. J. (1989). Informal and formal health care systems for the rural elderly. *Health Services Research, 23*(6), 785–806.

Crittenden, F. J. (1983). *Discharge planning for health care facilities.* Bowie, MD: Brady.

Daly, G. M., & Mitchell, R. D. (1996). Case management in the community setting. *Nursing Clinics of North America, 31*(3), 527–534.

Ervin, N. E., & Young, W. B. (1996). Model for a nursing center: Spanning boundaries. *Journal of Nursing Care Quality, 11*(2), 16–24.

Evans, R. G., Barer, M. L., & Marmor, T. R. (1994). *Why are some people healthy and others not? The determinants of health of populations.* New York: Aldine de Gruyter.

Gilbert, R. N. (1983). Competition spurs ambulatory choices. Hospitals, 57(10), 67–68.

Halverson, P. K., Kaluzny, A. D., & McLaughlin, C. P. *Managed care and public health.* Gaithersburg, MD: Aspen.

Institute of Medicine. (1988). *The future of public health.* Washington, DC: National Academy Press.

Krout, J. A. (Ed.). (1994). *Providing community-based services to the rural elderly.* Thousand Oaks, CA: Sage.

Leutz, W. M., Greenlick, M. R., & Capitman, J. (1994). Integrating acute and long-term care for the elderly: A key piece of the health reform puzzle. *Health Affairs, 13*(3), 59–74.

Levin, L. S. (1981). Self-care in health: Potentials and pitfalls. *World Health Forum, 2*(2), 177–184.

Little, C. (1992). Health for all by the year 2000. Where is it now? *Nursing and Health Care, 13*(4), 198–201.

Morrow, H. (1982). The fundamental influence of political, social, and economic factors on health and health care. *International Nursing Review, 29*(6), 183–186.

Orem, D. E. (1991). *Nursing: Concepts of practice* (4th ed.). New York: McGraw-Hill.

Ornish, D. (1998). *Love & survival: The scientific basis for the healing power of intimacy.* New York: HarperCollins.

Parker, M., Quinn, J., Viehl, M., McKinley, A. H., Polich, C. L., Hartwell, S., Van Hook, R., & Detzner, D. F. (1992). Issues in rural case management. *Family and Community Health, 14*(4), 40–60.

Shreffler, M. J. (1996). An ecological view of the rural environment: Levels of influence on access to health care. *Advances in Nursing Science, 18*(4), 48–59.

Sommers, A. R. (1983). The geriatric imperative. *Hospitals, 59*(9), 77–81.

Storfjell, J. L., Mitchell, R., & Daly, G. M. (1997). Nurse-managed healthcare: New York's community nursing organization. *Journal of Nursing Administration, 27*(10), 21–27.

Supplitt, J. T. (1982). Swing beds. *Hospitals, 56*(22), 67–72.

Wilkinson, R. G. (1992). Income distribution and life expectancy. *British Medical Journal, 304*, 165–168.

World Health Organization. (1978). *Primary health care.* Geneva, Switzerland: Author.

CHAPTER

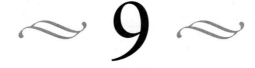

9

Organizational Culture

Harriet V. E. Coeling

Active work is required to develop, sustain, and deepen relationships within a group or culture. (Koerner, 1997, p. 66)

Chapter Highlights

- Definitions of organizational culture
- Corporate, work group, and interdisciplinary cultures
- Sources of organizational culture
- Value of understanding organizational culture
- Changing organizational culture
- Work redesign and cultural change
- Acquisitions and mergers
- Cultural assessment
- Ethics related to organizational culture

Recent years have witnessed the sudden and widespread popularity of a concept called organizational culture. The purpose of this chapter is to present the concept of culture and its importance in nursing administration practice. The concept of culture, developed by the discipline of anthropology, was embraced by both management theorists and organizational practitioners in the 1980s (Smircich & Calás, 1987). Nurse executives today are increasingly concerned with the culture of their organizations. Several conditions have contributed to this interest in organizational culture.

One condition was the shift in thinking in the human sciences. For many decades positivistic science dominated scientific fields (Smircich & Calás, 1987). An important goal of positivist science was control. It was believed that the process of positivistic science, involving construct validity and the measurement of dependent variables, would lead to findings that could be generalized. Scientists who used these processes were considered superior to scientists who sought understanding by looking at the creation of meaning within an organization and who did not seek generalizations.

In the late 1970s, however, management theorists began to value understanding, in addition to control, as a goal of management research. They began to study organizational culture in an attempt to understand what was happening as people interacted together within an organization. This new path of inquiry allowed them to ask radically different questions about the environments in which people worked. It allowed management theorists to study some of the more expressive aspects of organizational life. Part of this desire to find new ways to study organizations was a response to the realization that previous studies focusing on the measurement of variables in organizations had yielded few definitive findings (Starbuck, 1982). This shift in the goal of research has also occurred in the study of nursing management.

Another factor contributing to the study of organizational culture was the economic success of industry in Japan, along with increased foreign competition in steel, electronics, and other markets that the United States and Europe had dominated for years. The realization that other cultures did things differently, yet very successfully, prompted an openness to new ways of thinking and doing things among those who manage organizations. The loss of market share to other countries prompted managers to grasp any concept that promised help. Organizational culture offered such help. As a concept, organizational culture can be studied at the corporate level, where it is referred to as corporate culture, or at the department or unit level, where it is called work group culture.

PERSPECTIVES ON ORGANIZATIONAL CULTURE

Because the study of organizational culture has been advanced by three different traditions, namely, anthropologists, management theorists, and organizational practitioners, the organizational culture literature represents diverse and often conflicting recommendations. It is important for nurse executives to recognize the basic assumptions from which recommended management strategies are derived. Sackmann (1989) provides a comparison of these three traditions, or sets of assumptions, which reflect different goals and offer different rewards.

The goal of the cultural anthropologist is to understand a group's behavior. Because anthropologists are interested in understanding human variation, their goal is to describe unique situations, rather than to establish universal laws. The product of such research is a description of a cultural pattern that enables the manager to better recognize how the group works. Anthropologists do not see culture as power, nor do they see culture as causing behavior; rather, culture is the situation in which behavior occurs.

The goal of the organizational theorist is to revitalize organizational theory and develop a better conceptualization of organizational life. This research, which increases our understanding of all organizational participants, facilitates the prediction of both worker and manager responses.

The goal of the organizational practitioner or manager is to guide and control what goes on in organizations. The practitioner desires to find managerial formulas for success. The practitioner seeks to "master" the organization to make it function more effectively. Managing culture is seen as a powerful activity that enhances organizational effectiveness and financial success. It should be noted, however, that this effectiveness is defined by those who hold power. It is effectiveness as seen from management's perspective, not necessarily the worker's perspective.

Each perspective has its limitations for the nurse executive. The weakness of the anthropologist's approach is that it is limited to describing. Mere descriptions of group behavior are generally not associated with increased corporate profitability or a better style of organizational life.

The theorist has somewhat the same weakness as that of the anthropologist. By using an understanding of culture to predict behavior, however, the theorist can guide the nurse executive by predicting what outcomes might flow from certain interventions. The theorist, however, recognizes that multiple factors play a role in any organizational outcome and makes no promises of success if a certain strategy is used.

The culture controlling perspective, which seeks to identify the excellent culture, is intuitively appealing to the nurse executive because it offers strategies for success through the effective exercise of cultural levers. However, it has several potential pitfalls that the nurse executive would do well to recognize (Sackmann, 1989). First, this perspective advocates cultural-value engineering where administrators hold the power to prescribe certain values the employee must accept. Not all of today's nurses may want to give this power to their employers; nor is giving such power necessarily consistent with nursing practice excellence. Clinical leaders thrive more in a supportive environment than in a controlling environment. Second, it is questionable whether human behavior can be controlled to the extent that all nurses can be made to accept certain values and to follow a given set of organizational rules. Culture, based on survival strategy, is not easily manipulated. Change occurs most effectively when it responds to a changing environment while maintaining some of the organization's most cherished cultural values. Third, research has not yet proved what is the "best" culture for a health care organization. Finally, the assumption often associated with this perspective, namely, that a "good" culture is stable and homogeneous, is problematic in that such a culture has a negative effect on innovation and adaptation and robs the practitioner of some degree of autonomy and creativity. Sackmann (1989) notes that when the concept of culture is used by anthropologists, management theo-rists, or organizational practitioners, they are usually not aware of their different interests and expectations. Each group uses culture to meet its own needs. Yet, it remains important for nurse executives to differentiate the goal of understanding a culture from the goal of controlling the culture. Schein (1985) highlights these differences by disputing any inevitable link between culture and effectiveness and encourages practitioners to be more cautious about management's ability to manipulate culture. Nurse executives can profit from his advice.

DEFINITIONS OF ORGANIZATIONAL CULTURE

Considering the variety of perspectives that address the concept of organizational culture, it is not surprising that there is an even greater variety of definitions of organizational culture. Anthropologists define culture broadly to include knowl-edge, beliefs, artifacts, values, and customs. This broad definition is reflected in descriptions of organizational culture as "the way we do things around here" (Deal & Kennedy, 1982). However, more specific definitions of organizational culture are also common in the literature.

One approach is cognitive in nature. It focuses on what goes on inside of people. It focuses on the values (basic assumptions about what is desirable to do) and beliefs (basic assumptions about how the world actually works) people share in common. Schein (1984) typifies this school of thought by defining organizational cultures as the pattern of basic assumptions that a given group has invented, discovered, or developed in learning to survive by coping with its problems of external adaptation and internal integration, and that has worked well enough to be considered valid and, hence, should be taught to new members as the correct way to perceive, think, and feel regarding these problems. Quinn (1988), too, de-fines culture as the underlying assumptions and values present in the organiza-tion. This cognitive approach focuses on culture as a set of values.

In contrast, other writers take a more behavioral approach toward defining orga-nizational culture. They focus on what organizational members actually do. They study behavioral norms, behavioral rules, and what the organizational member is expected to do. Van Maanen and Barley (1985) characterize this line of thought. They define organizational culture as a set of solutions devised by a group of people to meet specific problems posed by the situations they face in common. This behavioral approach describes culture as a set of norms.

Many writers approach culture as including both basic values and behavioral norms and emphasize that culture is an integrated whole. Hall (1990), for exam-ple, describes a culture as a group of people who interact in a specific environ-ment, recognize common behavioral norms and values, have relatively similar beliefs, and use a common language. Figure 9.1 suggests a way to picture culture.

All culture scholars emphasize that culture emerges as a response to situations faced by the group members. Over time, these responses become entrenched in a

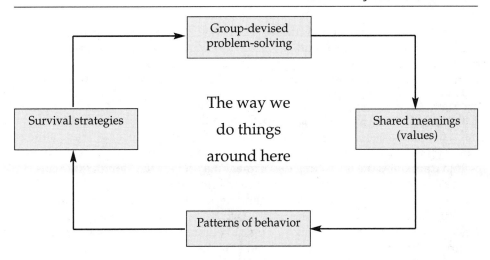

Figure 9.1 Unit culture: the ways people communicate, interact, and work with each other.

group behavior. These responses can be seen clearly in health care organizations that have existed for many years. Culture provides its members with a sense of unity and helps make their lives predictable.

Both groups also recognize that although culture is passed on to new members, it is done so in an informal manner. Work group rules are seldom if ever written down or presented formally to newcomers; they are inferred from what members say and do. Denison (1990) notes that culture is a form of internal control. Thus, culture stands in contrast to externally controlled, power-dependent activities, such as clearly stated goals, consciously derived strategies, carefully drawn organizational charts, codified policies and procedures, and consistently applied sanctions. Culture is what nursing has often called the informal organization. An organization's culture may or may not coincide with the formal management activities or it may do so to a greater or lesser extent.

CORPORATE, DEPARTMENTAL, WORK GROUP, AND INTERDISCIPLINARY CULTURES

Culture was originally studied by anthropologists. Their focus was on ethnic and national cultures. When management scholars began to investigate culture, they brought the study of culture to the organizational level. Early on, the culture of the organization was studied at the corporate level. The culture was identified by observing the norms and values of members of top management. It was assumed that the culture at the corporate level penetrated down to all levels of the organization. Peters and Waterman (1982) suggested that well-run companies have a unitary culture, that is, one common culture shared by both workers and management. Hence, the terms organizational culture and corporate culture became almost synonymous.

As the study of organizational culture progressed, however, the belief that well-run companies have only a unitary culture was questioned. Van Maanen and Barley (1985) recognized that even the best run companies have a variety of cultures. Subsequent research has identified subcultures at the department level, the work group level, and the interdisciplinary level.

Although Deal and Kennedy (1982) focused on the unitary culture of each company, they did suggest that most companies are actually a mix of different cultures. They described the cultures of different departments by proposing that within companies the marketing department may reflect the "tough guy" culture, sales and manufacturing are often characterized by working and playing hard, research and development frequently typify the "bet-your-company" culture, and the accounting department tends to be more process-oriented in nature. Vestal and Fralicx (1997) identify cultural differences in the various segments that comprise the U.S. Department of Veteran's Affairs.

Research also supports the existence of differing cultures at the work group level. Coeling and Wilcox (1988) described different nursing unit cultures within the same hospital. Coeling and Simms (1993b) found larger differences between nursing work group cultures within the same health care agency than between overall nursing department cultures between hospitals. Specific differences between nursing work group cultures can include differences in important sources of directives for nursing care (Coeling, 1997) and differences in accountability, authority, and autonomy (Webb, Price, & Coeling, 1996). Cultural differences between shifts on nursing units have also been observed and reported by a variety of staff nurses (Figure 9.2).

In health care Coeling and Wilcox (1990) identify cultural differences among different health care professionals within a hospital. Physicians focus on maintaining life above all else, nurses emphasize individualizing patient care, and respiratory therapists strive to get oxygen into the cells. Jones, DeBaca, and Yarbrough (1997) describe the importance of recognizing these interdisciplinary differences in work redesign efforts such as cross-training and patient-focused care. Simms, Coeling, and Rosemann (1998) present a model for work redesign that includes breaking down the walls that have previously separated professional groups so as to promote flexible, interdisciplinary work groups.

Expanding the concept of organizational culture outside of the specific organization, the national culture has been noted to determine in part the culture of the organizations existing within that nation. Newman and Nollen (1996) encourage multinational enterprises to recognize the value of adapting their management practices to the national cultures in which they operate to achieve high business performance. They provide evidence that work units that are managed consistent with national cultural expectations will be better performing than work units whose management practices do not fit the national culture.

Schein (1985) recommends that culture be viewed as a property of any independently defined stable social unit. If one can demonstrate that a given set of people

	Unit A		Unit B		Unit C		Unit D	
	C	P	C	P	C	P	C	P
Policies and procedures	50%	25%	25%	25%	13%	4%	46%	46%
Individual judgment	25	75	25	25	44	57	23	46
Physician's orders	25		50	50	39	35	31	8
Peer pressure					4	4		

	Unit E		Unit F		Unit G		Unit H	
	C	P	C	P	C	P	C	P
Policies and procedures	13%	27%	30%	35%	13%	18%	5%	5%
Individual judgment	47	40	25	40	36	51	73	90
Physician's orders	40	33	35	25	49	29	11	5
Peer pressure			10		2	2	11	

C = Current first-ranked source of directives   P = Preferred first-ranked source of directives

Figure 9.2 Differences between work groups. From *The Executive Nurse* by S. Byers, 1997, Albany, NY: Delmar, a division of Thomson Learning.

have shared a significant number of important experiences in the process of solving external and internal problems, one can assume that such common experiences have led them, over time, to a shared view of the world. Recognizing that different groups within a health care agency will have different cultures is important for the nurse executive to help groups work together to meet the needs of the client.

Culture researchers have studied the relationship of different cultures within an organization. Coeling and Wilcox (1988) looked at two nursing unit work group cultures in a health care organization. They found that group A emphasized teamwork and a sense of family, whereas group B focused on innovation and moving ahead professionally. Mullins (1989) subsequently studied the corporate level culture of that same organization. A comparison of the two studies suggests that the corporate values identified were general and broad in scope. Important organizational values included innovation, teamwork, and a feeling of family. Although both nursing units valued these cultural elements of innovation, teamwork, and a feeling of family, the groups differed in the emphasis given to the various behaviors. Group A was relatively less concerned with innovation and more inclined to emphasize teamwork and a sense of family than was group B. In contrast, group B spent a considerable amount of the time innovating and much less time promoting teamwork and a sense of family. Although the culture of the work groups did not conflict with corporate level cultural elements, the emphasis given to different behaviors varied between the groups within the organization.

SOURCES OF ORGANIZATIONAL CULTURE

A variety of factors contribute to the formation and continual shaping of a culture. These factors include group leaders, group members, the internal environment, and the external environment. A consideration of the variety of factors that impact on the culture reveals the difficulty of changing the culture by changing only one of these factors. It is the wise nurse executive who, in attempting to change a culture, considers all the forces that affect the culture.

Early studies of organizational culture focused on the corporate level of culture. Early theories about the source of culture gave considerable attention to the influence of the organizational founder on the current culture (Ott, 1989; Schein, 1985). Because the founders have considerable influence on the organization, their values, goals, and preferences often become those of the organization, and their approaches to matching a particular technology with a market opportunity prevail.

Another source of culture, where applicable, is the institution that founded the organization. This may be especially true in health care institutions, which often are founded by an established community or a religious organization. In such cases, the values of these founding groups impact on the nature of the culture because the purpose of the facility is to further the goals of the founding organization.

Although administrators have considerable power over members, they do not have total power. Workers bring to the organization their own values, goals, and customary behaviors. Over time, workers' norms are incorporated into the group culture. This is especially likely to occur when a large number of new employees who have similar values join the group at the same time. This might occur in nursing when several new graduates from the same school join a unit together.

If there is an acceptable fit between the new member and the group, the new member will reflect the values of the group. If, however, the new member's values and norms are dissimilar from the group, the new member will have to choose whether to adopt the norms and values of the group, remain an outsider, or leave the group. Groups differ in the extent to which they are willing to tolerate members whose behaviors deviate from that of the group's culture. Nursing units can often predict whether a new nurse will fit in with the unit after the new nurse has worked only a few days.

Various forces influence the shape of the culture (Table 9.1). One force is that of the technology of the work. In a health care setting, a group whose primary focus is to improve the client's physiological functioning may develop a different culture than a group whose focus is to assist the client with interpersonal processes. Also the acuity of the client determines the culture. Many nurses today are reporting changes in their culture that they attribute to the increased acuity of their clients.

Another force is critical incidents that have occurred within the history of the group. A strike that occurred 10 years ago may still determine how people inter-

Table 9.1 Factors that Form and Shape a Health Care Work Group Culture

Leaders	A nursing manager who has led a particular nursing work group for a long period of time and who is well liked and respected by the group members can influence the culture of a group. One may observe staff nurses imitating the manager's work patterns such as style of communicating with staff, families, and other departments both while the manager is the current leader and long after the manager has left the institution.
Staff	Group members themselves continually shape the culture of the group. This often occurs when a group of nurses who socialize together all work in the same work group. The norms of friendship group, such as honesty and loyalty, often become cultural norms of the work group.
Founding Agency	The original social calling of the institution can influence the manner in which clients are treated long after the institution is taken over by another organization. Nurses working in a hospital originally founded to minister to the underserved may continue to value offering special help to homeless clients long after the institution is taken over by a for-profit organization.
Technology	Different clinical specialties mandate different time orientations which in turn shape the group culture. A rehabilitation unit demands considerable patience on the part of the nurses; in contrast an emergency department often demands speed.
Focus of Prevention	The focus of prevention (primary, secondary, or tertiary) determines what types of care are rewarded. A primary care setting rewards nurses who can motivate clients to adopt a healthy lifestyle; in contrast a tertiary setting rewards nurses who can problem solve ways to maintain a client's usual life-style despite severe handicaps.
Critical Incidents	One-time events that are extremely stunning remain in the collective memory of the group, thus shaping the group culture. A work group that experiences a major fire in a client's room will be especially sensitive to potential fire hazards and fire prevention for years to come.
Physical Structure	The layout of the work area influences group behavior. A work area that includes a room with table, chairs, and a shelf on which to attractively store current professional journals can establish a work group norm of basing care on current professional guidelines.
Surrounding Community	The cultural makeup of the surrounding community can influence the care given to clients of diverse cultural backgrounds. Nurses in an agency located in a culturally diverse community may place a high value on culturally sensitive care.

act and who talks to whom. Unusual behaviors reinforced by the leaders and talked about by the members also shape the culture. For example, when one or two nurses are positively reinforced for taking initiative in an emergency situation and performing "medical" functions to save a client's life, the behavior may quickly become a group norm.

Physical facilities have an impact on group culture. The furniture provided will affect the formality of the atmosphere, which can, in turn, affect how group members interact with each other and do their work. The layout of the nursing station and client rooms may determine how closely co-workers interact to help each other, socialize with each other, and criticize each other.

Conditions in the external environment also influence a group's culture. If the organization is to successfully function in a given community, the value system of the surrounding community will have to be incorporated into that of the organization. The economic environment of the surrounding community is also very powerful in shaping a group's culture. If money is scarce and the community is unwilling or unable to purchase the hospital's services, the organization will have to adapt their services to what the client will buy.

THE VALUE OF UNDERSTANDING ORGANIZATIONAL CULTURE

Understanding organizational culture is important to nursing management theorists. The goal of the management theorist is to find new, more effective ways to study organizations. A qualitative culture study can be used in conjunction with a quantitative study to help interpret or place in context results from a statistical analysis of an organization. An organizational culture approach can also provide both a managerial and a nonmanagerial (worker) account of sense making in a particular organization by describing organizational life in all its fullness and thus enhance understanding of the work context. In short, organizational culture research has theory-generative, theory-contextualizing, and theory-testing functions for the nursing management researcher.

Understanding organizational culture also has practical benefits for employees. This understanding is useful for nurses who are looking for a new position, being oriented to a new position, or seeking to change an aspect of their organizational culture. If nurses both know the essential cultural elements for a given group and are aware of their preferences regarding each of these elements, then during the interview, they can inquire about the typical behaviors and values of the group and thereby decide if they would be compatible with this group. Furthermore, if new orientees understand how groups may differ in their responses to a situation, orientees will know what to watch for and what to ask about to learn about the job. This knowledge can help new members understand why things happen the way they do. Also knowing how to assess a group's culture will guide the nurse who wants to change the group. Being aware of the established way of doing things will help nurses appreciate the impact a change would have on the group and develop some tentative plans for the best way to bring about the change on the unit. Coeling and Simms (1996) and Fulton (1996) offer examples of how understanding a culture can facilitate the change process.

Coeling and Simms (1996) describe how cultural values of the nurses hindered the introduction of unlicensed assistive personnel (UAP) on a unit. Nurses on this unit communicated with each other in an indirect manner. They avoided assertive behaviors, such as telling others directly what to do and assuming the charge nurse role. What the nurses enjoyed was working directly with clients, understanding what the clients were feeling and seeing life from the clients' viewpoint. This valuing of perspective-taking facilitated another behavior important to these nurses, namely, educating clients and helping them cope with their disabilities. When the nurses first heard talk of a UAP coming to their unit, they feared two things. They feared they would not be able to guide and monitor the care given by the UAP because they did not like telling others how (and what) to do. They also feared they would lose their opportunity to talk with clients while providing daily care such as bathing and feeding clients, thus losing their ability to understand how to counsel clients in coping with their functional loses. This fear of needing to give up some of the behaviors they valued most led them to reject the idea of UAP on their unit. This fear could be overcome by helping nurses reframe the situation so as to see themselves as being responsible for the clients' adaptation to their disabilities, but not necessarily for doing all the teaching needed for this adaptation. The fear could also be overcome both by helping the nurses tailor the change to fit their values, for example, developing a communication pattern with the UAP that would allow for some indirectness and also by increasing some of the nurses' own assertiveness skills.

Fulton (1996) identifies the importance of supporting nurses' strongly held values when introducing new technologies. While studying the process of adoption of patient-controlled analgesia (PCA), he noted that nurses, who valued individual control, adopted PCA more readily if they perceived themselves as having some control and input into planning the implementation of PCA on their units as well as having input into patient selection for PCA. Additionally, when the nursing value of accountability was supported, by providing nurses the opportunity to acquire an in-depth understanding of the theory, processes, and psychomotor skills related to PCA, acceptance of this new technology increased.

In the same manner, an understanding of organizational culture is beneficial to nurse executives and management consultants for hiring, orienting, integrating a new technology, decreasing conflict, and merging groups. An understanding of the culture, along with the ability to determine the preferred culture of a potential employee, will assist the interviewer in determining whether a prospective employee would be a good match for the group. Early identification of an incompatible match can prevent premature resignation and the financial loss associated with such an event. A conscious awareness of the group culture can also assist in orienting a new employee. The faster new members learn the culture, the more quickly they will be productive for the organization. Knowledge of the culture also helps integrate a new technology. If the technology, such as a new piece of equipment or information processing system, supports the group culture, one can expect the innovation to be quickly adapted by the group. If the innovation conflicts with the culture, it will probably be resisted. Sathe (1985, p. 383) has developed the following formula to predict resistance to culture change:

Resistance to culture change = Magnitude of the change in the content of the culture, i.e., radical versus incremental change in the culture's content × Strength of prevailing culture, i.e., strong versus weak culture

This formula suggests that decreasing the magnitude of the change can facilitate its acceptance (Coeling & Wilcox, 1990). Understanding culture can also help alleviate group conflict. Sometimes, some nurses on a unit attempt to develop or sustain one cultural pattern, whereas other nurses support a different response to the problem at hand. Bringing these differences to conscious awareness will enable the nurses to make more conscious choices regarding the resolution of the conflict. Finally, an awareness of organizational culture is beneficial when merging units within a hospital or when merging two hospitals. Conflict, rather than acceptance, can be expected when groups merge and one of the two cultures expects or attempts to dominate the other. A conscious awareness of the cultural differences can enable the two groups to work together.

CHANGING ORGANIZATIONAL CULTURE

Organizational practitioners, such as nurse executives, are under intense pressure to bring about organizational change. In today's environment, where there is tremendous pressure on managers and managerial consultants to find new ways to increase productivity and ensure organizational survival, changing culture has been billed as the new solution on the horizon. Early studies of organizational culture suggested that having the right culture is the key to organizational success (Deal & Kennedy, 1982; Peters & Waterman, 1982).

However, nurse executives are wise to be cautious and resist rushing forward to try to change a culture. Although there is considerable agreement on the value of understanding organizational culture, there is not consensus on the value of changing the culture. Scholars coming from the anthropological tradition are slow to encourage culture change. They argue there is currently little evidence to support the belief that one culture is better than another (Hall, 1990). They ask not whether a culture is a good culture, but rather what the culture is good for; that is, what does it accomplish for the group and does this correspond to the group's goal?

Organizational theorists and practitioners alike have also questioned the effectiveness of using organizational culture as a means of control for organizational survival. Schein (1985) advises that we do not assume culture can be manipulated like other matters under the control of managers. He adds that culture controls the manager more than the manager controls culture. The motivation for employee change does not come from the power of the manager, but rather from the fact that some change may be needed for continued survival. Denison (1990) writes that culture changes occur more readily in response to an outside threat, a change in leadership, or a high turnover of personnel. Kilmann, Saxton, and Serpa (1986) also warn against seeing culture as a quick single remedy to a complex problem. They add that it is virtually impossible to improve the functioning of a complex organization by any quick fix, no matter how appealing this is.

Culture can indeed be changed, and in fact is always changing in an evolutionary manner as the surrounding environment changes. Schein (1996) emphasizes that leaders cannot arbitrarily *change* culture in the sense of eliminating dysfunctional elements, but they can *evolve* culture by building on its strengths while letting its weaknesses atrophy over time. Hence, the manager cannot manipulate culture by decreeing a new work redesign. The mental models developed by an organization through doing things in a successful way over time cannot be quickly given up. However, these mental models can be broadened and enlarged. This change in mental models (cultural evolution) is enhanced by leaders, themselves, who change their own behaviors and thus role model desired cultural behaviors to organizational members. Additionally these cultural changes can be encouraged by specific organizational activities discussed below.

Work Redesign and Cultural Change

Factors that facilitate work redesign and culture change include clear goals, organizational reward systems, a desire by participants to change, and alignment of change/redesign with the group culture. Clear goals are necessary to make explicit the desired change and enable the participants to see what they and their clients are gaining from the change. Early signaling and the use of symbols by leaders warn the members of upcoming changes and allow some early testing of responses. Wilkins and Patterson (1985) recommend the formulation of a plan to avoid costly mistakes related to change by asking the following questions:

1. Where do we need to be going strategically as a group?
2. Where are we now as a culture?
3. What are the gaps between where we are and where we should be?
4. What is our plan of action to close those gaps?

A thorough assessment and a clear plan of action involving participants at all levels of the organization are essential for successful change. Strong committed leadership that is able to clearly articulate the new vision and culture is needed to coordinate this effort (Vestal & Fralicx, 1997).

A reward system that supports the culture change is also critical. Culture change is an attempt to alter firmly entrenched values and behaviors. This often involves the loss of rewards associated with former behaviors. Hence, the reward for the new behavior must be great enough to compensate for the incurred loss. That it is easier to reinforce changes in behavior than changes in values suggests to the nurse executive that an initial focus on changing behaviors, rather than values, may be the most productive approach. Reinforced behaviors will eventually change values (Vestal & Fralicx, 1997).

Support by staff members for the change can be encouraged by prompting them to question their own values, by pointing out the conditions in the environment that necessitate changed behavior, and by changing behavior one step at a time. Brown (1985) recommends the use of participatory research for changes involving values, ideologies, and possible conflicts with power holders. Participatory research is a way to promote people-centered development in political and economic systems that encourage local empowerment. Participatory research involves having participants identify and analyze the problem as they see it and clarify their common vision for the future. The cultural assessment tools described in the following section, which assist nurses to identify both current and preferred culture, are especially suitable for this process.

Finally, it is essential to align work redesign with the culture of the group involved in the change. Reger, Mullane, Gustafson, and DeMarie (1994) suggest that implementation of organizational change is more likely to be successful if the process is perceived by individuals to build on the existing identity (culture) of the organization. Boston (1995) as well as Leatt, Baker, Halverson, and Aird (1997) also emphasize the importance of redesigning strategies and processes in a manner that fits the existing organization whenever possible. This involves tailoring the redesign to fit the norms and values of the group (Table 9.2). Rizzo, Gilman, and Mersmann (1994) describe how they incorporated an understanding of each nursing unit's unique culture into redesign plans for the nursing unit. Linking (aligning) new structures or processes (or both) to the current culture increases the probability of successful implementation of the work redesign. Leatt et al. (1997) advise that where the current culture of the organization already contains appropriate core values, leaders attempt to identify and protect these values. When such values are absent, new work processes involving cultural change are necessary. Clarity of goals, strong reward systems, and worker participation are especially important when new values need to be established.

CULTURAL CONSIDERATIONS IN ACQUISITIONS AND MERGERS

A different but equally important cultural challenge arises when one seeks to join two work groups or two health care agencies, as might occur in an acquisition or merger. It is important to address the cultural implications of an acquisition or merger very early in the acquisition/merger process. Voglewede (1996) notes that cultural factors account for a high percentage of the less-than-successful mergers, partnerships, and joint ventures that are occurring in today's health care marketplace. Nash and Everett (1996), in developing a model for facilitating organizational mergers, add that the cultural fit is at least as important as is the strategic

Table 9.2 Elements Needed to Make Successful Culture Change

Clear Explanations of Expectations	Helping nurses understand the need for a cultural change and delineating the way in which future work needs to be completed can speed the rate at which the change occurs. When nurses understand that the agency is in financial difficulty to the extent that their jobs may ultimately be lost if costs are not controlled, cost-cutting measures, such as limiting all lunch breaks to 30 minutes, so as to avoid hiring another person, even though that alters the group norm of providing extensive social support to each other, will be much more readily accepted by the staff.
Organizational Reward Systems	Rewarding new behaviors is a powerful way of facilitating change. The nurse executive can enhance documentation that ensures appropriate third-party reimbursement by personally complimenting nurses who do exceptionally complete charting, placing a commendation in their personnel files, and moving them into positions of increased responsibility.
Participant Involvement in Change	Allowing nurses to have input into the work redesign plans encourages them to participate more fully in the change process. As staff are allowed to invest themselves in deciding the requirements and training needed to serve as an UAP within a given work group, they feel a greater responsibility for the successful integration of UAPs into the work group.
Alignment of Work Redesign with the Group Culture	Maintaining as much of the current culture as possible during a period of work redesign facilitates internalization of the redesign plan. Nurse executives can assist groups with a long-established norm of helping a busy fellow-worker to transfer that norm to a plan for cross training of personnel, showing how cross training is an extension of their current value system of helping each other, and thereby enhancing the strength of this cultural change.

UAP, unlicensed assistive personnel.

fit between two merging organizations. Sherer (1994) goes so far as to advise decision-makers to ensure a cultural fit between the two organizations before discussing the economic aspects of a possible merger. McKibbin (1995) adds that mergers should be avoided if the cultural values of two organizations are not compatible.

Learning about the cultures of the two organizations may take even more time than performing the economic analysis because the cultural elements of organizations are seldom written down. In merger situations the culture is most commonly assessed by the act of listening to people as they talk about what goes on in their organization and watching to see what actually happens in a given setting. While listening to this talk the nurse executive will want to pay special attention to the content of the message, because content indicates what activities and values are attended to in the agency, compliments because they describe behaviors that are rewarded, and complaints because they point out behaviors to avoid. Behaviors that are repeated are important to note because they are especially valued and may be the most resistant to change. Additionally, a significant part of any organization's culture is the history and the heritage from which this culture arose. Understanding this heritage early on, too, will pay dividends down the road (Hanser, 1997).

Attention to the culture of the joining organization is important not only in planning the merger; it is also essential for success once the merger becomes official. Executives are urged to quickly move in and clarify the new vision for the newly formed entity. The values, behaviors, and structures that support the vision also need to be shared early on with all employees so they know how to direct their efforts. Helping the organizational members understand what they must do to succeed in the new culture can decrease their anxiety and build their commitment to the new work situation. Just as in work redesign, it is desirable to build the vision and the new culture on the existing cultures, incorporating the best of both cultures into the new vision (Fitzpatrick, 1996). Essential in all of this, however, is the recognition that joining two cultures takes time. Those who have gone through this process report it takes 2 to 10 years for cultural consolidation to occur (Kennedy, 1996).

ASSESSING ORGANIZATIONAL CULTURE

Early studies of organizational culture used the traditional anthropological method of analysis, namely, participant observation and questioning. The goal was to understand organizational life. Just as the anthropologist is interested in the workways, folk tales, and ritual practices of a culture, so also these early organizational culture scholars were interested in the workways, folk tales, and ritual practices of an organization.

Although observation and questioning provide the richest information regarding a given culture, they do require substantial time and skill on the part of the person who seeks to analyze that culture. In an attempt to assist the manager or worker who is relatively untrained in assessing a culture and who has a limited amount of time to assess a group's culture, several culture scholars have developed either specific categories of behaviors and values to investigate or tools designed to assess organizational culture.

Schein (1985) lists five categories of behaviors and values that provide important descriptors of an organization's culture: *(1)* the organization's relationship to its environment; *(2)* the nature of reality, truth, time, and space; *(3)* the nature of human nature; *(4)* the nature of human activity; and *(5)* the nature of human relationships. These content areas are based on the categories developed by the anthropologists Kluckhohn and Strodtbeck (1961) to study culture at any level. Grzyb-Wysocki and Enriquez's (1996) Cultural Assessment Survey (CAS) examines how people "fit in" and work together on the unit, what changes are desired, and what is most valued in this work group.

Early researchers have developed survey tools to assess organizational culture in a variety of work places. One early tool that can be used to describe a culture is the Work Environment Scale by Moos and Insel (1974). This tool, which provides a numerical score on the three dimensions of relationships, personal growth, and system maintenance and change, was developed to describe the social climate of a work place. Halpin and Croft devised the Organizational Climate Description Questionnaire (Halpin, 1966). This tool was later modified by Duxbury, Henly, and Armstrong (1982) for use in a neonatal intensive care unit. These tools were developed before organizational culture became a popular topic in the literature. Although some of these tools purport to describe organizational climate, the questions are similar to those on more recently developed tools designed to assess organizational culture. Denison (1996) identifies the many similarities between the concepts of organizational climate and organizational culture and notes the undesired consequences of continued separation of these two literatures.

Hofstede (1991) has developed a survey tool used primarily to assess organizational cultures in multinational organizations. Hofstede's tool provides a numerical score on the five dimensions of power distance, uncertainty avoidance, individualism-collectivism, masculinity-femininity, and long-term orientation.

More recent instruments include those developed by Cameron (Quinn, 1988), Kilmann and Saxton (1991), and Cooke and Lafferty (1994). Cameron's instrument provides a score on six dimensions of corporate culture. These dimensions include the organization's dominant characteristics, leader, glue, climate, criteria of success, and management style. The nurse executive can use the scores on these dimensions to describe the nursing culture in terms of its internal/external orientation and its flexibility/control orientation. The Kilmann-Saxton Culture-Gap Survey provides a numerical score on the dimensions of task support, social relationships, task innovation and personal freedom. It assesses both current and desired work group norms. Differences between the actual and desired norms are referred to as "Culture-Gaps." Identifying these gaps can motivate nurses to change their culture. Cooke and Lafferty's Organizational Culture Inventory (OCI) lists 96 statements that describe some of the behaviors and "personal styles" that might be expected or implicitly required of members of an organization. Participants are asked to describe the way people within their organization are expected to deal with one another. The OCI describes how organizational members perceive their culture along 12 dimensions of behaviors.

Coeling and Simms (1993a) have designed a tool specifically to assess the culture of a nursing work group. This Nursing Unit Cultural Assessment Tool (NUCAT) is broad in scope. It assesses a variety of behaviors that, through a series of qualitative and quantitative studies, have been found both to be important to practicing nurses and to differ between nursing units. All items on the tool assess different elements of culture and, hence, vary independently. This allows the tool to assess a unit culture in its fullness and gives a broad description of life on the unit. Table 9.3 portrays the relevant cultural factors used in the NUCAT.

However, this variety and breadth preclude its being divided into different dimensions with scores for each dimension. It is intended to be used as an initial scanning tool. It can be followed by tools that will provide a more definitive measure of a certain element if the need arises. Because it assesses the group's typical behavior and the individual's preferred behavior, it, too, can be used to identify

Table 9.3 Ten Cultural Factors Relevant to Nurses

1. Following orders:
   - Following policies and procedures
   - Following the organizational chain of command
   - Attending in-service meetings
2. Growing professionally:
   - Seeking promotions
   - Attending college
   - Discussing new nursing-care ideas
3. Valuing technical skills:
   - Handling emergencies competently
   - Working efficiently
   - Making patients comfortable
4. Using professional judgment:
   - Using individual judgment
   - Understanding patient's feelings
   - Being creative in providing nursing care
5. Preferring one's own way:
   - Trying to change someone's behavior by joking about it
   - Telling a peer how they should do a certain procedure
   - Competing with co-workers
6. Caring for co-workers:
   - Offering to help others
   - Providing emotional support for co-workers
   - Socializing with co-workers outside of the agency
7. Maintaining traditions:
   - Going along with peer pressure
   - Maintaining life when death is inevitable
   - Preferring old ways of doing things
8. Communicating directly:
   - Trying to change behavior indirectly
   - Asking for help directly
9. Working under difficult conditions:
   - Calling in sick when physically ill
   - Calling in sick when one needs a day off to rest
10. Assuming responsibility:
    - Having one nurse, rather than many nurses, develop the plan of care
    - Documenting what you have done

From *The Executive Nurse* by S. Byers, 1997, Albany, NY: Delmar, a division of Thomson Learning.

work group behaviors that might be producing group conflict, cultural differences between groups proposing a merger and work penetration points at which innovations can be introduced.

ETHICS RELATED TO ORGANIZATIONAL CULTURE

Although assessing a group's culture can have great value, some dangers are also associated with a cultural assessment. One danger is that the assessment may be inaccurate. Because culture is really a wholistic concept, a description of a pattern, one can never "measure" it in its full complexity. The best one can do is measure discrete elements of it as research variables and then attempt to describe the pattern these variables portray. Another danger is that conscious awareness of the culture might prompt a change to meet a specific standard when this change is not in the group's best interest. This phenomenon occurred as Americans gained world power and then tried to impose the American culture on natives in other lands and even on native Americans. This same phenomenon could occur if a nurse executive responsible for care provided by agencies from the United States and another country tried to impose U.S. work patterns on nurses from another nation and culture. Nurse executives will do well to ensure a change is indeed needed before expending time, money and energy on a given change.

It has also been questioned whether administrators have the right to change the behaviors, values, and beliefs of employees. As May (1993) notes, overriding of personal values by mandated organizational values could thwart the operation of conscience so that health care employees come to believe that what they are doing is morally right, even as their work efforts bring harm to others. An example might include a high degree of organizational emphasis on speed and efficiency that over time results in negative changes in the attitudes of health care employees toward the goals of caring and compassion. It is important to maintain awareness of this potential danger.

Another danger is the attempted change of a culture of such great magnitude that organizational members feel their work culture is being destroyed. Such conditions are extremely costly on a human level because large numbers of people have to face the fact that the way they have been thinking and feeling is no longer functional. Large-scale cultural change, such as may be associated with organizational mergers and work redesign, requires nurse executives to manage the emotional process involved in redefining beliefs, structures and practices. Maintaining trust is essential to this process. Johns (1996) describes a high-trust organization as one in which values such as personal worth, respect, and integrity prevail. The nurse executive is in a key position to promote a high-trust organization and in so doing enhance the quality of life for clients and employees alike.

SUMMARY

Organizational culture has become a major focus of management studies. It emphasizes the importance of understanding people, individually and collectively, to facilitate organizational success. Because it is a broad concept and one that derives from a variety of traditions, it is important for the nurse executive and the nurse researcher to clarify their working definition of culture and their basic assumptions and goals regarding culture. An understanding of culture can facilitate organizational hiring, orientation, work redesign, and mergers. Hasty attempts by the nurse executives to change the culture are ill-advised. Rather the current culture should be assessed and thoughtful decisions made regarding what aspects of the culture to change and what supports should be in place before the changes begin.

STUDY QUESTIONS

1. Compare and contrast three perspectives on organizational culture, namely the anthropological perspective, the management theorist perspective, and the organizational practitioner perspective.
2. Identify five sources of organizational culture and describe how each source may have contributed to the culture of a work group with which you are acquainted.
3. Think of three characteristics of your organizational culture that would be important to share with newcomers during their orientation period.
4. Identify three behaviors or strategies that facilitate cultural change and describe how you could incorporate these strategies into an upcoming change you will be directing.
5. How could you assess the organizational culture of an organization with whom you are considering a merger?

REFERENCES

Boston, C. (1995). Cultural transformation. *Journal of Nursing Administration, 25*(1), 19–20.

Brown, L. D. (1985). People-centered development and participatory research. *Harvard Educational Review, 55*(1), 69–75.

Coeling, H. V. (1997). Organizational subcultures: Where the rubber meets the road. In S. R. Byers. *The executive nurse* (pp. 184–206). Albany, NY: Delmar.

Coeling, H. V., & Wilcox, J. R. (1988). Understanding organizational culture: A key to management decision-making. *Journal of Nursing Administration, 18*(11), 16–24.

Coeling, H. V., & Wilcox, J. R. (1990). Using organizational culture to facilitate the change process. *American Nephrology Nurses' Association Journal, 17,* 231–236.

Coeling, H. V., & Simms, L. M. (1993a). Facilitating innovation at the nursing unit level through cultural assessment, part 1. *Journal of Nursing Administration, 23*(4), 46–53.

Coeling, H. V., & Simms, L. M. (1993b). Facilitating innovation at the unit level through cultural assessment, part 2. *Journal of Nursing Administration, 23*(5), 13–20.

Coeling, H. V., & Simms, L. M. (1996). Understanding work group culture on rehabilitation units: The key to facilitating group innovation and promoting integration. *Rehabilitation Nursing 21*(1), 7–12.

Cooke, R. A., & Lafferty, C. (1994). *Organizational culture inventory.* Plymouth, MI: Human Synergistics.

Deal, T. E., & Kennedy, A. A. (1982). *Corporate cultures.* Reading, MA: Addison-Wesley.

Denison, D. R. (1990). *Corporate culture and organizational effectiveness.* New York: Wiley.

Denison, D. R. (1996). What is the difference between organizational culture and organizational climate? A native's point of view on a decade of paradigm wars. *Academy of Management Review, 21*(3), 619–654.

Duxbury, M. L., Henly, G. A., & Armstrong, G. D. (1982). Measurement of the nurse organizational climate on neonatal intensive care units, *Nursing Research, 31*(2), 83–87.

Fitzpatrick, M. S., Sr. (1996). Sharing your culture with a new partner. *Health Progress, 77*(6), 54–57.

Fulton, T. R. (1996). Nurses' adoption of a patient-controlled analgesia approach. *Western Journal of Nursing Research, 18*(4), 383–396.

Grzyb-Wysocki, T., & Enriquez, M. G. (1996). The influence of organizational culture on patient care restructuring. *Seminars for Nurse Managers, 4*(1), 49–54.

Hall, P. (1990). *A cultural basis for cultural equality.* Paper presented at the Annual Convention of the International Communication Association, Dublin, Ireland.

Halpin, A. W. (1966). *Theory and research in administration.* New York: Macmillan.

Hanser, J. (1997). Finding new strength in unity. *Health Progress, 78*(1), 56-58.

Hofstede, G. (1991). *Cultures and organizations.* London: McGraw-Hill.

Johns, J. (1996). Trust: Key to acculturation in corporatized health care environments. *Nursing Administration Quarterly, 20*(2), 13–24.

Jones, K. R., DeBaca, V., & Yarbrough, M. (1997). Organizational culture assessment before and after implementing patient-focused care. *Nursing Economic$, 15*(2), 73–80.

Kennedy, M. (1996). Creating a new postmerger culture. *Health System Leader, 3*(5), 4–11.

Kilmann, R. H., & Saxton, M. J. (1991). *Kilmann-Saxton Culture-Gap Survey.* Tuxedo, NY: XICOM and Organizational Design Consultants.

Kilmann, R. H., Saxton, M. J., & Serpa, R. (1986). Issues in understanding and changing culture. *California Management Review, 28*(2), 87–94.

Kluckhohn, F. R., & Strodtbeck, F. L. (1961). *Variations in value orientations.* Evanston, IL: Row, Peterson and Company

Koerner, J. G. (1997). Cocreation of culture through choice. In J. A. Dienemann (Ed.). *Cultural diversity in nursing: Issues, strategies and outcomes* (pp. 63–69). Washington, DC: American Academy of Nursing.

Leatt, P., Baker, G. R., Halverson, P. K., & Aird, C. (1997). Downsizing, reengineering, and restructuring: Long-term implications for health care organizations. *Frontiers of Health Services Management, 13*(4), 3–37, 52–54.

May, L. (1993). Institutions and the transformation of personal values. *Clinical Laboratory Management Review, 7*(3), 191–93, 196–99.

McKibbin, S. (1995). The soul of a corporation. *Hospitals & Health Networks, 69*(10), 20–24.

Moos, R. H., & Insel, P. N. (1974). *Work environment scale.* Palo Alto, CA: Consulting Psychologist Press.

Mullins, D. G. (1989). Messages of values inculcation in a hospital organization. (Doctoral dissertation, Bowling Green State University, 1989). *Dissertation Abstracts International, 50,* 10A.

Nash, M. G., & Everett, L. N. (1996). Cultural cohesion versus collision. *Journal of Nursing Administration, 26*(7/8), 11–18.

Newman, K. L., & Nollen, S. D. (1996). Culture and congruence: The fit between management practices and national culture. *Journal of International Business Studies, 27,* 753–776.

Ott, J. S. (1989). *The organizational culture perspective.* Chicago: The Dorsey Press.

Peters, T. J., & Waterman, R. H., Jr. (1982). *In search of excellence.* New York: Harper & Row.

Quinn, R. E. (1988). *Beyond rational management.* San Francisco: Jossey-Bass.

Reger, R. K., Mullane, J. V., Gustafson, L. T., & DeMarie, S. M. (1994). Creating earthquakes to change organizational mindsets. *Academy of Management Executive, 8*(4), 31–42.

Rizzo, J. A., Gilman, M. P., & Mersmann, C. A. (1994). Facilitating care delivery redesign using measures of unit culture and work characteristics. *Journal of Nursing Administration, 24*(5), 32–37.

Sackmann, S. A. (1989). Managing organizational cultures: Dreams and possibilities, *Communication Yearbook, 13,* 114–148.

Sathe, V. (1985). *Culture and related corporate realities.* Homewood, IL: Richard D. Irwin.

Schein, E. H. (1984). Coming to a new awareness of organizational culture, *Sloan Management Review, 25*(2), 3–16.

Schein, E. H. (1985). *Organizational culture and leadership.* San Francisco: Jossey-Bass.

Schein, E. H. (1996). Leadership and organizational culture. In F. Hesselbein, M. Goldsmith, & R. Beckhard (Eds.). *The leader of the future* (pp. 59–69). San Francisco: Jossey-Bass.

Sherer, J. L. (1994). Dealing with that 'corporate culture thing'. *Trustee, 47*(6), 8–10.

Simms, L. M., Coeling, H. V. E., & Rosemann, M. A. (1998). An action approach to redesigning a patient-centered unit. *International Nursing Review, 45*(2), 58–60.

Smircich, L., & Calás, M. B. (1987). Organizational culture: A critical assessment. In F. M. Jablin (Ed.). *Handbook of organizational communication* (pp. 228–263). Newbury Park, CA: Sage.

Starbuck, W. H. (1982). Congealing oil: Inventing ideologies to justify acting ideologies out, *Journal of Management Studies, 19*(1), 3–27.

Van Maanen, J., & Barley, S. R. (1985). Cultural organization: Fragments of a theory. In P. J. Frost, L. F. Moore, M. R. Louis, C. C. Lundberg, & J. Martin (Eds.). *Organizational culture* (pp. 31–53). Beverly Hills: Sage.

Vestal, K. W., & Fralicx, R. D. (1997). Organizational culture: The critical link between strategy and results. *Hospital & Health Services Administration, 42*(3), 339–365.

Voglewede, R. (1996). The application of faith-based principles. *Health Progress, 77*(1), 46–50, 56.

Webb, S. S., Price, S. A., & Coeling, H. V. (1996). Valuing authority/responsibility relationships. *Journal of Nursing Administration, 26*(2), 28–33.

Wilkins, A. L., & Patterson, K. J. (1985). You can't get there from here: What will make culture-change projects fail. In R. H. Kilmann, M. J. Saxton, R. Serpa, & Associates (Eds.). *Gaining control of the corporate culture* (pp. 262–291). San Francisco: Jossey-Bass.

CHAPTER

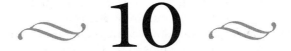

10

Nursing as a Business

Judith Lloyd Storfjell • Christine M. Smith

Business savvy is something we were never taught in nursing school. So, becoming a nurse entrepreneur has meant learning a whole new world— usually on your own, by trial and error. (Norris, 1991, p. vii)

Chapter Highlights

- Creating a niche
- Criteria for success
- Measurement and decision-making
- Examples of nursing businesses
- Steps in planning a nursing business
- The business plan

Because nursing is a service profession, nurses may find it incongruous to think that the *art and science of caring* can be a business or have a monetary connotation. In fact, provision of nursing care includes all the elements of a business—customers, money, staff, supplies, equipment, management, records, controls, planning, etc. Nurses provide services to meet specific needs—they provide value to a variety of customers. And, whether a nursing entity is large or small, whether it is for-profit or not-for-profit, it requires finances to operate.

CREATING A NICHE

Starting a new business can be exciting and full of risk. New ventures are all about hard work, creativity, and innovation (ideas explored in detail in Chapters

5 and 12). Creating a niche or unique specialization starts with idea development and involves determining what product you want to sell. Intrapreneurships are businesses developed within existing companies or health care systems; entrepreneurs enjoy the same characteristics as intrapreneurs but prefer to develop their own enterprise in an independent setting (Puetz & Thomas, 1998). The same personal, financial, and legal resources are required in either case. Nursing entrepreneurs are truly the change agents in nursing says Sullivan (1999). Entrepreneurs have a "can-do" spirit that captures the "imaginization," creativity, and enthusiasm essential for coping with new ventures. Entrepreneurs have learned to cope and do not give up easily.

What is a Small Business?

Christine Smith (Appendix A-F) describes a small business as one in which one or two persons are required to make all of the critical management decisions—finance, accounting, personnel, purchasing, processing, servicing, marketing, and selling—without the aid of internal specialists, and with specific knowledge in only one or two functional areas. Most nurses who manage their own business are sole owners; only a few employ other nurses and some may employ a part-time bookkeeper or clerical assistant.

Features that distinguish a small business from a larger organization include a small management team with strong owner influence; centralized power and control; a close and loyal work team; low employee turnover; lack of specialist staff; informal planning and control; education, experience, and skills that are practical but narrow. Small businesses are not just smaller versions of large companies. They have to be managed quite differently.

A Nursing Practice as a Business

A nursing practice is a small business when the nurse chooses to be self-employed and practices on a freelance or fee-for-service basis outside the parameters of traditional employment. The focus of the practice may be in any or all domains of nursing, that is, clinical, education, management, or research. A nurse choosing to function in the latter three areas will frequently be called a nurse consultant. The nurse in private practice may employ staff in the business or may choose to subcontract work to others. Nurses are also increasingly practicing in a wide variety of clinical areas and it is expected that this trend is likely to increase significantly over the next few years.

There are no limits on where a nurse may practice; rather the limits lie in the realm of competence of the individual nurse and the ability to deliver a professional service to the client within the scope of the nurse's registration. Every business owned and operated by a nurse is different for a number of reasons. One reason is the way we find ourselves in the situation of even thinking about such a notion. For some it may be that they are looking for some excitement because of boredom or lack of motivation in the present job or that there is the offer to do a 'project' outside the present role and employment and it seems like a good idea to try something different. For others it is a calculated decision planned with precision and launched with a defined promotion strategy and publicity. And for others still it may be an opportunity that appears at just the right time. These opportunities may come about as a result of significant changes in the life or career of a nurse, such as retrenchment, children growing up and no longer needing so much attention, or a marriage break-up, any of which may require that the nurse seek a new direction in life and nursing practice.

A few indicators point to success: having drive and energy; commitment to and total immersion and concentration on the goal; willingness to take a risk with a good chance of success; capacity to accept feedback on performance; a desire to take initiative; operating from an internal locus of control; a tolerance for ambiguity; and endurance, especially when things do not go according to plan. Nurses have to be strategic about the planning and decision to start their own business. The more time put into the planning the greater the chances of success, however that may be defined by each nurse. Some say that their success at running their own business is luck, that is, *when opportunity and preparation come together.*

CRITERIA FOR SUCCESS

Nurses are usually concerned about delivering services to clients or patients that will improve their well-being. However, although the provision of quality services is critical to a successful program or service, quality alone will not guarantee success. In fact, three interrelated factors are critical to the success of any health care business:

- Quality—provision of effective services
- Cost—efficient, cost-competitive service delivery
- Access—meeting the needs of customers, flexibility, ease of entry into the service delivery system

The ability to accomplish these three criteria is directly related to the success of any venture—the provision of high-quality, low-cost, customer-responsive services. As clinicians, nurses have more experience in providing and measuring the quality of services, but much less knowledge about managing costs and meeting customer needs.

Quality Services

The most important element of a successful business is the service itself—without the service or product, the business would not exist. Unless the standard of service is high, it will not survive for long. Therefore, considerable attention must be given to developing systems that will promote the delivery of services designed to achieve the appropriate goals. The measurement of this success is also important—to identify areas for improvement and to promote the business.

Service quality has a number of dimensions depending on who is evaluating it. According to Donabedian (1980), quality can be viewed according to structure, process, and outcome. For the nurse manager, this framework can be extremely useful. It is assumed that a well-structured program with appropriate processes will promote the delivery of quality services. Therefore, the evaluation of the organizational structure and the service delivery processes may serve as a proxy for evaluating the quality of the services themselves. Of course, it is ultimately best to measure the outcomes directly whenever possible.

Cost and Efficiency

Understanding and managing the cost of services is not as familiar to nurses as actually providing them. Because pressure on health care entities is increasing to reduce costs, long-term viability requires that services be cost competitive. Nurses do not need to be accountants, but as managers of service programs, they do need to understand what affects costs and know how to control them.

Financial plans, or budgets, are developed for services, programs, and businesses to forecast the financial future of the entity. These plans (budgets), however, are only as good as the assumptions on which they are based—service volume, reimbursement rates, labor costs, staffing, and other expenses. Considerable attention must be given to researching and validating these assumptions. In the simplest form, a budget consists of two parts: revenue (income) and expense. Expenses can be divided into three major categories: labor, occupancy, and other expenses. These expenses can be further divided into direct and indirect expenses. Direct expenses are those directly related to providing care to patients (e.g., nursing wages, clinical supplies); indirect expenses are costs incurred to support the direct delivery of care (e.g., management wages, space costs).

Once the budget is established, it should be used as a management tool. Regular financial statements should monitor variances to the budget, both revenue and expense. Each line item should be compared to the budget and variances explained. It can often be extremely useful to monitor changes in unit costs—the cost of delivering a unit of service (e.g., a clinic visit, a home nursing visit, an in-patient day). Because revenue is usually received according to the amount of service delivered, the unit cost can then be compared to the revenue per unit. This can be done on a simple spreadsheet that can be updated monthly or quarterly (Table 10.1). The most important part of this monitoring process is to explain any variances and make the necessary management adjustments.

To manage costs, it is sometimes useful to ascertain the costs of certain processes or activities. By using activity-based costing and management techniques (ABC/M), it is possible to monitor the costs of specific activities or processes such as admitting patients or billing payers, or treating a specific type of patient. Waste and inefficiency are much easier to identify and eliminate with this type of costing approach (Storfjell & Jessup, 1996). ABC/M should become part of the nurse-managers tool-kit.

Table 10.1 Sample Budget for *Well Planned Home Care*

ASSUMPTIONS:

Payer mix:		Nursing	PT	OT	SP	MSW	HHA	Totals
Medicare	75%	28,875	13,050	3,825	1,050	1,875	16,275	64,950
Medicaid	8%	3,080	1,392	408	112	200	1,736	6,928
MCO	12%	4,620	2,088	612	168	300	2,604	10,392
Private pay	5%	1,925	870	255	70	125	1,085	4,330
Total visits:	100%	38,500	17,400	5,100	1,400	2,500	21,700	86,600
Charge per visit		105	105	105	105	130	50	
Reimbursement:								
Medicare caps		103.00	102.00	101.00	102.00	128.00	49.00	
Medicaid		52.00	49.80	49.00	49.20	68.40	32.00	
MCO		70.00	70.00	70.00	70.00	70.00	35.00	
Bad debt (private)		4%	2%	2%	2%	5%	5%	
Hourly wages		20	21	20	20	18	9	
Contract fees			45	40	40			
% staff visits		100%	60%	50%	20%	100%	100%	
% contract visits			40%	50%	80%			
Visits per FTE		1,250	1,300	1,300	1,200	900	1,200	
Hours worked per year		2,080	2,080	2,080	2,080	2,080	2,080	
FTEs required		30.80	8.03	1.96	0.23	2.78	18.08	
Fringe benefit %	22%	22%	22%	22%	22%	22%	22%	
Per visit costs:								
Mileage		3.50	3.50	3.50	3.50	3.50	3.50	
Medical supplies		0.35						
MC Reimburseable supplies	1.50							

continued

Table 10.1 (continued)

Administrative wages:	Annual	# FTEs	Totals		Other admin costs:	
Executive Director	80,000	1	80,000		Administrative travel	8,000
Clinical Director	73,000	1	73,000		Occupancy (rent, etc.)	80,000
Financial Director	68,000	1	68,000		Telephone/postage	75,000
Clinical Managers	58,000	5	290,000		Conf/dues/meetings	40,000
QA/Medical records	56,000	2	112,000		Depreciation	40,000
Billing/acctg mgrs	48,000	2	96,000		Equip maintenance	25,000
Marketing/liaisons	48,000	5	240,000		Office supplies	85,000
Clerks	24,000	14	336,000		Legal/consulting	35,000
Total admin wages:			1,295,000		Miscellaneous	10,000

COST ANALYSIS:

	A&G	Nursing	PT	OT	SP	MSW	HHA	MC Supplies	Totals
REVENUE									
Medicare		1,998,900	936,802	256,262	71,881	158,416	571,087	202,298	4,195,646
Medicaid		160,160	69,322	19,992	5,510	13,680	55,552		324,216
MCO		323,400	146,160	42,840	11,760	21,000	91,140		636,300
Private pay		202,125	91,350	26,775	7,350	16,250	54,250		398,100
(Less bad debt)		(8,085)	(1,827)	(536)	(147)	(813)	(2,713)		(14,120)
Net Revenue:		2,676,500	1,241,807	345,333	96,355	208,533	769,317	202,298	5,540,142
EXPENSES									
Direct Expenses:									
Wages		1,281,280	350,784	81,600	9,707	104,000	338,520		2,165,891
Fringe benefits		281,882	77,172	17,952	2,135	22,880	74,474		476,496
Contract fees			313,200	102,000	44,800	8,750			460,000
Mileage		134,750	60,900	17,850	4,900		75,950		303,100
Medical supplies		13,475						129,900	143,375
Total direct expense:		1,711,387	802,056	219,402	61,542	135,630	488,944	129,900	3,548,862
Percent		48.22%	22.60%	6.18%	1.73%	3.82%	13.78%	3.66%	100.00% 64%

continued

Table 10.1 (continued)

COST ANAYLYSIS:

	A&G	Nursing	PT	OT	SP	MSW	HHA	MC Supplies	Totals
Indirect Expenses:									
Wages	1,295,000								1,295,000
Fringe benefits	284,900								284,900
Administrative travel	8,000								8,000
Occupancy (rent, etc.)	80,000								80,000
Telephone/postage	75,000								75,000
Conf/dues/meetings	40,000								40,000
Depreciation	40,000								40,000
Equip maintenance	25,000								25,000
Office supplies	85,000								85,000
Legal/consulting	35,000								35,000
Miscellaneous	10,000								10,000
Total indirect expense:	1,977,900								1,977,900 36%
Allocation		953,813	447,013	122,280	34,300	75,591	272,505	72,398	1,977,900
Total Expense		2,665,200	1,249,070	341,682	95,842	211,221	761,450	202,298	5,526,762
Gain (Loss)		11,300	(7,263)	3,651	513	(2,688)	7,867	—	13,381
Cost per visit		69.23	71.79	67.00	68.46	84.49	35.09	3.11	63.82
		Nursing	PT	OT	SP	MSW	HHA	Supplies	Total

Access to Service

A nursing business can be cost effective (high quality, low cost) and still not be successful if the services are not accessible to its customers. This means that success also requires that the services meet the needs of targeted customers and that they are easily available. Access may be even more complex to determine than cost of quality. Determining customer need may require surveying potential clients through written or telephone surveys or focus groups, analyzing demographic and utilization data, and conducting trials or tests. Customer responsiveness requires flexibility and the ability to change. It is important to see your business through the eyes of the customer—what is important to them, what are they willing to pay for, and what do they value?

For example, several years ago I (Storfjell) was required to provide total parenteral nutrition at home to my 2-year-old grandson while his parents attended a family funeral. Although I had worked in almost all aspects of home health care—staff nurse, supervisor, and manager—I had not provided clinical care for several years. I needed the services of a home health nurse. Through this role change I discovered that what I thought was important as a provider of care differed now that I was a consumer. To my surprise, it was extremely important to me that the nurse called before she came to my home, was exactly on time, and her attire was neat, that she was technically competent, and that she did not expect me to be an expert. Also, the fact that I was given a number to call 24 hours a day relieved me considerably. When the nurse called each day, just to check, my apprehension nearly vanished. I thought of all the home visits I had made without establishing a specific appointment and how few times I had followed up afterward.

MEASUREMENT AND DECISION-MAKING

To keep an organization successfully moving forward, some mechanism is needed to monitor the achievement of its vision and strategy. Decisions need to be made based on good information—something often rare in health care entities. Several years ago Robert Kaplan and David Norton (1996) looked at successful businesses and developed a balanced scorecard (BSC) approach to measure key indicators of success.

The Balanced Score Card Approach

The BSC translates a business unit's mission and strategy into tangible objectives and measures four areas:

- Financial—to succeed financially, how should we appear to our stakeholders?
- Customer—to achieve our vision, how should we appear to our customers?
- Internal business processes—to satisfy our stakeholders and customers, what business processes must we excel at?
- Learning and growth—to achieve our vision, how will we sustain our ability to change and improve?

The BSC emphasizes that financial and nonfinancial measures must be part of the information system for employees at all levels of the organization. Not only must nurses understand more than clinical service delivery, but also all employees must understand the financial and other consequences of their decisions and actions. By determining and monitoring key indicators in these four areas, attention is focused at all levels on the critical success factors. Change occurs in areas that are measured and rewarded.

NEW BUSINESS DEVELOPMENT

Although nurses are often managers of units or specific programs within established health care entities, they are also recognizing the potential for developing new services and businesses. Actually, who is better positioned to plan and operate health care entities than nurses? As providers and managers, nurses have an opportunity to observe first-hand the health care needs of their clients. They are in a unique position to identify early trends, to observe gaps in service, and to recognize when access to care is less than optimal. As providers of health care services, nurses are at the front line of market research. In addition, they are in a better position than most to develop client-focused processes and systems of care. Finally, their use and understanding of the nursing process has provided them with good problem-solving skills.

Nurses are ideal entrepreneurs and intrapreneurs. They can identify unmet needs, plan customer-friendly services, and evaluate outcomes. Other disciplines may have financial, marketing, planning skills, but they usually lack the in-depth knowledge of the client and the service process that nurses possess, the most important ingredient in developing and managing a successful business. All that remains for most entrepreneurs is to become familiar with tools and processes related to business development—things much easier to learn than the intimate knowledge of the client and product. Chapter 32 provides many examples of assistive technologies that are natural products for a nursing business.

The key is to use knowledge about client needs to design a service that meets these needs efficiently and effectively. A program or business will not achieve long-term success without focusing on cost, quality, and access. High-quality, low-cost services that do not meet customers' needs will not attract or maintain a dedicated clientele. Low-quality services at any price will not continue to attract customers over time. High-cost services, no matter the quality, may price themselves out of business. Therefore, planning for a successful venture must include mechanisms for ensuring the quality of services, for managing cost, and for meeting customers' ever-changing needs.

EXAMPLES OF NURSING BUSINESSES

Start-ups are frequently launched within existing entities—such as an adult day care center affiliated with a hospital, a day surgery program, or a birthing center. They can also be freestanding enterprises. Nursing businesses range from an independent practitioner providing services in a clinic or client's home, to a national chain of nursing service providers. The oldest form of nurse-owned agencies (or businesses) are in the community—home health, hospice, private duty, case management, or nurse staffing businesses. But this is only the beginning. For example, nurses can contract with health care facilities to manage specific inpatient or outpatient units such as dialysis or critical care units. Freestanding nurse practitioner practices are growing in number. Appendix A provides detailed examples of nursing businesses as described by the nurses who started them, including obstacles they have encountered.

Nurses have also developed occupational health service businesses and consulting practices. It is not unusual for a nurse entrepreneur to contract with a public health department for the management and provision of government-funded programs such as well-child clinics, immunization clinics, or family-planning clinics. In fact, the potential for different types of nursing businesses is as broad as the variety of services nurses provide.

For instance, Mariah Taylor, a pediatric nurse practitioner, established a clinic in Portland, Oregon, to serve the working poor (1999). Melodie Chenervert turned frequent moves into the motivation for developing her own business promoting professional pride (1999). Inventor Kathleen Vollman, a clinical nurse specialist, turned a search for equipment to better meet her patients' needs into a design and development company (1999). In fact, the founder of public health nursing, Lillian Wald, was actually as much an entrepreneur as she was a nursing visionary.

Nurses are also developing programs that demonstrate the cost effectiveness of nursing care. A good example of this is the Community Nursing Organization (CNO). Four CNOs were developed in 1994 as part of a Health Care Financing Administration (HCFA) demonstration project (Storfjell et al., 1997). Specific home-based and community-based services were bundled together (e.g., home health care, medical equipment, outpatient therapy, ambulance service) into one capitated payment to be managed by nurses. The purpose of the CNO was to test the impact of both a model of nurse-managed health care and a capitated reimbursement system.

The four CNO sites (New York, Arizona, Minnesota, and Illinois) spent considerable time defining their purpose and their philosophy of practice. They all determined that nursing case management was essential to success. Nursing case management was determined to be the key to improved health of the elderly participants and, therefore, reduced costs of health care services. Each site had to establish its own approach, develop processes, recruit participants, and monitor the costs and quality of services. Findings from these nursing businesses will not only affect their clients, but may have a more far-reaching impact on health care delivery and reimbursement models. Other examples of nursing businesses by intrapreneurships and entrepreneurships are provided in Figure 10.1.

Intrapreneurships

Home Town Nurse Program (Julie Morath)	Abbott Northwestern & United Hospitals, Twin Cities, Minnesota
Doulas for Women in Labor (Cynthia Patrick and Cindy Crosby)	Salem Hospital, Salem, Oregon
Center for Caring (Barbara Balik)	United Hospital, St. Paul, Minnesota
Hos Tech, Inc. (Kathleen Vollman)	Henry Ford Hospital, Detroit, Michigan

Entrepreneurships

Creative Healthcare Management (Marie Manthey)	Minneapolis, Minnesota
Pro-Nurse (Melodie Chenervert)	Gaithersburg, Maryland
North Portland Nurse Practitioner Community Health Clinic (Mariah Taylor)	Portland Oregon
Van Slyck & Associates (Ann Van Slyck)	Phoenix, Arizona

Data compiled from Marion, J. (1999). Change from within. *Reflections*, 25(2), 10–12; Manthey, M. (1999). I never saw myself as a change agent. *Reflections*, 25(2), 19–21; Taylor, M. A. (1999). The clinic of last resort. *Reflections*, 25(2), 24–30; Van Slyck, A. (1999). The stamina to succeed. *Reflections*, 25(2), 13–15.

Figure 10.1 Examples of Nursing Intrapreneurships and Entrepreneurships

Business Versus Nursing Discipline

An idea or concept is only the first step. Nurses get ideas all the time. Transforming a good idea into a viable business is not automatic. Too many entrepreneurs go into business thinking it is something it is not. The same discipline required to be an effective nurse is also necessary to develop a successful business. Both nursing and business require careful assessment, the ability to analyze data, attention to detail, and sound decision-making. It is a common misconception that entrepreneurs are risk takers. The truth is that successful entrepreneurs know how to understand and manage risk. In fact, the parallels between success in both nursing and business are striking.

STEPS IN PLANNING A NURSING BUSINESS

The key principles of the Community Health Accreditation Program (CHAP) standards provide an excellent framework for designing a viable venture (Mitchell & Storfjell, 1989). These four principles and the supporting standards are one of the best guides to organizational viability:

- The organization's structure and function consistently support its consumer-oriented philosophy and purpose.
- The organization consistently provides high-quality services and products.

- The organization has adequate human, financial, and physical resources effectively organized to accomplish its stated goals.
- The organization is positioned for long-term viability.

The first step in planning a business is to identify the product or service and to define or develop the need. The importance of this step cannot be underestimated. Frequently, creative individuals will come up with "good ideas" and will proceed to develop businesses without first establishing that there is a real need or market for the service or product—one of the reasons for the high number of business closures each year. Establishing need will involve some market research to determine if the product is viable—who the potential customers are, how much they are willing to pay for the service, and how the service can best be presented to meet their needs. This market analysis needs to be approached from several perspectives:

- Review of data—demographic data and utilization patterns for similar services.
- Surveys or interviews—the "purchasers" and "users" of the planned service need to develop a profile and some means of obtaining their opinions and input. For instance, telephone interviews can be conducted or written surveys distributed. Other effective methods of clarifying service needs include interviewing key informants or conducting focus groups.

Once the service is defined and the market identified, the organizational vision and strategy need to be developed and then specific planning regarding organization and structure can occur. Legal and regulatory requirements need to be researched and plans made for compliance. The legal structure of the business needs to be established—corporation, partnership, or sole proprietorship; business licenses or certifications obtained; and a name reserved.

A plan for operations needs to be developed including planned work flows and processes, policies and procedures, necessary controls, and a plan for collecting and managing necessary data. Resources that will be required to develop and operate the business should be determined carefully. These include necessary staffing, finances, and physical requirements. Budgets need to be developed and sources of financing obtained. Detailed plans for implementing and evaluating the new business should be outlined carefully.

Actually, all of these necessary steps are best summarized in a business plan—a compilation of specific plans for planning and implementing a new business.

The Business Plan

Numerous books and articles have been written on how to write a business plan, with various approaches. However, business plans in themselves do not guarantee success. In fact, according to Sahlman (1997), business plans do not predict the success of a new venture. They often overlook four critical success factors:

(1) the people involved—their skills and experience; *(2)* the opportunity—what the business will sell and to whom; *(3)* the context or external environment—regulations, demographic trends; and *(4)* risks and rewards—everything that can go right or wrong with anticipated responses. Both intrapreneurial and entrepreneurial ventures require systematic planning and analysis.

Although a business plan may be necessary to obtain financial support for a specific venture, it should be viewed most importantly as a tool for the entrepreneur. It provides a framework for effective planning. Business plans (Figure 10.2) should include at least the following areas:

- Background and rationale
- Marketing analysis and plan
- Description of services to be provided
- Resources required (staffing, facilities, equipment)

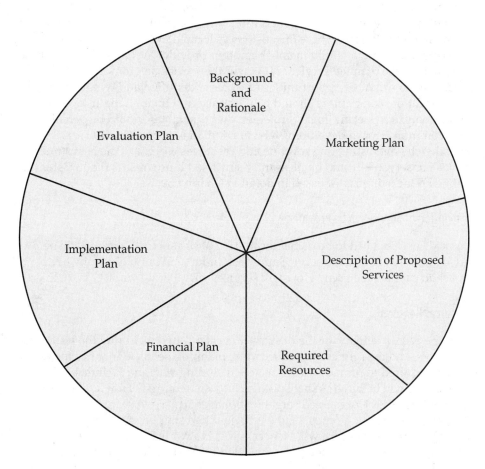

Figure 10.2 Components of a business plan

- Organization and management
- Financial plans—operating, capital, and cash flow budgets
- Implementation plan
- Evaluation plan

Background and Rationale

The first step in developing a business plan is to establish the need for the service or business—the opportunity. Why is it important? Who are the customers? What specific need does it meet? Who are potential competitors? What geographic area will be served? What are the unique qualifications of the developers—the people involved?

Marketing Analysis and Plan

Once the need for a service has been established, a plan must be developed to identify and reach potential customers. What is the size of the potential market? What is the anticipated market penetration (what percent of potential customers do you hope to attract)? Where are customers located? Who will make the "buy" decision—the client, a family member, another provider? What will attract these customers to the planned service? How will the service be promoted with each market segment? What opportunities have been identified and what threats exist? In addition, competitors should be identified and their strengths and weaknesses analyzed. Specific goals, strategies, and timetables should be detailed. The most common error in developing a business plan is to overestimate service volume, thereby overestimating revenue and resources required. The best strategy is to plan conservatively and be pleasantly surprised if progress is made faster than planned. Marketing is discussed in detail in Chapter 30.

Description of Services to be Provided

Planned services need to be detailed carefully. What specific services will be provided and what makes the service approach unique? What philosophy or approach to care will be used? How will services vary? How will they be delivered?

Resources Required

Once the basic premises for the business are established including the need, the customers, and the services to be provided, planning needs to identify the resources required to provide these services including staff and facilities. What type of staff will be hired? What specific skills are required? How will the program or business be organized (organizational chart)? How many staff will be necessary (e.g., staffing ratios)? How will qualified staff be recruited and retained? What type of space will be necessary? How much space is required? What equipment is necessary (e.g., clinical, office)? How will appropriate facilities be located and obtained?

Organization and Management

The corporate structure, either a separate entity or an intrepreneurial program, should be described. The composition and qualifications of the board of directors needs to be detailed; the internal organizational structure and the responsibilities of officers should be explained. Of particular importance is a description of the experience and background of principals and key employees including the status of employment agreements. Internal controls, accountability systems, and management reporting systems should be planned and described carefully.

Financial Plans

Adequate financial planning is critical including anticipated start-up and operational costs, sources of funding, and cash flow requirements. Three-year operational, cash flow, and capital budgets should be developed including detailed assumptions for each. Financial measures should be identified including unit costs and reimbursement, planned days in receivables, and other pertinent financial indicators.

Implementation Plan

This section should describe the steps planned for implementing the project or business including a schedule that shows the timing of activities for the major implementation events. Often entrepreneurs underestimate the time required to complete various tasks so consider the implications of potential delays. In addition, describe potential barriers and anticipated responses to unexpected events.

Evaluation Plan

How will you know if the project/business is successful? What quality, customer, internal processes, and financial indicators—the BSC—will be monitored? How will this information be collected and analyzed? How will changes be made based on evaluation findings?

SUMMARY

Because nurses understand client needs and effective processes of care, they are in an ideal position to manage and develop cost-effective programs and services that are in every respect a business. A key requirement is creativity and innovation. But this is only the beginning. Success requires that the vision be coupled with a disciplined approach to planning and decision-making—actually very similar to the nursing process. When an intimate knowledge of the client and a comprehensive understanding of service delivery methods are combined with careful planning and astute management techniques, businesses owned and managed by nurses should excel.

STUDY QUESTIONS

1. Review the descriptions of small businesses in the Appendix. Compare and contrast the steps taken in building each business with those undertaken in this chapter. What obstacles were encountered by the nurse entrepreneurs?
2. Select an area of practice in which you would like to establish an entrepreneurship or business. Write a business plan and develop a time chart for establishing your business.
3. What factors are critical to the success of any business?
4. What assistive devices are used by you or family members. How would you market and sell these products in a nursing business?

REFERENCES

Chenervert, M. (1999). My portable career. *Reflections, 25*(2), 22–23.

Donabedian, A. (1980). *Explorations in quality assessment and monitoring: Vol. I.* Ann Arbor, MI: Health Administration Press.

Kaplan, R. S., & Norton, D. P. (1996). *The balanced scorecard.* Boston: Harvard Business School Press.

Manion, J. (1999). Change from within. *Reflections, 25*(2), 10–12.

Manthey, M. (1999). I never saw myself as a change agent. *Reflections, 25*(2), 19–21.

Mitchell, M. K., & Storfjell, J. D. (Eds.). (1989). *Standards of excellence for home care organizations.* New York: National League for Nursing.

Norris, D. A. (1991). *How I became a nurse entrepreneur: Tales from 50 nurses in business.* Petaluma, CA: National Nurses in Business Association.

Puetz, B. E., & Thomas, K. J. K. (1998). What's your niche? Starting a new venture. In J. A. Dienemann (Ed.), *Nursing Administration* (pp. 225–241). Stamford, CT: Appleton & Lange.

Sahlman, W. A. (1997). How to write a great business plan. *Harvard Business Review, 75*(4), 98–108.

Storfjell, J. L., & Jessup, S. (1996, December). Bridging the gap between finance and clinical with activity based cost management. *Journal of Nursing Administration, 26*(12), 12–17.

Storfjell, J. L., Mitchell, R., & Daly, G. M. (1997, October). Nurse-managed healthcare: New York's Community Nursing Organization. *Journal of Nursing Administration, 27*(10), 21–27.

Sullivan, E. J. (1999). The can-do spirit. *Reflections, 25*(2), 4.

Taylor, M. A. (1999). The clinic of last resort. *Reflections, 25*(2), 24–30.

Van Slyck, A. (1999). The stamina to succeed. *Reflections, 25*(2), 13–15.

Vollman, K. (1999). My search to help patients breathe. *Reflections, 25*(2), 16–18.

PART

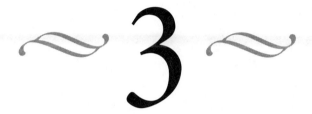

3

Essential Competencies in Practice Settings

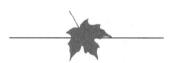

CHAPTER

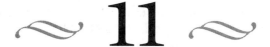

~ 11 ~

Strategic Planning

Eunice A. Bell

*Nurse executives are primary players in institutional strategic planning . . .
and must strike a balance between the nursing mission and the business
plan. (Martin, 1998, p. 30)*

Chapter Highlights

* The concept of strategic planning
* From strategic planning to strategic thinking
* The process
* Critical elements of external assessment
* Internal assessment
* Defining the business-centered mission
* Role of nursing administration

The purpose of this chapter is to examine the concept and process of strategic planning as a critical function of nursing administration. The advent of the 21st century
requires health care institutions to address both economic forces and future trends
to remain competitive in a sea of change. Strategic planning provides the process
for achieving goals in a dynamic environment. Health care providers are adopting
business strategies based on a proactive approach. Foremost among the current crisis strategies is the use of strategic planning to address expected macro changes in
the population profile and biomedical and information technology.

THE CONCEPT

Drucker (1974) defines strategic planning within the context of business and industry as "a continuous systematic process of making risk-taking decisions today with the greatest possible knowledge of their effects on the future, organizing efforts necessary to carry out these decisions and evaluating the results of these decisions against expected outcomes through reliable feedback mechanisms" (p. 125).

Domanico (1981) presented one of the earliest descriptions of the strategic planning process in hospitals as "the process whereby hospitals assess the total health care market and their true competitive position within the market to determine future directions while at the same time addressing community needs and satisfying regulatory requirements" (p. 25). The application of strategic planning to nursing administration was first reported by Jones (1988). She suggested that the nursing department's strategic plan is developed in the context of the needs of the total institution and describes its newly defined missions. Departmental strategic plans may include goals of productivity, cost containment, revenue increases, and quality enhancement.

FROM STRATEGIC PLANNING TO STRATEGIC THINKING

Strategic planning is the starting point for strategy-driven management of health care organizations. Whythe and Blair (1995) suggest that it is essential that health care managers conceptualize their organizations in terms of systems, as each decision needs to be made in terms of its ramifications in and on the environment. This conceptualization is the basic component of strategic thinking. Loveridge and Cummings (1996) described the transition in organizational focus from developing strategic plans to learning how to think and manage strategically. Vail (1989) comments that the "implementing of a plan is the hardest—the doing of the strategizing" and refers to strategy as "the conduct of some whole unit in relation to its environment" (p. 162). He further suggests that strategies, as acts of leadership, are initiatives, conspicuously thought out choices, that when operationalized become a change process.

The Process

Whythe and Blair (1995) identified the following steps in the strategic planning process (Figure 11.1):

1. Planning the process
2. Developing and/or assessing the mission statement
3. Conducting the external assessment
4. Conducting the internal assessment
5. Setting goals and objectives
6. Formulating strategic options

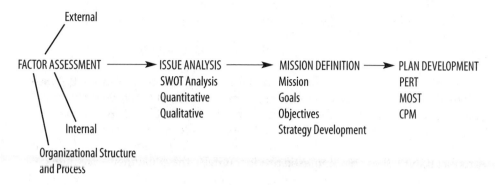

Figure 11.1 Strategic planning process. CPM, critical path method; MOST, management operations systems technique; PERT, program evaluation and review technique; SWOT, strengths, weaknesses, opportunities, threats.

  7. Selecting and developing strategies
  8. Developing the implementation plan

Step One: Planning the Process

The first step includes deciding on committee structure, the method of data collection, time frames for tasks, schedules for meetings, and the expected time required for the strategic planning process.

Step Two: Developing and/or Assessing the Mission Statement

The statement is developed in response to the needs of major stakeholders of the organization. Senior management and the governing body of the organization collaborate in an assessment of the mission determining that there is a shared set of values and purpose.

Step Three: Conducting the External Assessment

Dienemann (1998) indicated a major player in the strategic plan process is the marketing division of the organization. Their contribution is the analysis of external factors offering opportunities and threats. Analysis techniques include consumer analysis, both customer satisfaction and market segmentation and competitor analysis. The *critical elements of the external assessment* are:

  • Economic factors
  • Political factors
  • Market trends
  • Technology trends
  • Social/life-style trends
  • Regulatory factors

- Competition/institution image
- Manpower trends

Economic Factors

Both a macro and a micro examination of economic factors is essential. Because of the globalization of the economy, macro analysis should include the national and international economic climate and the effect on health care providers and consumers, the manpower supply, and the payers (governmental, business, and private). Economic markers important in this analysis include the gross national product (GNP), the gross domestic product (GDP), the consumer price index (CPI), and the rate of inflation/recession. At the micro examination level, assessment of state and local business climate, unemployment rates, and addition or loss of business/industry is needed. Changes in payer demands, which reflect pressure from employer groups and consumers to reduce costs, should be assessed. Assessment of change in payer mix based on changes in the business profile or the community would be helpful in the assessment process. Because economic factors are the key to the fiscal health of health care organizations and their ability to deliver care efficiently, assessment of the economic environment is a critical first step in the strategic planning process.

Political Factors

Political issues are a direct reflection of political party differences; thus, national, state and local elections may result in changes in priorities and directly affect health care delivery. Health care-related political issues that could affect strategic planning are abortion services, contraceptive services, and sex education for teenagers. States and localities vary in their response to these issues. Some issues such as time off for childbirth, adoption, and the care of acutely or terminally ill family members have been addressed by legislation at the national level. However, it is generally not comprehensive in scope and subject to change as the political climate changes. Local political issues that affect care delivery include access to care for the indigent and the homeless and care of increasing numbers of clients who are positive for the human immunodeficiency virus.

Market Trends

Market trends at the national, state, and local level should be examined with care. Trends in alternate care delivery modes currently being tested in other geographic areas could provide important data for strategic planners looking for a new service/program to address local needs. Investigation of new areas of marketing focus may be conducted using the following categories:

1. Payer marketing—promoting services and fee structures to business groups
2. Packaged services marketing—packaging all services in one center, for example, childbirth services, gynecologic surgery, mammography, and bone density studies

3. Program-focused marketing—addressing broader concepts as children's hospitals and health services and health promotion centers

Close examination of the directions and strength of market trends as well as the diversity of market focus will provide the assessors with important data for strategic planning.

Technology Trends

Strategic planning requires an in-depth knowledge of advances in biomedical and information systems as they affect quality of care and the competitive position of the organization. This information may be obtained from local practitioners, researchers, professional groups, and commercial sources. In the assessment, it is important to determine the risks (medical and economic) in adoption of a new technology.

Social/Life-style Trends

Changes in society that affect health care delivery should be assessed. The "baby boomer" population reaching middle and old age, increasing numbers of single parents and full-time working mothers, the returning-to-the-nest syndrome, the increasing housing options for older adults, and the disabled are social changes that have a direct impact on how, where, and when health care is delivered.

Regulatory Factors

Assessment of the impact of governmental regulation on the delivery of health care is crucial to the planning process. Changes in Occupational Safety and Health Administration (OSHA) rules may affect both the patient/consumer and health care personnel. Environmental Protection Administration (EPA) regulations regarding hazardous waste and water, air, and soil pollution may profoundly influence the plans for new services. The Food and Drug Administration's (FDA) control of diagnostic and treatment procedures and substances is an important regulatory function that must be addressed in planning new endeavors. Further, regulations at the state and local levels may affect new programming. Health services agencies (HSAs), which review utilization and confirm the need for new equipment and facilities, and state laws affecting reimbursement for services, are significant forces in strategic planning.

Competition/Institution Image

An assessment of the competitive position of the institution in both the community and the region may be based on utilization data, such as the number of patient-days, percent occupancy, physician specialty mix, and case mix. Fiscal data to be compared might include current ratios, operating margins, and long-term debt to equity ratios. Changes in services, administrative teams, and facilities of competing hospitals provide further data for assessment for the competitive position.

The institutional image may be assessed via qualitative measures, such as patient satisfaction surveys, community focus groups, interviews with physicians and employees, and media coverage. Quantitative data may be obtained from retention rates for physicians, nurses, and allied health personnel, hospital report cards, and reports from the Joint Commission on the Accreditation of Healthcare Organizations (JCAHO).

Manpower

Information about local, state, and national manpower trends is needed for the external assessment. Nationally, the supply of physicians continues to be maldistributed to specialties, despite the focus of health maintenance organizations (HMOs) on a generalist gatekeeper. Supply and demand of nurses remains cyclical. There is a demand for increasing numbers of RNs in nonacute community settings at the same time that higher nurse/patient ratios are needed in acute care facilities. Educational institutions recruiting young adults for nursing programs find this segment of the population decreasing in size. Planning for new services, new care delivery systems, and new programs requires an in-depth knowledge of the manpower available to staff proposed changes. Information is available locally from schools of nursing and medicine, manpower studies, and professional practice groups. At the state and national level, manpower information is available from governmental agencies and professional organizations. In addition, national initiatives funded by foundations have identified workforce issues requiring planning (Lewis, Sechrist, Schultz & Keating, 1997).

Step Four: Conducting the Internal Assessment

Whythe and Blair (1995) list the internal assessment components as management, human resources, finance, marketing, clinical systems, organizational structure, organization culture, physical plant, information systems, and leadership abilities. Again, the institution's marketing department can provide the planners with information on internal strengths and weaknesses.

Internal Assessment

An internal assessment by strategic planners would illustrate strengths and limitations and the areas open to development. The assessment should include organizational culture, the communication process, and institutional demographics. The organizational culture can be examined via behaviors, norms, values, rules, and the philosophy. Organizational behavior is based on a common language, terminology, and rituals. This is reflected in the interactions between and among groups. The perceived worth of groups to the organization is reflected in the relationships of such groups as physicians and nurses. Norms about work behaviors (how hard to work) may agree or disagree with the philosophy of the institution and organizational values of efficiency, quality of work, and dependability. Rules for getting along in the organization provide a framework for the climate, that is, a feeling that is derived from patient/worker interaction and that indicates the openness of employees to change. These data will be crucial to planners wishing to predict the success of proposed programs. (See Chapter 9 for further discussion of cultural assessment.)

Effective organizational communication is crucial in developing new programs and, thus, assessment of the process is a primary need for strategic planning. Factors for examination are the patterns and channels of formal and informal communication, the efficiency and effectiveness of communication, and the nature of communications. An assessment of the organizational demographics will determine the human resources available as employees, volunteers, consultants, and collaborators. Further, data on age, gender, race, education, and experience will provide a detailed profile of the hospital resources.

Step Five: Setting Goals and Objectives

Goals are time specific end points in the strategic plan. Whythe and Blair (1995) describe them as reachable, verifiable, specific, and explicit. They flow from the matching of organizational strengths and weaknesses with environmental threats and opportunities.

Step Six: Formulating Strategic Options

After goal setting, means for relating them to the environment are developed. Several techniques are available for this step. They include statistical forecasting, Delphi activities, brainstorming, scenario building, and dilemma construction. The end game is to form a list of realistic strategies for the completion of each goal. Whythe and Blair (1995) propose three types of alternate strategies:

1. Practical alternates—readily available
2. Incremental alternates—may follow in some sequence
3. Radical alternates—require significant changes

Step Seven: Selecting and Developing Strategies

Strategies are selected independently of the option development stage to allow that time to design a variety of alternates and prohibit emphasis on the first option. At this point, stakeholder responses should be anticipated and efforts made to increase support and minimize opposition to the final selections.

Step Eight: Developing the Implementation Plan

The final step in strategic planning is the development of the plan. The problems have been defined, alternate strategies identified and evaluated, and the best strategies selected. A detailed comprehensive model is presented. Each strategy is assigned to a responsible individual or group and a time line confirmed and a completion date set. Check points are established for assessing the rate of progress. Tools such as the program evaluation review technique (PERT) or critical path method (CPM) are used to graphically present planning, scheduling, and costing in a network model. Nursing departments are most familiar with the CPM, which parallels the clinical use of critical paths as quality measures. Evaluation of strategy effectiveness follows and leads to minor adjustments, major adjustments, or abandonment of the current strategy and adoption of a new strategy. Figure 11.2 summarizes the strategic planning scenario.

Defining the Business-Centered Mission

The planners must also articulate a business-defined mission that is goal oriented, action focused, and strategically advantageous to the organization. The business-defined mission represents the broad purpose of the institution, reflecting needs, wants, resources, and restrictions. Goals are set to exploit the opportunities and avoid the threats identified in the analysis. Optimizing goals, which are set at appropriate intervals, motivate action and reflect organizational risk taking.

Your health care institution is conducting a strategic planning project. The Vice President of Patient Care Services (Nursing Administrator) is a member of the institutional team. She has directed nurse managers of departments/units to develop a unit strategic plan. Your manager has appointed you to the unit strategic planning team. Following the process below (based on your experience on this unit) describe your contribution to each step. If you need other information, make an appointment with your nurse manager to review what you have and add needed information.

Unit Strategic Planning Process

Step One: Planning the process. Develop committee structure, methods, time frame, meeting schedules.

Step Two: Developing the mission statement. Build unit statement from institutional mission.

Step Three: Conducting the external assessment. Determine external factors affecting your unit.

Step Four: Conducting the internal assessment. Assess unit structure, clinical care delivery, culture, and leadership.

Step Five: Setting goals. Set unit goals with time specific end points.

Step Six: Formulate strategic options. Brainstorm with the unit team to develop several alternate strategies to reach each goal.

Step Seven: Selecting strategies. Choose strategies that address the needs of unit stakeholders and are practical, incremental, or radical.

Step Eight: Developing the implementation plan. Assign strategies, develop time lines and completion dates. Design evaluation measures.

Figure 11.2 Strategic planning scenario.

A primary strategy for addressing the business-defined mission has been diversification, which is a strategy that attempts to spread financial risk by taking advantage of new market opportunities. Two major concepts of diversification are vertical and horizontal integration. Vertical integration can be forward directed (developing programs or services for health care beyond the hospital acute care focus): health screening and wellness centers are examples. Backward integration addresses raw materials or precursors needed in acute care delivery, for example, intravenous solutions and pharmaceuticals.

Horizontal integration strategies seek to enlarge the scope of practice by acquiring like institutions in the area, linking several acute care agencies, or joining acute and nonacute facilities. The strategy seeks advantage from economics of scale, concentration of management, and increased access to capital.

THE ROLE OF NURSING ADMINISTRATION

Nurse executives are primary players in the institutional strategic planning function. They collaborate with other executives on the institutional planning team. Jones (1988) describes their role in relation to the nursing department as a communicator of departmental needs and accomplishments to the team, a controller of cost in service delivery, and an operational decision-maker. Martin (1998) proposes that nurse executives find a balance between nursing and business administration. They can contribute a nursing perspective to the business-defined mission and assist in the development of appropriate goals. They are the prime movers in operationalizing the strategies. When selecting among alternate strategies, they exercise political acumen to promote the best possible outcome. They use negotiation to win approval of programs that will be most successful. When final decision-making occurs, they use highly developed skills of analysis for the selection of appropriate strategies. At the divisional level, nurse executives lead the nurse managers in the strategic planning process and mentor them as they develop unit-based plans. Rowland and Rowland (1997) report that departmental planning efforts result in "higher quality of care, greater staff satisfaction, lower patient costs, and higher contribution to the profit margin of the health care facility" (p. 33). Jones and Beck (1996) assert that strategic planning can be stimulating and challenging for all levels of nursing staff. Dynamic planning in a positive environment joins staff in meeting common goals. Beyond the institution, nurse executives are often involved as strategic planners in national grant-funded initiatives to strengthen hospital nursing (Taft, Minch, & Jones, 1992). The contributions of nursing administration to strategic planning at national, organizational, divisional, and unit levels makes it a critical player in the success of health care organizations of the 21st century.

SUMMARY

Strategic planning has been discussed as the basis for strategic management of health care delivery. The movement from business to health care and to nursing is described. Major subconcepts include strategic thinking and management. The planning process encompasses developing the mission statement, assessing external and internal environments, setting goals, formulating options, selecting strategies, and developing the implementation plan. Nursing administration is involved in the strategic planning process at the organizational, departmental, and unit levels. Further, nurse administrators play a major role in national strategic planning initiatives to improve patient care delivery.

STUDY QUESTIONS

1. Review changes that have occurred on a nursing unit where you have worked as a student or staff member. Relate this change to an organizational strategic plan.
2. Select two of the external factors/trends in this chapter and assess the impact of those factors/trends on your organization.
3. Referring to the internal assessment, describe the nursing culture in your organization and discuss its effect on strategic planning.
4. Referring to the change in question 1, describe two other strategic options that might have been considered in addressing the change.
5. Compare the use of critical path method in patient or client care with critical paths in strategic planning. Discuss the primary concept shared by both.
6. List the four levels in which nursing executives contribute to strategic planning. Describe how the nursing executive's role differs at each level.

REFERENCES

Dienemann, J. A. (1998). *Nursing administration: Managing patient care.* (2nd ed.). Stamford, CT: Appleton & Lange.

Domanico, L. (1981). Strategic planning: Vital for hospital long-range development. *Hospital and Health Services Administration, 26*(4), 25–40.

Drucker, P. (1974). *Management tasks, responsibilities, politics.* New York: Harper & Row.

Jones, K. R. (1988). Strategic planning in hospitals: Applications to nursing administration. *Nursing Administration Quarterly, 13*(1), 1–10.

Jones, R., & Beck, S. (1996). *Decision making in nursing.* Albany, NY: Delmar.

Lewis, E. M., Sechrist, K. R., Schultz, M. A., & Keating, S. B. (1997). California Strategic Planning Committee for Nursing: Experiences and challenges. *Journal of Nursing Administration, 27*(3), 3–5.

Loveridge, C. E., & Cummings, S. H. (1996). *Nursing management in the new paradigm.* Gaithersburg, MD: Aspen.

Martin, M. (1998). Achieving the right balance in strategic planning. *Nursing Management, 29*(5), 30–31.

Rowland H. S., & Rowland, B. L. (1997). *Nursing administration handbook* (4th ed.). Gaithersburg, MD: Aspen.

Taft, S. H., Minch, E. L., & Jones, P. K. (1992). Strengthening hospital nursing: Part I, the planning process. *Journal of Nursing Administration, 22*(5), 51–63.

Vail, P. B. (1989). *Managing as a performing art.* San Francisco: Jossey-Bass.

Whythe, E. G., & Blair, J. D. (1995). Strategic planning for health care provider organizations. In L. F. Wolper (Ed.), *Health care administration: Principles, practices, structure and delivery* (2nd ed.). Gaithersburg, MD: Aspen.

CHAPTER

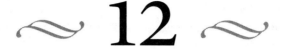

~ 12 ~

Receptivity to Change and Innovation

Sylvia A. Price

Change and innovation are closely related concepts. In our society, change is inevitable and innovation is a necessary component of our culture.
(Author)

Chapter Highlights

- Change and innovation theories and models
- Stages of change
- Organizational behavior model
- Strategies for change
- Resistance to change

The field of nursing administration is continually undergoing change. Changes in the health care delivery system, in science and technology, and in government regulations have made a significant impact on professional nursing administrative practice. Innovation is often perceived as threatening because it usually is accompanied by change while individuals tend to seek stability within their internal or external environment. In many health care institutions nurse executives have added responsibility for patient care-related services in addition to nursing that reflects both cost and quality issues. They must facilitate receptivity to change and innovation. In addition, these nurse executives are often responsible for planning, initiating, and implementing change within nursing and patient care services by converting new ideas or thoughts into action.

Drucker (1985) indicates that innovations may spring from a "flash of genius." However, most innovations, especially the successful ones, result from a conscious, purposeful search for innovation opportunities that are found in only a few situations. He suggests that every organization needs strategies for innovation. These include *(1)* Be the firstest with the mostest. Be first in the market and be first to improve a product or cut its price or both, which discourages prospective competitors. *(2)* Be the second with the mostest strategy. Let someone else establish the market. Be able to satisfy markets with narrow needs and specific capabilities. Provide excellent products for narrow market segments, that is, big purchases with narrow needs. Offer few features. *(3)* Use the niche strategy. Locate a finite market and establish yourself so that it is not worthwhile for others to enter because the market cannot be expanded. *(4)* Make the product your carrier. Develop one product to carry another.

Pearson (1988) also asserts that successful innovations require the following key components: "*(1)* a champion who believes that the new idea is really critical and who will keep pushing ahead, no matter what the roadblocks; *(2)* a sponsor who is high up enough in the organization to marshal its resources—people, money, and time; *(3)* a mix of bright, creative minds (to get ideas) and experienced operators (to keep things practical); *(4)* a process that moves ideas through the system quickly so that they get top-level endorsement, resources, and perspective early in the game—not in the bottom of the ninth inning" (p. 101).

Nurse executives at all organizational levels must be committed and personally involved in the processes of change and innovation. Leaders and members of successful organizations generally set demanding goals for themselves, are more innovative, take more risks, and change at a more accelerated rate. Change has a dominant role within any organizational enterprise. The survival of health care organizations within our society largely depends on their responding appropriately to the forces of change. These forces include such things as science and technological innovations, the knowledge explosion, and social changes. Managing change is a critical element of the nurse executive role. Nurse executives need and use their skills in orchestrating change. Therefore, they must be knowledgeable about the theoretical basis of the change process, understand the reasons for resistance to change, and pursue opportunities for innovation.

CHANGE AND INNOVATION THEORIES AND MODELS

One of the major influences in the early development of change theory was Kurt Lewin (1951), a social scientist. He managed situations where tensions and conflicts were evident by focusing on the cooperative humane element within the situations and by devising ways of managing and improving them. He was a founder of the group dynamics movement; he established the first organization devoted to research on group dynamics in 1945.

Lewin's Force Field Theory

Lewin described the phenomenon of force field theory as a state in which equilibrium is maintained in an organization by the existence of both *driving* and *restraining* forces. Organizations may be experiencing equilibrium with forces pushing for change, while at the same time, there are forces resisting a change to maintain the status quo. For change to occur, the driving forces increase as a result in some movement. These driving forces tend to facilitate change because they push individuals in the desired direction. However, this alteration may also increase resistance by adding strength to the restraining forces. An effective approach might be to reduce or eliminate the restraining forces, thus reaching a new level of equilibrium.

Lewin described changing as a three-step process by *(1)* unfreezing the existing equilibrium or present level. It is in this stage that motivation for change occurs. The group must first make a diagnosis of the problem. Active participation in the identification of the problem and generation of alternate solutions helps to modify attitudes; *(2)* change itself. The emphasis is on moving to a new level of equilibrium in which participants agree that the status quo is not gratifying to them. The actual change or moving requires that new responses be developed based on collected information; *(3)* refreezing or stabilizing the change. The involved individual(s) in this stage integrate new concepts into their own value system that are congruent with the individual's existing self-concept and values. Reinforcement of the new behavior is essential to a successful implementation of the change.

Planned change theory can be envisioned from various perspectives that have their foundations in the Lewinian approach. Changes that are conscious, deliberate, and intended, at least on the part of one or more agents of change, are planned changes. The process of planned change involves a change agent, a client system, and a collaboration to resolve the clients' problems.

Lippitt's Theory

Lippitt (1973) expanded Lewin's theory to a seven-phase planned-change model. His focus was on what the change agent must do, rather than on the evolution of the change. However, he did emphasize the importance of participation of members of the target system. Problem identification, communication, and rapport building are key aspects of the change process. The phases of the model include:

1. Diagnosis of the problem. This is an important step. Involve key individuals in data collection, analysis, and problem identification.
2. Assessment of the motivation and capacity to change. The success of any change program is based on accurate assessment of the potential for change

in individuals, groups, and the environment. Awareness of the need to change must be translated into a desire to change and also requires a readiness and capacity to change. Assess factors such as the availability of resources (human, financial, and physical), organizational climate, structure and function of the organization, timeliness, and the credibility of those initiating the change.

3. Assessment of the change agent's motivation and resources. It is important that the initiator of change clearly assess his or her role in a particular situation. The change agent may be external or internal to the client system. Whether to have an external or internal change agent depends on the identified problem and the environmental conditions in which the change occurs. The external change agent must have credentials and expertise and must gain acceptance with the client system. The internal change agent can usually determine the organizational climate, readiness of the participants to change, and the power bases of key individuals in the organization. A combination of both an external and internal change agent may also be effective.

4. Selection of progressive change objectives. Formulate an action plan, strategies for the change, and establish criteria for evaluation with key individuals participating. The change is usually implemented for a trial period, evaluated, and modified.

5. Identification of the appropriate role(s) for the change agent. The change agent can act as an expert, consultant, facilitator, coordinator, leader, or a combination of these roles. It is important that whichever role(s) is (are) designated, the participants involved understand the expected outcomes.

6. Maintenance of the change. Emphasis on this phase is on the communication process with continuous feedback on progress to all those involved in the change process.

7. Termination of the helping relationship. The change agent gradually withdraws from the situation, allowing the client system to maintain or operationalize the change.

There are limitations to the planned change approach to organizational change. For example, how effective or realistic is the planned change model in today's complex, changing environment? Because health care organizations deal with a high degree of uncertainty, is it realistic to assume that change is conscious, deliberate, and intended as depicted in the planned change model? Can individuals change their behavior if they do not anticipate that this change will give direction and meaning to their work within the organization?

Nurse executives who manage innovative organizations must condition themselves to look for change and innovative opportunities within their organization. They must search for clues on ways to change without disruption. Change must be seen as a challenge, not a threat. Drucker (1990) emphasizes that one should refocus and change the organization when one is successful. Put your efforts into successes, improve the area of success, and change them. He stresses that innovative organizations systematically look both outside and inside for clues to innovative opportunities.

Rogers' Diffusion of Innovation Theory

Another way of examining innovation is to focus on personal characteristics of the individuals involved. Rogers (1983) reviewed studies and used summative techniques to identify personality and demographic characteristics associated with innovativeness. The following discussion illustrates his diffusion of innovation theory.

Rogers envisioned the change process as having antecedents that included both the background of individuals involved in the change and the environment where the change occurred. His five-phase innovation-decision model is a mental process that describes *(1)* how an individual (or other decision-making unit) passes from first knowledge of an innovation, *(2)* forming an attitude toward it, *(3)* making a decision to adopt or reject it, *(4)* implementing the new idea, and, *(5)* confirming the decision (p. 20). He emphasizes the reversible nature of change because participants may initially adopt a proposal or at a later date *discontinue* it; whereas, the reverse may occur, that is, initially reject the proposal but adopt it at a later date.

Rogers conceptualizes the following five-step process to the diffusion of innovation:

1. Knowledge occurs when the individual (or other decision-making unit) is exposed to the innovation and begins to understand how it functions.
2. Persuasion occurs when the individual (or other decision-making unit) forms a favorable (or unfavorable) attitude toward the innovation.
3. Decision occurs when the individual (or other decision-making unit) participates in activities that lead to a choice to adopt or reject the innovation.
4. Implementation occurs when the individual (or other decision-making unit) operationalizes the innovation and reinvention or alterations may occur.
5. Confirmation occurs when the individual (or other decision-making unit) seeks reinforcement that the decision was correct. If there are conflicting messages about the innovation, the original decision may be reversed.

Rogers emphasizes that two important components to a successful change process are that key individuals and policymakers must not only be interested in the innovation but committed to making it happen.

Tornatzky, Eveland, and Fleischer (1990) assert that individual characteristics of innovators do seem to make some difference. In any given setting in which innovation-related activities occur, the personal attributes of participants may be equal to or more important than the group or organizational factors. They state that "no matter what pains are taken to provide the right decision-making processes or reward system, and no matter how pressing and persuasive the external economic environment is, if rigid and timid people are employed in jobs that are key to fostering an innovation process, it will likely fail" (p. 35). However, they note that the best and brightest people do not guarantee success. In many cases, the promise of desirable individual characteristics of participants may be "smothered" by organizational or environmental context.

There are also limits to the use of individual characteristics in relation to making a difference in innovating systems. Certain individual characteristics such as sex or personality tend to be difficult to change. The authors state that the only practical way to use this information is through the selection of participants, which is difficult to do, because we usually have a workforce to start with and rarely have freedom to select at will.

THE 10 STAGES OF CHANGE

Perlman and Takacs (1990) imply that organizations rarely deal consciously or constructively with the human emotions associated with organizational change. Yet, these are the resources and energy from within individuals that are necessary to help accomplish change. They emphasize that to cope with and work through the changes that affect the organization, members must deal with the emotional processes of letting the past die and of experiencing depression. The model presented by Kuebler-Ross (1969) in her book, *On Death and Dying*, is useful in dealing with a major aspect of change: grief. Although she deals with death and dying on an individual level, the stages she presents are compatible with those encountered in organizational change. Perlman and Takacs added five phases to Kuebler-Ross's original five to more fully explain the problems associated with change.

The purpose of the model is to enable practitioners to face some of the more personal and emotional issues that change produces, and to offer tools that will assist them in making conscious choices about dealing with change in the organization.

Phase Equilibrium

1. High energy level. State of emotional and intellectual balance. Professional and personal goals are in harmony.
   Intervention: Inform employees of any change in the environment that will have impact on status quo.
2. Denial. Energy is drained by the defense mechanism of rationalizing or denying of the reality of the change. Employees experience negative changes in physical health, emotional balance, logical thinking patterns, and normal behavior patterns.
   Intervention: Use active listening skills; for example, be emphatic, use reflective listening techniques. Focus on impact of the change.

3. Anger. Energy used to ward off and actively resist the change by blaming others. Frustration, anger become visible.
Intervention: Recognize symptoms, legitimize employee feelings, focus on positive aspects of change.
Active listening, problem-solving skills needed by managers.

4. Bargaining. Energy used in an attempt to eliminate the change. Talk is about "if only." Others try to mediate the problem. Bargains can compromise the needed change.
Intervention: Explore ways of achieving desired changes through conflict management techniques.

5. Chaos. Diffused energy, feeling of powerlessness, sense of insecurity.
Intervention: Quiet time for reflection and listening. Recognition of being in state of flux.

6. Depression. No energy left to produce results. Self-pity, remembering past, expressions of sorrow, and feeling nothingness and emptiness.
Intervention: Provide necessary information in a timely fashion. Allow sorrow and pain to be expressed openly.

7. Resignation. Energy expended in passively accepting change. Lack of enthusiasm.
Intervention: Hold employees accountable for their own behavior, but allow them to move at their own pace.

8. Openness. Availability of renewed energy. Willingness to expend energy on what has been assigned to individual.
Intervention: Patiently explain again in detail the desired change.

9. Readiness. Willingness to expend energy in exploring new events. Reunification of intellect and emotions begins.
Intervention: Assume directive management style: assign tasks, monitor; provide direction/guide.

10. Reemergence. Rechanneled energy produces feelings of empowerment, employees become more proactive.
Intervention: Mutual answering of questions; mutual understanding of role and identity. Employees will take action based on their own decisions.

The generators of change and recipients of change in an organization must work through the various stages to deal effectively with the emotional dimensions of change. If those involved work through the intellectual and emotional issues in each phase, Perlman and Takacs indicate that the organization and its employees will become stronger and the change is more likely to be successful and lead to success.

REAL-TIME STRATEGIC CHANGE

Jacobs (1994) proposes real-time strategic change, which is a contemporary approach to change theory. He stresses that too many organizational change efforts result in frustrated leaders, disillusioned workers, and few, if any, positive lasting changes. The fast-changing pace of our environment leaves organizations struggling to institutionalize new strategies and ways of working, some of which are no longer relevant at the time of implementation. Jacobs believes that the majority of these efforts fall short because the key individuals who are interested in and affected by these changes are not included in planning and implementing them.

He emphasizes that organizations need a better way of changing, that is, to involve large percentages of their employees in shifting from a "business as usual" scenario to a scenario of real-time strategic change. In the real-time scenario, all members of the organization are meaningfully involved in deciding on and responsible for delivering the organization's results.

Real-time strategic change is an overall process, accompanying technology, and the type of results organizations achieve by engaging in the process and applying the technology. It outlines a complete approach to the business of change including the specific phases involved and the various roles required. As a technology it provides a method referred to as a set of principle-based practices and processes that are used in different ways at various phases of a change effort. It is important to note that real-time strategic change defines the results achieved, which are fundamental, far-reaching, and fast-paced change.

Jacobs defines *real time* as "the simultaneous planning and implementation of individual, group, and organization-wide changes. Participants in large group gatherings experience, experiment with, refine, and institutionalize these new ways of doing business in the events themselves and continue to do so over time as they respond to an ever-changing environment" (p. 21). The total organization including individuals, work teams, functional groups, and the organization as a whole practice new ways of doing business as individuals communicate, make decisions, and collaborate in productive and satisfying ways. These individuals leave interactive, organization-wide events clear about why the change is needed, are committed to creating a successful future for themselves and their organization, and are aligned with the organization's overall strategic direction.

Real time emphasizes the importance of current reality as a main driver throughout the process. Jacobs states that real time is a change approach that emphasizes working through real issues with the real people affected by them, and getting results.

ORGANIZATION DEVELOPMENT MODEL

A contemporary approach to the management of change and the development of human resources in organizations has become known as organization development (OD). Davis and Newstrom (1985) emphasize that OD is an intervention strategy that uses group process to analyze the characteristics and features of the organization to focus on change. French and Bell (1990) assert that OD is a top management-supported, long-range effort to improve an organization's problem-solving and renewal processes, particularly through a more effective and collaborative diagnosis and management of organizational culture. They stress that special emphasis must be on the formal work team, temporary team, and intergroup culture—with the assistance of a consultant-facilitator and the use of theory and technology of applied behavior science, including action research.

The OD model is an intervention strategy that uses the group process to achieve planned change by concentrating on the organization's culture. It is based on the assumption that change involves a systematic diagnosis of the total organization, the development of a strategic plan for improvement, and the mobilization of resources to carry out the effort. Changing beliefs, attitudes, values, and structures will be necessary for the organization to grow as well as to survive.

There were two major reasons that OD became an important tool in organizations. First, the reward structure on the job did not provide adequate reinforcement for conventional training programs and it often failed to carry over in the job (Ehrenberg, 1983). Second, technological advances and the acceleration of change requires flexibility in organizations. OD can encourage the organization to foster and respond to change by opening channels of communication, increasing the amount and accuracy of information, and building trust and rapport through a process of group problem-solving at all levels of the organization.

In OD, the emphasis is on the total system and the creation of a climate that fosters learning, creativity, and innovation opportunities that permeate the total enterprise. Change agents, either internal or external, function to stimulate and coordinate change within the group. The experiential learning techniques used include training, role-playing, problem-solving, discussion groups, and lectures. It is important to note that with regard to the methodologies used, emphasis is placed on gaining competence in dealing with interpersonal relationships. Goals often are concerned with developing skills in areas such as communication processes and decision-making. The value system includes an integration of individual needs and management goals, enhanced learning opportunities, and encouragement of more open human relationships.

Action research is the critical element for most OD interventions. It is a process describing a series of events and actions. French and Bell (1990) define it as "the process of systematically collecting research data about an ongoing system relative to some objective, goal, or need of that system; feeding this data back into the system; taking actions by altering selected variables within the system based both on the data and on hypotheses; and evaluating the results of actions by collecting more data" (p. 99).

Davis and Newstrom (1985) describe an action research approach used in OD:

- Initial diagnosis. A decision by management to use and support OD is followed by selection of a change agent or consultant. This individual meets with top management to outline a process to examine the nature of the organization's problems and, subsequently, to develop the series of OD approaches.

- Data collection. Surveys or interviews may be undertaken to determine organizational climate and existing and potential managerial problems. The consultant usually meets with specified work groups within the organization to develop information. Questions to be addressed include: What conditions contribute to or interfere with your job effectiveness? What would you most like to change in the way you function in the organization? What would you most like to change in the way the organization functions?
- Data feedback and confrontation. Small groups are selected to analyze the data collected. Areas of disagreement are mediated and priorities for change established.
- Action planning and problem-solving. Groups use the data analysis and report to develop specific recommendations for change. The discussion focuses on issues in their department, group, or activity. Plans are specific, including specifying who is responsible, and deadlines for completion of action taken.
- Team building. During the entire period of group meetings, the consultant encourages the groups to examine how they work together. The consultant helps them to value open communication and trust as prerequisites for improved group functioning. Team building may be encouraged further by having individual managers and their subordinates work together as a team in OD sessions.
- Intergroup development. After development of small group teams, there may be development among larger groups comprising teams from all levels of the organization.
- Evaluation and follow-up. The consultant helps the organization evaluate the result of the OD efforts and develops additional programs in areas where additional results are needed.

The OD model appears to be a beneficial organizational intervention. Its focus is on a behavioral approach to problem-solving within the total organization. OD is time consuming and costly. Factors such as invasion of privacy and psychological harm must be considered in some of the methods used. The potential for contribution for redesigning work groups to yield productive teams is critical to a successful OD approach.

ORGANIZATIONAL BEHAVIOR MODEL

Organizational behavior emphasizes the nature of individuals and organizations. It is the study of how individuals perform within an organization. The key elements include individuals, structure, technology, and the environment in which the enterprise operates. The role of management is to provide a climate in which organizations function effectively. A major tenet of the organizational behavior approach is understanding of both individual and group behavior. Understanding of this behavior is a complex process. Nadler and Tushman (1980) stress that organizational behavior must be managed despite this complexity. Ultimately, the organization's work is accomplished through people, individually or collectively, on their own or in collaboration with technology. They believe that the management of organizational behavior is central to the management task. This task involves the capacity to *understand* the behavior of individuals, groups, and organizations to *predict* what behavioral responses will be elicited by managerial actions and, finally, to use this understanding and these predictions to achieve control.

Nadler and Tushman have developed a congruence model of organizational behavior that reflects the basic systems concepts and characteristics. This model specifies four critical inputs: *(1)* the environment of all factors outside the organization being examined including such areas as markets, suppliers, governmental and regulatory bodies, labor unions, and competitors; *(2)* organization's resources referred to as a range of different assets to which it has access—employees, technology, capital, and information. One concerns the relative quality of those resources of value in light of the environment; *(3)* the organization's history is important because there is growing evidence that the way organizations function today is influenced by past events; and *(4)* a fourth derivative input, strategy, including the issue of matching the organization's resources to its environment or making the fundamental decision of "What business are we in?" Strategy is a critical input because it determines the work to be performed by the organization and it defines desired organizational outputs.

The major outputs are what the organization produces, how it performs, and how effective it is. One needs not only to be concerned about system's basic output—the product—but to think about other outputs that contribute to organizational performance. When evaluating organizational performance three factors to consider are *(1)* goal attainment, or how well the organization meets its objectives; *(2)* resource utilization, or how well the organization makes use of available resources; and *(3)* adaptability, or whether the organization continues to have a favorable position vis-à-vis environment. In other words, whether it is capable of changing and adapting to its environmental changes.

The last element is the transformation process. Given an environment, a set of resources, and history, the question is "How do I take a strategy and implement it to produce effective performance in the organization, in the group/unit, and among individual employees?" Their model is based on how well components fit together, that is, the congruence among the components; the effectiveness of this model is based on the quality of these "fits" or congruence. These component parts are the fundamental means for transforming energy and information from inputs into outputs.

As depicted in the Nadler-Tushman transformation model, organizations are composed of the following four major components:

1. Task is the basic or inherent work to be done by the organization and its subunits or the activity the organization is engaged in. Emphasis is on the

specific work activities or function that need to be done and their inherent characteristics. For example, analysis of the task would include a description of the basic work flow and function (knowledge or skills demanded by the work, kinds of rewards provided by the work). It is assumed that the reason for the organization's existence is to perform the work (task) consistent with strategy.

2. Individuals who perform organization tasks. Identify the nature and characteristics of the organization's members (individual skills and knowledge, different needs or preferences that individuals have, perceptions or expectancies that they develop, other background factors that may influence individual behavior).

3. Formal organizational arrangements. These include the structures, methods, procedures that are explicitly and formally developed so that individuals will perform tasks consistent with organizational strategy. This activity encompasses a number of factors, including the way jobs are grouped together in units, internal structure of those units, and the coordination and control mechanisms used to link the units together. Other factors to consider are job descriptions, and the work environment which characterizes the immediate environment where work is done, and the organization's formal systems for attracting, placing, developing, and evaluating human resources.

4. Informal organization. Informal arrangements are usually implicit and unwritten but may influence behavior as they include the structures, processes, and arrangements that emerge from within the organization. These adaptations may either aid or hinder the organization's performance (pp. 43–45). (See Figure 12.1.)

The steps in the problem-analysis process of the model are *(1)* to identify symptoms and list data indicating possible existence of problems; and *(2)* to specify inputs by identifying the system and determine the nature of its environment, resources, and history. Identify critical aspects of strategy. Then, identify outputs by indicating data that define the nature of outputs at various levels (individual, group/unit, organizational). This specification should include desired outputs (from strategy) and actual outputs being obtained.

Problems are then identified by indicating areas where there are significant and meaningful differences between desired and actual outputs. To the extent possible, identify penalties; that is, specific costs (actual and opportunity costs) associated with each problem. The basic components of the organization are described in relation to the basic nature of each of the four components with emphasis on their critical factors.

Assess congruence (fits). Conduct analyses to determine relative congruence among organizational components. Generate, identify, and analyze causes to fit with specific problems. Identify action steps and indicate the possible actions to deal with problem causes.

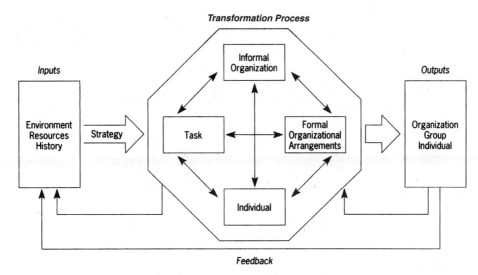

Figure 12.1 A congruence model for organizational analysis. Reprinted from *Organizational Dynamics,* Autumn 1980. Copyright © 1980 American Management Association International. Reprinted by permission of American Management Association International, New York, NY. All rights reserved. http://www.amanet.org.

This congruence model and the problem-analysis process are tools for structuring and dealing with the reality of the complexities of organizational life. It must be noted that there is no one best way of handling a particular situation. Nadler and Tushman emphasize that the model and process could assist the manager in making a number of decisions and evaluating the consequences of them.

STRATEGIES FOR CHANGE

Chin and Beene (1976) propose a three-way classification of the strategies of change. *Empirical-rational* strategies of change are based on the assumptions that humans are guided by reason and follow their rational self-interest once it is disclosed to them. A change is proposed by some person or group that knows of a desirable solution. It is assumed that the individual or group will adopt the proposed change if it can be rationally justified and if it can be demonstrated that the individual or group will gain by the change.

The basic tenet of this strategy is that trust in the scientific method is the predominant motivator by which to change human behavior. Change agents using this model will use research methods to scientifically study the organization to determine the need for change, how it should be carried out, and whether the change, once initiated, has improved the effectiveness of the organization.

Elements of empirical-rational strategies include such areas as recruitment and retention. For example, personnel selection and replacement: there may be an incongruence between the people occupying positions and the job responsibilities. Improving performance requires the development of scientific testing of potentialities and attitudes. Use of applied research and linkage systems for diffusion of research results is another element in this model.

The objective of the *normative reeducative* strategies of change is to improve the problem-solving capabilities of a system. A problem-solving process must affect both the human problems of the organization as well as the system's task requirements set by its goals of production and distribution. Problem-solving processes must be developed to deal with sociotechnical difficulties by converting them into identifiable problems and organizing the relevant processes of data collection, planning, intervention, testing of solutions, evaluation, feedback to results, and re-planning. All of these processes are required in the solution of a problem. Intervention by outside agents is used extensively in implementing this approach to change.

The assumption of this model is focused on human motivation; individuals are motivated primarily by unsatisfied needs. Employees do not passively wait for an administrator to suggest changes. They are in the pursuit of realizing their potential and will initiate changes on their own, if possible.

The person is the basic unit of the social organization. Intervention methods are designed to assist people to discover themselves as "persons" and achieve commitment to continuing personal growth in their interrelationships. People must learn from their experiences if self-directed change is to be maintained and continued. The elements of normative-educative strategies imply that the emphasis is on the client system and involvement in programs of change and improvement. The role of the change agent is to implement the change by intervening mutually and collaboratively with the client system.

Power-coercive change strategies approaches to effecting change are based on the assumption that power is part of all social interactions. The differences among social interactions lie in the sources of power on which the strategies of change depend and the ways in which power is generated and applied in the processes of effecting change. The application of power results in a state wherein those with greater power alter the behaviors of those who have less power. The ingredients of power that power-coercive strategies use are the political and economic sanctions in the exercise of power. Political power carries with it legitimacy and the sanctions associated with those who break the law. Economic power exerts coercive influence over the decisions of individuals to whom it is applied.

The objective of power-coercive strategies of change is to increase political and economic power for the goals that the strategists of change have determined to be desirable. The elements of this model focus on the use of nonviolent strategies for indicating value conflicts and specifying the inequities in existing patterns. Sit-ins and other types of nonviolent demonstrations are also used. Political power is essential to achieving changes in institutional life; normative reeducative strategies must be combined with political coercion before and after the political action so that the public is adequately informed and accepts the changes in practice.

Beckard and Pritchard (1992) suggest developing a commitment plan and implementing strategies that will achieve desired results. Some of the strategies they recommend are:

- Establishing a mechanism to identify problems
- Instituting educational activities for managing organizational change and helping individuals understand the reasons for change
- Ensuring that the organizational leadership demonstrates its own commitment to change
- Encouraging collaboration even when individuals have widely different ideas and knowledge bases
- Improving communication strategies (pp. 79–84)

Successful Change Strategies

An example of a successful change effort is illustrated in the professional nursing practice model at Sioux Valley Hospital (SVH), a 475-bed tertiary care hospital, that implemented a patient care delivery system based on differentiated practice on five demonstration units. The project was designed to position nurses as true business partners with other major individuals in the health care industry (Koerner, Bunkers & Nelson, 1991; Koerner, Bunkers, Nelson, & Santema, 1989). In an effort to recognize and use the abilities of the nurse, SVH selected factoring as the mechanism for placing nurses in their respective roles. RNs on each model unit were factored into either the ADN (Case Associate) or BSN (Case Manager) job description in collaboration with their head nurse. Individuals were "frozen" into their selected job description for a minimum of 3 months. Then, positions were reopened, allowing for transfer to the alternate role if a staff nurse or manager felt uncomfortable with the job description originally selected.

Staff were requested to be more autonomous and accountable and management to change their behavior from directing and controlling to one of facilitating staff to manage their own practice. Koerner et al. (1989) imply that a critical factor in the success of implementing differentiated practice lies in adequate and repeated staff development programs. This differentiated nursing practice model has shown that factoring allows currently licensed nurses to use the competencies they have developed through professional activities and experience since graduation. The differentiated nursing practice model is discussed in more detail in Chapter 4.

Beer, Eisenstat, and Spector (1990) state in a provocative article that although senior managers understand the necessity of change to cope with new competitive realities, they often underestimate what it takes to bring it about. They tend to assume that promulgating company-wide programs that include mission statements, "coporate culture" programs, training courses, quality circle programs, and new pay-for-performance systems will transform organizations and change employee behavior. In their study of organizational change at six large corporations, they found the opposite to be true: the major obstacle to revitalization is the idea that it comes about through company-wide change programs, especially when a corporate staff group such as human resources is the sponsor. They believe successful change efforts focus on the work itself, that is, by aligning employee roles, responsibilities, and relationships to address the organization's most important competitive task, or "task alignment." It is their belief that any approach to change starting at the periphery and moving steadily toward the corporate core is the most effective way to achieve enduring organizational change. Managing change involves process over specific content, recognizes organization as a unit-by-unit learning process rather than a series of programs, and acknowledges the payoffs that result from persistence over a long period of time are superior to quick fixes.

This change strategy could be applicable to health care organizations because of the need to make changes in providing programs that address issues in cost containment and involve consumers in their choice of health care options.

Resistance to Change

A significant aspect of the change process involves an alteration in the status quo. Often when any change is proposed, resistance may surface. Organizational change efforts frequently encounter human resistance.

Argyris (1992) emphasizes that anyone who has planned major organizational change realizes how difficult it is to foresee accurately all the major problems that occur. This includes the enormous amount of time needed to iron out the kinks and get individuals to accept the change and the apparent lack of internal commitment to help make the plan work. This is manifested partly by individuals at all levels resisting taking the initiative to make modifications that they envision are necessary so that the new plan can work. He reviewed his notes regarding implement change from 32 major reorganizations in large organizations where he was a consultant or had a research role. He found that not one could be labeled as fully completed and integrated 3 years after the change had been announced, that is, individuals were still fighting, ignoring, resisting, and blaming the reorganization without feeling a strong obligation personally to correct this situation.

Argyris believes the reasons for this delay are embedded in the change strategy typically used by management. The basic strategy has been for top management to take the responsibility to overcome and outguess the resistance to change. This strategy does not tend to succeed because management works hard, applies pressure, which creates resisting forces that are costly to the organization's effectiveness, its long-run viability and flexibility as well as to individuals at all levels. He suggests that management experiment with the strategy of reducing the restraining forces by involving, at least, the management employees at all levels in the diagnosis, design, and execution of the change program.

Nurse executives must assess those individuals in the organization who are likely to resist the change initiative and attempt to ascertain their reasons for resisting. Individuals or groups can react very differently to change—from being apathetic to it, to aggressively opposing it, or to quickly adopting it, or sabotaging it. Nurse executives need to be aware of the most common reasons people resist organizational change. Kotter and Schlesinger (1979) present the following reasons:

- People think they will lose something of value because they focus on their own best interests and not those of the total organization.
- People misunderstand the change and its implications, and they perceive that it is likely to cost them more than they will gain.
- People assess the situation differently from those initiating the change and believe that greater costs than benefits will result from the change for themselves as well as for the organization.
- People have low tolerance for the change because they fear they will not be able to develop the new skills and behavior that are required of them.

Resistance to change may be caused by errors on the part of the change agent or consultant who may not communicate trust or may not understand the nature of the advocated change and its relevance to the client system. Resistance should be viewed constructively by change agents.

Rubin, Plovnick, and Fry (1974) point out that by resisting change, whether actively or passively, an organization is communicating a message—it is providing data. In a very real sense, an organization is telling us something about "who it is"—its major resources, and limitations, its attitude toward outsiders and change, its important internal norms and values, and the nature of its relationship to other systems in the environment.

Zaltman and Pinson (cited in Zaltman and Duncan [1977]) state that resistance is not simply lack of acceptance or the reverse of acceptance of a proposed change. It may reflect clients' attitudes toward innovation itself. For example, when an innovation is incompatible with a particular norm, it may be accepted by one person as a symbol of defiance and rejected by another who fears social disapproval. An innovation may be a source of attraction to visionaries and a source of resistance to more conservative clients.

One of the most important sources of resistance to change is the perception that the change will be a threat to the power or influence of various parts of the organization. When two or more organizations merge, a difficult problem to overcome is the feeling on the part of the individual organizations that they are going to lose, or have diminished control, over decision-making. Change should be presented in a way that minimizes the degree to which it is perceived as threatening.

Members of the merged organizations must be informed about the need and consequences of the change. They must be active participants in the change process. Nurse executives and unit nurse managers need to assist their staff in accepting change by providing necessary information, emotional support, and an educational environment for upgrading skills.

The structure and climate within an organization can effect resistance to change. individuals should be able to experience a need for change, accept the reality of change, and be committed to it. Finally, there must be a potential for change in the system and some control or influence over the anticipated change.

Carr, Hard, and Trahant (1996) state that real change succeeds only in the presence of a compelling need for it. Currently, there are four types of forces that are driving organizations to change. These include:

- **Market forces.** Global competition, new market opportunities, and changing customer needs.
- **Rapidly changing technologies.** Technology changes almost as rapidly as the weather and long-term forecasts have similar reliability. The rapid pace of technological change is relevant to organizations that use the technologies. They offer the potential for competitive advantage or parity, but only when an organization changes to create new ways of doing business using the high-tech tools. The days of gaining lasting advantage from simply automating current processes are over.
- **Changing political institutions and societies.** Putting business and services in private hands has long been a factor of increased activity and productivity. The two most significant trends are the privatization of organizations that were once run by the government or a monopoly and the need for government organizations to become more efficient and less costly to operate.
- **Internal need to improve performance and competitive situations.** Although the external world creates many compelling needs for change, the internal one is the daily reality for most organizations. Shareholder dissatisfaction, falling profits or market share, and threats to corporate survival itself command the most immediate attention (pp. 30–34).

SUMMARY

Receptivity to change and innovation can be envisioned from various perspectives. Innovation can be a flash of genius or changes that are conscious, deliberate, and intended—at least on the part of one or more agents of change. Lewin's theory of change involves three stages of change that are referred to as unfreezing, moving, and refreezing. Lippitt expanded Lewin's theory to a seven-phase change-process model. Rogers model focuses on the innovation-decision process. Jacobs proposes real-time strategic change, which is a contemporary approach to change theory.

Proponents of an organizational behavior model believe that it is the management of organizational behavior that is central to the management task. Organizational development (OD), on the other hand, is an intervention strategy that uses group processes in an attempt to modify or change beliefs, attitudes, values, and structures for the organization to adapt and survive in our changing society.

For change to succeed in an organization, whether through planned change, OD, the application of organizational behavior models, the individuals must be supportive of or agreeable to the change. Significant components of the nurse executive role include continually pursuing sources of opportunities for innovation and being a facilitator in providing a learning environment that enhances the change process. Organizations must constantly search for ways to innovate and change to survive in today's competitive marketplace.

STUDY QUESTIONS

1. Change and innovation within an organizational enterprise are resourceful ideas or approaches to existing challenges. They are usually proposed to improve some aspect of the operative units of the organization. You are to propose an innovation that should be responsive to an existing need or problem in a health care organization. What change or innovation theory would guide your planned change?
2. Describe a situation and identify the existing problem, the need for change, and the appropriate rationale. Specify the design of your plan including the change model you propose to use, the process for implementation, projected timetable for each phase, proposed budget (estimate of costs for human and physical resources), evaluation process, and all possible resources, values, cultural climate, or organizational conflicts.
3. Why do people resist change in any practice setting? Describe at least three reasons why people resist organizational change.

REFERENCES

Argyris, C. (1992). *On organizational learning.* Cambridge, MA: Blackwell.

Beckard, R., & Pritchard, W. (1992). *Changing the essence: The art of creating and leading fundamental change in organizations.* San Francisco: Jossey-Bass.

Beer, M., Eisenstat, R., & Spector, B. (1990). Why change programs don't produce change. *Harvard Business Review, 68*(6), 158–166.

Carr, D. K., Hard, K., & Trahant, W. (1996). *Managing the change process: A field book for change agents, consultants, team leaders, and reengineering managers.* New York: McGraw-Hill.

Chin, R., & Beene, K. (1976). General strategies for effecting changes in human systems. In W. Bennis, K. Beene, & K. Corey (Eds.). *The Planning of Change* (3rd ed., pp. 22–45). New York: Holt, Rinehart & Winston.

Davis, K., & Newstrom, J. (1985). *Human behavior at work: Organization behavior* (7th ed.). New York: McGraw-Hill.

Drucker, P. F. (1985). The discipline of innovation. *Harvard Business Review, 43*(3), 67–72.

Drucker, P. F. (1990). *Managing the nonprofit organization.* New York: HarperCollins.

Ehrenberg, L. (1983). How to ensure better transfer of learning. *Training and Development Journal, 2,* 81–83.

French, W., & Bell, C. (1990). *Organization development: Behavioral science interventions for organization improvement* (4th ed.). Englewood Cliffs, NJ: Prentice-Hall.

Jacobs, R. W. (1994). *Real time strategic change.* San Francisco: Berrett-Kohler.

Koerner, J., Bunkers, L., & Nelson, B. (1991). Change: A professional challenge. *Nursing Administration Quarterly, 16*(1), 15–21.

Koerner, J., Bunkers, L., Nelson, B., & Santema K. (1989). Implementing differentiated practice: The Sioux Valley Hospital experience. *Journal of Nursing Administration, 19*(2), 13–20.

Kotter, J., & Schlesinger, L. (1979). Choosing strategies for change. *Harvard Business Review, 57*(2), 106–114.

Kuebler-Ross, E. (1969). *On death and dying.* New York: MacMillan.

Lewin, K. (1951). *Field theory in social science: Selected theoretical papers.* New York: Harper & Brothers.

Lippitt, G. (1973). *Visualizing change: Model building and the change process.* Fairfax, VA: NTL Learning Resources Corporation.

Nadler, D., & Tushman, M. (1980). A model for diagnosing organizational behavior, *Organizational Dynamics, 9*(4), 35–51.

Pearson, A. (1988). Tough-minded ways to get innovative. *Harvard Business Review, 67*(3), 99–106.

Perlman, D., & Takacs, G. (1990). The 10 stages of change. *Nursing Management, 21*(4), 33–38.

Rogers, M. (1983). *Diffusion of innovations* (3rd ed.). New York: The Free Press.

Rubin, I., Plovnick, M., & Fry, R. (1974). Initiating planned change in health care systems. *Journal of Applied Behavioral Science, 10*(1), 107–124.

Tornatzky, L., Eveland, J., & Fleischer, M. (1990). Technological innovation as a process. In L. Tarnatzky & M. Fleischer (Eds.), *The processes of Technological Innovation* (pp. 27–50). Lexington, KY: Lexington Books.

Zaltman, G., & Duncan, R. (1977). *Strategies for planned change.* New York: Wiley.

CHAPTER

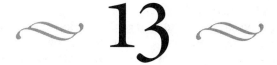

13

Effective Communication

Lillian M. Simms • Phyllisis M. Ngin

Without regular communication with others, we are limited to knowing only what is happening in our own environment. (Authors)

Chapter Highlights

- Communication with self
- Anger as an impediment
- Revitalization of self
- One-to-one communication
- Group communication
- Formal and informal groups
- The computer as a communication tool
- Public speaking

The purpose of this chapter is to present communication as a concept and a basic management skill with emphasis on the personal aspects of communication. Anger is discussed as an impediment to communication with self and others. Levels of communication with self and others are explored and the computer is presented as the key to your second self and expanded communication capabilities. Communicating clearly and effectively is always difficult and anger creates a distinct barrier to communication. Learning to observe and change our part in relationship patterns is important in practicing new behavioral responses to anger. According to Lerner (1997), we cannot make other people change their steps to an old dance but we can change our own steps and then the dance will no longer continue in the same pattern.

What messages do I convey about myself to others? Everyday we convey our thoughts and ideas to others through our work and behavior. Gold (1978) describes communication as both a cause of consternation and an enigma. Bordon and Stone (1976) describe it as a contact sport, our only way of contacting others. Communication is the hub of existence and a basic self-tool for survival.

Everything written about communication would consume volumes. A meaningful distillate emerges in the words of Gold: "Whatever else communication is, its definition, scope and purpose, it is a process, and not simply one of language and all its component parts" (Gold, 1978, p. 72). It is a process with a purpose that an individual consciously or unconsciously uses to affect others.

Each of us has a personality and an appearance like that of no one else in the world. This uniqueness is our most valuable attribute, and it represents a balance between our personal role identities and our professional role identities. All communications between nurses and others involve the two role identities, and they may come into conflict when personal goals conflict with organizational expectations (Bradley & Edinberg, 1982). In the fully functioning administrator, the two personalities merge.

Communication is the central part of everything done in administration. Words are powerful tools because they enrich life by expanding the range of human experience. Without regular communication with others, we are limited to knowing only what is happening in our own environment. Communication is thus a key to creativity and the creative experience (Csikszentmihalyi, 1996). Communication, or lack of it, is one of the most frequently mentioned problems in a division of nursing. Nurse executives write for others to read and read what others have written. Everyday communication flows to and from the nurse executive by virtue of telephone, written materials, computer printouts, and meetings. The basic purpose of communication is to effect change in our environment, in others, and in ourselves. Spheres of communication and related skills are portrayed in Figure 13.1.

COMMUNICATING WITH SELF

Building on earlier work by McGregor and Robinson (1981) Simms, Price, and Ervin in 1994 present communications with self as the element of first importance in communication matrix, followed by communication one-to-one and in small and large groups. The most valuable tools for handling criticism and blame are the confidence and perspective one gains by knowing and communicating with oneself. To communicate with oneself necessitates taking time to think and dream. It involves introspection and self-awareness. It mandates coming to grips with oneself regarding who one is, how one presents oneself, what one thinks is

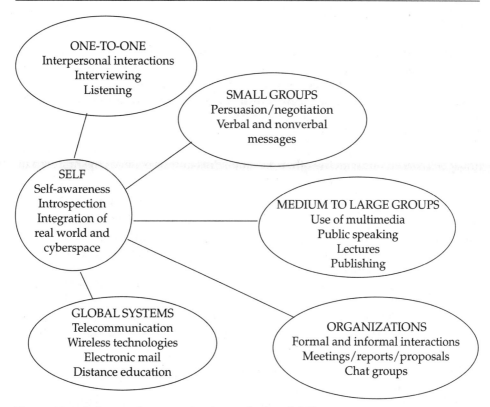

Figure 13.1 Spheres of communication and related skills.

important in life, and, in doing this, determining one's own philosophy of life. It means knowing one's own energy cycle and knowing what place at home or work provides the solitude needed for creative thinking. To be comfortable with oneself in solitude can be energizing.

Time for communication with oneself can be misused if spent in self-blame. Self-criticism is important and an important part of self-renewal if used appropriately. Set aside time on your calendar to think and dream. Take a walk, putter in the kitchen or garden, or sit in a rocking chair and stare engrossed in your own thoughts. Develop a curiosity about your own thoughts, ask yourself questions about an idea. Try to extract a logical decision from intuition. Recognize your brewing times—times when no ideas come forth and you know you are unconsciously mulling over an idea.

Read literature other than that required for your work. Read novels that will help you fantasize. Read science fiction. Above all, take the time to appreciate your surroundings and environment. Come to know yourself and understand how you perceive your environment. The ability to think clearly in abstract terms emanates from the ability to communicate with yourself.

Anger

One area in which communication with oneself is very important is anger. Duldt (1981a) states that health professionals frequently encounter anger in their daily practice, yet it is rarely studied. Anger interferes with communication with others and above all with the self. Anger turned inward is a self-destructive process that can lead to depression and burnout (Figure 13.2 presents Duldt's description of the process of anger) (1981b). One needs to recognize the source of anger and explore the underlying reasons for it. Although many authors assume that anger must be worked out with the other person(s), this author believes the first step in resolution of angers is to talk to oneself.

Anger is but one of numerous emotions that may be experienced during communication. The term *active listening* is commonly advocated in discussions on effective communication and anger can seriously impede listening. The relationship between anger and communication has always been noted in the psychiatric nursing literature under topics related to therapeutic communication and anger (Janosik & Davies, 1996). Generally, these discussions are related to nurse-client interactions not with nurse-nurse or nurse-health professional. Other links have been made with violence in the workplace (Noer, 1993), but few authors other than Duldt (1981a) have targeted anger as a barrier to everyday communication in the workplace.

Duldt's description of the process of anger (see Figure 13.2) published in 1981 is still relevant in today's organization and various replications by other authors have not changed the basic steps in the process. Duldt's work on anger has recently been rediscovered in Minneapolis at the University of Minnesota Health System as the nursing department developed characteristics and behaviors of a healthy work environment (Kreitzer et al., 1997). The project team concluded that effective interpersonal relationships are based on open communication, trust, and mutual respect; recognition of and dealing with anger are an essential part of creating a healthy workplace.

Nurse executives should pay attention to both the facts and emotions conveyed in various encounters of conversation. Eye contact, touching, handshakes, activities that tend to be forgotten in human interactions, help bridge the gaps in communication and counteract anger. Noer (1993) addresses the need to deal with anger of survivors of severance in organizations who perceive unfairness in top management severance and bonus payments at the expense of employees and retirees. The related anger is widespread in downsizing organizations and profoundly affects the employees who remain. A thirst for information stimulates the need for more and improved communication at all levels—up, down, laterally, oral, written, formal, informal, verbal, and nonverbal. Anger can be detrimental to learning. Feelings of helplessness trigger feelings of anger and even rage, which interferes with effective communication. In receiving information, nurse executives should pay attention to both the facts and emotions conveyed. Paraphrasing for clarification and understanding is important. In giving information/feedback, communication should be specific and not judgmental. Embedded in these precepts is the

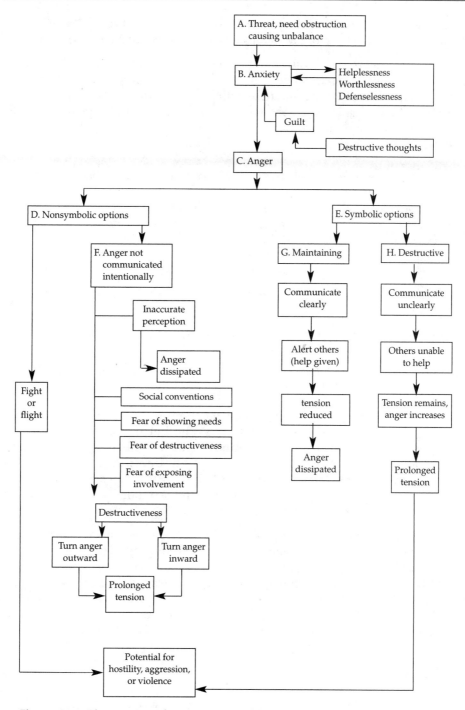

Figure 13.2 The process of anger. From Duldt, B. W. (1981). Anger: An occupational hazard for nurses. *Nursing Outlook, 29*(9), 514. Copyright 1981 by Mosby-Yearbook, Inc. Reprinted with permission.

attempt to address emotions. Employers and employees contribute to anger in the workplace in the form of low self-esteem and ineffective coping strategies.

According to Allcorn (1994), anger and accompanying aggression can contribute to innovation and productivity or be major blocks of work and change. Non-adaptive expressions of anger interfere with personal judgment and lead to self-defeating communication and behavior. The communication of anger may range from open, direct communication to passive and covert communication. Allcorn recognizes seven angry types:

1. Big talkers who monopolize conversations and make unrealistic promises and statements
2. Blamers who believe others are responsible for their anger
3. Creators who exhibit behaviors that include projection, denial, rationalization, and displacement and find many covert ways of communicating their anger
4. Day dreamers who remain detached or removed from ongoing events and conversations
5. Doers who are overly energized workers, often motivated by an unhealthy need to achieve
6. Saboteurs who withhold participation, information, and effort and are resistant to change
7. Stuffers who have learned to suppress their feelings and seek to hide conflict rather than deal with it

It is important to recognize that anger is an emotion, a state of arousal. Look at yourself in a mirror. Ask yourself what factors contributed to your state of anger. What did you do to bring about the condition? What did others do? What is the pattern of your anger? At whom is it most frequently directed? In what other ways could you react to the same situations? Most organizations recognize excess stress and burnout as interferences with good administration. Few realize the importance of understanding and using anger.

Venting your anger with yourself can occur in various ways. Talk to yourself. Write to yourself. Explain why you are angry. View yourself as objectively as you can. Pretend your best friend is in the same situation. What would you advise him or her to do? Map out a strategy for resolving the anger in the most constructive and least constructive ways. Set a time and date for resolving the problem. Allocate a set time each day for communicating with yourself about the problem, but do not allow yourself to spend more than the allotted time. Continual reworking of the problem can also be destructive.

Revitalization of Self

Another period of communicating with oneself is the special time between jobs when one has time to introspect and revitalize oneself. This may be an enforced period because opportunities did not develop as planned or because a position was phased out because of funding changes or reorganization. Increasingly, nurse executives are subject to severance because of conflicting philosophies with medical staff or hospital administration. This period of time can be productive or depressing, depending on one's approach.

Do not make excuses for what went wrong. Analyze the situation in terms of what you learned. Attempt to reopen your mind to all the facts that contributed to the situation. Use this time to sort out your thinking and make decisions about new goals. This can be a fruitful period for self-analysis and self-assessment in terms of personal history. Organize your thoughts and plan to speak to others regarding your experiences. This will not only force you to redirect yourself in a positive manner but will also allow you to share your expertise with others.

The following questionnaire is designed to give you tentative insight into your current tendencies toward nonassertiveness (passivity), assertiveness, or aggressiveness. The Assertiveness Scale (Figure 13.3, pages 234–35) is primarily a self-examination and discussion device.

ONE-TO-ONE COMMUNICATION

Nurse executives play a complex, intertwined combination of interpersonal, informational, and decisional roles. Mintzberg (1975) describes the administrator as the nerve center of the organizational unit. Administrators require "soft" information as well as "hard" data. Soft information can be **gossip, hearsay, or speculation.** It may be acquired on the telephone, in the office, in the coffee shop, in the restroom, or by the water cooler. First-rate soft information greatly enhances the quantity and quality of information stored in the brain of the nurse executive. Mintzberg (1975) stated that the executive may not know everything, but he or she typically knows more than any member of the staff.

One-to-one communication may be thought of in terms of giving and receiving information. The inexperienced executive may not fully realize the value of listening and may perceive one-to-one communication only as an opportunity for disseminating information and delegation. The effective executive spends more time listening than talking. Regularly scheduled one-to-one conferences with subordinates create a positive, healthy climate for interaction—a time for the executive to get to know the staff and a time for staff to understand the executive as a person with goals and ideals for change.

These conferences would be scheduled on a regular basis with all workers who report directly to the nurse executive. In addition to getting to know each other, the one-to-one conference serves several other purposes:

- Updating each other on projects, problem areas, and other pertinent topics
- Educating each other about clinical or administrative areas
- Joint problem-solving
- Working on written material
- Guiding and coaching staff

Are You Passive, Assertive, or Aggressive?

The following questionnaire is designed to give you tentative insight into your current tendencies toward nonassertiveness (passivity), assertiveness, or aggressiveness. The Assertiveness Scale is primarily a self-examination and discussion device. Answer each question mostly true or mostly false as it applies to you.

	Mostly True	Mostly False
1. It is extremely difficult for me to turn down a sales representative when that individual is a nice person.	___	___
2. I express criticism freely.	___	___
3. If another person were being very unfair, I would bring it to that person's attention.	___	___
4. Work is no place to let your feelings show.	___	___
5. No use asking for favors; people get what they deserve on the job.	___	___
6. At work is not the place for tact; say what you think.	___	___
7. If a person looked like he or she were in a hurry, I would let that person in front of me in a supermarket line.	___	___
8. A weakness of mine is that I'm too nice a person.	___	___
9. If my restaurant bill is even 25 cents more than it should be, I demand that the mistake be corrected.	___	___
10. I have laughed out loud in public more than once.	___	___
11. I've been described as too outspoken by several people.	___	___
12. I am quite willing to have the store take back a piece of furniture that has a scratch.	___	___
13. I dread having to express anger toward a co-worker.	___	___
14. People often say that I'm too reserved and emotionally controlled.	___	___
15. Nice guys and gals finish last in our business.	___	___
16. I fight for my rights down to the last detail.	___	___
17. I have no misgivings about returning an overcoat to the store if it doesn't fit me properly.	___	___
18. If I have had an argument with a person, I try to avoid him or her.	___	___
19. I insist on my spouse (roommate or partner) doing his or her fair share of undesirable chores.	___	___
20. It is difficult for me to look directly at another person when the two of us are in disagreement.	___	___
21. I have cried among friends more than once.	___	___
22. If someone near me at a movie kept up a conversation with another person, I would ask him or her to stop.	___	___
23. I am able to turn down social engagements with people I do not particularly care for.	___	___
24. It is poor taste to express what you really feel about another individual.	___	___
25. I sometimes show my anger by swearing at or belittling another person.	___	___
26. I am reluctant to speak up in meetings.	___	___
27. I find it relatively easy to ask friends for small favors such as giving me a lift to work when my car is being serviced or repaired.	___	___

continued

28. If another person was smoking in a restaurant and it bothered me, I would inform that person. ____ ____
29. I often finish other people's sentences for them. ____ ____
30. It is relatively easy for me to express love and affection toward another person. ____ ____

Scoring and Interpretation

Score yourself plus 1 for each of your answers that agrees with the scoring key. If your score is 10 or less, it is probably that you are currently a nonassertive individual. A score of 11 through 24 suggests that you are an assertive individual. A score of 25 or higher suggests that you are an aggressive individual. Retake this test about 30 days from now to give yourself some indication of the stability of your answers. You might also discuss your answers with a close friend to determine if that person has a similar perception of your assertiveness. Here is the scoring key.

1. Mostly false	11. Mostly true	21. Mostly true
2. Mostly true	12. Mostly true	22. Mostly true
3. Mostly true	13. Mostly false	23. Mostly true
4. Mostly false	14. Mostly false	24. Mostly false
5. Mostly false	15. Mostly true	25. Mostly true
6. Mostly true	16. Mostly true	26. Mostly false
7. Mostly false	17. Mostly true	27. Mostly true
8. Mostly false	18. Mostly false	28. Mostly true
9. Mostly true	19. Mostly true	29. Mostly true
10. Mostly true	20. Mostly false	30. Mostly true

Figure 13.3 Self-assessment tool on personal communication style. DuBrin, A. J. (1988). *Contemporary applied management* (2nd ed., pp. 50–52). Plano, TX: Business Publications. Reprinted with permission.

This last purpose is perhaps the most important function of the nurse executive who is interested in improving the functioning of the staff. The nurse executive will need to assess each worker's strengths and areas for improvement and to encourage self-assessment. Part of each conference time is then spent on providing guidance in the areas for improvement. Various approaches will be needed in providing guidance, for example, discussion about options for problems, role-playing assertiveness, and suggesting literature to read. One-to-one conferences are reduced over time as individual workers assume more responsibility for their own development and creative behavior.

"Imaginization" is about creativity and is related to communication and shared understandings. One of the functions of leadership says Morgan (1993) is to generate a sense of shared visions and shared values (see Chapter 5). The coffee corner, the computer work station, the water fountain, and various other points of human interaction are important to breaking down old communication lines. As dysfunctional departments are replaced by decentralized decision-making work units, information can flow effectively using all the communication tools available to humans and in interesting and new patterns.

The Interview

Interviews are golden opportunities to assess the quality of another's attributes and determine the potential for fit with the organization. It is also a time for the interviewer to present himself or herself as an administrator with a sense of direction and enthusiasm for a creative, stimulating work environment. The interview is a special form of one-to-one communication, allowing for both concentrated presentation of self and listening. As with any one-to-one conversation, the participants are particularly vulnerable to overdisclosure of information. The interaction mandates participation, for no others are present.

The skilled interviewer prepares in advance, giving attention to topics to be covered or omitted. One important ingredient for preparation is a careful review of the applicant's resumé. The development of a list of questions can be started from this review, noting such inquiries as major responsibilities in the last position, recent content of continuing education programs attended, presentations, and focus of graduate study. In addition to review of the resumé, the interviewer will want to gather written information about the position and organization, if this was not previously sent to the applicant.

The major goal of a job interview is to determine the best match of individual with a specific position at a given point in time. Another goal of an interview is to make a friend for the organization. Even if the applicant is not eventually offered a position, the skilled interviewer is able to conclude the interview on a positive note and convey appreciation for interest in the organization. An applicant who feels good about the interview and organization is more likely to make positive statements and refer others for jobs.

Verbal Communication

Verbal communication may be thought of as the transmission of human ideas through either the spoken or the written word. Verbal communication can therefore be first or second hand, direct or indirect. First-hand, or direct, verbal communication comes out of the oral cavity without opportunity for editorial changes. Second-hand communication—in the form of reports, bulletins, schedules, rumors, assorted papers, and other media—has the potential for tampering with and editing the original data.

Administrators constantly have the problem of putting their words on paper. As Swift (1973) states, the administrator's words in memos and letters are almost always designed to change the behavior of others in the organization. Intelligent written communications are the result of thinking well, composing ideas, writing down the message, editing, and rewriting. Many nurse executives dictate the first draft and then edit and rewrite as needed.

Effective written communication is hard work. Swift (1973) suggests that, to write effectively, administrators must isolate and define the critical variables in the proposed message and then scrutinize the message for clarity, simplicity, and time. He describes writing as feedback and a way for the administrator to discover the self. It is the evidence of one's thinking. In other words, if administrators write well, they think well. If they learn to think well, it will be more likely that they will write well. There is no better way to foster creative thinking habits than to develop message-writing skills.

Fielden (1982) suggests that, to get messages across, one must vary writing style to suit each situation. Expert writers select a style that fits a particular reader and the particular writing situation. Situations are described as positive or negative, conveying good or bad news. Or they may convey a directive or information. Whatever the case, the writer chooses the appropriate words and format to produce the desired result.

The nurse executive must determine the desired effect and select a writing style that will achieve that purpose. Fielden (1982) suggests the following styles as examples:

1. Forceful: direct and active
2. Passive: low power and ambiguous
3. Personal: friendly and positive
4. Impersonal: nonuse of personal names
5. Colorful: flowery, many adjectives and verbs

In addition, nurse executives should develop a vocabulary that personalizes all their messages.

Nonverbal Communication

Nonverbal communication emanates from each person in personality style, choice of food, housing, office arrangement, priorities for appointments, and social habits. In other words, one's behavior travels as an advance guard every time one speaks in public or attends public activities. Everything an executive does is open for discussion, either positive or negative. Does one always go along with the crowd, or does one favor individualized activities? How much does the executive value personal privacy? Overemphasis on personal privacy may be viewed as detrimental to the organization. The effective executive uses nonverbal communication deliberately.

Nonverbal messages are also conveyed through dress, body postures, gestures, facial expressions, and voice intonations and are just as important as verbal communication. In fact, less than 10% of a message's impact is from its verbal content. The rest of the impact is nonverbal, from vocal inflections and content, and facial expressions. Our voice intonations and facial expressions are revealed subconsciously but they nevertheless display our feelings, communicating our emotions as well. When the nonverbal message contradicts the verbal message, more weight is placed on the nonverbal content of our overall communication.

It is perhaps useful to also note that just as words have different meanings in different cultures or communities, so do most forms of nonverbal communication. Displays of affect (e.g., sadness, joy, or anger) vary in their forms and meanings (Trompanaar, 1993) and as such can lead to embarrassment at best and misunderstanding and communication breakdown at worst.

GROUP COMMUNICATION

Nurse executives spend most of their time in communication, and committee meetings are increasingly becoming the most frequent group activity. The executive is also involved in large-group, formal presentations within or outside the organization. Public speaking as a special form of group communication is addressed later in this chapter. Small and medium-sized groups are usually task forces or committees established to advance management objectives and facilitate the work of the organization.

A critical problem is wasted time through unproductive committee work. Chronically unproductive committees should not exist simply because participants enjoy themselves. Perhaps the committee does not need to exist or it consists of the wrong people. The nurse executive needs to decide which groups should exist and whether they should be standing or ad hoc groups. Different purposes for group meetings are generally to:

- Transmit information
- Promote harmony
- Solicit information from group
- Seek new ideas
- Mobilize a group (Costello-Nickitas, 1997)

All contribute to the database of the nurse executive and are assistive in decision-making or implementing decisions. Although other skills are important in group meetings, those of listening, persuasion, and debate are especially important for the practicing nurse executive.

Organizing for a committee meeting is a skill that all nurse executives must possess and must teach by example. An organized agenda should include the topic, person responsible, action to be taken, and allotted time. If problem-solving is the action to be taken, sufficient time must be allocated for discussion and debate. The executive will be aware if the group is not moving to resolution and can adjust the agenda. Another key factor in having productive meetings is to have members come to the meeting prepared. If materials are to be discussed, they should be distributed well enough in advance.

Persuasion

McGregor and Robinson (1981) define persuasion as any effort to influence or change the beliefs, attitudes, or feelings of another person. The principal purpose of persuasion is to influence change in a planned direction. An individual or group will be persuaded more quickly if the speaker has the group's attention and has personal and professional credibility. The nurse executive will attempt to persuade individuals as well as groups. In both cases, familiarity with concepts and evidence is crucial. Repetition of key words and phrases needs to occur with group members both inside and outside of scheduled meetings.

Nurse executives can learn through practice and appropriate workshops to be highly skilled persuaders. Attention to interpersonal skills, dressing to match the meeting environment, and the ability to argue without abrasiveness contribute to the effectiveness of the persuader. Dress for both comfort and personal style. The image one conveys is another message of persuasion.

Negotiation

Negotiation is the highest level of persuasion (Simms et al., 1994). Successful negotiation provides satisfaction to both parties and is termed partnering. Both participants emerge as winners in the "I win, you win" relationship. Other levels of persuasion include:

Persuasion:	I win, you lose.
Accommodation:	I lose, you win.
Compromise:	I lose, you lose.

Successful negotiation is the result of:

- Clarity of proposal
- Timing (date and time of day)
- Graphic and textual supporting materials
- Attention to verbal and nonverbal communication
- Advance orientation to topic (seeding an idea and nurturing its growth and development before final negotiation)

Skilled administrators develop the style of negotiating that is best for them. Testing and evaluating different approaches facilitate this development.

According to Lewicki, Hiam, and Olander (1996), there are five basic approaches to negotiating: collaborative (win-win), competitive (win at all cost), avoiding (lose-lose), accommodating (lose to win), and compromise (split the difference). These five approaches to negotiation are influenced by the importance of maintaining the relationship relative to the importance of achieving one's desired outcomes (Figure 13.4).

Prior to the negotiation encounter, there should be consideration and selection of the right strategy. During preparation:

1. Analyze your own position. (What would you like to get out of the process? What outcomes are desirable to you? Is maintaining the relationship important?)

High	Accommodating		Collaborative
Importance of RELATIONSHIP		Compromise	
Low	Avoiding		Competitive
	Low	Importance of OUTCOME	High

Figure 13.4 Negotiation strategies.

2. Understand the position of the other party. (What does the other party wish to get out of the process? What are their desired outcomes?)
3. Assess the contextual issues. (How much can I trust the other? Do you have organizational support for your position?)

Debate

Effective nurse executives are comfortable in leadership roles, have the ability to deal with conflict, and can engage in effective dialogue while presenting data in support of their position. It is increasingly important to be able to support and defend a position, even if it is unpopular. The ability to defend no cutbacks of the staff is a good example of administrative activity requiring intelligent and creative persuasion. Giving testimony for an organization and negotiating with other interest groups is another example (Byers, 1997).

Debate involves persuasion and argument at their best. Until recent times, debate was thought to be relegated to politicians. Budget meetings, curriculum meetings, in fact, all meetings resulting in controversial decisions benefit from hearty debate of the issues. Debate can also be used as an important teaching and learning strategy in leadership role seminars. Effective debating requires that the speakers learn to select, conceptualize, and analyze a topic. They must further be able to gather supportive materials and prepare to deliver a talk that will convince others that an idea is sound.

Formal and Informal Groups

To create a climate in which the nurse executive can maintain a flow of communication to and from staff, among staff, and to and from the rest of the organization is a major challenge. Useful information is everywhere, and the excellent nurse executive must access it either directly or indirectly. Get out and be seen, move around, listen to the grapevine, talk some but do not give away too much, listen a lot. Schedule and hold regular staff meetings. Attend required meetings most of the time.

Direct information generally is obtained through meetings of formal groups such as standing committees, boards, and other institutional groups requiring the presence of the nurse executive. The formal group situations also allow the nurse executive time for informal exchange with members of other disciplines.

Informal groups are characterized by irregularly occurring meetings between two or more persons without agendas. These tend to deal with immediate concerns, but often the topic is content for a larger range of problem resolutions. The nurse executive may find the informal group occupying a good deal of time if formal groups do not meet regularly with agendas to which everyone has a chance to contribute. Informal groups can bring out valuable information that does not always fit in the format of a formal meeting with a tight agenda. Informal, casual encounters may be arranged to break communication barriers with members of established formal groups.

Dialogue

Anyone doing serious work with groups and team learning must be familiar with the art and practice of dialogue. The word *dialogue* comes from two Greek roots, *dia* meaning through or with each other and *logos* meaning the word (Senge et al., 1994). People have always gathered in small groups to talk about ideas and events. In organizations, there is the same need to create productive conversations. Systematic blocks to communication must be identified if a true learning organization is to be created. In designing forums to move rapidly toward a shared vision, the use of dialogue rather than discussion and decision-making take the forefront. Facilitators (the new nurse executives) must bring people out of their shells who have not spoken so their views are also heard. Such dialogue invites people to treat each other as colleagues rather than as managers and workers.

Senge draws heavily on the theory of dialogue in making his arguments and describes dialogue as a form of conversation which allows effective communication to occur. Effective dialogue becomes a mode of exchange among human beings that kindles the flow of meaning and builds the appreciation of one another as genuine human beings with divergent points of view. Senge et al. (1994) further notes that dialogue becomes skillful discussion in a learning environment—the core of common meaning. During the dialogue process, people learn to think together, not just to solve problems. They come to know what they are supposed to do, building on a common vision and sense of alignment with the organization. Thus dialogue is emerging as a key component of team learning in learning organizations.

THE COMPUTER AS A COMMUNICATION TOOL

The key to using computers in nursing administration is understanding them. According to Worthley (1982), the basis of the problems encountered in using computers is the unenlightened use of technology. Although the technology is well developed, the management and use of computer technology is underdeveloped. No administrator would think of running an office without a computer or a copying machine. Yet many nurse executives are not comfortable using computers.

In 1984, Turkle (as described by Holloway, 1998) explored the subjective computer—the machine as it enters social psychological development of the human mind—and concluded that computers are becoming the machine to extend oneself beyond ones own environment to nurture the development of the second self. She notes that a relationship with a computer can influence people's conceptions of themselves, their jobs, their relationships with other people, and with their ways of thinking about social processes.

By 1998, Turkle was known as the Margaret Mead of Cyberspace, the ethnologist who has been able to link the real world with cyberspace in a meaningful way. She sees the computer as a tool for expanding one's interactions, just as the telephone did when it appeared as the latest communication tool on the horizon. For over 20 years, she has studied the psychology of human interactions with particular attention to children and their ease with blending digital objects and virtuality with real-world phenomena. She calls it bricolage or tinkering, a genuine integration of real and unreal realms with a fluidity that needs adoption in adults.

In various studies, nurses have been found to be skeptical, anxious, and even resistant to computer use (Ngin & Simms, 1996). These authors concluded from their own research on patterns of computer use that nurse managers had significantly greater access to computers and technical support than staff nurses and spent twice the amount of time using computerized information systems. The advent of computerized clinical records for all patients in most health care settings demands computer literacy for all the workers including nurses with various titles and job descriptions. Using computers as a second self and the tool for communication and record keeping can potentially achieve the linkage Turkle describes as essential for accomplishing work in the new age.

Historically, most new inventions have caused consternation and fear. People tried to stop the use of the first Model T Fords. The telephone was much feared, as were the first electric lights. Understanding nuclear technology is almost as difficult as understanding computer technology for many individuals. Both technologies have the capacity for easing human work, but both are constantly under challenge.

Harnessing computer technology in nursing has the potential for freeing professional nurses to practice nursing in its most humane form. Time-consuming record-keeping activities and the ordering of supplies can be extensively simplified using computers. Patient classification and care audits and staffing and scheduling activities are just a few of the communication activities that can be facilitated with computers. The most sophisticated systems establish patient files in computer memory and have provisions for adding information to those files on an on-line, real-time basis. The able nurse executive should rate a computerized nursing information system as a high priority and take full advantage of institutional computer experts in planning implementation. Chapter 24 presents a detailed discussion of computerized information systems.

Importance of Computer Literacy

Every office in every organization has used paper for all manner of communication such as memos, forms, and procedures. Once the infrastructure of personal computers and networks is in place and each employee has a work station, local, national, and global information can be accessed easily. The electronic mail system promotes rapid and timely communication of relevant information. Electronic voice mail further assists functionality of workers. The management of information by electronic computers is providing the ability for rapid decision-making leading to improved responsiveness of organizations. According to Reddy (1990), organizations mapped for controlling information exchange have led to dinosaurs and inertia in decision-making.

Modern computers have revolutionized the amount of information available in an organization and the time it takes to move it within the organization. Information once available only to top and middle managers is now accessible at all levels leading to decentralized structures that promote decision-making close to the front line. This has created unprecedented communication across levels and demise of middle managers (Bolman & Deal, 1991). The information-based organization needs far fewer traditional command and control managers, if any, and could lead to increased organizational effectiveness.

Nurses have always been responsible for generating and sharing clinical, patient-related information. Nurse executives gather data, write reports and proposals, and continuously keep in touch with relevant constituencies. The means by which these information activities are carried out include shift reports, progress notes, flow charts, telephone calls, electronic mail, patient conferences, meetings, letters, and presentations. In the last decade, information technology has made tremendous inroads into delivery and management. Health care delivery settings rely on information technology and computers to manage their business, administrative as well as clinical needs. It is now possible to capture, retrieve, and disseminate all kinds of patient and systems information on-line. Every health care employee (including cooks, materials handling, unit clerk, lab technician, nurse, physician, dietitian, social worker, nurse aide, administrator, etc.) will be expected to use computers as part of their daily routine by the year 2000.

Computers and information technology are no longer *alternative* tools for nursing practice. They are *essential* tools. Nevertheless, the effectiveness of computers depends on how well they are able to meet the needs of users and how well users are able to use them. Nurse executives should be informed about the range of information systems available that can assist in meeting their information needs as systems and clinical managers. Nurse executives appreciate systems that manage staff scheduling and bed occupancies, assess patient acuity, and collect quality care data; they find access to disease and drug information useful for themselves and for patient education. Systems are deemed useful when they assist in providing timely information (e.g., lab reports, infection rates, diet changes) and offer alternative means of instant communication to all units via electronic mail.

Use of the computer is significantly associated with ability to use the computer (Ngin & Simms, 1996). Nurses' use of computers is also associated with their perception of the technology and their role orientation. Computer use is regarded favorably among nurse executives partly because the image of computer use is consistent with the image of managers as indirect caregivers. The image of a staff nurse at the computer rather than at the bedside has been perceived as incongruent with their professional role. With the arrival of the pocket computer, this image is changing and the pocket computer is rapidly replacing the scissors of old as an essential part of personal equipment in any setting. Computing technologies have become an undeniable extension of nursing practice.

PUBLIC SPEAKING

Public speaking is an important and expected part of the nurse executive's role. Fully functioning administrators need to be able to speak in public forums, panel discussions, social gatherings, open board meetings, and various other formal gatherings. Impromptu talks and requests for one's opinion are part of the job. The ability to deliver formal scholarly papers is often a qualification for the job and also one of its duties.

Clear, effective public speaking can be mastered. It emanates from the ability to think clearly and set objectives. It emanates from a curiosity about the world of work and the world at large. It emanates from a strong internal sense of eagerness to share knowledge about a topic. One cannot present a topic that one is not interested in; one cannot present a talk of merit if one lacks self-confidence.

To prepare to be a speaker of worth, it is important to read, absorb, and create files for "bits" of information about a topic of interest. Several weeks before a scheduled presentation, communicate with yourself as to what you want to present. Write an outline for your talk, and edit and revise it until you are sure it meets the needs of your audience. Learn how to use Power Point™, Page Maker™ or other graphic software so that you can generate new slides or overheads easily. Be comfortable with making changes as additional information causes you to believe changes are necessary. Until one becomes a practiced, accomplished, self-confident speaker, one should tape a practice session and review for clarity and tone.

Pay attention to clothing, for one's attire will convey a message, as will the speech given. Public speaking is a human-to-human process. The speaker must develop a sense of responding to cues in the audience. Are they listening? Can they understand you? Are you delivering a message? All effective communication implies messages sent and messages received.

Most nurse executives are expected to be able to give a variety of public presentations, ranging from orienting new staff, to progress reports, to scholarly papers based on research or literature review. All types of communication convey a message from the administrator and the institution and need to be thoughtfully prepared.

SUMMARY

This chapter has presented communication as a concept and a basic management skill. Anger is presented as a major impediment to communication and must be dealt with in oneself and others before a learning organization can be implemented. The importance of communication with oneself and others in formal and informal groups is especially emphasized. Although computer technology is well developed elsewhere, the use of computerized information systems is not widespread in nursing practice. Harnessing this technology has the potential for freeing nurses to practice nursing in its most humane form. The idea of a computer as a second self is proposed.

STUDY QUESTIONS

1. To what extent do you communicate with yourself about work-related problems or issues?
2. How do you personally prepare for small group interactions?
3. Select a recent situation in which you interacted with several people in a formal group structure. How did you communicate verbally and nonverbally?
4. Considering your immediate peers, whom do you consider an effective communicator? Why?
5. How do you plan to nurture your computer utilization skills over the next 5 years?
6. Describe your public speaking style.
7. How computer literate are you? Do you use a computer in your everyday life?

REFERENCES

Allcorn, S. (1994). *Anger in the workplace.* Westport, CT: Quorum Books.

Bolman, L. G., & Deal, T. E. (1991). *Reframing organizations.* San Francisco: Jossey-Bass.

Bordon, G. A., & Stone, J. D. (1976). *Human communication.* Menlo Park, CA: Cummings Publishing Co.

Bradley, J. C., & Edinberg, M. A. (1982). *Communication in the nursing context.* New York: Appleton-Century-Crofts.

Byers, S. (1997). *The executive nurse.* Albany, NY: Delmar.

Costello-Nickitas, D. M. (1997). *Nursing leadership.* Albany, NY: Delmar.

Csikszentmihalyi, M. (1996). *Creativity.* New York: HarperCollins.

DuBrin, A. J. (1985). *Contemporary applied management* (2nd ed.). Plano, TX: Business Publications.

Duldt, B. W. (1981a). Anger: An alienating communication hazard for nurses, *Nursing Outlook, 29*(11), 640–644.

Duldt, B. W. (1981b). Anger: An occupational hazard for nurses, *Nursing Outlook, 29*(9), 510–518.

Fielden, J. S. (1982). What do you mean you don't like my style? *Harvard Business Review, 60*(3), 128–138.

Gold, H. (1978). Communicating with others: One to one. In L. M. Simms & J. Lindberg (Eds.), *The Nurse Person.* New York: Harper & Row.

Holloway, M. (1998). An ethnologist in cyberspace. *Scientific American, 278*(4), 29–30.

Janosik, E. H., & Davies, J. L. (1996). *Mental health and psychiatric nursing,* (2nd ed.). Boston: Little, Brown.

Kreitzer, M. J., Wright, D., Hamlin, C., Towey, S., Marko, M., & Disch, J. (1997). Creating a healthy work environment in the midst of organizational change and transition. *Journal of Nursing Administration, 27*(6), 35–41.

Lerner, H. (1997). *The dance of anger.* New York: HarperCollins.

Lewicki, R. J., Hiam, A., & Olander, K. W. (1996). *Think before you speak.* New York: Wiley.

McGregor, G. F., & Robinson, J. A. (1981). *The communication matrix.* New York: AMACOM.

Mintzberg, H. (1975). The manager's job: Folklore and fact. *Harvard Business Review, 53*(4), 49–61.

Morgan, G. (1993). *Imaginization.* Newbury Park, CA: Sage.

Ngin, P. M., & Simms, L. M. (1996). Computer use for work accomplishment. *Journal of Nursing Administration, 26*(3), 47–55.

Noer, D. M. (1993). *Healing the wounds.* San Francisco: Jossey-Bass.

Reddy, R. (1990). A technological perspective on new forms of organizations. In P. S. Goodman, L. S. Sproull and Associates. *Technology and organizations.* San Francisco: Jossey-Bass.

Senge, P. M., Kleiner, A., Roberts, C., Ross, R. B., & Smith, B. J. (1994). *The fifth discipline fieldbook.* New York: Doubleday.

Simms, L. M., Price, S. A., & Ervin, N. E. (1994). *The professional practice of nursing administration* (2nd ed.). Albany, NY: Delmar.

Swift, M. H. (1973). Clear writing means clear thinking means. . . . *Harvard Business Review, 51*(1), 59–62.

Trompanaar, F. (1993). *Riding the waves of culture.* London: Nicholas Brealey.

Turkle, S. (1984). *The second self-computers and the human spirit.* New York: Simon & Schuster.

Worthley, J. A. (1982). *Managing computers in health care.* Ann Arbor, MI: Health Administration Press.

CHAPTER

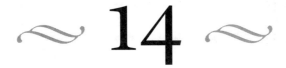

14

Conflict Management

Sylvia A. Price

Conflict is a part of life, at least as we know it. How we deal with the fact of conflict has much to do with how we express our being. (Bugental, 1965, p. 23)

Chapter Highlights

- Conflict management
- Characteristics of conflict
- Types of conflict
- Sources of conflict
- Functional and dysfunctional conflict
- Strategies for conflict resolution
- Techniques of conflict resolution

Conflict and conflict resolution within the framework of professional nursing administrative practice will be addressed in this chapter. Nurse executives must cope with the competing pressures and demands of health care administrators for cost effectiveness, of medical staff for competent nursing assistance, and of nursing personnel for improved wages, benefits, and working conditions. Although continued conflict can and does produce stress in nurse executives, it can also provide an opportunity for the individual and organization to change and grow.

Conflict is an inherent part of an individual's personal and professional life. It is inevitable. Conflict may result from divergence of opinion, incompatibility, transmission of erroneous information, or competition for scarce resources. Although often envisioned as a negative manifestation of human interaction, conflict can have positive as well as negative aspects. How conflict is perceived and managed is the essence of whether the process is productive or unproductive to the individual or organizational system. The concepts, theories, and processes related to conflict and conflict resolution have been the subject of extensive and intensive study.

Conflict has a variety of definitions. Robbins and Coulter (1997) depict conflict as "perceived incompatible differences resulting in some form of interference or opposition. Whether the differences are real or not is irrelevant. If people perceive that differences exist, then a conflict state exists" (p. 631).

Leininger (1974) views conflict as "opposing viewpoints, forces, issues, and problems which confront individuals, groups, and institutions, having been generated from a variety of internal and external personal and group forces" (p. 18). In their definition, Polzer and Neale (1994) emphasize resource scarcity as a source of conflict because "members of an organization will not be able to receive the level of resources they desire. Therefore, conflict arises between organizational members regarding the distribution of desired resources" (p. 116).

PHILOSOPHICAL AND HISTORICAL BACKGROUND OF CONFLICT MANAGEMENT

Early classical writers on management, the traditionalists, considered conflict a destructive force and believed it was the role of the manager to eliminate conflict from the organization. This philosophy dominated the literature until the 1940s. Traditionalists felt that if a staff member created a conflict situation by disagreeing with the views of management or co-workers, then that person must be discharged from the organization. Because the reason for dismissal was rarely discussed, others were encouraged to abide by rules and regulations.

In contrast with the traditional view of conflict, the human relation's view of conflict stressed that, although harmful, conflict was inevitable. In the human relation view, conflict in complex organizations was accepted, and an attempt was made to rationalize its existence. This was done by devising measures to reduce, rather than to eliminate conflict. Such measures focused entirely on the development of conflict resolution techniques. This reasoning eventually led to the view that conflict could be turned to beneficial use. Robbins and Coulter (1997) espouse that conflict can be a positive force in an organization and that some conflict is absolutely necessary for an organization to perform effectively. This approach is that of the interactionist view of conflict.

Interactionists recognize the need for conflict and encourage opposition as a creative force that must be stimulated as well as resolved. Indeed, they are concerned when conflict is inadequate or absent and in need of greater intensity. The interactionists believe that organizations that do not encourage conflict increase the probability of or lack of motivation, creative thinking, and effective decision-making. They point out that companies have failed because few staff members questioned decisions made by management; in such cases, apathy allowed inadequate decisions to remain in effect because of a conflict-free management group.

Social scientists and humanists have studied conflict and conflict behavior, particularly since World War II. They have identified four major approaches to understanding conflict:

1. The study of interpersonal conflict is spearheaded by psychiatrists, psychiatric social workers, and psychiatric nurses. This type of conflict can and does occur within the individual. Ambivalence as well as disordered perception, feeling, and behavior are usually evident. These symptoms are associated with psychiatric problems.
2. The interactional-sociological approach focuses on group behavior and interactional phenomena in decision-making within a group.
3. The anthropological approach emphasizes the stresses of culture acclimatization, value and cultural conflicts, and conflicts related to personality and the social environment.
4. The economic-political approach emphasizes conflicts related to political concerns, power games, coalitions, and political and economic processes.

In the health care arena, nurse executives need to be knowledgeable in identifying, managing, and resolving conflict. They must not only deal with conflict effectively and use it constructively, but they must also stimulate it if none is apparent.

CHARACTERISTICS OF CONFLICT

Baldridge (1979) noted that the situations that provoke conflict can be described by four general characteristics. The first is known as the iceberg phenomenon, in which an apparent problem draws attention to other critical issues under the surface. The superficial problem is raised as a pretense for bringing more fundamental issues to light. For example, an initial problem related to staffing, such as nurse assignment patterns, may actually be merely the externalization of a much more basic issue: the wish to gain participation in decision-making at the staff nurse level.

The second characteristic situation is related to issues that cause large-scale conflict that tends to have a unifying effect on diverse interest groups. This has occurred in almost all campus resistance movements, in which individuals usually have no common interest other than being bound by the current conflict situation.

Third, conflict is often the result of rising expectations, rather than the presence of intolerable conditions. Nurse executives need to be cognizant that major concessions and improved conditions can induce a high level of expectation and thus actually provoke new conflict with the repetition of a similar pattern.

Fourth, the issue in conflict often has moral overtones that justify and legitimize radical action. Individuals use issues such as sex discrimination and nurse power as ultimate goals to justify almost any short-range excesses. At the other end of the organizational spectrum, however, the same tactic is used by nurse executives when they demand autonomy in their negotiations with the governing boards of health care agencies.

TYPES OF CONFLICT

Although conflict situations have similar characteristics, the forms of conflict are highly diverse. They may be categorized as intrapersonal, interpersonal, intergroup, or interorganizational in nature. *Intrapersonal conflict,* which was mentioned earlier as a psychiatric phenomenon, is incongruous to an individual's role; there is lack of conformity between people's goals and what is expected within the framework of their roles. "Intrapersonal conflict exists in the cognitive and affective realms of an individual's mind. Thus, an individual may perceive that he or she is in conflict with the organization or other employees, but the conflict, in fact, exists only in that person's mind, not at a behavioral level" (Zey-Ferrell, 1979, p. 299).

However, intrapersonal conflict can be the underlying cause of *interpersonal conflict.* For example, emotionally distressed persons bring to their jobs feelings that relate to their private lives. Preoccupation with personal problems can produce less concentration on work-related responsibilities and decision-making. The behavior due to mental processes, especially for the nurse executive, can be the source of interpersonal conflict among peers, subordinates, and co-workers of other disciplines.

Interpersonal conflict arises between two or more individuals or within a group. For example, withholding information may create a conflict between a nurse executive and her assistant. Conflicts among division heads, staff nurse and physician, and committee members may occur for the same reason.

Interpersonal conflict may be inherent in a person's role when there is disagreement between the values and beliefs of the occupant of the role and the expectations set forth by others. In many health care institutions in the 1990s, the nurse executive is accountable and responsible for the practice of nursing. However, disagreement can occur if one professional challenges the practice decisions of a member of another profession. Kalisch and Kalisch (1977) refer to a common source of conflict in the traditional behavior pattern between physicians and nurses as "physician's dominance and nurse's deference." This hierarchical attitude and expectation is found not only at the practice level but extends through executive-administrative levels.

In the capacity of executive-level administrator, Kelley (1977) maintains that the role of nurse executive is extremely difficult to enact because "that role is often stereotyped and contradictory, with multiple split opinions on its power and authority. A top-level nurse administrator . . . . [is] surrounded by different sets of behavioral expectations to satisfy from groups higher up, lower down, and on the same level in the structure" (p. 157). Studies conducted by Arndt and Laeger (1970) and Halsey (1978) both concluded that conflict and role strain existed for the nurse executive resulting from pressure to respond to role prescription from a variety of sources.

It is vital that nurse executives examine their role conception. Executives should take an activist's position in regard to that role, making it the sort of role they perceive it to be, rather than merely fulfilling the role others expect or anticipate. An attempt to subscribe to the latter philosophy can be a source of intrapersonal conflict.

Intergroup, or *interorganizational, conflict* arises between two groups, such as in the form of interdepartmental issues. Disagreements and the transmission of erroneous information between departments, such as between medicine and nursing, are common sources of this type of conflict. Such conflicts are depicted as harmful by management, but Argyris (1976) points out that "instead of trying to stamp out intergroup conflict as bad and disloyal, the executives must learn how to manage it so that the constructive aspects are emphasized and the destructive aspects deemphasized" (p. 23).

SOURCES OF CONFLICT

Power, defined as the ability to influence others, may be a major source of conflict. Frost and Wilmot (1978) emphasize that, because it is always interpersonal, power exists only in a human context and is, in a sense, "given from one party to another in conflict" (p. 52). Within this context, power is not an actual show of force, but it is the perceived potential of one party to exert influence on another party, depending on the values and nature of the relationship of those involved. Individuals and groups have power when they have access to information and have control of resources and support services to carry out tasks.

In their classic studies French and Raven (1968) described situations in which one person has power over another. These five bases of social power are reward power, coercive power, legitimate power, referent power, and expert power. Raven and Kruglanski (1975) added a sixth power base, information power. The basis of *reward power* is the ability to offer rewards. Thus, an individual is made to perceive that compliance with the wishes of another will lead to positive rewards. *Coercive power,* the opposite of reward power, is exercised in such a way that one individual perceives that another can mete out punishment. *Legitimate power* is based on agreement and values held in common, enabling one individual to exercise power over the other by consent. *Referent power* is based on identification with the ideals of an individual and the wish to emulate that person. *Expert power* is present when a person is perceived to have superior knowledge or skill in a particular field. *Information power* refers to a person's ability to use explanations or other persuasive communication to modify the behavior of others; it is based on the individual's knowledge of or access to information.

Because of position, knowledge, profession, and organizational context, the nurse executive may acquire and use all of the types of power described. The nurse executive should neither avoid nor overplay the use of power, not fail to use it for ethical and legitimate purposes. Others are aware of potential resources of power, and the administrator who uses overkill in a power conflict risks loss of effectiveness. Thus, the administrative nurse must frequently come to terms with conflicts between personality, professional ideals, and the needs of the institution.

By position and title, the nurse executive's legitimate power and authority is generally recognized throughout the organization. However, the precise scope of this power and authority may be an area of conflict. An issue in many health care facilities is who controls the practice of nursing. The administrator of nursing has the authority, but the extent of power may be limited to resolving problems that occur within the department. Unless the director has other powers to augment his or her legitimate power, legitimate power may not be sufficient for the administrator to decide a nursing practice issue related to the overall organization or to other disciplines.

The nurse executive also has substantial reward and coercive power based on the right to hire, evaluate, promote, and discharge individuals. The nursing administrator needs to be sensitive to the fact that power is only a part of the continuing relationship between the supervisor and the supervised and that power is not an acceptable substitute for skillful leadership and motivation.

The nurse executive has expert power derived from two sources: professional nursing knowledge and administrative skills. In the past, these two types of power were not always compatible and were a source of intrapersonal conflict. With the acceptance of nursing administration as a legitimate area of nursing practice this should not be an important source of conflict. Simms, Price, and Pfoutz (1985) explored the role of the nurse executive in acute, home, and long-term care and educational settings. Results of this study yield the postulation that a new administrative role, the nurse executive, is emerging in acute, home care, and educational settings. The role requires advanced education and a high degree of leadership and management competence intricately linked with clinical nursing knowledge and research.

The role also demands teacher/learner skills with the nurse executive modeling behaviors that can be learned by others. Because conflict is almost always personalized by all participant parties it seems essential for personal behavioral change to occur if a state of dynamic conflict fluidity is to be achieved. In a healthy organization, conflict is stimulating and scientific debate of diverse ideas can lead to multiple creative ventures.

Charisma, which describes the "magnetic" personality of the nurse executive, is an influential element of this power base. Referent power may or may not be strong enough to induce others to emulate the nurse executive. However, it can be diminished when the nurse executive develops hostile, defensive personality patterns.

Nurse executives who are knowledgeable about the various types of power and power bases and how they are applied are better able to function in an enlightened position and provide a climate for more effective leadership. They need to make informed and high-risk decisions that may be potential sources of conflict. As members of the executive team in health care delivery settings, these nurse executives must take risks and move into positions of power. Much of the power that executive gains is derived from their access to information. The nurse executive who is knowledgeable about the information network of the organization realizes there are formal channels that transport information to the decision-makers. Legitimate access and the authority to command information are important tools for the nurse executive.

ASSESSMENT OF FUNCTIONAL AND DYSFUNCTIONAL CONFLICT

Health care organizations are often classified as complex organizations. In complex and highly diversified organizations, conflict is inevitable and even desirable. Inappropriate responses to conflict can be unhealthy for individuals and groups within the organization. It is imperative that nurse executives reduce or increase conflict and tension to tolerable levels and channel the energy created by conflict situations toward constructive goals.

Conflict in and of itself can be a positive or negative force. It is the use or misuse of this force that determines its effect and relative value. Robbins and Coulter (1997) imply that the demarcation between functional and dysfunctional conflict is neither clear nor precise. When some conflicts support the goals of the organization, they are functional conflicts of a constructive nature. If the conflicts prevent an organization from achieving its goals, they are dysfunctional and are of a destructive nature. The authors stress that no level of conflict can be adopted as acceptable or unacceptable under all conditions.

A conflict may be dysfunctional at one time in a given setting, as perceived by individuals in the organization, or may be considered functional at another time in a different setting by individuals at the top level in the organization. For example, a conflict may occur over an administration decision to implement a computerized information system in a home health care setting, especially if the staff nurses were not involved in the decision, and they perceive this change as an increase in their work load. However, management's rationale for the change was that data on the population served by the home health care agency would be more readily available and accessible and would facilitate planning for needed services.

Characteristics do exist that assess actual conflict and functional from dysfunctional conflict. MacFarland, Leonard, and Morris (1984) propose an assessment guide that can be used to determine interpersonal or intergroup conflict within the organization and whether a given conflict is functional or dysfunctional (Figure 14.1). They emphasize that conflict assessment can help formulate a conflict diagnosis in the organization or subsystem or both. They also emphasize

Interpersonal or intergroup?

1. Who?
   - Who are the primary individuals or groups involved? Characteristics (values; feelings; needs; perceptions; goals; hostility; strengths, as past history of constructive conflict management; self-awareness)?
   - Who, if anyone, are the individuals or groups that have an indirect investment in the result of the conflict?
   - Who, if anyone, is assisting the parties to manage the conflict constructively?
   - What is the history of the individuals' or groups' involvement in the conflict?
   - What is the past and present interpersonal relationship between the parties involved in the conflict.
   - How is power distributed among the parties?
   - What are the major sources of power used?
   - Does the potential for coalition exist among the parties?
   - What is the nature of the current leadership affecting the conflicting parties?

2. What?
   - What is (are) the issue(s) in the conflict?
   - Are the issues based on facts? Based on values? Based on interests in resources?
   - Are the issues realistic?
   - What is the dominant issue in the conflict?
   - What are the goals of each conflicting party?
   - Is the current conflict functional? Dysfunctional?
   - What conflict management strategies, if any, have been used to manage the conflict to date?
   - What alternatives in managing the conflict exist?
   - What are you doing to keep the conflict going?
   - Is there a lack of stimulating work?

3. How?
   - What is the origin of the conflict? Sources? Precipitating events?
   - What are the major events in the evolution of the conflict?
   - How have the issues emerged? Been transformed? Proliferated?
   - What polarizations and coalitions have occurred?
   - How have parties tried to damage each other? What stereotyping exists?

4. When/Where?
   - When did the conflict originate?
   - Where is the conflict taking place?
   - What are the characteristics of the setting within which the conflict is occurring?
   - What are the geographic boundaries? Political structures? Decision-making patterns? Communication networks? Subsystem boundaries?
   - What environmental factors exist that influence the development of functional versus dysfunctional conflict?
   - What resource persons are available to assist in constructive conflict management?

continued

Functional or dysfunctional?

	YES	NO
Does the conflict support the goals of the organization?	[ ]	[ ]
Does the conflict contribute to the overall goals of the organization?	[ ]	[ ]
Does the conflict stimulate improved job performance?	[ ]	[ ]
Does the conflict increase productivity among work group members?	[ ]	[ ]
Does the conflict stimulate creativity and innovation?	[ ]	[ ]
Does the conflict bring about constructive change?	[ ]	[ ]
Does the conflict contribute to the survival of the organization?	[ ]	[ ]
Does the conflict improve initiative?	[ ]	[ ]
Does job satisfaction remain high?	[ ]	[ ]
Does the conflict improve the morale of the work group?	[ ]	[ ]

A yes response to the majority of the questions indicates that the conflict is probably functional. If the majority of responses are no, then the conflict is most likely a dysfunctional conflict.

Figure 14.1 Guide for assessment of conflict. From MacFarland, G., Leonard, H., & Morris, M. (1984). *Nursing leadership and management.* Albany, NY: Delmar, a division of Thomson Learning. Copyright 1984 by Delmar, a division of Thomson Learning. Adapted with permission.

that at times the level of conflict may be either too low or too high within the work group. If the level of conflict is too low, it may be necessary for the nurse executive or manager to stimulate conflict. If the conflict is too high, the executive must apply conflict resolution strategies. The authors propose an assessment guide that may indicate "too low or too high conflict levels" (Figure 14.2). An affirmative response to the questions can be indicative of such conflict states. First, one should analyze the data collected from the assessment guide for actual conflict to formulate a conflict diagnosis. The data are then analyzed to determine the nature of conflict, whether it is too high or too low. The authors imply "that the conflict diagnosis can be stated to include the type of conflict and the related source, for example, dysfunctional interpersonal conflict related to differences in values, functional intergroup conflict related to differing subgoals, or too-high interpersonal conflict related to unequal access to resources" (p. 318). These conflict diagnosis statements along with an understanding of the nature of conflict can give direction to the selection of appropriate conflict management strategies.

As nurse executives attempt to identify the issues and sources of conflict, the next logical step is to select the strategy or strategies for managing conflict and to revisit their influence on and participation in the conflict.

STRATEGIES FOR CONFLICT RESOLUTION

A number of strategies can be used in an attempt to reduce conflict. It is important to select the conflict resolution strategy that is most appropriate for the

Is conflict too low?

	YES	NO
Is the work group consistently satisfied with the status quo?	[ ]	[ ]
Are no or few opposing views expressed by work-group members?	[ ]	[ ]
Is little concern expressed about doing things better?	[ ]	[ ]
Is little or no concern expressed about improving inadequacies?	[ ]	[ ]
Are the decisions made by the work group generally of low quality?	[ ]	[ ]
Are no or few innovative solutions or ideas expressed?	[ ]	[ ]
Are many work-group members "yes-men"?	[ ]	[ ]
Are work-group members reluctant to express ignorance or uncertainties?	[ ]	[ ]
Does the nurse manager seek to maintain peace and group cooperation regardless of whether this is the correct intervention?	[ ]	[ ]
Do the work-group members demonstrate an extremely high level of resistance to change?	[ ]	[ ]
Does the nurse manager base the distribution of rewards on "popularity" as opposed to competence and high job performance?	[ ]	[ ]
Is the nurse manager excessively concerned about not hurting the feelings of the nursing staff?	[ ]	[ ]
Is the nurse manager excessively concerned with obtaining a consensus of opinion and reaching a compromise when decisions must be made?	[ ]	[ ]

A yes response to the majority of these questions can be indicative of a too-low conflict level in a work group.

Is conflict too high?

	YES	NO
Is there an upward and onward spiraling escalation of the conflict?	[ ]	[ ]
Are the conflicting parties stimulating the escalation of conflict without considering the consequences?	[ ]	[ ]
Is there a shift away from conciliation, minimizing differences, and enhancing goodwill?	[ ]	[ ]
Are the issues involved in the conflict being increasingly elaborated and expanded?	[ ]	[ ]
Are false issues being generated?	[ ]	[ ]
Are the issues vague or unclear?	[ ]	[ ]
Is job dissatisfaction increasing among work-group members?	[ ]	[ ]
Is the work-group productivity being adversely affected?	[ ]	[ ]
Is the energy being directed to activities that do not contribute to the achievement of organizational goals (e.g., destroying opposing party)?	[ ]	[ ]
Is the morale of the nursing staff being adversely affected?	[ ]	[ ]
Are extra parties getting dragged into the conflict?	[ ]	[ ]
Is a great deal of reliance on overt power manipulation noted (threats, coercion, deception)?	[ ]	[ ]
Is there a great deal of imbalance in power noted among the parties?	[ ]	[ ]

continued

	YES	NO
Are the individuals or groups involved in the conflict expressing dissatisfaction about the course of the conflict and feel that they are losing something?	[ ]	[ ]
Is absenteeism increasing among staff?	[ ]	[ ]
Is there a high rate of turnover among personnel?	[ ]	[ ]
Is communication dysfunctional, not open, mistrustful, and/or restrictive?	[ ]	[ ]
Is the focus being placed on nonconflict relevant sensitive areas of the other party?	[ ]	[ ]

A yes response to the majority of these questions can be indicative of a conflict level in a work group that is too high.

Figure 14.2 Guide for assessment of level of conflict. From MacFarland, G., Leonard, H., & Morris, M. (1984). *Nursing leadership and management.* Albany, NY: Delmar, a division of Thomson Learning. Copyright 1984 by Delmar, a division of Thomson Learning. Adapted with permission.

nature and type of conflict. Feldman and Arnold (1983) summarize four major strategies for intergroup conflict.

Avoidance

This type of strategy attempts to keep the conflict from surfacing at all. Examples would be to ignore the conflict or impose a solution. This conflict is temporary where concern for people and production is low. This may be appropriate if the conflict is trivial or if quick action is needed to prevent the conflict from occurring.

Defusion

Under this strategy, an attempt is made to deactivate the conflict and cool off the emotions and hostilities of the groups involved. Examples would include trying to "smooth things over" by playing down the importance and magnitude of the conflict or of established superordinate goals that need the cooperation of the conflicting groups to be accomplished. This strategy is appropriate where a stop-gap measure is needed or when the groups have a mutually important goal.

Containment

Under this strategy, some conflict is allowed to surface, but it is carefully contained by spelling out which issues are to be discussed and how they are to be resolved. To implement this strategy, the problems and procedures may be structured, and representatives from the conflicting parties may be allowed to negotiate and bargain within the established structure. This is appropriate when open discussions have failed and the conflicting groups are of equal power.

Confrontation

Under this strategy, which is at the other end of the continuum from avoidance, all the issues are brought into the open, and the conflicting groups directly confront the issues with each other in an attempt to resolve the conflict. This is most appropriate when there is a minimum level of trust, when time is not critical, and when the groups need to cooperate to get the job done effectively (pp. 526–528).

Three basic strategies that individuals can use in interpersonal conflict, as well as intergroup and organization conflict resolution approaches are identified by Filley (1975) for dealing with conflict according to outcome—lose-lose, win-lose, and win-win.

Lose-Lose

In a lose-lose approach to conflict resolution, neither party wins. One common approach is to compromise or take the middle ground in a dispute. Another is to pay off one of the parties in the conflict that may take the form of a bribe. A third approach is to use a third party as an arbitrator. Another lose-lose strategy is when the parties in a conflict resort to bureaucratic rules or regulations to resolve the conflict. It is important to note that in all of these approaches, both parties lose. It is sometimes the only solution to the conflict, but it is generally a less desirable one.

Win-Lose

This strategy is commonly used for resolving conflict. In a competitive type culture one party in a conflict attempts to assemble its forces to win and the other party loses. Examples of win-lose strategies can be observed in a supervisor and subordinate and line and staff relationships, and labor-management disputes. In a win-lose strategy someone always loses, which may make the loser bitter and revengeful.

Characteristics that are common in the win-lose and lose-lose situations include:

- The conflict is a personal "we-they" conflict rather than a problem-centered focus. This is very likely to occur when two cohesive groups that do not share common values or goals are in conflict.
- Parties direct their energy toward total victory for themselves and total defeat for the other. This can cause long-term problems for the organization.
- Each sees the issue from her or his own viewpoint rather than as a problem in need of a solution.
- The emphasis is on outcomes rather than definition of goals, values, or objectives.
- Conflicts are personalized.
- Conflict-resolving activities are not differentiated from other group processes.

- There is a short-run view of the conflict, with settlement of the immediate problem as the goal rather than resolution of differences (Filley, 1975, p. 25).

Win-Win

A win-win strategy of conflict resolution is the most desirable especially from an organizational perspective. Innovation, creativity, and energies are expended at solving the problems rather than demeaning the other party or parties involved. The needs and desires of both parties in the conflict situation are achieved, and both receive rewarding outcomes. These win-win strategies are usually associated with a favorable organization experience, improved decision-making, and satisfaction to both parties in the conflict situation.

TECHNIQUES OF CONFLICT RESOLUTION

As Kelley (1983) stresses, "accomplishing organizational objectives according to an established timetable with a minimum of resources while influencing resolution of conflict is a major basis upon which nursing service administrators are evaluated and retained or released" (p. 427).

Negotiation

Negotiation is an indispensable tool for the nurse executive. However, the knowledge and skill to use this tool effectively has been limited to a degree in the health care field and in nursing in particular. Nevertheless, the responsibility of negotiating on behalf of the nursing division is a responsibility of the top level nursing executive. Negotiation is given different meaning by various theorists. Strauss (1979) views negotiation as a cyclic interactional process that can be analyzed by three interacting elements. The first, process elements, includes such strategies as persuasion, trade-offs, appeals, demands, compromises toward middle positions, and mutual agreements. The second is the structural element, which incorporates the interacting parties in the negotiation process, the environmental setting, the timing of meetings, and the balance of power of the two parties. The last element is the negotiating situation itself. The interactive element comprehends the complexity and number of issues to be resolved, the experience of the negotiators, and the alternatives available to ensure the continuance of negotiations.

Cohen (1980) presents another perspective on negotiation. He views it as a process of information, timing, power, and pressure to secure a commitment to change behavior. Power, the ability to use resources to achieve worthwhile goals, may include risk taking, competition, and persistence. Cohen stresses that successful negotiation is based on accurate and sufficient information gathered by critical listening, questioning, and reading cues. It is important to note that, to achieve agreement in negotiations, group tension must be reduced. Stress relief may be achieved by the following steps: *(1)* the maintenance of time limitations by both parties and *(2)* the application of pressure on the negotiator to take or avoid risks.

General guidelines to effective negotiations include belief in oneself as an able negotiator; willingness to seek assistance in problem-solving, in the recognition that the objective is collaborative settlement as commitments made to individuals, not necessarily organizations; encouragement of an exchange of information; and the ability to assess and validate changing circumstances in the negotiating process.

Collaboration

I-win-you-lose collaboration as a strategy or technique is closely related to negotiation, and the terms are sometimes used interchangeably when conflict resolution is discussed by different authors. However, collaborative theory supports the belief that people should bring their differences to the surface and delve into the issues to identify underlying causes and to find an alternative mutually satisfactory to both parties. The approach is based on the assumption that people will be motivated to invest time and energy in such problem-solving activity. The conflict is viewed as a creative, positive force that will lead to an improved state of affairs to which both sides are fully committed. When progress can no longer be made, a mediator (third-party consultant) may be used to assist the parties to arrive at a win-win position.

Collaborationists further argue that theirs is the preferable strategy for the good of an organization because *(1)* open and honest interaction promotes authentic interpersonal relations; *(2)* conflict is used as a creative force for innovation and improvement; *(3)* the process enhances feedback and information flow; and *(4)* the solution of disputes in itself serves to improve the climate of the organization by enhancing openness, trust, risk taking, and feelings of integrity (Likert & Likert, 1976).

Collaboration has been most effective in situations in which there is *(1)* a high degree of required interdependence; *(2)* power parity, allowing the parties to interact openly, using all of their resources to further their beliefs and concerns regardless of their superior-subordinate status; *(3)* potential for mutual benefits; and *(4)* the expectation of organizational support.

Team Approach to Resolving Conflict

Amason, Hochwarter, Thompson, and Harrison (1995) stress that conflict is a natural part of a team environment. Teams must be able to manage that conflict and how they do so brings out the best or worst of employee involvement. Teams have proved useful in improving the equality of decision-making assisting to build a cooperative goal-oriented culture (see Chapter 7).

Amason et al. conducted on-site interviews with teams from 10 diverse organizations. These teams were responsible for making important strategic decisions for their companies. The researchers found that although some types of conflict can be detrimental to a team's success, other forms of conflict generate a more open, creative, and ultimately more productive team. In other words, how the teams managed conflict was the crux of team effectiveness. Conflict is a natural part of the process that makes team decision-making so effective in the first place. These effective teams realized how to manage conflict so that it made a positive contribution, whereas less effective teams avoided conflict or allowed it to produce negative consequences that hampered their effectiveness.

Although disagreements among team members occur, so long as they are substantive, issue-related differences of opinion, they tend to improve team effectiveness. Conflict theorists refer to these types of disagreements as cognitive conflict, or what the researchers call C-type conflict. The elements of C-type conflict are:

- Team members examine, compare, and reconcile these differences. This process is to reach high-quality solutions that are understood and accepted by all team members.
- The majority of the managers believed C-type conflict improves overall team effectiveness. It focuses attention on the all-too-often-ignored assumptions that may underlie a particular issue.
- It facilitates frank communication and open consideration of different alternatives.
- Encourages innovative thinking and promotes creative solutions to problems.
- Improves quality of team decisions. Seems to promote acceptance of the decision by team members.

Disagreements over personalized, individually oriented matters are largely detrimental to team performance. Conflict theorists refer to these type of disagreements as affective conflict—or what the researchers call A-type conflict. A-type conflict lowered team effectiveness by provoking hostility, distrust, cynicism, and apathy among team members. The characteristics of A-type conflict are:

- Focus on personalized anger or resentment, usually directed at specific individuals rather than specific ideas.
- It undermines team effectiveness—fosters cynicism, distrust, and avoidance, thereby obstructing open communication and integration.
- The quality of decisions declines. Members who are hostile or cynical are unlikely to understand decisions that were made largely without their participation.
- Commitment to the team erodes because team members no longer associate themselves with the team's actions.

Amason et al. (1995) emphasize that conflict can improve team effectiveness. If they are to reach their full potential, teams must accept conflict. However, by allowing conflict teams are at risk of provoking destructive conflict or A-type conflict. As Figure 14.3 depicts, teams become more effective when they encourage good conflict and restrain the bad conflict.

Strategies for the team leader to use to build an effective culture before, during, and after the team interactions include:

- Disseminate a full agenda early. The agenda provides focus and should have an itemized list of proposals with their rationale.
- State the philosophy for the team and back up that philosophy. Stating the philosophy behind team decision-making would be helpful.
- Provide the right environment for the meeting. Providing the appropriate environment can increase the team's performance and reduce A-type conflict (e.g., seating location, shape of the meeting table).
- Have behavioral strategies to run the meeting in mind before the meeting begins. The behavior of the team leader is central to keeping the meeting productive. The leader has to have strategies that ensure a climate of openness and cooperation.
- Keep a sense of where the discussions are going. The team leader may need to facilitate and monitor team discussions to limit personalized statements made during heated debates.

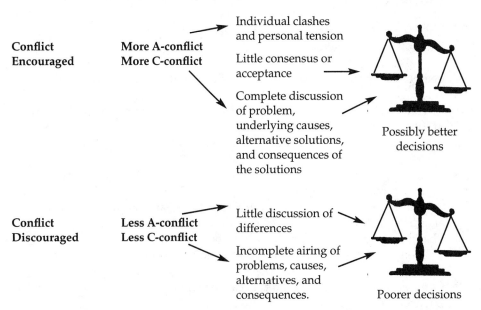

Figure 14.3 The outcomes of encouraging or suppressing conflict. Reprinted from *Organizational Dynamics,* Autumn 1995. Copyright © 1995 American Management Association International. Reprinted by permission of American Management Association International, New York, NY. All rights reserved. http://www.amanet.org

- Channel discussion from A-type conflict to C-type conflict. The leader must act to keep the group focused on the positive aspects of open discussion. The leader is trying to draw people out to get their opinions such that they will not personally attack others in the process.
- Support the team. A leader must continually exhibit behavior that shows support for the team. There is a need to focus the team so it is functioning as a team and not a collection of individuals. This team focus increases the caring nature of each member toward each other and builds support for the team decision.
- Be proactive and reactive, not passive. The team leader must actively support a positive culture for the team. The leader's behavior needs to focus on building the team and the culture that will support active debate that is positive and constructive (pp. 29–33).

Nurse executives are frequently encouraged to develop leadership skills that emphasize the resolution or suppression of conflict. At the same time, they often find that power is necessary to direct and coordinate day-to-day activities, compete for scarce resources, and attain goals. To perform these tasks effectively, however, nurse executives must understand and be able to plan strategies for dealing with conflict. They need to know how power is distributed within the organization and where they stand within the power structure to determine how to acquire the leverage needed to fulfill their role.

In the organizational hierarchy of a hospital, the two major power structures are the administration and the medical staff. These two groups are often inherently in conflict because of differences in their goals: the goal of the administrators is to realize an efficient, cost-effective organization, and that of the physicians to obtain optimum resources for their patients. In most hospitals, physicians do not have formal organizational authority over hospital employees, including nurses; yet, they do have power. Thus, an important task of the nurse executive is to increase the power of nursing without aggravating organizational conflict.

One route by which this objective can be attained is to emphasize the dependence of other organizational units of the hospital on nursing. For example, if the chief of pediatrics wants to open an intensive care unit for newborns, he or she must rely on the nursing director to staff it. The nursing executive in turn must provide personnel not only in sufficient numbers but also with the necessary critical care skills for quality patient care, ready and fully trained on the day that the unit accepts its first patient. Rather than treating this accomplishment as a routine assignment to be expected of the position, the executive should use the opportunity to make the hospital community aware of the importance of the nursing role to the realization of a goal. Further, the executive should convey the idea that he or she has resources—that is, power—and is ready to use them to help or hinder the attainment of an objective of a member from another area in the hierarchy. Moreover, power may be augmented by gaining support from subgroups within a high-power group. Thus, by supporting the physicians, nurses can gain leverage in dealing with administrators who may be more interested in satisfying physicians than nurses.

SUMMARY

Because conflict is an inherent part of an individual's personal and professional life, it is inevitable. Conflict, often viewed as a negative manifestation of human interaction, can have positive as well as negative aspects. How individuals perceive conflict may be influenced by the definition and theory they accept. There are three major philosophical views of conflict: the traditionalist, who views conflict as a destructive force that should be eliminated from organizations; the behavioralist, who views conflict as an inevitable occurrence that should be reduced or controlled; and the interactionist, who views conflict as a creative force that must be stimulated as well as resolved.

Four approaches to understanding the nature of conflict are *(1)* the interpersonal-psychological approach, *(2)* the interaction-sociological approach, *(3)* the anthropological approach, and *(4)* the economic-political approach. Each approach assumes different sources of conflict.

Various situations provoke conflict, such as the use of an apparent problem, which evokes a more critical issue to the surface; large-scale issues that tend to unify a diverse interest group; rising expectations; and moral overtones that justify radical action. The types of conflict that may be encountered are intrapersonal, or role conflict, interpersonal, and intergroup, or interorganizational. Power is viewed as one of the primary sources of conflict. This is particularly true when the disposition of power is seen as a "have" or "have-not" situation.

Many techniques or approaches may be used effectively for conflict resolution. Avoidance, defusion, containment, and confrontation are four major strategies that may be used for intergroup conflict. Three basic strategies that individuals can use in interpersonal, as well as in intergroup, for dealing with conflict include lose-lose, win-lose, and win-win approaches. Negotiation and collaboration are common techniques applied in conflict resolution. Each has its own advantages and disadvantages. Selection of the appropriate technique of conflict resolution strategy should be contingent on the characteristics of the situation.

The nurse executive must be cognizant of the particular circumstances underlying the presence of personal or organizational conflict. Rigorous analysis is essential before managerial intervention to facilitate conflict resolution.

STUDY QUESTIONS

1. Formulate a definition of conflict. Explain your rationale for this selection.
2. Compare and contrast the approach to conflict of traditionalists, behavioralists, and interactionists. Which approach do you favor. Why?

3. From your perspective, cite at least two examples and sources of conflict. What strategies or techniques for conflict resolution would you likely use? Explain.

4. Briefly describe a situation involving a nurse executive in which conflict involves power and elements of the use of power. What is the actual or potential power base(s) of the participants? Describe the factors that influence the power base of the participants. Analyze ways in which an increase in power would either sustain or resolve the conflict situation.

5. Practice diversity by sincerely trying to listen to persons with whom you always seem to be in conflict. What do you learn from listening attentively?

6. What is the difference between C-type conflict and A-type conflict? As a team leader in a home health care agency where dysfunctional conflict is evident, what strategies would you use to stimulate C-type conflict?

REFERENCES

Amason, A., Hochwarter, W., Thompson, K., & Harrison, A. (1995). Conflict: An important dimension in successful team management. *Organizational Dynamics, 24*(2), 20–35.

Argyris, C. (1976). *How tomorrow's executives will make decisions. Think, 33*(6), 22–35.

Arndt, C., & Laeger, E. (1970). Role strain in a diversified role set: The director of nursing service. *Nursing Research, 19*(3), 253–259.

Baldridge, J. (1979). *New approaches to management.* San Francisco: Jossey-Bass.

Bugental, J. F. T. (1965). *The search for authenticity: An existential-analytic approach to psychotherapy.* New York: Holt, Rinehart & Winston.

Cohen, H. (1980). *You can negotiate anything.* Secaucus, NJ: Lyle Stuart Publishers.

Feldman, D., & Arnold, H. (1983). *Managing individual and group behavior in organizations.* New York: McGraw-Hill.

Filley, A. (1975). *Interpersonal and conflict resolution.* Glenview, IL: Scott Foresman.

French, J., & Raven, B. (1968). The bases of social power. In D. Cartwright & A. Zander (Eds.), *Group dynamics: Research and theory.* New York: Harper & Row.

Frost, J., & Wilmot, W. (1978). *Interpersonal conflict.* Dubuque, IA: William C. Brown.

Halsey, S. (1978). The queen bee syndrome: One solution to role conflict for nurse managers. In M. Hardy & M. Conway (Eds.), *Role theory: Perspectives for health professionals.* New York: Appleton-Century-Crofts.

Kalisch, B., & Kalisch, P. (1977). An analysis of the sources of physician-nurse conflict. *Journal of Nursing Administration, 7*(1), 50–57.

Kelley, J. (1977). The role of the top level nurse administrator. *Proceedings, Nursing Administration: Issues for the 80s—Solutions for the 70s.* University of Minnesota, Battle Creek, MI: W. K. Kellogg Foundation.

Kelley, J. (1983). Negotiating skills for the nursing service administrator. *Nursing Clinics of North America, 18*(3), 427–438.

Leininger, M. (1974). Conflict and conflict resolution: Theories and processes relevant to the health professions. *The American Nurse, 6*(12), 17–22.

Likert, R., & Likert, J. (1976). *Ways of managing conflict.* New York: McGraw-Hill.

MacFarland, G., Leonard, H., & Morris, M. (1984). *Nursing leadership and management.* Albany, NY: Delmar, a division of Thomson Learning.

Polzer, J. T., & Neale, M. A. (1994). Conflict management and negotiation. In S. Shortell, A. Kaluzny, and Associates, *Health care management: Organization design and behavior* (3rd ed.). Albany, NY: Delmar.

Raven, B. H., & Kruglanski, W. (1975). Conflict and power. In P. C. Swingle (Ed.), *The structure of conflict.* New York: Academic Press.

Robbins, S., & Coulter, M. (1996). *Management* (5th ed.). Englewood Cliffs, NJ: Prentice-Hall.

Simms, L., Price, S., & Pfoutz, S. (1985). Nurse executives: Functions and Priorities, *Nursing Economic$, 3*(4), 238–244.

Strauss, A. (1979). *Negotiations: Varieties, contexts, processes and social orders.* San Francisco: Jossey-Bass.

Zey-Ferrell, M. (1979). *Dimensions of organizations.* Santa Monica, CA: Goodyear Publishing.

CHAPTER

~ 15 ~

Humor in Administration

Lillian M. Simms • Sylvia A. Price

Humor provided a continuous thread as the team struggled to accomplish its formidable task. (Bolman & Deal, 1991, p. 298)

Chapter Highlights

- State of the comic art
- The nature of comedy
- Theories of humor
- Humor as a coping mechanism
- Humor as a management skill
- Humor as a clinical skill
- Managing creativity and humor

The purpose of this chapter is to call attention to the relationship between humor and management, a topic rarely discussed in nursing. Examination of the relationship will not make you laugh, but a comic outcome may be achieved: a restructuring of your perception of comedy and management. This chapter develops the thesis that the qualities inherent in good management are similar to those of good comedy. This classic review of the comedy literature extends the discussion of humor as an essential leadership skill, first introduced in Chapter 5.

There has been a virtual explosion of information in the field of management since the early 1980s. These same decades have seen a parallel emergence of comedy in literature, theater, research, and the information media with the unique combination of management and comedy coming out in the 1990s in the works of Gareth Morgan. Current conferences on humor and laughter are playing to full houses across the country, just as conferences on management thrive and proliferate. However disparate the two arenas appear, they share a basic theme: how people behave, both as individuals and as members of organizations. Managers and comedians have much in common. Managers focus on the survival of the organization, namely, on improving productivity, ensuring quality, and reducing costs through people. Comedians focus on the survival of people and their attitudes and values for dealing with the content and context of their environments.

Humor can be used constructively to influence human behavior in health service organizations. In particular, nurse executives, like comedians, can be bearers of a special kind of wisdom and grace: the wisdom to see humor as a rich and versatile source of new knowledge and the grace to create the comic vision. Appreciating humor, even recognizing it, requires human skills of the highest order, as does managing enterprises of human service.

Humor serves an important function in organizations (Bolman & Deal, 1991). Along with metaphors and play, humor illustrates the "as if" quality of symbols. All three provide ways of grappling with issues that are too complex or threatening to deal with directly. Humor also has several important functions in organizations such as integrating, expressing skepticism, and nurturing flexibility and adaptiveness. Humor can be a distancing device but more often can be used to socialize, include, and convey membership. Most of all, humor provides a way to break frames of thinking to help illustrate that any single definition of situations is arbitrary. According to Bolman and Deal (1991), effective work groups encourage both play and humor. The authors cite examples of surgical teams and cockpit crews who have learned that joking is an essential source of creative invention and team spirit. Humor relieves tension and helps to resolve issues that arise in everyday work.

Morgan (1993) uses humor to great advantage as he writes about "imaginization" as a new way of thinking about organizations (see Chapter 6). His book *Imaginization* is deadly serious but full of humor and good fun. The book is an excellent example of how humor can be used to improve our abilities to understand situations in new ways. *Imaginization* comes as a surprise to those who wish to understand organizational and leadership theories and offers a path to demystifying good management. Morgan represents the first scholar to link management and comedy in a meaningful way and his book should be required reading for nurse executives in education and practice. Viktor Frankl (Dunn, 1999a) described humor and meaning as avenues to help transcend life circumstances. The uniquely human capacity of self-distancing thus allows one to view organizations and one's work humorously and objectively.

STATE OF THE COMIC ART

There was widespread ignorance among scientists and professionals of our humor heritage and the potential for the positive use of the comic tradition. Interest in the serious study of humor by scholars, educators, scientists, and therapists is a fairly new phenomenon that has only recently captured popular attention. Cummings (1979) noted that the pioneers in developing constructive use of humor in therapy in the treatment of retarded children, alcoholics, and drug addicts have been greeted by a majority of their professional colleagues with a lack of enthusiasm not dissimilar to that demonstrated by many members of the medical profession when innovators in that field insisted that nutrition be recognized as an important factor in physical and emotional well-being.

Recently, innovations in the teaching field have intentionally demonstrated the use of humor in textbooks to enhance learning; not a new idea, as the Talmud instructs its readers to "begin a lesson with humorous illustrations." Vera M. Robinson (1991) was the first nurse to legitimize humor as a fruitful concept and tool in communication and intervention with clients in *Humor and the Health Professional*. Norman Cousins' article "Anatomy of an Illness" in *The New England Journal of Medicine* (1976) stirred immediate and persistent controversy in the medical world. The publication of his book by the same title became popular literature, with its message that human beings possess remarkable powers of self-healing both of the body and mind. Cousins' use of humor to enhance his self-healing has become a modern legend.

Comedy has two essential ingredients: incongruity and surprise. Surprise and incongruity are exemplified in the unlikely perspectives of two students of comedy: Conrad Hyers and John Allen Paulos. Conrad Hyers (1981) presents an engaging interpretation of the religious dimensions of laughter, humor, and comedy in *Comic Vision and the Christian Faith*. John Allen Paulos (1980) has comprehensively studied the formal properties of humor by mathematical analyses in *Mathematics and Humor*. The ubiquity of humor is seen in the diversity of studies currently under the umbrella of the Workshop Library on World Humor, a nonprofit organization headquartered in Washington, D.C., which serves as a clearinghouse for the humor movement. Among topics under study are psychological theories of humor, the shaping power of comic strips, stand-up comedy, the holy fool, construction and implications of ethnic and disparagement humor, children's humor, and the comedy styles of humorists such as Rabelais, Chaplin, Robin Williams, and Patch Adams.

All of these examples illustrate the range and depth of the humor revolution. The promise of the comic viewpoint in the affairs of people and their organizations is a sudden insight, a fresh and accommodating change in viewpoint, an ability to see things in a new way, as Thoreau would say, to affect the "quality of the day." Beyond each day, "the importance of the comic vision in our time is amplified by the unparalleled knowledge and technological power available to us for dehumanizing and destroying as well as benefiting one another" (Hyers, 1981).

THE NATURE OF COMEDY

The plea for the comic vision begins with understanding the nature of comedy and an appreciation of the comedic rules. Finding a universal definition of comedy is as difficult as finding a universal definition of nursing. Our authorities on comedy speak from a heritage accumulated over the past several thousand years. No one of the following observations tells the whole story; neither do all of them together; none of them, you will observe, is good for much of a laugh:

- Plato first noted that the genius of comedy and tragedy were the same: a true artist in tragedy was also an artist in comedy.
- Aristotle reflected the attitude of the classical writers who considered comedy base and ignoble. Comic heroes were smaller than life. Audiences looked up to tragic heroes and looked down on comic heroes.
- In Roman comedy, the characters who are comic are from real life, are common people. The emphasis is on the physical, on social problems, and on the community setting of the city. Roman comedy established that catastrophe in comedy is never permanent. There are those whom we laugh at and those whom we laugh with.
- Satire results from moral indignation. It seeks to reform or at least expose vice and stupidity by attacking with sarcasm, wit, irony, or ridicule. It is not always fun or funny. There are basically two categories: Horatian and Juvenalian. The satire of Horace presents folly and lets it be its own worst enemy through accurate reproduction, only subtly exaggerated. The satire of Juvenal attacks folly full tilt; its contempt and anger are undisguised and overt.
- Moliere's play *Tartuffe* was banned as immoral and blasphemous when he attacked the vices of the age by depicting them in ridiculous guises.
- Schiller, poet and dramatist, declared that high comedy is the greatest of literary forms. The more comedy tends to be physical, the lower it is; the more it tends to be intellectual, verbal, concerned with the play of ideas, the higher it is. George S. Kaufman once defined high comedy as "a show that closed last Saturday."
- Meredith (1918) instructed us that true comedy is not contempt as is satire, but seeks thoughtful laughter.
- Kronenberger (1952) compared tragedy and comedy: both comedy and tragedy are about human limitations and human failure. Tragedy is idealistic and says, "The pity of it." Comedy is skeptical and says, "The absurdity of it." Tragedy laments the flaws of humanity; comedy looks for them. In tragedy, humans aspire for more than they can achieve; in comedy, they pretend to it. Comedy is criticism. It does not deny idealism but shows how far human beings fall short of it.
- Bergson (1911) observed that comedy is based on our sense of the full, rich, spontaneous variety of human nature. When the human becomes nonhuman and acts mechanical, we laugh. Comedy is social.
- Freud (1961) proposed that laughter is the surplus energy released when fear is appeased. Jokes release the anger or fear resulting from stress. All jokes release bottled-up anger or fear by presenting them in disguise so that we can laugh at stress; the disguise protects us from direct personal pain.

We laugh for two reasons: *(1)* the catharsis of relief ("thank God this has not happened to me") and *(2)* the warding off of suppressed anxiety ("by God, this might happen to me").

- Grotjahn (1966) refined the concept of comic distance. A joke is funny according to the efficiency of its disguise. The better the disguise, the better the joke. The disguise gives the audience the safety of comic distance or protecting objectivity.

- Frye (1956, 1958) speaks of mature comedy and comic grace. Comedy is designed, not to condemn evil, but to ridicule a lack of self-knowledge. "The essential comic resolution . . . is an individual release which is also a social reconciliation. The normal individual is freed from the bonds of . . . society, and a normal society is freed from the bonds imposed on it by . . . individuals." Comic grace is the grace of acceptance. A fundamental principle of comedy is to include rather than exclude, to soften and reduce distance between people.

- A cartoonist is a sit-down comic. The cartoonist Scott Adams (1996a) observes that we laugh when we feel superior to the comic figure. The more secure one feels, the more ready one is to laugh. Thus Dilbert has become the poster boy for organizational America. No matter how bad off we are with reengineered or down-sized workplaces, Dilbert is in a worse place.

- Arthur Koestler (1964) links creativity and comedy on the principle of connectivity. A good joke connects two unrelated things in an unexpected surprise. Koestler cites humor as one of the most basic forms of "bisociative" thinking—two different frames of reference collide to produce the surprising result.

- Pollio's study (Pollio & Talley, 1991) of the language of comedy suggests that whenever there is comedy, there is originality, spontaneity, superiority, and social significance. The comic event is best considered as a coherent gestalt—it does not seem reducible to any single principle.

- Kets DeVries (1993) speaks of humor as a balance to power. He further suggests that historically the person who assumed a stabilizing role in relation to an arrogant leader was the fool or clown.

- The stand-up comedians of our time still serve the basic function that court jesters did in times of yore. We expect, as did kings, that comedians be in touch with the chaotic forces in the universe, to protect and assure us that all will turn out all right, eventually (Adams, 1996b).

From the abundance of these random observations on the nature of comedy over time, one can readily see that comedy is a wide roof under which every man and woman can find shelter. The brotherhood of comedy and tragedy is significant and clear. Comedy is serious business. It is also clear that comedy is relative, a matter of opinion.

Vera Robinson (1991) provides us with a generic definition. She views humor as any "communication which is perceived by any of the parties as humorous and leads to laughing, smiling, or a feeling of amusement." Robinson notes that within health care settings, most of the humor is spontaneous or situational in nature, unlike the formal humor of literary work or the planned inclusion of jokes in speeches or lectures. Humor as a communication that results in certain observable behavior is an operational definition that serves the researcher's need for measurement. To the humor researcher, measurement is the riddle to be solved. Humor depends on so many emotional, social, and intellectual facets of human beings that it appears immune to quantitative analysis.

THEORIES OF HUMOR

We have seen that comedy defies definition, resists measurement, is a matter of opinion, is an ancient art enjoying a modern lifestyle. Humor may be a contemporary phenomenon of inquiry, but it has a natural history that is instructive. The ancient conception of comedy was narrower than ours, confined to farce, burlesque, and slapstick. This conception persisted until 1651, when the English philosopher Thomas Hobbes introduced a theory of laughter referred to as the superiority or disparagement theory. A sense of satisfied superiority and self-satisfaction are factors in many kinds of humor and play a prominent role in sick and ethnic jokes. Superiority is the primitive base on which humor theory was developed.

In 1776, James Beattie identified incongruity as a comic principle. Incongruity as oddness, or inappropriateness, was further developed in the 18th and 19th centuries by the philosophers Schopenhauer and Kant. Schopenhauer was so funny that countless adherents to his pessimistic philosophy committed suicide. Kant in 1790 called attention to the element of surprise, the unexpectedness of incongruity: "laughter is an affection arising from a sudden deflation of a strained expectation into nothing" (Paulos, 1980). Herbert Spencer and Charles Darwin observed the physiological bases of laughter, laughter as a release of energy, an observation that influenced later theorists, in particular, Freud.

In the early 20th century, the critic George Meredith (1918) emphasized a different aspect of humor: the social regulatory function. He wrote that the comic spirit is a sort of social corrective and springs into action whenever men wax out of proportion—whether they are planning short-sightedly or plotting dementedly. Meredith noted that humor, societal health, and the social equality of men and women were closely related.

The French writer Henri Bergson crafted a celebrated phrase in 1911 when he attributed laughter to the mechanical encrusted on something living. In other words, when humans become rigid, machinelike, and repetitive, they become comic, because the essence of humanity is its flexibility of spirit.

A well-known theory was developed by Freud in 1905. Through jokes and witticisms, a person vents his or her aggression or sexual anxieties in a disguised or playful manner. Max Eastman (1936) emphasized the relationship of humor and play as well as the requirement of an objective disengagement to appreciate humor. Eastman developed the derailment theory of humor. Humor is context dependent; that is, normal events are derailed by the situation. Humorous events are not incongruous per se but become incongruous given their situation. Perhaps this theoretical insight is the origin of the popular situation comedies rampant in the television media.

In 1964, Arthur Koestler compared the continuity of creative insights in humor with the creative insights of science and poetry: the logical pattern of the creative process is the same in all three fields: creativity consists of the discovery of hidden similarities, but the emotional climate is different . . . the comic smile has a touch of aggressiveness, the scientist's reasoning by analogy is emotionally detached, that is, neutral; the poetic image is sympathetic or admiring, inspired by a positive kind of emotion. Koestler's principle is that creative insight in all fields share the same logical patterns. Koestler's theory synthesized incongruity theory with the psychological theory of humor. Laughter is the discharge of emotional energy resulting from the "biociation" of two incompatible frames of reference. Koestler has a disciple in John Allen Paulos (1980).

Paulos explores the operations and structures common to humor and in the formal sciences of logic, mathematics, and linguistics. He develops a mathematical model of jokes using the mathematical theory of "catastrophe." Paulos exemplifies the universality of humor across disciplines and promises a humorous continuity in the age of information and its computer technology.

This chronology is admittedly incomplete, but the common ingredients of humor emerge despite the different approaches of theorists of humor. An essential ingredient of humor is the juxtaposition of two or more incongruous ways of viewing events, ideas, people, and their roles. For something to be funny, some unusual, inappropriate or odd aspect of it must be perceived and compared with the norm. Another essential ingredient of humor is the proper psychological and emotional climate. The proper emotional climate is both subjective and objective and, in the current understanding of comedy theory, an undefined conjecture.

Vera Robinson (1991) provides a cogent description of theories of humor in an overview of humor as a complex cognitive, emotional, psychological, and physiological phenomenon. She chooses to approach theories of humor by disciplinary categories (Table 15.1).

HUMOR AS A COPING MECHANISM

Chapter 5 presented coping as an essential skill for leadership. Without a doubt, humor is one of the most needed and least understood coping skills. Robinson (1991) describes humor as a way of coping with aggression and anger and a psychological, adaptive defense mechanism. She points out that humor is one of the important ways to deal with the burdens of everyday reality. The rules of logic, time, place, and proper conduct are suspended. There is obviously a range of

Table 15.1 Disciplinary Perspectives on Humor

Perspectives	Theory
Humanities	Comedy reveals human imperfections, makes people more tolerant, and stimulates courage to face life.
Philosophical	Laughter, a physical activity, results from a pleasant change in psychological state and is a natural expression of amusement.
Psychoanalytical	Humor is a relief mechanism allowing people to deal more readily with negatives in their lives.
Anthropological	Humor is a cognitive experience which must have a cultural niche, a "permitted disrespect" with a combination of friendliness and antagonism.
Biological	A survival instinct, developed as an evolutionary process—a way to deal with untoward or attack situations.
Sociological	Humor promotes group cohesion and initiates relationships, minimizing stress in organizations.
Play	Enjoyment of the laughable emerges from a play mood or refusal to take a situation seriously.
Superiority	Asserts our own superiority by laughing at the inferiority, stupidity, or misfortunes of self or others.
Surprise	A classic theory that laughter emerges from sudden insight or perception—the concept of surprise at the incongruity of a situation or action.

healthy or unhealthy behaviors. However, emotionally, humor is healthy when it helps individuals handle the realities of downsizing, work redesign, and position elimination. Humor becomes destructive and dysfunctional when it becomes a pathologic denial of reality, a force for running away from difficulties.

Schechtman (1998), an international change consultant, explains that our work-related problems are almost always rooted in our past, which leads us to be stuck in the same jobs and the same relationships. He proposes that people in all professions and work need new skills and knowledge. The Fifth Wave challenge for both individuals and organizations is to connect knowledge to self-growth. Instead of holding onto the past, we can choose to grow. Chapter 22 presents a path to personal empowerment. We are suggesting that one way to upgrade your path to self-growth and personal empowerment is to add humor to your "bag" of coping skills.

Robinson (1991) proposes that you can increase your humorous perspective in several ways: *(1)* analyzing your current sense of humor and *(2)* understanding the techniques of comedy and comedy styles. Open yourself up to humor by looking for absurdities in life, seeing comedy films, becoming more playful, and expanding your humorous attitude. We further suggest adding humor analysis to your self-analysis by determining what makes you laugh and what made you laugh in childhood.

Robinson (1991) has concrete suggestions for increasing one's humorous perspective. In addition to giving yourself permission to laugh at work, she proposes that you seek out humorous items. Start collecting cartoons, jokes, funny sayings, and humorous incidents and stories. We suggest buying new books like Moore's (1996) *Downsize This* and Shelton's (1997) *You Might as Well Laugh* to help you see humorous ways of looking at organizations and home life. Simms has for years posted humorous items on her office door and delighted in listening to the chuckles of passers-by. It is amazing what wonderful relevant cartoons can be found in the *New Yorker* magazine, *Harvard Business Review,* the *Humor & Health Journal,* and the daily newspaper. Adding humor to your everyday relationships can strengthen your coping skills at home and at work.

HUMOR AS A MANAGEMENT SKILL

Humor and laughter can improve business relationships. Feigelson (1998) asserts that you are more likely to be with and interact with someone with whom you have shared laughter. When we share laughter together, we create a foundation of positive feelings that can help balance the effects of negative situations. Laughter is a good releaser of tension. It also stimulates creativity in the workplace. Noer (1993) describes the widespread anger that occurs with layoffs. Employees feel fatigued and drained with the downsizing and continuing reductions. Those remaining need coping mechanisms to help them recover from the "layoff survivor sickness" that invariably occurs with downsizing. The anger and frustration are frequently manifested as deteriorating physical and psychological health in workers and managers.

At the 1999 American Organization of Nurse Executives Annual Meeting in Charlotte, North Carolina, Schechtman (1998) shared that he no longer teaches management theories in his change workshops. Instead, he teaches coping and grieving skills as more relevant to modern organizations. We propose that humor is one of the best coping mechanisms to be mastered by nurse executives.

Feigelson (1998) discusses the importance of bringing laughter into business meetings. When people are smiling they are more able to have positive interactions. She describes four different kinds of business meetings, all of which are relevant for nurse executives: *(1)* decision-making, *(2)* networking, *(3)* learning, and *(4)* celebration. She then goes on to describe the role of humor in the four types of meetings (Figure 15.1).

HUMOR AS A CLINICAL TOOL

Although it is hard to pinpoint what humor is, it is easy to define what it does. Humor causes pleasant feelings and enjoyment. Humor makes us smile, laugh, or feel amused or amazed. It alerts our senses and makes us responsive as well as resilient. Barry (1999) notes that humor undoubtedly has positive health benefits. Studies have confirmed that hearty laughter can provide exercise by increasing

	Decision-Making	Networking	Learning	Celebrating
What is the primary purpose of the meeting?	• To solve problems • To make decisions • To plan and review	• To meet other people • To build relationships	• To raise awareness • To share information • To learn new information • To increase skills	• To recognize accomplishments • To honor someone • To enjoy the event and each other's company
What kinds of groups meet?	• Teams • Staffs • Task forces • Boards and councils • Committees	• Professional associations • Business and civic groups • Support groups • Social clubs	• Students • Adult learners • Trainees • Employees • Team members	• Work groups • Colleagues • Friends • Neighbors • Families
What are primary sources of tension at meetings?	• Having to make a decision • Needing to accomplish a task • Not trusting others • Being unclear of the task • Not knowing the consequences • Not having criteria for success	• Meeting new people • Fearing the unknown • Feeling shy • Not having credentials • Lacking credibility • Lacking experience	• Worrying • Feeling bored • Being annoyed by the teaching style • Feeling uncertain	• Ensuring that each person enjoys himself or herself • Helping everyone share in the joy • Not feeling comfortable in the group • Not knowing what to expect
What is the primary role of humor and laughter?	• To reduce tension • To enliven the meeting • To promote creative thinking • To re-energize • To unify	• To create a pleasant atmosphere • To put people at ease • To create connections • To build cohesiveness	• To reduce stress • To gain and maintain attention • To communicate more easily • To improve memory • To refresh or provide a break	• To relax • To allow people to help each other have a good time • To enhance good feelings • To entertain • To increase the joy of being together

Figure 15.1 Four types of meetings and the role of humor. From Energize your meetings with laughter, by Sheila Feigelson, 1998, Alexandria, VA: Association for Supervision and Curriculum Development (ASCD). p. 21. Copyright 1998 by Sheila Feigelson. Reprinted with permission fromt the author.

the heart rate, stimulating blood circulation and breathing, and improving muscle tone. Barry describes other benefits of humor, which has been found to:

- Reduce pain, probably through the release of endorphins, the body's natural painkillers
- Reduce stress by lowering levels of cortisol, a stress hormone
- Stimulate the immune system
- Stimulate mental functions, such as alertness and memory

Within the world of health and illness, humor serves three major functions, states Robinson (1991). Humor serves to communicate important messages, promote social relations, and diminish the discomforts that occur in an illness setting. In times of illness, patients and health professionals are strangers who are suddenly thrown together in very intimate relationships. Schechtman (1998) espouses the importance of the familiar. Robinson (1991) has long discussed the importance of the familiar in establishing continuing relationships, noting that humor quickly provides a sense of the familiar, is easily facilitated, and does not offend.

Dunn (1999b), based on an interview with James A. Thorson, a humor researcher, describes six elements that comprise a sense of humor:

- Humor creativity
- Humor appreciation
- Coping humor
- Humor as a social lubricant
- Appreciation of humorous people
- Joy of life (happiness)

Older people who are coping well have a terrific sense of humor. There are marked gender differences. Most hospitals will tell you that the cancer patients are the funniest. Nurse executives need to understand theories of humor to create healthy workplaces and great places to work in which patients not only cope but are encouraged to recover. To our knowledge, humor has never been taught as an essential skill in schools of nursing. Vera Robinson has been unique in her steadfast efforts to stimulate recognition of humor as a valuable leadership and clinical skill.

Patch Adams (1998) believes that humor is an antidote for all ills. A social revolutionary in the health care world, Adams has initiated a unique and positive approach to health and healing. Adams believes that healing should be a creative, loving, and humorous interchange. His Gesundheit Institute built in Northern Virginia in 1971 is the base for Patch's dream of a yet to be built 40-bed free hospital on 310 acres in a medically underserved area of West Virginia.

For years, clowns have been part of therapy for children. Adams brings the importance of humor to all ages, believing that laughter has a positive effect on cardiovascular and respiratory problems as well as being the foundation for good mental health. Adams is not alone in his convictions and many health professionals are indicating a willingness to work with him and support his efforts.

HOW TO BE A COMEDIAN

To humorize management in constructive and productive ways requires awareness, accumulation of comic knowledge, and the progressive mastery of comic skills. A generous appreciation of comedy, its relative nature, and its rules is developed in individuals and in organizations by the same process of developing and using new knowledge and new technology from other relevant fields. Currently, nurse executives are addressing the business of nursing, establishing the economic rationality of practice, and integrating complex information technology into their professional practice. The arguments for an economic framework for nursing practice, whether clinical or administrative practice, carries the urgency of survival. Similarly, if no other argument can be made that will convince nurse executives of the value of the comic perspective, humor as a conferment of survival skills, is the most compelling.

Vera Robinson has developed guidelines for increasing a humor conscience, identifying appropriate uses, and establishing a knowledge base for comedy and comic techniques for the health professional. Another survival manual for administrators is Carolyn L. Vash's book, *The Burnt-out Administrator,* which is written with insight and humor (1980). Assuming an informed student of the comic tradition, what possibilities are at hand for nurse executives and their staffs to step outside themselves and their bureaucratic systems, to see themselves and their organizations from a comic perspective? Just as humor and jokes have at least two levels of meaning, organizational theory has two levels of conceptualization, normative and descriptive, what ought to be and what actually is. The organizational chart and job description are two handy hooks with which to begin practicing humor. What insights might emerge if a humorist designed an organizational chart that truly reflected organizational decision-making, actual power centers, and patterns of information flow? Is there a department of applied humor, a committee on utilization of humor, or a consultant on comedy? Is there a locus for maintaining an organizational sense of humor? What would a job description reveal about the reality of nursing, if actual work performed were described instead of work expected? Would a recognition program change if humor or the ability to create laughter were among the criteria of achievement? How would a humor break affect the work of committees? Would instruction or policy be followed more willingly if formulated in a comic vocabulary? Would the graffiti of disenchantment that peppers the walls of a unit or department in crisis or under threat change from rage to more accommodating slogans? If humor were legitimized, what would happen to the relationship between management and labor? Would communication failures persist if subject to comic analysis?

The folklore of an organization and the ambiguous context of organizational reality is a dazzling lode for the comedian. Humor ranges in a continuum from healthy to unhealthy. It is healthy when it deals with immediate issues and helps the individual or the organization handle reality. It is dysfunctional or unhealthy when it denies reality.

In an entirely different context from that of the inherent absurdities of organizational endeavors, humor has the potential for enriching nursing diagnostic and therapeutic practice. The American Nurses Association's Social Policy Statement (1997) expands the 1980 definition of nursing, "the diagnosis and treatment of human responses to actual or potential health problems" to include a list of human phenomena that call for nursing intervention, such as self-care limitations, impaired functioning, and pain and discomfort. Laughter is a human response, inherent in humanness. It is also a functional ability amenable to nursing assessment and nursing treatment. Inability to laugh or to respond appropriately to the comic is a health problem. Recent research on the relationship of the right and left sides of the brain promises diagnostic criteria in brain-damaged patients such as in stroke. "Only when the brain's two hemispheres are working together can we appreciate the moral of a story, the meaning of metaphor, words describing emotion, and the punch lines of jokes" (Gardner, 1981).

Using the sense of the ridiculous has also been posited as a memory enhancing device; the more ridiculous the image created in terms of association, the more likely the name, place, or event will be remembered. Laughter presupposes a system of shared values and beliefs. Laughing with someone enfolds him or her in a system of support and care. The therapeutic use of humor treats the people in pain, not the pain in people. Recognizing laughter as evidence of a positive patient care outcome expands opportunity to collaborate with patients in their own self-regulation.

MANAGING CREATIVITY AND HUMOR

Within the economic dynamics of the 1990s, nursing service organizations that purposefully and persistently manage the generation and development of new ideas will have a significant competitive edge in the future marketplace. Dennis D. Pointer (1985), senior research fellow at the Rand Corporation, prophesied "organizational creativity and innovation will become 'the high ground' of the health care industry." To varying degrees all organizations resist creativity, innovation, and change, particularly large scale organizations and those dependent on complex routines such as hospitals. "An organization's climate and culture are among the most important barriers to or facilitators of creativity and innovation," declares Pointer.

It is within the climate and the culture of an organization that a friendly sense of humor, the comic vision, and healthy laughter play constructive roles. Humor experiences such as having humor consultants or workshops that entertain, even energize, the participants are temporary in effect if there are no sustaining or organizational values that integrate humor into the daily grind of work. Humor in the workplace connects our shared experiences of organizational life. It connects things in a way we never suspected. Most of us operate from only one frame of reference at a time. A new frame of reference gives a new center of gravity. Discovery of surprising relationships among the ordinary and mundane startles our imagination out of habit and cliché. The catapult of humor is an effective yet frequently neglected pathway to creative and innovative behavior. Many corporations are beginning to take serious interest in humor to be used in training, employee relations, and other day-to-day activities.

The manager's use of humor is purposeful—to help pace, lighten, and highlight the content and context of work. Humor brightens the corner where you are. The manager is not an entertainer, but a role model and facilitator who seeks and empowers a natural and healthy sense of organizational humor. For instance, Ben and Jerry's Ice Cream in Vermont has a joy committee. The concept of a sense of humor residing in an organization humanizes the organization and allows a fresh orientation from which to see how to make conflict manageable and goals clear. Given the popular advocation of humor in management evident in current literature (Kushner, 1990; Paulson, 1989; Ross, 1989), humor is acknowledged as one of the easiest and most accessible and most effective ways to stimulate new ideas and new approaches to old problems. The spontaneity of humor frees us to step outside one's own discipline and traditional behavior to seek new sources of knowledge to serve the organization. In particular, humor demands originality and creativity in thought and action.

Both humor and creativity are boundary free and have a natural connection. They are kissing cousins. Both are nonlinear phenomena characterized by divergent thinking through which many solutions to address problems become possible. Both share wide ranging knowledge sources and a repertoire of language and conceptual skills. Howard Gardner's (1982) psychological research on various types of intelligence has shown that the best predictor of creativity is an active sense of humor, not intelligence as currently measured. Koestler (1964) in the first chapter titled "The Jester" in his book *Act of Creation,* makes a convincing argument for the basic nature of creativity as expressed in the process of humor. For Koestler, the studies of creativity and humor are inseparable—sharing a common cognitive pathway. The commonality is the same process of appreciating a joke, for solving a problem and for having an artistic, high experience.

Alice M. Isen's (1987) research on creativity and states of mind or mood found that 70% of students put into a cheerful mood by a comedy film correctly solved problems; on the other hand, only 20% of those who watched a math film came up with a correct answer. Isen speculates that positive mood influences creativity by changing the way cognitive material is organized—being in a happy mood may cue you into a cognitive context that could significantly affect your creativity. An aspect of Isen's work is the implication that creativity can be manipulated, can be fostered, can be enticed by laughter—therefore, learned.

The author of *Uncommon Genius,* Denise Shekerjian (1990), believes creativity can be learned but not through a formula or recipe slavishly followed. "The phenomenon of the creative spark is larger than any of my findings can suggest. But I do firmly believe that if we cultivate a consciousness about the way we think and work and behave, improvement in our creative abilities is possible—and improvement is not something to be taken lightly." Her computer search in preparation for her book produced 6,821 "hits" on creativity in print from 1967 to date—and those are just the ones in English. Shekerjian interviewed 40 winners of the MacArthur Foundation Fellowships to write her guide to creativity. She blends her conversations with the 40 awardees with theory and literature and life and shows us how to nurture creativity in our lives.

Researcher David Perkins of Harvard University is codirector of Project Zero, a project studying cognitive skills of scientists and artists. Perkins (McAleer, 1989) contends "there is no justification for assigning abilities such as math or music or general faculties like intuition and rationality to the left or right hemispheres of the brain. The two hemispheres interact and cooperate in a variety of complex ways not yet fully understood." According to Stanford University neurologist, Karl Pribrim (McAleer, 1989) the frontal lobe is more verbal on the left and more visual on the right. "If there is an important simple anatomical way of dividing the brain in relation to creativity it's a front/back, not a right/left division."

Not since the post-Sputnik years has there been such a surge of creative research about creativity and innovation. As creativity and innovation shape the template of the 21st century, nurse executives have a profound and joyful resource in humor.

Csikszentmihalyi (1996) presents another vital link to understanding creativity, the creative process, and how creativity can enrich our personal and work lives. Creative individuals tend to have a playfully light attitude. Linked with perseverance, playfulness and a willingness to bounce ideas around are important and fun in science. Csikszentmihalyi's (1996) discussion of personality traits that are essential to creativity includes "playfulness" or playfully light attitude that has the lightness of joking. This quality of creative people is always combined with discipline and hard work. Cultivating curiosity and interest (surprise) can lead to higher level creativity. Surprise can be nurtured through humor and other daily activities. Csikszentmihalyi suggests that one can practice "surprise" by *(1)* trying to be surprised by something every day, *(2)* surprising at least one person every day, and *(3)* writing down each day what surprised you and others. These activities also nurture the sense of humor advocated by Robinson (1991).

It is hard to imagine more anxious scenes than those in acute care settings. However, more and more health professionals are beginning to accept the value of mirth as a vital force in care and recovery and among health care workers themselves. In general, doctors have been slower than nurses to use humor. Much of the advocacy for today's humor surge began with Norman Cousins' (1976) *Anatomy of an Illness* in which he accounts how he fought pain and disease by dosing himself with humorous books and reruns of "Candid Camera."

THE PUNCH LINE

At this time in this routine, a disquieting question should be raised and resolved. Is there a comedy of management or a management of comedy? Is there a distinction here that makes a difference? A Soviet diplomat was asked what in his mind was the difference between capitalism and communism. With a straight face he responded that in capitalism, humans exploit humans and in communism, it is the other way around. The alignment of management and comedy demonstrates two key characteristics of humor: opposition and relational reversal. Opposition is the articulation of contrasts: expectation versus surprise, the mechanical versus the spiritual, superiority versus incompetence, balance versus exaggeration. Reversal is cognitive restructuring that produces a change in perspective. It is the setting up of a premise, an expectation or a process that suddenly shifts direction and meaning (for example, "that is not dirt in your soup; it is earth"). Like a relational reversal, a pun forces one to perceive in quick succession two incongruities or unlikely sides of an idea.

The comedy of management resides in the response to the dynamics of unruly oppositions common in administrative practice: predictability versus surprise, control versus freedom, stability versus chaos, full knowledge versus inevitable ignorance. Comedy of management is keeping the people who dislike you from the people who are undecided.

The management of comedy is exemplified in the dynamics of relational reversal, in securing a new way of looking at the mundane to find the marvelous or beyond the marvelous to find the mundane. Through the management of comedy, human resources of imagination and creativity are liberated for invention and experimentation. Responding to events is the comedy of management, whereas shaping events is the management of comedy.

SUMMARY

Humor is a distinct universe of discourse with its own logic and its own reason. Constructive humor integrates, combines into one view or framework, the best of two worlds: nursing and management. Humor makes possible new connections between two dissimilar theory and practice universes. Good management is the constructive and creative use of human resources. Good comedy enlightens and informs us about our self-concept and our organizational concept. A comic perspective leads an organization toward greater awareness of its strength and weaknesses and allows an organization to respond to one of the most powerful human drives: the urge to try something new. When you have a hammer in hand, you look for nails. When you have a comic perspective, you look for new ways to respond and express creativity.

STUDY QUESTIONS

1. What value does humor have in your personal and professional life? Examine what makes you laugh. Do you initiate and create humor?
2. What do you mean when you say someone has a sense of humor? Can you specify or qualify your definition of a sense of humor?

3. Select an organization with which you are familiar and analyze it according to a comic perspective. What kind of humor is characteristically expressed? What patterns of joking relationships characterize the organization? How does the organization use comic framework and techniques to accomplish organizational work or goals? How much fun or playfulness is tolerated or sanctioned by the organization?

4. Read the comic strip Dilbert for examples of humor that are relevant for your workplace.

REFERENCES

Adams, P. (1998). *Gesundheit*. Rochester, VT: Healing Arts Press.

Adams, S. (1996a). *The Dilbert principle*. New York: HarperCollins.

Adams, S. (1996b). *Dogbert's management handbook*. New York: HarperCollins.

American Nurses Association. (1997). *Nursing: A social policy statement*. Kansas City, MO: Author.

Barry, P. (1999, April). It's no joke: humor heals. *AARP Bulletin, 40*(4), 14–17.

Bergson, H. (1911). *Laughter: An essay on the meaning of the comic*. New York: Macmillan.

Bolman, L. G., & Deal, T. E. (1991). *Reframing organizations*. San Francisco: Jossey-Bass.

Cousins, N. (1976). Anatomy of an illness. *New England Journal of Medicine, 295*(26), 1458–1463.

Csikszentmihalyi, M. (1996). *Creativity*. New York: Harper Perennial.

Cummings, H. (1979). *The importance of not being earnest in the arts, sciences and professions*. Address presented at the Second International Conference on Humor. Los Angeles.

Dunn, J. R. (1999a). The wit and wisdom of Viktor Frankl. *Humor & Health Journal, VIII*(1), 1–9.

Dunn, J. R. (1999b). What is a sense of humor? *Humor & Health Journal, VIII*(2), 1–8.

Eastman, M. (1936). *Enjoyment of laughter*. New York: Simon & Schuster.

Feigelson, S. (1998). *Energizing your meetings with laughter*. Alexandria, VA: Association for Supervision and Curriculum Development (ASCD).

Freud, S. (1961). Jokes and their relation to the unconscious. In J. Strachey (Ed.), *The complete psychological works of Sigmund Freud* (p. 8). London: Hogarth Press.

Frye, N. (1956). *The anatomy of criticism*. Princeton, NJ: Princeton University Press.

Frye, N. (1958). The structure of comedy. In S. Barnett (Ed.), *Eight great comedies*. New York: New American Library.

Gardner, H. (1982). *Art, mind and brain: A cognitive approach to creativity*. New York: Basic Books.

Gardner, H. (1981). How the split brain gets a joke. *Psychology Today, 15*(2), 74.

Grotjahn, M. (1966). *Beyond laughter: A psychoanalytical approach to humor*. New York: McGraw-Hill.

Hyers, C. (1981). *The comic vision and the Christian faith*. New York: Pilgrim Press.

Isen, A. (1987). A creative muse. *Journal of Personality and Social Psychology, 52*, 1122–1131.

Kets deVries, M. F. R. (1993). *Leaders, fools and imposters*. San Francisco: Jossey-Bass.

Koestler, A. (1964). *The act of creation*. London: Hutchinson.

Kronenberger, L. (1952). *The thread of laughter*. New York: Knopf.

Kushner, M. (1990). *The light touch: How to use humor for business success*. New York: Simon & Schuster.

McAleer, N. (1989). On creativity. *Omni, 11*(7), 42–44.

Meredith, G. (1918). *An essay on comedy.* New York: Scribners.

Moore, M. (1996). *Downsize this.* New York: Crown Publishers.

Morgan, G. (1993). *Imaginization.* Newbury Park, CA: Sage.

Noer, D. M. (1993). *Healing the wounds.* San Francisco: Jossey-Bass.

Paulos, J. (1980). *Mathematics and humor.* Chicago: University of Chicago Press.

Paulson, T. (1989). *Making humor work: Take your job seriously and yourself lightly.* Menlo Park, CA: Crisp Publications.

Pointer, D. (1985). Responding to the challenges of the new health care marketplace: Organizing creativity and innovation. *Hospital and Health Services Administration, 30*(6), 10–23.

Pollio, H., & Talley, J. (1991). The concepts and language of comic art. *Humor, 4*(1), 1–20.

Robinson, V. (1991). *Humor and the health professions.* Thorofare, NJ: Slack.

Ross, B. (1989). *Laugh, lead and profit: Building productive workplaces with humor.* New York: William Morrow.

Schechtman, M. R. (1998). *The internal frontier.* Los Angeles: New Star Press.

Shekerjian, D. (1990). *Uncommon genius.* New York: Viking Penguin.

Shelton, S. K. (1997). You might as well laugh. Baltimore: Bancroft Press.

Vash, C. (1980). *The burnt-out administrator.* New York: Springer.

PART

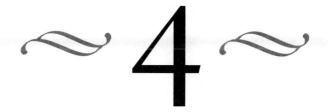

4

Facilitating Professional Nursing Practice

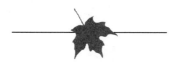

C H A P T E R

~ 16 ~

Ethical Decision Making and Moral Judgments

Charlotte McDaniel

A critical component to the study of ethics is a systematic approach that involves rational thinking; it implies an ability to think critically about moral and ethical issues. (Author)

Chapter Highlights

- Ethics defined
- Ethics and quality care
- Ethics and current practice
- Ethics and benefits
- Generic decision models
- Ethical decision models
- Ethics and professional practice

Ethics as a basis for clinical practice is important to nursing and to health care. The importance of ethics for the delivery of nursing care, however, is receiving increasing attention in nursing administration because of the contribution that ethics can make to a positive work environment and to the organizational culture of nursing practice.

Nursing administration as a professional practice for the delivery of health care is fundamentally a moral practice. Nursing administration is fundamentally moral because the delivery of nursing care is based on the interaction and interrelationships of patients as human beings and on decisions about them and their care (Beauchamp & Childress, 1994). Because morals and ethics are intertwined, nursing care is also an issue of ethics. Nurses make decisions in the daily implementation of their practice and in the management of patient care that affect and influence human beings and their lives. These important and often critical decisions are significant to nursing administration because nurse executives shape and sustain the practice environment of those nurses who are delivering patient care.

ETHICS DEFINED

Although ethics is variously defined, it is recognized as a branch of philosophy that addresses questions of right or wrong. Generically, ethics is a term that refers to the ". . . various ways of understanding and examining the moral life." (Beauchamp & Childress, 1994, p. 4). It explores, in a systematic way, what persons should do by encouraging individuals to address usual actions, or decisions. Ethics, as a discipline and an endeavor, provides a framework for exploring human conduct, including not only our behavior, but our motivations and our objectives in a rational systematic way. Ethics, therefore, is the rational and systematic examination of issues pertaining to right and wrong. "Ethics systematically explores what we ought to do by asking persons to consider . . . our ordinary actions, judgments, and justifications" (Beauchamp & Childress, 1989, xii).

A critical component to the study of ethics is a systematic approach that involves rational thinking; it implies an ability to think critically about moral and ethical issues. Essentially, this process is ethical decision-making. Although distinctions can be made between morals and ethics, because the focus of this chapter is on decision-making in applied ethics for the administration of nursing care, for the purposes of this chapter the two terms will be used synonymously. This is appropriate because nursing administration is based on decision-making, and ethics pertains to rational decisions about ethical issues.

ETHICS AND QUALITY CARE

A sound sense of ethics, conveyed by ethical decisions, is essential to quality nursing care. It is important not only to professional nurses and to nursing, it is also important to the patient as the health care consumer. Patients understand and perceive an ethical system by the nature, the competency, and the quality of the care that they receive. Consumers formulate their understanding of the ethical nature of nursing by those individual and patient care dimensions of nursing practice.

Ethical practice is also important to nurse executives who are responsible for those nurses and, in turn, to other administrators to whom nursing reports. This is not to imply that current practices are unethical, but, simply that applied ethics is fundamental and important to quality nursing care and administration. Ironically, a well-grounded and ethically based administration frames nursing practice, which, in turn, supports the professional practice of nursing administration. Thus, the interrelationship of these two—care and administration—are not only necessary to each other, they are essential to each other.

ETHICS AND CURRENT PRACTICE

Nurse executives experience ethical dilemmas in their daily administration of health care services and patient care. Unfortunately, the reality is that in the current administrative practice of contemporary health care ethical dilemmas and challenges develop in the management of those services. For this reason, an equally realistic perspective regarding ethical dilemmas is to be thoughtful about and prepared to address them. Among several that occur often are four that are most frequent: resource allocation, support of nursing staff, patients with compromised quality of life, and noninsured or underinsured patients.

One of the ethical dilemmas most frequently encountered is the allocation of scarce resources. This issue raises the concept of justice or rationing in health care. As we all know, there are never enough resources; consequently, the ability to rationally and ethically distribute scarce resources is an important, and frequent, administrative function. Those resources may be, for instance, personnel, finances, or high-acuity beds. Regardless of the substance, the process and the issues are similar for decision-making regarding resource allocation.

Another common encounter is the need to support one's own nursing staff, yet be challenged with the need to retain a financially viable endeavor, such as the nursing department or the clinical patient care service. Nurses on staff may not understand the need for executives in nursing to retain a holistic perspective and to view the patient care system within its larger context. The dilemma is supporting one's own staff in the face of conflicting choices.

Common ethical challenges also pertain to patients who are at the end of life, or the quality of their life may be dramatically reduced. In these situations, the ethical challenge pertains to such nationally recognized issues as euthanasia, it raises the prospect of assisted suicide, or it raises the probability of a triage in which another patient may benefit more from the technology or care that is under the jurisdiction of the nurse administrator. Nursing staff may have different perspectives among themselves, as well as between them and other practitioners. Providing guidance in these situations is one of the nurse executive's administrative arts.

An increasingly contemporary situation is the need to provide care for patients who may not be insured, or they may be underinsured for the care needed. Nurses in the clinical setting typically would want to treat or care for patients. In today's market the need for coverage has never been greater, and the tension between the mandate for provision of care, especially to needy or underserved individuals, and the need for financially viable organizations is marked with ethical challenges. Here, too, assisting the nursing staff in understanding the various perspectives on this ethical dilemma is, in itself, challenging.

Of course, nurse executives and administrators face numerous other ethical challenges in today's health care. However, many of them have ramifications emerging from a specific situation or patient care case, but they may illustrate more common ethical concepts or issues in health care. Resource allocation and quality of life are two examples. Nurse administrators face these ethical challenges not only in their direct decision-making, but also in aiding and empowering clinical nursing staff to address them as well. Both of these common ethical decisions require administrative acumen that nursing executives illustrate in their daily management of health care services.

Faced with an ethical dilemma, what do nurse executives do? How do administrators make decisions? Studies on ethics and administration in nursing report several general findings. Among them is information that nurse administrators experience conflicts of an ethical nature that emerge from tensions among various components of the facility (Aroskar, 1998), and that administrators may use nonsystematic means to resolve dilemmas or conflicts (Haddad, 1997). Another finding is that nurse administrators and managers, as well as practicing nurses, continue to use professional codes as guides for decision-making in nursing (Esterhuizen, 1996). These ethical decisions could include, for example, but are not limited to allocation of nursing staff, downsizing, reimbursement rationing, aiding staff in decisions regarding futility, genetic screening, or do not resuscitate (DNR) orders, as well as the many intra- and interdisciplinary decisions to which nurse administrators contribute. However, these findings suggest that models commensurate with the definition of ethics as a systematic and rational approach are needed by nurse executives to sustain them in their professional practice of nursing administration.

ETHICS AND BENEFITS

Applied ethics also benefits the nursing personnel and the administrators as well as the patients. Several examples illustrate how nursing personnel benefit from ethics applied to the clinical setting. For example, ethics provides a framework and language that spans interdisciplinary groups, providing a common language for enhanced communication. It can assist in examining the ever-present issues of authority, power, and collegial relationships in health care (Aroskar, 1998) retaining a balance in clinical practice. Ethics applied to the work environment and illustrated in behavior of personnel provides a more positive work setting, one that clinical nurses prefer (McDaniel, 1998a). Understanding the contributors to a positive work setting or to satisfaction of the work of nurses can be fruitful to nurse administrators (McDaniel, 1995). Administrative strategies that enhance ethics may counter turnover or burnout in nurses, thereby, improving nurse retention and work, the latter reducing costs of personnel turnover and training. Studies report that registered clinical nurses prefer an ethical environment, an environment that is strongly related to nurse retention and reduced turnover (McDaniel, 1998a). It may assist in the understanding of, and ethics decisions inherent in, downsizing among employees (Hinderer, 1997). Applied ethics is inherent to quality leadership; it is important to professional administration (Greene, 1997). Applied ethics not only improves the work setting, the work of personnel, and the work decisions, it also may contribute to enhanced patient outcomes. For these reasons, and as these six examples suggest, strategies that use applied ethics, enhance ethical practice, and support nursing care in health care settings are critical to the professional practice of nursing administration.

DECISION-MAKING IN NURSING ADMINISTRATION

Nurse executives must balance clinical and organizational imperatives in managing the professional practice environment. It is clear that the quality of the decision is critical to the well-being of an organization. Although the information required for patient care or administrative decision-making may vary, the nature of the underlying decision process and its use in health care organizations is similar.

Alternative choices of action bridge the gap between a problem and a goal. The generation of alternative problem solutions assists in formulating a plan of action. Rarely, does a problem have only one solution. In fact, the challenge of administrative decision-making in health care is to arrive at one best alternative among several competing ones. Basically, decision-making is a cognitive process of selection that precedes the chosen behavior.

In thinking about decisions, it can be useful to differentiate the decision process from the decision itself. Although heuristic in nature, decision-making can be divided into two parts, the process of the decision-making and the content about which the decision will be made. This section examines general decision-making as a foundation for ethical decision-making. The focus is on the decision process.

The decision process is a series of interrelated steps for systematically and logically coming to a decision. It is analogous to other systematic processes that guide intellectual work, such as the scientific method or the research process. Decision-making is the point in the process at which the choice, or selection of alternatives, is made and is often viewed as the culmination of the decision process.

Referring to the model by Burkhardt (Figure 16.1), one can see that gathering data and identifying moral claims is a first step and represents process. Once completed, one can move to the identification of major participants, which is gathering of content, then on to how these participants think: do they use a particular philosophical orientation, for instance? The desired outcome is clearly stated to make sure that all information is gathered to aid in attaining that outcome. Some decision-makers would put outcomes as the second step, to ensure that all information is gathered. Continuing along on the figure, the next step is to discuss possible options or other alternatives available, again, to attain the

Gather data and identify conflicting moral claims

- What makes this situation an ethical dilemma? Are there conflicting obligations, duties, principles, rights, loyalties, values, or beliefs?
- What are the issues?
- What facts seem most important?
- What emotions have an impact?
- What are the gaps in information at this time?

Identify key participants

- Who is legitimately empowered to make this decision?
- Who is affected and how?
- What is the level of competence of the person most affected in relation to the decision to be made?
- What are the rights, duties, authority, context, and capabilities of participants?

Determine moral perspective and phase of moral development of key participants

- Do participants think in terms of duties or rights?
- Do the parties involved exhibit similar or different moral perspectives?
- Where is the common ground? The differences?
- What principles are important to each person involved?
- What emotions are evident within the interaction and with each person involved?
- What is the level of moral development of the participants?

Determine desired outcomes

- How does each party describe the circumstances of the outcome?
- What are the consequences of the desired outcomes?
- What outcomes are unacceptable to one or all involved?

Identify options

- What options emerge through the assessment process?
- How do the alternatives fit the lifestyle and values of the person(s) affected?
- What are legal considerations of the various options?
- What alternatives are unacceptable to one or all involved?
- How are alternatives weighed, ranked, and prioritized?

Act on the choice

- Be empowered to make a difficult decision.
- Give oneself permission to set aside less acceptable alternatives.
- Be attentive to the emotions involved in this process.

Evaluate outcomes of action

- Has the ethical dilemma been resolved?
- Have other dilemmas emerged related to the action?
- How has the process affected those involved?
- Are further actions required?

Figure 16.1 A guide for decision-making. From Burkhardt, M. A., & Nathaniel, A. K. (1998). *Ethics and issues in contemporary nursing.* Albany, NY: Delmar, a division of Thomson Learning.

desired outcome. The last two steps in this decision-making model are the implementation of the selected choice, followed by an assessment of that choice; these latter two steps are always conducted in light of the desired outcome. If, on assessment, the outcome is not met or not of the desired quality—a key issue in patient care—then the staff or nurse executive may need to return to the initial step, or to other possible alternatives. In any decision, there may be no perfect solution. In view of the outcomes administrators may select the one that attains the best solution to the identified problem.

To illustrate this process, if two clinical practicing nurses are in disagreement about whether to move a patient from the intensive care unit in favor of one who would, following triage, benefit more from the care, they could state their moral claims and desired outcomes, assess the participants including the family, attempt to determine which moral orientation they are each using, and then discuss possible alternatives and their probable outcomes. Once clear on these steps, they could implement a "trial" move for the patient and then assess the status of both patients.

As shall be seen, what differs most in these next two models of decision-making, the prescriptive and the descriptive models, is the components of the process. These components may vary depending on the underlying model because the process of decision-making is prescriptive or prescribing an outcome, or descriptive or describing an outcome that is acceptable.

Prescriptive Model

In the Prescriptive Model, which derives from economic theory, decisions rest on assumptions that a rational decision-maker strives to reach *optimal* outcomes and the information is available to determine those outcomes. A prescriptive process includes the following steps to arrive at a quality decision (Figure 16.2):

1. Recognition and analysis of the problem or situation requiring a decision
2. Identification of all feasible alternative solutions
3. Determination of potential favorable and unfavorable consequences and their likelihood for each alternative considered
4. Selection of the alternative that results in *optimal* outcomes

In the prescriptive model, for example, two nurses who disagree on DNR orders can state the problem in their own words, identify their feasible solutions, state the favorable and unfavorable consequences of each decision, and select alternative *optimal* outcomes that they could mutually agree on. It would be helpful to do this decision model in a group or a nursing ethics committee to ensure that all viable alternatives are explored. This is one advantage of a group discussion for ethics resolutions.

Descriptive Model

In contrast, a descriptive model for decision-making is based on how decisions are *actually* made. One of the most influential of these was formulated by Herbert

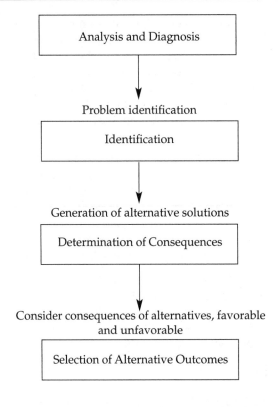

Figure 16.2 Prescriptive model for decision-making.

Simon (1976). This classic model acknowledges that decision-makers often have limited time or information on which to make a rational decision. This grounding in reality is particularly relevant to the busy nurse executive. Descriptive models lead to what Simon calls "satisficing" in which the decision-maker searches for alternatives until one is found that provides an *acceptable* solution, rather than an optimal solution. Steps in a decision process based on the descriptive model of satisficing include (Figure 16.3):

1. Recognition and analysis of the problem or situation requiring a decision
2. Development of criteria for an acceptable outcome
3. Identification of alternatives
4. Evaluation of whether the alternative will lead to acceptable outcomes
5. Selection of a *satisfactory* alternative

To explore the same situation but for the descriptive model, the two nurses would state the problem and proceed in a similar manner, use the group to process the information and to attain maximum viable alternatives, then evaluate

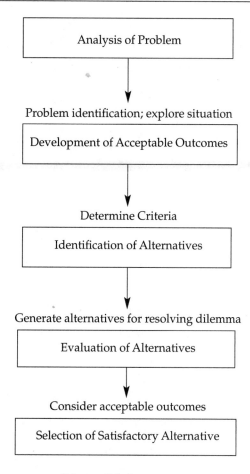

Select *satisfactory* outcome

Figure 16.3 Descriptive model for decision-making.

using the group to assess and discuss acceptable outcomes. Finally, the nurses would select a satisfactory, rather than an optimal, alternative to the initially stated solution. This will result in the descriptive *satisficing* alternative.

Other and less well formulated models are also used but are considered less likely to consistently produce good outcomes. For that reason this discussion will be limited to these two. However, two additional steps are often included as components of the decision process: implementation of the decision and the evaluation of the decision outcome. No decision process is considered complete without these final steps (Figure 16.4).

Ethical Decision Models

Applied ethics implies decision-making. Generically, decision-making in applied ethics involves the content of ethical theory applied to situations in a systematic,

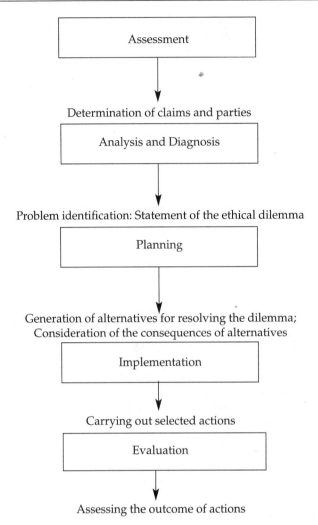

Figure 16.4 Ethical decision-making model: complete process. Adapted from DeLaune, S., & Ladner, P. (1998). *Fundamentals of nursing: Standards & practice.* Albany, NY: Delmar, a division of Thomson Learning.

rational, and critical manner. In this particular discussion those relevant situations pertain to health care. The situations emerge out of the nursing administration of health care delivery. The aim is to analyze the situation to determine an ethically sound administrative solution. This process is fundamental to applied ethics in nursing administration.

Although applied ethics relies on the process of decision-making, the content will differ and it may influence the process. To some extent, the content of ethics can influence the process of decision-making. In most cases, however, a model of applied nursing ethics will be similar to the generic model discussed earlier.

Nursing Model for Process

A widely used model of ethical decision-making for nursing has been formulated by Mila Aroskar (1980). It proposes three steps for ethical decisions: *(1)* obtain information or data, *(2)* consider questions from decision theorists, and *(3)* articulate the ethical theories (Figure 16.5).

Other models of decision-making in nursing ethics are in the nursing literature. Although it is beyond the scope of this chapter to examine them all in detail, models address ethical decision-making and moral judgments. However, there are common themes among the models. One of them is that a systematic and rational approach would be fruitful. Another implication is that there is no *one* way to resolve an ethical dilemma.

Ethical Content—Principles and Theories

The content of ethics can influence the process of the ethical decision-making. The relationship between the process and the content of ethics is more sensitive than with generic decision models. The influence would depend on the choice of principles or theories as potential content. One may also combine and use both of them.

When philosophers have attempted to determine common features of a problem or case, they are often stated as principles (Beauchamp & Childress, 1994). Nursing has borrowed from biomedical ethics in its application of key principles as a "framework" or a set of parameters for examining ethical situations. Administrative decisions concerning, for example, allocation of resources, can be examined in the light of ethical principles it poses for the decision-maker. Justice is a principle relevant to allocation.

There is no agreement on the exact number or set of principles; however, several emerge as major ones. They are beneficence, justice, and autonomy (Beauchamp & Childress, 1994). Briefly defined, *beneficence* is doing good, *justice* is also called fairness or equality, and *autonomy* refers to rights of self or others. Administrative

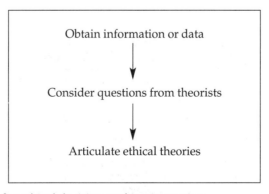

Figure 16.5 Steps for ethical decision-making in nursing.

situations can be examined in light of the principle that emerges as the central one in that situation. In many instances, a case may illustrate more than one principle. The principle becomes, then, a means of examining the situation and exploring its alternatives. Principles become a framework for examining ethical situations (Table 16.1).

Theories of ethics can also provide content for ethical decision-making. Although a variety of theories are used, several appear frequently. These are the utilitarian, the deontological, and the egoist theories (Aroskar, 1980). Briefly, the utilitarian focuses on the consequences of a decision, the deontological addresses the act itself, and the egoist would be concerned with the best solution for oneself (Figure 16.6).

The theory selected for ethical examination can influence the process because the alternatives may need to be reexamined in light of the outcome. Also, the type of ethical situations confronted by nurse executives are often vastly troublesome with no clearly defined right or wrong answers. That is why a decision framework for ethics is so important to the professional practice of nursing administration.

ETHICS AND PROFESSIONAL PRACTICE OF NURSING ADMINISTRATION

Confounding ethical situations that need nursing administration attention typically occur in the relationships among personnel. Ethical situations for nursing administration usually emerge out of the intra- or interdisciplinary relationships in health care settings.

Today's health care environment is changing rapidly, creating a turbulent and more ambiguous context for nursing practice. Major contributors to this constant change are, among others, the increasing amount of technology that nurses are required to understand and use in their work, the restructuring of health care with increasing integration of health care systems, and the significant changes in the reimbursement of health care services. Although increased technology is advancing health care and extending life, a side effect of these advances is the increasing number of ethical issues that the use of technology creates. The exten-

Table 16.1 Overview of Ethical Principles

Principle	Explanation
Beneficence	The duty to do good to others and to maintain a balance between benefits and harms
Justice	The equitable distribution of potential benefits and risks
Autonomy	Respect for an individual's right to self-determination; respect for individual liberty

Adapted from DeLaune, S., and Ladner, P. (1998). *Fundamentals of nursing: Standards & practice.* Albany, NY: Delmar, a division of Thomson Learning.

THEORY	EXPLANATION
Utilitarian	Focuses on the consequences of a decision
Deontological	Addresses the act itself
Egoist	Concerned with best solution for self

Figure 16.6 Comparing common ethics theories.

sion of life, for instance, provides both opportunity and challenge for ethics decision-making ranging from issues such as futility and intensive care of the young (Penticuff, 1998), to decisions about organ procurement and nurses' role (Siminoff & Sturm, 1998). Advancing technology also renders increasing numbers of and complexity about decisions that have ethical implications and in which nurses need to participate in an ethical environment (McDaniel, 1998a). Health care changes bring with them an increasing number of ethical situations that affect nurses, their work, and their professional relationships with those in health care. Those changes raise ethical issues for nursing work, affecting the relationships among nurses and among nurses and auxiliary personnel, physicians, and nurse executives.

Nursing Staff

Nurses face challenges in their daily practice that require decisions and judgments that are ethical in nature. Nurses also make ethical decisions about their work, their collegial relationships, and patient care (Corley, 1998), informed by professional, institutional, and group norms. These decisions require judgment about what is right and wrong and what is the best outcome in light of the ethical parameters.

Because one's ethical system is informed by the values of individuals, nurses may differ among themselves in the priority they place on a situation or they may differ in philosophy. There may be conflicts among nurses about the best way in which to resolve a conflict. These, in turn, create ethical conflicts of an intraprofessional nature. In these instances of ethical disagreement, the support and education provided by nurse executives is important to shape and sustain nurses, their practice, and their ethical decisions. It is here that a nurse executive can play an important role in facilitating resolution of ethical dilemmas.

Nurses and Auxiliary Personnel

Ethical situations also emerge in the interactions between nurses and auxiliary personnel. Ethical conflicts may occur among the nursing service personnel, referring to nurses and their auxiliary co-workers, support services, or health-related personnel. Ketefian (1981) found that moral reasoning differed according to educational level. If there are differences in educational background among nursing service personnel, one can anticipate differences in moral reasoning. Understanding these perspectives and their influence on ethical dilemmas can assist nurse executives in developing supports and strategies for arriving at an ethical solution.

When nurses are responsible for the delegation and implementation of care provided by those under nursing service but who are not professional nurses, the responsibility itself may take on ethical parameters. Nurses may be reluctant to assume responsibility for auxiliary functions (Cohen, 1991). In the face of mounting nurse shortage and increased demand for care, auxiliary personnel may be pressed into delivery of care that is beyond the scope of their education and experience. Nurses, who rightfully perceive their responsibility for other personnel in differentiated practice environments, may be unsure about the level of accountability that they as nurses assume. These situations can pose ethical conflicts surrounding the work relationships among personnel in nursing service.

Nurses and Physicians

The range of ethical dilemmas may also extend to nurse-physician interactions. Although the contemporary health care climate is changing rapidly, there are several reasons why tensions may occur. Nurses and physicians continue to have a differential relationship to the health care setting, even though an increasing number of physicians are shifting from the previous fee-for-service reimbursement method to a salaried one. These structural differences may lead to varied perceptions of accountability, responsibility, and power in the organization pertaining to their work and their respective patients. Such differences may lead to interdisciplinary tensions.

Other conflicts may occur. Physicians and nurses may place varying importance on aspects of the patient's treatment. Nurses and physicians may have different perspectives of patient care situations emerging from their different philosophical backgrounds and approaches (McDaniel, 1997). Nurses may assume an advocacy role for the patient, or they may select another priority for the allocation of increasingly scarce resources for patients, placing them in conflict with treatments advocated by a physician. On a constructive note, however, ethics can assist in providing a mutually recognized language and decision model that aids in resolving conflicts between nurses and physicians for their respective patient care. One avenue for these decisions is the interdisciplinary health care committee on which an increasing number of nurses contribute as full members (McDaniel, 1998b). These assist both the caregivers as well as the administrator in creating a positive work environment.

Nurses and Nurse Executives

Ethical conflicts can also occur between nursing staff and nurse executives. In many instances, these dilemmas occur because there are inherent differences in the perspectives that staff nurses and nurse executives hold. For example, staff nurses will usually assume what is termed a micro level perspective, illustrated by concern for an individual patient or case. This perspective is commensurate with their level of responsibility for individual patient care. In contrast, an executive will assume, by virtue of position, a macro perspective, illustrated by concern for a whole unit or facility. Staff nurses, delivering care at the bedside, will view their patient care situation differently than their nurse executive(s). Although often overlooked as an inherent distinction, different levels of responsibility contribute to differing perspectives about the situation and its outcome. These perspectives need to be explored to arrive at an ethical and mutual understanding of the situation.

A common difference is illustrated in the assignment of nursing staff. Staff nurses may experience a shortage of qualified co-workers to deliver the quality of desired care. Although staff may misunderstand the allocation for such situations, the shortage of competent personnel is always a difficult situation both for the nursing staff who deliver the care and for the nurse administrator who manages the care. Shortage of nursing personnel is an ethical issue of resource allocation and pertains to justice as a principle.

Nurse executives, too, experience ethical conflicts when they must allocate fewer available nursing staff across more patients than actually provides adequate coverage, or administrators may be restrained from providing the full complement of care by restrained reimbursement, a common issue in today's health care climate. This situation is especially troublesome because it has implications for quality of care for patients as well as quality of care for nursing staff. Nurse executives who experience this level of administrative and ethical conflict are often placed in a compromising situation with their own facility administrators as well. To support one's own administrator in the face of institutional constraints and the need also to support one's staff and their patients is an ethical conundrum. The resulting hierarchical ethical conflict is one of the most difficult for nurse executives and, thereby, affects the professional practice of nursing administration.

Given the fact that ethical conflicts occur with seemingly increasing frequency in today's health care climate, there are avenues to constructively address conflicts that have not been previously addressed. In addition to decision models and ethical processes, there also are two primary structures within which decision models may be placed. The structures are increasing both in frequency and in use. They are the nurse or intradisciplinary ethics committee and the institutional (facility) or interdisciplinary ethics committee in health care. Although there are differing perspectives about the need or use of nurse-only intradisciplinary and facility-wide interdisciplinary committees (Haddad, 1997), both have a purpose and a place in health care. Both serve as structured avenues for the resolution of ethical dilemmas in health care. For this reason, nurse administrators are encouraged to understand and to use both of them.

As an intradisciplinary committee, the nurse ethics committee provides an opportunity for nurses to engage in conversation, to model appropriate behaviors and decision-making, and, essentially, to learn about the resolution of ethical dilemmas in a setting among other nurse colleagues and workers. It is useful in the resolution of dilemmas among nurses about the allocation of nursing resources, for instance, or about differing treatment models. It may serve an educational purpose for nurses, and it may be a first step or a foundation for membership on an interdisciplinary committee.

In contrast, the interdisciplinary ethics committee as a facility-wide committee provides a structure in which decision processes and models can be used by a range of occupations in health care. It provides a positive avenue for nurses to engage in constructive resolution of ethical conflicts among a diverse range of health care workers, including caregivers, administrators, and patients (McDaniel, 1998b). As a committee formulating some of the health care policies that are implemented within an institution or setting, it is critical that RNs are members of these committees. Thus, within any health care setting, ethical dilemmas occur and structures and models can be used to aid in ethical decision-making (McDaniel, 1997, 1998b).

As illustrated by these two types of ethics committees, structural avenues are available for the constructive resolution of ethical dilemmas within which both ethical decision-making and moral judgments may occur. These avenues enhance professional nursing administration. As a means to support their nursing staff and the patients and families, nurse administrators can support and use any and all of these strategies of ethical decision-making in their professional practice.

SUMMARY

Decision-making is a cognitive process of interrelated steps for systematically and logically coming to a decision. It may be subdivided into the process and content of decision-making. The process can be based on a prescriptive or a descriptive model. In applied ethics for administration, nursing models and ethics content are used. Situations requiring ethical administrative decisions may emerge from relationships among personnel in the professional practice of nursing administration.

STUDY QUESTIONS

1. Describe an ethical issue in your work setting. How would you resolve this issue?
2. Some hospitals continue to ignore nurses' contributions to ethics committees. What can nurse executives do to ensure nursing participation on these committees?
3. Legalized assisted suicide is being considered in many states. What are the most important concerns for nurse executives regarding this decision? For patients? For physicians?

4. What structures are available in your setting to allow nurses' participation in ethics decision-making?

5. As a nurse executive, what can you do if disagreements occur between clinical nurses and physicians or other practitioners regarding an ethical situation involving patient care?

REFERENCES

Aroskar, M. (1980). Anatomy of an ethical dilemma: The theory. *American Journal of Nursing, 80*(4), 658–663.

Aroskar, M. (1998). Ethical working relationships in patient care: Challenges and possibilities. *Nursing Clinics of North America, 33*(2), 313–324.

Beauchamp, T., & Childress, J. (1989). *Principles of biomedical ethics* (3rd ed.). New York: Oxford University Press.

Beauchamp, T., & Childress, J. (1994). *Principles of biomedical ethics* (4th Ed.). New York: Oxford University Press.

Burkhardt, M. A., & Nathaniel, A. K. (1998). *Ethics and issues in contemporary nursing.* Albany, NY: Delmar.

Cohen, E. (1991). Nursing case management: Does it pay? *Journal of Nursing Administration, 21*(4), 20–25.

Corley, M. (1998). Ethical dimensions of nurse-physician relations in critical care. *Nursing Clinics of North America, 33*(2), 325–338.

Delaune, S., & Laudner, P. (1998). *Fundamentals of nursing: Standards & practice.* Albany, NY: Delmar.

Esterhuizen, P. (1996). Is the professional code still the cornerstone of clinical nursing practice? *The Journal of Advanced Nursing, 23*(1), 25–31.

Greene, J. (1997, August 5). 1997 *Hospital & Health Networks* leadership survey. *Hospitals & Health Networks, 71*(15), 26–30, 32–36, 38–40.

Haddad, A. (1997). Nursing ethics committees. *HEC Forum, 9*(1), 1–108, special issue.

Hinderer, D. (1997). Hospital downsizing: Ethics and employees. *Journal of Nursing Administration, 27*(4), 9–11.

Ketefian, S. (1981). Critical thinking, educational preparation, and development of moral judgment among selected groups of practicing nurses. *Nursing Research, 30*(3), 98–103.

McDaniel, C. (1995). Organizational culture and ethics work satisfaction. *Journal of Nursing Administration, 25*(11), 15–21.

McDaniel, C. (1997). The development and psychometric properties of the Ethical Environment Questionnaire. *Medical Care, 35*(9), 901–914.

McDaniel, C. (1998a). Ethical environment: Reports of practicing nurses. *Nursing Clinics of North America, 33*(2), 263–384.

McDaniel, C. (1998b). Hospital ethics committees and nurses' contributions. *Journal of Nursing Administration, 28*(9), 47–51.

Penticuff, J. (1998). Defining futility in neonatal intensive care. *Nursing Clinics of North America, 33*(2), 339–345.

Siminoff, L., & Sturm, C. (1998). Nursing and the procurement of organs and tissues in the acute hospital setting. *Nursing Clinics of North America, 33*(2), 239–252.

Simon, H. (1986). *Administrative behavior.* New York: Free Press.

CHAPTER

~ 17 ~

Integrated Quality Management

Marylane Wade Koch

Without theory, there are no questions; without questions, no learning; hence, without theory there's no learning. (W. Edward Deming, 1982)

Chapter Highlights

- Quality control: The industrial model
- Quality movement in health care
- Defining quality
- Components of integrated quality management
- Goals of quality management
- Trends in quality

America has a new measurement for products and services: "quality." Consumers ask for "quality" in food, cars, and education. "Quality" is a nebulous term often defined by the perception of the consumer. Many have tried to define "quality." One thing is sure: health care cannot escape this measurement by consumers. The expectation of "quality" is foremost in the minds of health care consumers including patients, insurance companies, and the federal government—anyone paying the bill for health care services.

The health care provider must face the challenge of the question: "Can quality health care be delivered at cost-efficient prices?" The nursing professional must meet this challenge by implementing a process that addresses the multifaceted issues in providing "quality" health care. Although other businesses have implemented quality control programs, health care has been slow to respond in this area. Now, regulatory groups as well as the consumers demand it.

A new paradigm for the nursing professional includes integrated quality management: improving health care services through quality assessment and improvement, utilization management, infection control, and risk/safety management. The goal is "quality" care in the appropriate setting at reasonable costs with positive patient outcomes. The challenge to the nurse executive is empowerment of the professional nurse to demonstrate positive patient outcomes through integrated quality management. This promotes excellence, boosting the image of professional nursing to consumers and third-party payers who decide what "value" health care service has in dollars. Professional nursing practice can make a difference in patient care outcomes, demonstrating "value" through integrated quality management.

QUALITY CONTROL: THE INDUSTRIAL MODEL

The history of modern quality control can be traced to Shewhart of Bell Laboratories. In the 1930s, Shewhart used the control chart to produce military supplies cheaply and in mass quantities. The applied statistics, called z-1 standards, were considered classified information (Ishikawa, 1985). Britain also adopted these standards.

When Japan was devastated by World War II, the equipment and communications were poor. The United States government stationed there required implementation of quality control. In 1946, modern statistical quality control began to grow in Japan. Various leaders, such as W. Edward Deming and J. M. Juran, moved the country of Japan from a reputation of inferior products to one of superior products.

Both Deming and Juran later came to the United States and assisted American companies in organizing quality programs. Deming is well known for his 14 points that are key to any quality management program:

1. Create a constancy of purpose for service improvement
2. Adopt a new philosophy
3. Cease dependence on mass inspection
4. End practice of awarding business on price alone
5. Find problems. Constantly improve every process for planning, production, and service.
6. Institute training on the job
7. Institute leadership for system improvement
8. Drive out fear for effective environment
9. Break down barriers between staff areas and departments
10. Eliminate slogans, posters, and numerical goals, asking for improved productivity without providing methods

11. Eliminate numerical quotas for workforce
12. Remove barriers to pride of workmanship
13. Institute a vigorous program of education and self-improvement for everyone
14. Create a structure in top management that will push every day for the above (Deming, 1982)

Juran has emphasized that quality must be implemented from the top down. He defined seven steps for management to follow for quality improvement:

1. *Awareness* of the competitive challenges and your own competitive position
2. *Understanding* of the new definition of quality and of the role of quality in the success of your company
3. *Vision* of how good your company can really be
4. *Plan* for action. Clearly define the steps you need to take to achieve your vision
5. *Train* your people to provide the knowledge, skills, and tools they need to make your plan happen
6. *Support* to ensure changes are made, problem causes are eliminated, and gains are held
7. *Reward and recognize* to make sure that successes spread throughout the company and become part of the business plan (Vasilash, 1988)

QUALITY MOVEMENT IN HEALTH CARE

Many nurse executives associate quality assessment and improvement with the Joint Commission for the Accreditation of Healthcare Organizations (JCAHO), created in 1952. Actually, the quality health care movement actualized much earlier with Flexner and Codman in the early 1900s. In 1912, Codman designed and implemented the first medical "audits," an early form of outcome monitoring. When the American College of Surgeons formed their accreditation body in 1919, standards development, education, and practitioner competence were included. This group later became JCAHO. Quality assurance standards were made mandatory in 1981 with revisions in 1984.

JCAHO (1987) announced plans to revise the accreditation process. This revision has become known as the Agenda for Change. This Agenda was a major research and development process to improve JCAHO's ability to assist and evaluate health care organizations in provision of daily quality improvement. The Agenda includes educational and communications initiatives. Standards are more descriptive and less prescriptive. In short, the Agenda moves JCAHO in the position to evaluate not *can* the organization provide quality health care (structure and process), but rather *does* the organization provide quality health care (outcome) (JCAHO, 1987).

In January 1990, JCAHO approved 12 principles for continuous quality improvement (CQI) described as "dynamic" in the preamble. The underlying principle is respect for the values, needs, and concerns of the consumers. These principles include such areas as philosophy and culture, mission, leadership, CQI systems, performance appraisals, education and training, and organizational relationships.

In recent years, JCAHO has expanded its role to include new strategies for quality and performance improvement. JCAHO does not mandate a specific model to accomplish quality improvement. The expectation is that the model used will include interdepartmental and interdisciplinary emphasis. JCAHO has standards that address organizational performance in specific areas. JCAHO surveyors assess not just what the organization can or says it does, but actually what it accomplishes. The standards define maximum achievable expectations of performance relating to patient care and management. The standard "Improving Organizational Performance" described the components as plan, design, measure, assess, and improve. The definition of performance is basically doing the things right and doing it well. The dimensions of performance that JCAHO has defined are efficacy, appropriateness, availability, timeliness, effectiveness, continuity, safety, efficiency, and respect and caring (JCAHO, 1997–1998) (Figure 17.1).

DIMENSIONS OF QUALITY PERFORMANCE

- **Efficacy**—degree to which the intervention has been shown to accomplish the intended outcome
- **Appropriateness**—degree to which the intervention is relevant to client needs
- **Availability**—degree to which appropriate interventions are available to meet client needs
- **Timeliness**—degree to which the intervention is provided at the most beneficial time to the client
- **Effectiveness**—degree to which the intervention is provided in the correct manner to achieve the intended client outcome
- **Continuity**—degree to which the interventions are coordinated between organizations, among care providers, and across time
- **Safety**—degree to which the risk of an intervention and risk in the environment are reduced for both client and health care provider
- **Efficiency**—degree to which care has the desired effect with a minimum of effort, expense, or waste
- **Respect and caring**—degree to which clients are involved in health care decisions and are treated with sensitivity and respect for their individual needs, expectations, and differences by health care providers

Figure 17.1 Dimensions of quality performance. Data from Joint Commission on Accreditation of Healthcare Organizations (1996). *1997 Accreditation manual for hospitals.* Oakbrook Terrace, IL: Author.

More agencies are in place to monitor and evaluate health care quality. The Agency for Health Care Policy and Research (AHCPR) was established in December 1989 under the Omnibus Budget Reconciliation Act of 1989. It is a part of the Untied States Department of Health and Human Services. AHCPR is the lead agency, given the charge of supporting research designed to improve health care quality, as well as reduce health care costs and broaden access to essential services (AHCPR Overview, 1999). Its research provides practical, science-based practice guidelines for health providers, consumers, and health purchasers.

The three strategic goals of the AHCPR are:

1. Support improvements in health outcomes
2. Strengthen quality measurement and improvement
3. Identify strategies to improve access, foster appropriate use, and reduce necessary expenditures (AHCPR Strategic Plan, 1998)

In June 1998, Vice President Al Gore formed the planning committee to create the Forum for Health Care Quality Measurement and Reporting with the private sector. Its charge is to develop a comprehensive national plan for quality improvement in health care. The Vice President supported the need for this group with the Department of Health and Human Services report "The Challenge and Potential for Assuring Quality Health Care in the 21st Century." It details the many and wide-ranging problems in the health care industry, including underuse of services, overuse of services, misuse of services, and variations of services. It also notes examples for improved delivery of care, reduced mortality and morbidity, and better quality of life that could be applied nationwide (Challenge and Potential, 1999).

Another group active in evaluating health care quality is the National Committee for Quality Assurance (NCQA). This group defined the first national standards for managed behavioral health care organizations. The mission of the NCQA is to provide information on health care quality in the marketplace, particularly to employers and consumers. They strive to "drive" quality improvement and reward managed accountability (NCQA Mission 1999).

DEFINING "QUALITY"

"Quality" has been defined in many ways. The Japanese Industrial Standards define quality control as "a system of production methods which economically produces quality goods or services meeting the requirements of consumers" (Ishikawa, 1985). Modern quality control combines this with the use of statistical methodology. Ishikawa (1985), a foremost authority, states, "To produce quality control is to develop, design, produce, and service a product which is economical, most useful, and always satisfactory to the customer." A definition that has received wide acceptance is "fitness for use" (Juran, 1989).

Donebedian (1980), a leader in medical quality assurance, initially defined quality as "that kind of care which is expected to maximize an inclusive measure of patient welfare, after one has taken account of the balance of expected gains and losses that attend the process of care in all its parts." JCAHO (1990) defines quality as "the degree to which patient care services increase the probability of desired patient outcomes and reduce the probability of undesired outcomes, given the current state of knowledge." Others contend that quality is consumer perception: the degree to which the customer is satisfied with the product or service. Quality, then, is meeting or exceeding customer expectations.

QUALITY MANAGEMENT

Today, more health care organizations have a Total Quality Management (TQM) program for Continuous Quality Improvement (CQI), the term used by JCAHO. Quality management is different from a "fire-fighting" philosophy because it is organized, systematic, planned, and proactive. Quality management, or improvement, must be a **planned** change. Juran (1989) describes quality improvement as "the organized creation of beneficial change; the attainment of unprecedented levels of performance . . . a break-through."

TQM, or CQI, is the process of continuously improving the quality of products or service in any business. The anticipated results are increased customer satisfaction, more profit and market share, better productivity, and decreased costs through better resource utilization. Whatever the term used, the goal is the same: to expand traditional quality processes to include all clinical, administrative, and support functions to improve the quality of health care.

Most health care organizations have a quality improvement (QI) program. This program provides systematic monitoring and evaluation of patient care delivery. Organizations may also have infection control, risk and safety programs, and utilization management in place. What is often missing is the integration of all quality management components into nursing practice in the clinical and administrative settings.

Components of Integrated Quality Management

Integrated quality management includes but is not limited to:

1. Quality performance and improvement
2. Infection control
3. Utilization management
4. Risk/safety management

These areas, although unique and separate in some ways, have many commonalities. It is believed that each area is so dependent on the other that the whole is enhanced by integration, resulting in synergy that produces more value than one area alone. An integrated QM program can be the competitive strength of any health care organization.

Quality and Performance Improvement

The organization may systematically address performance improvement through steps such as listing and prioritizing improvement opportunities, defining customer requirements, using measuring tools, displaying data, analyzing data, generating potential and selecting best solutions, implementing the solution, and evaluating and tracking effectiveness. Models used to achieve performance improvement may vary in number and name of steps, but all should use a systematic approach to improve the process reviewed. The key to success is data that create a baseline and continued measurement. Benchmarking with other similar organizations to identify best practices to improve work processes is important to continue to improve health care (Price, Koch, & Bassett 1998).

The foundation of all quality and performance processes is measurement. It offers a roadmap of where the organization has been and what improvement has occurred. JCAHO explains measuring performance as allowing people to establish acceptable criteria, judge the stability of existing process, and identify opportunities for improvement (JCAHO, 1997–1998). Organizational leaders should identify indicators that focus on major functions or processes. Some areas might be customer satisfaction and JCAHO dimensions of performance such as timeliness, effectiveness, and efficiency. To best use limited resources, the importance of the indicator and the ease of access to data must be considered.

Infection Control

Infection control is probably the oldest component of integrated QM, its beginnings dated B.C. Infection control has a basic tenet, the understanding of communicable disease as causing illness through specific agents or toxic substances. Basic transmission modes and causes of communicable disease are important concepts for the practicing health care professional.

Trending and reporting infection control information is necessary to integrated QM. The type of surveillance and its scope can be determined by QM reports such as nosocomial rates or clean wound infection rates. Incidence and prevalence data can be determined through QM studies with appropriate follow-up and actions taking place. Although infection control is a unique component, it is nonetheless a necessary one to an integrated QM program.

Utilization Management

Utilization management (UM) is the planned, organized directing of the health care resources in a cost-efficient manner, contributing to the quality of patient care and goals of the organization. In the past, UM was known as utilization review (UR) for, indeed, this process was just that—chart review for evaluating the use of medical services, procedures, and facilities against predetermined criteria. UM identifies and resolves problems that can cause inappropriate use of scarce health care resources.

Although required by the Social Security Amendments of 1965, UM gained a respected place in QM during the 1980s with the advent of diagnosis-related groups (DRGs). JCAHO developed an UM Standard in 1980. The Peer Review Organization (PRO) was established by the federal government to monitor the quality and appropriateness of patient care services. One example of UM is inappropriate scheduling of services that may cause a delay in patient treatment. Discharge planning is an important part of UM as is case management. UM complements the other components of QM by appropriate management of health care resources. UM has as its goal the appropriate level of care for each patient, thereby managing resources.

Risk/Safety Management

Risk Management (RM) is the part of QM that demonstrates ongoing assessment of potential and actual organizational losses. Often, these risks can be equated into dollars lost or saved for the organization. The RM program is designed to avert losses and minimize exposure. Trending of incident reports is one important way RM contributes to QM process.

Safety and security problems fall under RM. There must be emphasis on preventive maintenance programs and disaster planning for the health care organization. RM works with other areas to secure QM data that enhances the process, such as patient advocacy programs, patient education, and patient satisfaction surveys. RM is an important part of QM as it works with other QM processes to maintain a safe environment with minimal risk to both patients and health care providers.

The U.S. Department of Labor created the Occupational Safety and Health Administration (OSHA) to provide standards of safe practice through injury prevention in the workplace. OSHA is an important part of risk and safety management. OSHA staff are charged with establishing and enforcing protective standards as well as providing consultative assistance to 6.5 million employers with over 100 million working men and women. The vision of OSHA is "to be a world class leader in occupational safety and health, with a clear focus on protecting the safety and health of America's workers" (OSHA's Mission, 1999). To achieve this vision, OSHA has three goals:

1. Improve workplace safety and health as evidenced by fewer hazards, reduced exposures, illnesses, and fatalities.
2. Change workplace culture to increase employer and worker awareness of, commitment to, and involvement with safety and health.
3. Secure public confidence through excellence in the development and delivery of OSHA's programs and services (A High Impact Agency, 1999).

Each area of integrated QM is important and can stand alone for its unique purposes. As integration and consequent energy occurs, however, each builds on the strength of the other. QI trends are available to RM to reduce the chance of losses through adverse outcomes. UM uses the QA and RM reports to manage health care resources judiciously for better quality care. Infection control or safety concerns become indicators for QA and planned change can be evaluated. It is the interrelationship that gives such strength to the integrated QM concept.

Goals of Quality Management

The goal of most health care organizations is to provide "high-quality health care," as defined in the mission statement. QM strives to create a culture where positive, honest communication can occur. Processes are put in place to monitor and evaluate problems, decrease the spread of infection, use resources appropriately, guard the organization from loss, and protect the consumer from adverse outcomes.

Quality management shows the consumer he or she is getting equitable value for the cost. A quality reputation can mean increased market share from customer satisfaction. QM can also help educate the consumer to what is reasonable for affordable costs. The goal is to provide the appropriate level of care needed for the specific consumer at a reasonable cost with a positive outcome.

Strategies for Integrating Quality Management

Most nurses prefer one area of integrated QM to the others. Perhaps the nurse has had experience with QA and QI or infection control. Another likes RM and can readily point out patient and visitor needs. Still others seem "naturals" at finding ways to use resources more efficiently. To further integrate QM into the practice setting, however, each nurse must understand the basic principles of all areas and how they interrelate. This helps broaden the perspective of the individual nurse and improves the comprehensiveness of QM in nursing practice.

The accountability for QM rests at each level of nursing, from staff to nurse executive. To integrate QM into all practice settings, a new paradigm must be the vision of nursing administration. Early in the professional nurse's experience, the components of QM must be introduced and applied to basic nursing process. Educators and managers themselves must learn to value QM and become mentors for the nurse. Plans of care must address all components to produce positive patient care outcomes.

Nurse executives must recognize the impact of QM on advanced nursing practice. In JCAHO's Agenda for Change, the leadership standards hold the advanced practice nurse accountable for assessing and planning quality care. Nurse executives and advanced practice nurses can discuss the fears and positive outcomes that QM can bring with the staff and nurse managers. Staff and manager orientation can include the basics of QM, setting expectations for performance appraisals. Nurse executives must stay current with trends by reading and disseminating current literature related to QM. Research and publishing must be encouraged as nurses experience positive change with integrated QM.

Quality management can be interdepartmental and collaborative. Working with other professionals will bring more options for defined concerns with both patients and processes. Learning to value differences is an important part of integrated QM. Quality management offers many opportunities for collaborative practice both within and outside the practice of nursing.

Trends in Quality Management

The trends in health care for QM are numerous. Today's consumers are more educated and have more expectations. Some of the trends that nursing professionals face in the present and future practice environment are directly related to QM.

Nursing Research

The nurse executive has the professional responsibility to promote and support nursing research. Nurses are both consumers and producers of research. The nurse executive must make research for the cornerstone of professional decision-making.

Quality management interfaces well with nursing research. Data collection and analyses are important parts of QM as well as research. All components of QM—quality assessment and improvement, utilization management, infection control, and risk/safety management—have some elements of research. The monitoring and evaluation of integrated QM clearly complements nursing research.

Quality management research can assist the nurse in documenting the clinical impact of professional practice to the external payers and regulation groups. Nursing research can assess the effectiveness of nursing interventions in outcome monitoring of the patient care part of QM. This type of study, combined with risk management and infection control, can demonstrate that professional nursing can make a difference in patient care outcomes.

Nursing research done in the area of health promotion is another natural fit for QM. As nurses confirm the impact of healthy life-styles on disease prevention, third-party payers and consumers may spend their health care dollars in health promotion provided by nurses. Nurses can make a difference in prevention of infection, such as AIDS, by teaching universal precautions. Research on high-risk populations and necessary intervention may change the course of this devastating illness and produce positive outcomes. Again, QM has direct interface with nursing research.

Research dissemination and utilization is essential to quality health care in nursing practice. Research is concerned with the process and the outcome, as is QM. Nurse executives can foster the environment that encourages nursing research through integrated QM. Studies can include cost and effectiveness of nursing care and implications for patient safety. Agencies that use QM in nursing research will have a competitive edge in both staff retention and establishing preferred provider relationships.

Nursing Ethics

Bioethics is the term used to define the application of ethics to society and human life as discussed in Chapter 16. This is a major area of concern in the current health care environment and concerns that relate directly to QM include:

- Treatment of dying patients
- Mercy killing, mercy deaths, and euthanasia
- Organ transplants
- Birth control, sterilization, and abortion
- Genetics, fertilization, and birth
- Human experimentation and informed consent
- Allocation of limited health care resources
- Confidentiality of the professional relationships (Thiroux, 1986)

The right-to-die issue continues to face health care professionals. The Cruzan case brought the concern to Congress for legislative action. On June 25, 1990, the Supreme Court issued the first right-to-die decision in favor of Nancy Cruzan. From this landmark case came legislation to regulate health care providers who accept federal payments. They must explain and offer an advanced directive to patients admitted for any service in any setting. This initiative, the Patient Self-Determination Act, mandates the patient has every opportunity to receive information and understand all options while still competent. This must be documented in the patient record. It is only one example of the challenge of ethics that can be addressed through a QM process. This poses some interesting risk and safety issues in health care. The Act indirectly addresses efficient use of limited health care resources.

Mandatory testing and disclosure of HIV is a major concern in health care today. The American Nurses Association (ANA) has issued a statement that supports strict adherence to universal precautions and infection control measures as the only way to stop AIDS transmission. Because of cost and unreliable AIDS testing, it is not practical to mandate testing and disclosure. There is no way to police the AIDS virus. Only teaching and effective safe practices by humans will curtail this debilitating disease.

In all of the examples mentioned previously, there are definite *risks* and *safety* issues to both patients and health care providers. These ethical dilemmas will affect the utilization of health care resources, **utilization management.** Many involve **infection control** principles, such as organ transplants and AIDS transmission. Finally, both positive and adverse outcomes will be demonstrated through monitoring and evaluation of **quality assessment** and **improvement.** Quality management plays a major role in nursing ethics.

Information Systems

The nurse executive who wants to manage manpower effectively while integrating QM into practice will value computerization. Computers are useful in data management and analyzation. Risk management incident-report data can be trended more easily with computerization. QM and QI data can be stored on the computer for regular analysis. Infection-control surveillance reports are conveniently available to the practitioner for easy reference on computer. Computerization can improve the efficiency of trend reporting, an important part of QM.

Marketing

As health care reimbursement decreases, providers must compete with other providers for limited dollars. Marketing is an important part of strategic planning for the nurse executive. Marketing plans identify the needs, preferences, and perceptions of consumers. QM can assist the nurse executive in designing the marketing plan.

Integrated QM includes measuring a beginning, benchmarking, of preferences and perceptions. The improvement outcome is measured, providing guidance to the nurse executive for effectiveness of marketing strategies. Some common measures of marketing effectiveness are use of services, employee and consumer satisfaction, turnover rates, and revenues and expenses. The nurse executive who has the professional goal of providing quality health care services has initiated a marketing goal as well. Demonstrated quality can attract and retain customers and payers.

Nursing Agenda for Health Care Reform

More than 40 nursing agencies have joined ANA in support of the Nursing Agenda for Health Care Reform (1991). Nurses have always supported access, quality, and affordable costs in health care delivery. This agenda defines methods of immediate reform to relieve the many ills of the current health care delivery system.

The agenda outlines restructure of the health care system to use the most cost-effective providers and therapeutic options in an appropriate setting (UM). A public plan would be offered to the poor and individuals-at-risk because of pre-existing illnesses, such as AIDS (RM and infection control). Steps would be taken to reduce costs through case management and prudent resource allocation based on policies developed from outcome research (QA and QI).

In short, integrated QM supports the agenda through:

- Provider availability
- Consumer involvement
- Outcome and effectiveness monitoring
- Review mechanisms
- Managed care
- Case management

SUMMARY

Professional nursing and QM have compatible goals. The nurse is the health care professional nearest the consumer for the most consistent periods of time. Integrated QM empowers nurses to practice their professional philosophy. It gives nursing the image boost needed in today's environment, promoting research and professional autonomy.

A result of QM is increased organizational self-esteem, as professional nurses feel excited about the quality of care they provide. The increased morale makes retention and recruitment easier for nurse executives. Both the consumer and the provider benefit from QM.

The challenge to the nurse executive is to be a visionary in redefining the organizational culture that supports, encourages, and rewards professional excellence, demonstrated through QM in patient care delivery. The tools and principles of QM must be incorporated into daily nursing practice, whatever the setting. The time of opportunity for professional nursing has come; with integrated QM nurses can demonstrate their value and impact on positive patient care and organizational outcomes for health care into the present and future environment.

STUDY QUESTIONS

1. What are the implications for professional nurses in the evolving movement of quality and performance improvement?
2. What are the chief components of integrated quality management? Give an example in one practice setting.
3. What are some strategies the nurse executive might use to integrate quality management into nursing practice?
4. Describe how integrated quality management relates to trends in nursing research, nursing ethics, information systems, and marketing.
5. What are the implications for Nursing's Agenda for Health Care Reform and quality management?

REFERENCES

AHCPR Overview—online. (1999). Available: http://www.ahcpr.gov/about/overview.htm (June 8, 1999).

AHCPR Strategic Plan: Agency for Health Care Policy and Research—online (December 15, 1998). Available: http://www.ahcpr.gov/about/stratplan.htm (June 8, 1999).

A High Impact Agency: Goals for the Year 2000. (1999). Available: www.soah.gov/oshinfo/1pger1.html (June 8, 1999).

Agency for Health Care Policy and Research. (1996). Rockville, MD: Public Health Service.

American Nurses Association. (1991). *Nursing's agenda for health care reform*. PR-3, 220M.

Challenge and Potential for Assuring Quality Health Care for the 21st Century—online. (1999). Available: http://www.ahcpr.gov/qual/21stcena.htm (June 8, 1999).

Deming, W. E. (1982). *Quality, productivity, and competitive position*. Cambridge: Massachusetts Institute of Technology Center for Advanced Engineering Study.

Donebedian, A. (1980). *Exploration in quality assessment and monitoring: A definition of quality approaches to its assessment.* Ann Arbor, MI: Health Administration Press.

Ishikawa, K. (1985). *What is total quality control? The Japanese way.* Englewood Cliffs, NJ: Prentice-Hall.

JCAHO (1990). *Accreditation manual for hospitals, 1991.* Chicago: Author.

JCAHO (1987). *Overview of the joint commission's agenda for change.* Chicago: Author.

JCAHO (1997–1998). *JCAHO comprehensive accreditation manual for home care.* Chicago: Author.

Juran, J. M. (1989). *Juran on leadership for quality: An executive handbook.* New York: The Free Press.

NCQA Mission. (1999). Available: http://www.nahdo.org/frawley/sldo2.htm (June 8, 1999).

OSHA's Mission. Over 100 million Workers Count on OSHA—online. (1999). Available: www.osha.gov/oshinfo/mission.html (June 8, 1999).

Price, S., Wade Koch, M., & Bassett, S. (1998). *Health care resource management: Present and future challenges.* St. Louis: Mosby.

Thiroux, J. P. (1986). *Ethics: Theory and practice* (3rd ed.). New York: Macmillan.

Vasilash, G. S. (1988). Buried treasure and other benefits of quality. *The Juran Report, 9,* 30.

CHAPTER
18

Advancing Nursing Research in a Professional Practice Climate

Lillian M. Simms · Naomi E. Ervin

The overall purpose of research dissemination is to begin the process of getting new knowledge used for the good of society. (Cronenwett, 1995, p. 430)

Chapter Highlights

- Role of the nurse executive
- Researchable nursing problems
- Collaborative research
- Developing a nursing research emphasis
- Applications of research to practice
- Assimilation of innovations

Florence Nightingale's devotion to statistics paved the way for the development of modern research. Although she had no interest in the germ theory, she understood the impact of environment on disease and related mortality (Cohen, 1984).

The purpose of this chapter is to present nursing research as an essential component of a professional nursing practice climate. Nurse executives play a key role in promoting the application of nursing research to practice by stimulating staff involvement in research and promoting a climate in which research can occur. Executives are not necessarily researchers, but they must be knowledgeable about research methodology and must be willing to set the stage for research to occur. In other words, nurse executives must be willing to promote research-based nursing, for they are in key positions to influence the amount and nature of the research undertaken by nursing staff, faculty, and students (Simms, Price, & Pfoutz, 1987).

ROLE OF THE NURSE EXECUTIVE

Although increasing numbers of nursing departments are hiring nurse researchers, the role of the nurse executive is to foster a climate in which nursing studies can be conducted and nursing research findings can be applied to practice. The nurse executive who plans to establish a nursing research program is often faced with selling the concept to nursing staff. More recently, the emphasis has changed to utilization as more nurses graduate from educational programs with an appreciation for research. In many institutions a research program is often considered a nicety rather than an essential tool for data-based decision-making. Furthermore, nursing staff may still view those conducting research as away from practice and not reality based.

Nurse researchers are fostering nursing research and initiating creative ways to link research with practice (Bostrom & Wise, 1994). The models vary from agency-based programs to various types of collaboration with schools of nursing and other health-related schools. The particular model used should provide the best fit with the agency and the administrative style of the nurse executive.

The role of the nurse executive in promoting research-based nursing, therefore, is one of leadership. It may not be necessary to develop an in-house research program if abundant resources are available from other disciplines. Whether the nursing division is a research utilizer or a combined research conductor and utilizer, the steps of the research process must govern the decision to study, not to study, or to apply data from another study. Too many administrators attempt to match solutions with problems without fully understanding the problem to be solved or studied.

In selling the concept of research throughout the agency, the nurse executive must encourage staff to understand and participate in research-related activities (Hefferin, Horsley, & Ventura, 1982). Such activities include and are not limited to emphasis on nursing process and quality assurance, attendance of research conferences, and participation in ongoing studies, either as subjects or data collectors. To introduce research findings into practice, the nurse executive must be able to evaluate research, using self-skills or obtaining the expertise of a nurse researcher capable of evaluating research.

Sanders, Davidson, and Price (1996) studied the perception of unit nurse managers (head nurses/nurse executives) as to what constituted their role functions, activities, and responsibilities. Four major components were used to clarify this description: administration, clinical practice, education, and research. Facilitation, utilization, and development were the subcategories in the research component. In the facilitation subcategory only two items were of significant importance: collaboration with other departments on research projects (78%) and supporting the work of others (77%). Perhaps this is the most typical experience or contact these managers had with research. All of the other items ranked in the 30% to 40% range (i.e., provide access to populations, member research committee, delegate staff to research assignment). All the percentages in the utilization items ranked greater than 50%. In this category applying research to patient care standards and the use of innovation from nursing and related fields both ranked at 76%, whereas utilization of data for decision-making ranked 69%. In the research development category the following items ranked greater than 50%: stimulate development of projects, raise researchable questions, and develop own research.

In a similar study that examined the role of the chief nurse executive in the Veteran Affairs setting, Jaco, Price, and Davidson (1994) reported that the two research facilitation items identified as important included employment of a nurse researcher (72%) and joint research with other schools of nursing (75%). The majority of the respondents indicated that utilization of research items was an important aspect of their role. The only item on the scale that did not receive a majority of positive responses was participation in data collection. Only 35% of the respondents identified this item as important to their role. The other interesting item was publishing research findings. Although 73% responded that this item was important, only 41% believe they had the opportunity to implement it as part of their role. All of the items on the research development scale were identified as important, with the exception of involvement as a co-researcher. Respondents did not believe they had the opportunity in their position to be directly involved as a researcher. Although 55% believed this item was important, only 37% indicated that they did not have the opportunity to participate in research. These nurse executives support research activities, encourage a milieu conducive to research, and promote the inclusion of research findings in development of evidence-based practice.

The final role of the nurse executive is that of defender of practice changes. Many nurses see research as irrelevant to their practice, and the administrator often finds it necessary to justify decisions for changes in practice as well as to reallocate resources if necessary. Thus, the nurse executive is conceived to be the leader, the pacesetter, the climate creator, the evaluator, and the defender of research-based practice. It is necessary for administrators to have research skills, and doctorally prepared nurses are increasingly moving into administrative roles. To use the skills and work of others in orchestrating professional nursing practice, it has become essential for all nurse executives to have, at a minimum, data management and research appreciation skills.

RESEARCHABLE NURSING PROBLEMS

Nursing problems surface in many possible ways, but basically they are related to clinical and systems questions. Although most nursing staff will not have the qualifications to conduct research, they can be encouraged to participate in generating priority nursing problems. It is then up to the nurse executive to seek the most appropriate resources for studying problems.

Clinical, educational, and administrative problems can be brought into focus for study by using the research process. Elevating the area of concern from the mundane to the abstract is the first step in conceptualizing the area of study. This can be done by raising questions researchable within the areas of practice or questions that can be answered by other research.

The importance of using the expertise of qualified nurse researchers cannot be overemphasized. At least one doctorally prepared nurse is essential to the conduct and utilization of quality nursing research. As professional nursing practice becomes increasingly based on empirical research findings, it is important that rigorous studies be conducted or used in changing practice or making clinical decisions.

Nursing problems requiring investigation may be clinical, administrative, or educational. Agency needs for research may vary, but the nature of the nursing problems should have commonality across institutions. Clinical nursing problems requiring special emphasis within the field are those related to mobility, eating, continence, cognition, and skin integrity. New clinical studies may be generated, or developed studies from other settings may be replicated. Figure 18.1 suggests options for relevant research.

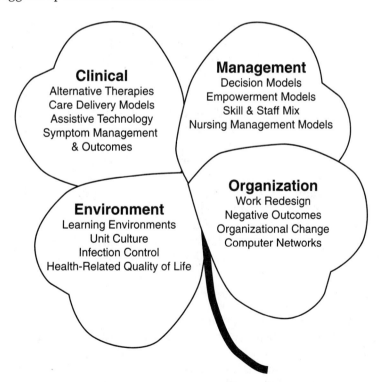

Figure 18.1 Options for nursing administration research.

Administrative studies of importance for nursing usually relate to the care given, as opposed to the nursing process or the activities investigated in clinical studies. Productivity and staffing pattern studies fall in this category, as do staff morale and satisfaction investigations. Another possibility for administrative study is the descriptive measure of technical and professional roles in nursing. Quality of care research overlaps both clinical and administrative questions.

The paucity of research on outcomes of organizational change and nursing administration issues has been identified by Jennings (1995) and Aiken, Sochalski, and Lake (1997). Contemporary health care is too complex to continue pursuing research from a narrowly defined clinical practice perspective only. An integration of clinical and administrative frameworks for investigation is needed. The void in knowledge development for nursing administration creates obstacles in linking nursing knowledge about patient care. The clinical research focus has prevailed even though nursing administration helps create the environment for care in all settings, manages patient care delivery, and contributes to the goals of clinical effectiveness and efficiency. There is a need to understand environment as it pertains to nursing as a process and health care delivery. We need to redirect our focus to include the environment of care delivery, outcomes of organizational change in health services, and outcomes of clinical practice.

A much neglected area for research within nursing divisions is that of evaluation of in-service educational programs. The questions arise as to whether continuing education makes a difference in behavior and whether it affects competency. Many types of issues are emerging today related to competency measures for re-licensure and institutional licensure. The correlation of basic educational preparation to job performance needs much study.

The American Nurses Association (ANA, 1997) has identified the following areas of nursing research priority for the 21st century, all of which reflect a high value for quality and affordable health care. They are:

- Develop and test models for health care delivery that are clinically effective, cost effective, and accessible.
- Develop culturally sensitive instruments to measure variables and outcomes sensitive to nursing interventions.
- Evaluate approaches to nursing education.
- Identify and test strategies that foster healthy behaviors and self-care.
- Identify and test interventions to minimize or prevent environmentally induced health problems.
- Evaluate the effects of health technologies in acute and chronic illness.
- Develop and test primary care nursing strategies.
- Test models of nursing management.
- Develop databases of health care use and critical health status in vulnerable populations.
- Investigate and test provider/patients collaborative decision-making models for their effect on improved patient/family outcomes.

- Analyze and evaluate home health care services and outcomes of care for elders living at home and in long-term care facilities.
- Test affordable models of health care that do not compromise quality.
- Identify quality indicators that reflect appropriate nursing skill and staff mix (ANA, 1997).

COLLABORATIVE RESEARCH

To be effective in any given setting, nursing research must be a collaborative effort using intra- and interinstitutional resources. Collaboration between nurses in practice and academic settings and integration of nurses into the broad scientific community are essential to a sound research focus (Buhler-Wilkerson, Naylor, Holt, & Rinke, 1998).

Horsley (Hefferin, Horsley, & Ventura, 1982) and Hinshaw and colleagues (Hinshaw, Chance, & Atwood, 1981) have pioneered collaborative research programs. A collaborative research development model requires clinicians and researchers to be equally functioning team members in the development of clinical nursing research proposals. Clinicians, administrators, educators, and researchers can collaborate and negotiate to produce sound, practice-based research that yields relevant, accurate information for practice decisions and contributes to nursing knowledge. Nurses in all of these roles are all responsible for making nursing professional.

Intra- and interinstitutional collaboration goes beyond nursing to include the expertise of physicians, health services-related engineers, biologists, psychologists, and sociologists as appropriate. Although nursing needs to develop its own knowledge base, it is apparent that, as an applied science, the profession can benefit from interdisciplinary and nursing-related research from other fields.

Positive and negative factors influence the development and maintenance of collaborative research programs. Positive factors include institutional commitment to quality, patient-centered care and widespread enthusiasm and interest with the nursing division for professional nursing practice. The support of hospital or agency administration and medical staff for a collaborative research program cannot be overestimated. The control of research subjects and resources clearly can influence the longevity and quality of any research programs.

In an ongoing analysis of the biomedical and health services research literature, Mitchell and Shortell (1997) have collaborated successfully in studying the linkage between adverse outcomes of care and variations in organization of care delivery. This work is leading to testing of outcomes related to patient functioning in everyday life and self-care. Both are important topics for nursing administration research.

DEVELOPING A NURSING RESEARCH EMPHASIS

Before the development of a nursing research emphasis or program, the preferred model must be selected. Although distinct models exist, each has different merit for different agencies based on available resources:

- Practice-based research networks: affiliation of clinicians interested in studying similar phenomena (Grey & Walker, 1998).
- University-based model: research is initiated and designed by scholars in schools of nursing, conducted in laboratories or health care agencies, and reported in research journals with opportunity for wide-spread application to practice (Loomis & Krone, 1980).
- Agency-based model: an agency hires a researcher to assist in developing a study or hires a permanent, full-time researcher to stimulate in-house research (Loomis & Krone, 1980).
- Collaborative university–agency-based model: the nurse researcher is director of both research programs and uses the skills of faculty researchers and agency staff.
- External consultant model: a nurse researcher is hired for specific studies.
- Nursing development unit model: a cluster of units on which clinical research can be tested (Ashurst, Clarke, Evitts, Lacey, & Snashall, 1990).
- Nursing sabbaticals: agency provides support to complete a research or publishing project (Sperhac, Haas, & O'Malley, 1994).

The attitude of the nurse executive is critical. Once the commitment is made to establish a research emphasis and the model selected, a nursing research and review committee needs to be established (Rempusheski et al., 1996). This group works closely with the nurse executive or nurse researcher in establishing a philosophy and goals consistent with ANA standards for nursing practice and with the orientation of the institution.

Obtaining funding for a proposed research emphasis depends on the creativity of the nurse executive. Depending on institutional receptivity to nursing research, the emphasis may be openly established. Other approaches include linkages with a quality assurance role, research consultation, or adjunct appointments for faculty researchers.

APPLICATIONS OF RESEARCH TO PRACTICE

A commitment to research is not enough to maintain an in-house research emphasis. Conducted or utilized nursing research must be seen as validating the effectiveness of nursing care and as an important means of improving nursing practice. If research is relevant to practice, it will be accepted and used by practicing nurses.

Tranmer, Kisilevsky, and Muir (1995) discuss the effectiveness of a research utilization strategy for staff nurses in a neonatal intensive care unit of a community teaching hospital. Specific objectives for staff nurses involved in the project were to increase job satisfaction by expanding research activities, to learn to critique research literature, and to gain an understanding and appreciation of research through participation in a research study. The project demonstrated that with appropriate organizational and individual support, research utilization can occur in the acute care setting. Individual and organizational strategies that support, recognize and legitimize nursing research activities as an integral component of nursing practice require further development.

According to Cronenwett (1995), two forms of research are important to practitioners:

1. Decision-driven models, in which knowledge is used when it is implemented as part of a new practice, protocol, or intervention; generally leads directly to some course of action, e.g., clinical intervention studies.
2. Conceptual utilization models, in which the purpose of research is to influence thinking instead of action, e.g., work excitement research.

Application to practice can occur through data-based decision-making or clinical practice activities. Decisions to alter staffing patterns can be based on research. Selection of nursing care delivery models can and should be based on research. The continuation or abandonment of decubitus care methodologies should be based on results of investigative studies. Quality of patient care must be evaluated in terms of outcomes as well as processes. Patient classification systems have little use unless linked with clinical and administrative decision-making. Systematic evaluation of practice modes not only improves the quality of practice but also the quality of patient life.

Perhaps the best application of research to practice is the establishment of the testing, questioning, thinking environment in which professional nurses feel comfortable in asking, "Is this the best way, is there a better way?"

UTILIZATION OF NURSING RESEARCH

Fawcett (1980) suggests that only when professional nursing practice is based on knowledge validated by research will nursing gain independence as a profession. As long as nursing is viewed as an occupation, institutional policies and politics will keep nurses second-class citizens. The only way to generate nursing knowledge, so essential to professional status, is through scientific nursing research: the study of nursing phenomena. Moch et al. (1997) propose an effective mechanism linking research and practice as the result of a 4-year case study of staff nurses/researcher using semistructured group discussions. The authors describe the process and outcomes of researcher-initiated discussion groups with nurses in clinical practice. The discussions were organized to use the expertise of practicing nurses to provide feedback on a program of research. Practicing nurses were asked to comment on research findings based on their clinical experience. Discussion served as a means for researchers and clinicians to understand each others' expertise.

As research is increasingly linked to practice, nursing research review committees will play a more important role in promoting pragmatic studies of scientific merit that are related to clinical practice (Rempusheski et al., 1996). Collaborative linkages between service and education will further nurture research utilization when faculty members serve on hospital research review committees and clinical nurses are invited to serve on university research review boards and nursing faculty research teams. White, Leske, and Pearcy (1995) describe three other collaborative models that link research with practice. The CURN model encourages staff participation in research-related activities. The Stetler model encourages individual practitioners to become involved in research utilization and evaluation on a routine basis. The Iowa model addresses the identification of frequently encountered clinical problems as triggers that initiate assembling relevant research literature and evaluation protocols.

ASSIMILATION OF INNOVATIONS

Research in isolation is meaningless, and theory in and of itself is irrelevant. If nursing research is to be palatable in practice, it must be presented in terms that are understandable and useful for implementation. Nursing theories developed and tested through research must become part of the language of nursing. As nursing practice becomes increasingly based on empirical research findings, it is important to conduct rigorous studies to assess current nursing practice or to evaluate changes in practice. A systematic review of existing nursing research and the assimilation of innovation protocols for nursing practice have been described by Bostrom and Wise (1994), who describe the gap that exists between discovery of potential innovations and implementation into practice. Their Retrieval and Application of Research in Nursing (RARIN) is a project that is helping to reduce this gap in a western hospital. The goal is to improve the quality of nursing care by facilitating the transfer of new and clinically relevant nursing information to practice. A protocol for implementing nursing research was established on four experimental units, which included:

1. Installing computer terminals that are linked electronically through a local area network (LAN). The LAN is linked to over 100 information databases supported by local and national institutions including the Library of Medicine's MEDLINE citation retrieval system.
2. Creating two nursing research databases for local system users.
3. Training nurses in the target units in using the network, local databases, and MEDLINE.
4. Providing consultation and support for nurses to use existing research and to conduct their research.

Stages in the assimilation of innovation are knowledge awareness,evaluation/ choice, and adoption/implementation.

The goal of research-based practice is important to professional nurses (Barnsteiner, Ford, & Howe, 1995). Research is best disseminated by integrating it into standards, procedures, and patient/family education materials. Dissemination efforts are for naught if knowledge is not used by practitioners. Clinical advancement programs are best implemented when clinical practice levels include research competencies. Research then becomes the base for quality clinical practice (Figure 18.2). The participatory action research approach described in Chapter 22 also offers much promise for stimulating participation in and utilization of research.

SUMMARY

In the final analysis, it is left to the nurse executive to use nursing research and introduce research findings into practice. This is accomplished through the establishment of a professional practice environment that promotes involvement of staff in research activities and demands that clinical nursing policies and procedures are research based. Once the environment of research-based practice is established, it is no longer necessary to treat the concept as a separate goal, for, as in all professions, it becomes internalized in behavior.

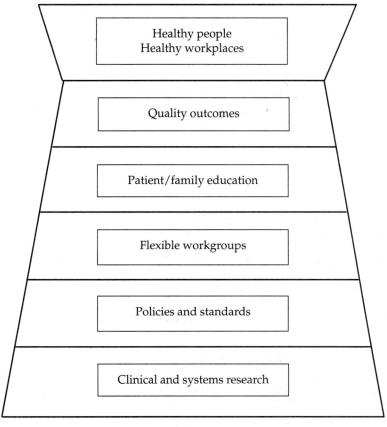

Figure 18.2 The research utilization process.

STUDY QUESTIONS

1. Identify three clinical or systems problems on your unit(s).
2. Develop a collaborative research approach for studying these problems.
3. Explain the difference between process and outcome research.
4. Describe three models for developing a nursing research emphasis.

REFERENCES

Aiken, L. H., Sochalski, J., & Lake, E. T. (1997). Studying outcomes of organizational change in health services. *Medical Care, 35*(11), NS6–NS18, supplement.

American Nurses Association. (1997). *Directions for nursing research: Toward the twenty-first century.* Washington, DC: American Nurses Publishing.

Ashurst, A., Clarke, D., Evitts, A., Lacey, J., & Snashall, T. (1990). Creating a climate for the development of nursing. *Nursing Practice, 4*(1), 18–20.

Barnsteiner, J. H., Ford, N., & Howe, C. (1995). Research utilization in a metropolitan children's hospital. In M. G. Titler & C. J. Goode (Eds.), *The Nursing Clinics of North America* (Vol. 30, No. 3, 447–456). Philadelphia: Saunders.

Bostrom, J., & Wise, L. (1994). Closing the gap between research and practice. *Journal of Nursing Administration, 24*(5), 22–27.

Buhler-Wilkerson, K., Naylor, M. D., Holt, S. W., & Rinke, L. T. (1998). An alliance for academic home care: Integrating research, education, and practice. *Nursing Outlook, 46*(2), 77–80.

Cohen, I. B. (1984). Florence Nightingale. *Scientific American, 250*(3), 128–137.

Cronenwett, L. R. (1995). Effective methods for disseminating research findings to nurses in practice. In M. G. Titler & C. J. Goode (Eds.), *The Nursing Clinics of North America* (Vol. 30, No. 3, 429–438). Philadelphia: Saunders.

Fawcett, J. (1980). A declaration of nursing independence: The relation of theory and research to nursing practice. *Journal of Nursing Administration, 10*(6), 36–39.

Grey, M., & Walker, P. H. (1998). Practice-based research networks for nursing. *Nursing Outlook, 46*(3), 125–129.

Hefferin, E. A., Horsley, J. A., & Ventura, M. R. (1982). Promoting research-based nursing: The nurse administrator's role. *Journal of Nursing Administration, 12*(5), 34–41.

Hinshaw, A. S., Chance, H. C., & Atwood, J. (1981). Research in practice: A process of collaboration and negotiation. *Journal of Nursing Administration, 11*(2), 33–38.

Jaco, P., Price, S., & Davidson, A. (1994). The nurse executive in the public sector. *Journal of Nursing Administration, 24*(3), 55–63.

Jennings, B. M. (1995). Nursing research: a time for redirection. *Journal of Nursing Administration, 25*(4), 9–11.

Loomis, M. E., & Krone, K. P. (1980). Collaborative research development. *Journal of Nursing Administration, 10*(12), 32–35.

Mitchell, P. H., & Shortell, S. M. (1997). Adverse outcomes and variations in organization of care delivery. *Medical Care, 35* (11), NS19–NS32, supplement.

Moch, S. D., Robie, D. E., Bauer, K. C., Pederson, A., Bowe, S., & Shadick, K. (1997). Linking research and practice through discussion. *IMAGE, 29*(2), 189–191.

Rempusheski, V. F., Wolfe, B. E., Dow, K. H., & Fish, L. C. (1996). Peer review by nursing research committees in hospitals. *IMAGE, 28*(1), 51–53.

Sanders, B., Davidson, A., & Price, S. (1996) The nurse executive: A changing perspective. *Nursing Management, 27*(1), 42–46.

Simms, L. M., Price, S. A., & Pfoutz, S. K. (1987). Creating the research climate: A key responsibility for nurse administrators in acute, long-term and home care settings. *Nursing Economic$, 5*(4), 174–178.

Sperhac, A. M., Haas, S. A., & O'Malley, J. O. (1994). Supporting nursing research. *Journal of Nursing Administration, 24*(5), 28–31.

Tranmer, J. E., Kisilevsky, B. S., & Muir, D. W. (1995). A nursing research utilization strategy for staff nurses in the acute care setting. *Journal of Nursing Administration, 25*(4), 21–29.

White, J. M., Leske, J. S., & Pearcy, J. M. (1995). Models and processes of research utilization. In M. G. Titler & C. J. Goode (Eds.), *The Nursing Clinics of North America* (Vol. 30, No. 3, 447–456). Philadelphia: Saunders.

CHAPTER

~ 19 ~

Mobilizing Nursing Resources

Lillian M. Simms • Naomi E. Ervin

No organizational system can perform at its peak unless enough individual members are willing and able to perform at their peaks. (Adams, 1998, p. 231)

Chapter Highlights

* Human potential and motivation
* High-performing systems
* Competency and relicensure
* Traditional practice patterns
* Redesigning nursing practice patterns
* The flexible work group
* Energizing responsibilities of the nurse executive

The new world of work entails the radical redesign of every aspect of an organization (Hammer & Champy, 1993). Nurses who once did what they were told now make decisions on their own. The purpose of this chapter is to discuss an approach to mobilizing nursing resources according to levels of expertise, considering human potential. Practice patterns are discussed in terms of organizational variables, nursing resources, and patient care needs and a flexible work group model is proposed.

Trying to understand recruitment and retention in nursing today is like looking for a straw in the wind and trying to describe its path. The wind keeps shifting, and a tornadic gust threatens to blow the whole issue out of our sphere of influence, if not out of nursing's area of responsibility. Retention concerns viewed as major problems in the 1980s have become opportunities for work redesign in the 1990s. Many hospitals and health care agencies have moved in the direction of nonnursing control of nursing recruitment and retention through the establishment of human resource departments that control hiring and firing of all health personnel.

In the mid-1990s, recruitment and retention issues in nursing gave way to work redesign and downsizing issues. Understanding human potential becomes critical in rebuilding a workforce after downsizing and layoffs. Managers in a downsizing organization have a tremendously difficult task—not only with their own feelings but with the complex feelings of others who have survived. Noer (1993) speaks of survivor sickness. Downsizing and redesign that has not included employee participation can end up in an organization of depressed employees, an organization with failure to thrive syndrome, and a risk-averse workforce. In its 1996 Position Statement on Restructuring, Work Redesign and the Job Security of Registered Nurses, the American Nurses Association (ANA) supported participation of RNs as full partners in work redesign decisions. The model for practice patterns redesign presented in this chapter provides for continuous involvement of professional nurses in the redesign process.

Nursing is a focal point for the delivery of patient care in all health care delivery settings. Failure to change or implement professional practice patterns may be the result of a lack of understanding of nursing resources and of the appropriate use of nurses according to experience and expertise.

Differentiated practice distributes nursing work according to caregiver and care coordinator activities, and undifferentiated practice is a real barrier to full professional practice (Goertzen, 1991). This is frustrating to nurses who are often seen as focusing on menial tasks while their real, modern-day contribution is much more advanced. No recognition is given to the various educational levels for nurses and the expectations for performance are indistinguishable for AD and BSN nurses. The special skills of the master's and doctorally prepared nurses often go unrecognized and unused.

A serious barrier to professional practice in large, complex organizations is depersonalization. Until recently little consideration has been given to joint practice or to developing models for patient centered care. Nurses are often treated as elements of production rather than intelligent, dedicated professionals. Differentiated practice promotes more efficient and effective distribution of talent according to educational preparation and experiential competency. As a model for intelligent distribution of nursing resources, it serves as a catalyst for patient-focused care.

HUMAN POTENTIAL AND MOTIVATION

Nurses today want to be recognized as professionals. They want to be recognized for their contributions to patient care, and they want the right to control their professional practice within the limits of the law. Unquestionably, these rights always involve maximizing human potential. Human potential means all of one's potentialities: knowledge, talents, capacities, creativity, wisdom, character, and genetic makeup.

The acquisition of technical skill alone does not provide the necessary base for the independent thinking and action essential in today's nursing practice. Men and women have a great deal of unrealized potential, and helping staff discover that potential can be one of the most exhilarating experiences for the nurse executive.

The identification of needs for growth, development, and utilization of potential is an important part of Maslow's self-actualization. This concept was introduced in Chapter 5. The fully functioning administrator encourages the development of human potential in self, peers, and subordinates. Optimal biopsychosocial functioning, so carefully nurtured in patients, needs also to be nurtured in oneself and one's fellow workers.

Howard McClusky had a passionate belief in the power of education to improve the condition of people's lives and to liberate them from the meanness of intolerance and self-interest. Lifelong learning and the fulfillment of growth needs are indeed powerful tools in enhancing human potential. Lifelong learning can help individuals become the persons they are best able to become. In most people, there is a large domain of unexpressed and underexpressed talent that could be developed through educative means.

In his classic work, McClusky (1974) further theorized that failure to internalize the learner role as a central feature of the self is a major restraint in the adult's achievement of his or her potential. Studying, learning, and intellectual adventure must become part of one's life in both work and social environments. Senge (1990) has reconfirmed the power of learning and the importance of learning environments.

Striving to learn about employees and matching them with educational and work experiences can be one of the nurse executive's most stimulating and rewarding challenges. Because the power of education lies both in learning and in teaching abilities, the administrator needs to be a learner as well as a teacher. Satisfaction with work and assumption of responsibility for professional behavior flourish in an environment that fosters maximizing human potential through continued learning.

The role of the nurse executive as a teacher has been largely unrecognized (Pfoutz et al., 1987; Simms, 1991). In fact, in their efforts to stay away from educational roles, many administrators may lose sight of the fact that most education occurs in noncredit or nonformal learning environments. Achieving one's maximum potential involves learning new behaviors. Many administrators spend a great deal of time teaching others how to perform assigned tasks rather than delegating the responsibility for those tasks. How much better it would be to teach individuals how to approach tasks so that they can grow and develop while unleashing their own creativity in resolving problems that contribute to the need for the assigned tasks. Understanding the logic and rationale behind various administrative strategies encourages the learner to have positive feelings toward the ongoing project; as a result, the learner is less likely to resent and thus negatively influence change.

Motivation

Motivation is an internal force that incites a person to action; what motivates one person will not necessarily excite another. According to Herzberg's (Herzberg, Mausner, & Snyderman, 1959) research, rewards can be listed under two broad categories: hygienes, or extrinsic factors, and motivators, or intrinsic factors. The hygienes include:

- Company policy and administration
- Supervision
- Relationships with supervision
- Work conditions
- Salary
- Relationship with peers
- Personal life
- Relationships with subordinates
- Status
- Security

The motivators include:

- Achievement
- Recognition
- Work itself
- Responsibility
- Advancement
- Growth

If managers want to develop a highly motivated staff, says Herzberg, they should focus on the true initiators of action: the motivators, or intrinsic factors. These intrinsic factors are in keeping with the human need theory of Abraham Maslow (1962), which postulates that humans have the need to grow and develop beyond basic coping needs. A satisfied need does not motivate. If all basic and safety needs are met, one can move on to meeting belonging needs and so on up the ladder. Self-actualization needs are never fully met, and by definition, self-actualization is a self-perpetuating, ongoing, and never finished process.

The work of David McClelland (1961) must also be recognized as an important landmark in the field of motivation. He states that, to one degree or another, there are three basic human needs in all individuals:

- Achievement: the need to excel, to achieve in relation to a set of standards, to strive, to succeed
- Power: the need to make others behave in a way they would not have behaved otherwise
- Affiliation: the desire for friendly and close relationship

Although some individuals are motivated by the need to exercise power, others are motivated by the need to achieve. The nurse executive's challenge is to find avenues for these needs to be met. There is also a strong need in staff nurses for affiliation. Some observers suggest this motivation as the major reason why many more young women than men enter nursing.

Expectancy theory suggests that the strength of a tendency to action in a certain way is dependent on the strength of an expectation that an act will be followed by an attractive outcome (Robbins & Coulter, 1996). Attractiveness, performance-reward linkage, and effort-performing linkage are the key variables in this approach to developing human potential. Attractiveness is determined by what one would like to have, such as a promotion or merit increase. Performance-reward linkage is the individual's perception that certain actions will lead to a desired reward. Effort-performing linkage is the perception that a desired reward, such as a raise, is worth the effort to achieve.

Expectancy theory also presupposes the importance of intrinsic factors. The theory holds that workers attempt to complete jobs they know can be accomplished and expend energy on those that will result in personal benefit. In the world of nursing, however, employees may not consider many activities, such as care plans and patient classification systems, to be meaningful activities; thus, the question arises as to how one chooses meaningful activities that also meet the goals of the nurse executive to provide excellent nursing care.

Deci's theory (Deci, 1975) highlights the concept of competence as a strong motivator. Elaborating on Herzberg's work, Deci describes intrinsic motives as informing those activities for which there is no apparent reward. Most people will actively look for stimulation in their work. When there is overstimulation, the individual withdraws and seeks another area of competence. Understimulation results in less than minimal competency. The skillful administrator seeks an environment balanced between overstimulation and understimulation.

Overstimulation can result from the occurrence of numerous clinical projects and changes at one time. Because staff need time to incorporate changes into their functioning, three or four changes attempted at the same time may result in very little lasting change. Also, staff may feel guilty if they neglect their usual tasks for innovative endeavors.

Understimulation can be the result of an environment of no changes or of rigidity. At times, staff require a period of time to become comfortable with changes, but this must not continue indefinitely. A situation of heavy work loads and understaffing can also result in understimulation because staff are forced to give up the challenging tasks—for example, patient teaching, patient care conferences, and committee work—to meet minimal patient needs.

Having staff involved in setting objectives can contribute to arriving at a balanced environment. However, staff may tend to overestimate the amount of work and underestimate the amount of time required to accomplish objectives. Trial and error are sometimes important learning tools as a group of staff struggle to put a new clinical concept into place.

Another useful concept in developing human potential is found in the classic work in operant conditioning conducted by Skinner (1953). The classic operant conditioning process is portrayed as:

$$\text{Stimulus} \rightarrow \text{response} \rightarrow \text{consequences} \rightarrow \text{future response to stimulation}$$

Skinner's theory focuses on four variables: positive reinforcement, extinction, punishment, and avoidance learning. This theory provides guidelines for rewarding desirable behavior and for punishment as a negative reinforcer designed to stop negative behavior. The principles of reinforcement theory can be used to modify behavior in a desired direction. For example, consider the case of a nurse executive who wants to have the staff conduct group patient teaching sessions but none of the staff has enough confidence to volunteer. In such a situation, staff could be reinforced for learning and practicing skills that would lead to conducting group sessions.

A nonmotivating environment produces disillusionment, job dissatisfaction, and role conflict. Role theory is structured on the observable fact that there are prescribed relationships and activities for specified roles; for example, a traffic police officer is expected to direct traffic, and a secretary is expected to type the boss's letters. There is little agreement in our society as to the expectations for the role of a nurse. An ambiguous role, coupled with an abundance of diverse job descriptions, compounds the problem and interferes with the maximum development of potential.

Today's mobile, intelligent, aggressive, and talented nurses need leaders who can help them identify personal and professional goals. They need administrators with enthusiasm, sensitivity, and creativity in patient care and nursing administration; administrators who understand the difficulties involved in simultaneously pleasing patients, physicians, and administrators. The nurse leader with such qualities seeks to create a learning environment in which professional nurses are motivated to practice at their highest level (Simms, 1991).

HIGH-PERFORMING SYSTEMS

Peter Vaill (1982) proposed the following characteristics of high-performing systems:

- Clear on their broad purposes and on nearer term objectives for fulfilling these purposes. They know why they exist and what they are trying to do and members have pictures in their heads that are strikingly similar.

- Commitment to these purposes is never perfunctory, although it is often expressed laconically. Motivation is always high and energy focus is more important than energy level.
- Teamwork is focused on the task, and members have discovered the aspects of systems operations that require integrated actions and have developed related behaviors and attitudes. There are firm beliefs in a "right organizational form," and a noticeable amount of effort is devoted to attaining and maintaining this form. Once members have found a form that works, they cling to it.
- Leadership is strong and clear and it is not ambivalent. There is no question of the need for initiative or of its appropriate source, although it may not always be the same person. Leaders are experienced as reliable and predictable.
- Fertile sources of inventions and new methods are within the scope of the task they have defined and within the form they have chosen.
- They are clearly bounded from their environments, and a considerable amount of energy, particularly on the part of leaders, is devoted to maintaining these boundaries.
- Avoid external control, scrounging resources from the environment nonapologetically. They produce what they want by their standards, not what someone else wants.
- Above all are systems that have jelled, even though the phenomenon is difficult to describe. Demonstrate an intense interdependency and fit of the various elements and practices of the system.

Vaill has based his propositions on the intensive study of individual cases. His propositions have relevance for nurse executives as they attempt to improve productivity in various environments. The new world of work entails the radical redesign of every aspect of an organization (Hammer & Champy, 1993). People who once did what they were told now make choices on their own. Workers focus on customers' needs rather than their bosses.

In recent years, too much attention has been focused on the shortage of nurses, particularly in hospitals. For the following reasons, it is difficult to understand why a shortage was perceived to exist (if, indeed, one does any more):

1. Since 1950, the general hospital occupancy rate has declined significantly (Aiken, 1995).
2. Since 1950, the nation's nursing pool has increased with an excess of ADNs (Aiken, 1995).

Most evidence provided to support a shortage is based on anecdotal material. Over the past 10 to 15 years, there has been steady growth in the supply of nurses. There has also been an increase of newly licensed nurses. Seventy-five percent of all nurses are employed, an increase from 55% in the 1960s. Even though nurses may vacate positions temporarily during childbirth, they do return. The current supply of nurses should be visualized as a dynamic, constantly changing, constantly growing entity with a shortage only at the BSN and graduate levels.

Various reasons are cited for the perceived shortage of nurses. Aiken (1995) calls attention to the high probability that demand for professional nurses has been increasing and continues to increase at a rate faster than the supply of nurses is increasing. This may be due to the higher acuity rate in all settings, the technological revolution in the delivery of care, and the inability of ADNs to handle complex care.

If nurses are going to be part of high-performing systems, a transformation of the nursing workforce will be needed. Over the years, Aiken has repeatedly expressed concern about the lack of differentiation of nursing tasks but in 1995, she took a strong stand for transforming the nursing workforce and using nurses according to their level of education and expertise. She notes that the United States has an adequate supply of nurses but lacks a mix of talents that can meet present and future challenges in our health care system. Most nurses work in hospitals but it is unlikely that hospitals can continue to absorb the additional nurse graduates each year. With the dramatic increase in the employment of unlicensed assistive personnel, we are probably preparing too many AD nurses in this country. As hospitals continue to reduce the number of inpatient days, jobs for nurses in hospitals will continue to decline and the growth of jobs in ambulatory settings will increase.

If high-performing nursing systems are to prevail, nurses in today's settings need a better education. Increasingly sicker patients in hospitals require more complex nursing care. As medical education changes, there will be fewer medical residents in hospitals, creating another need for better prepared nurses at the baccalaureate and graduate levels. In the community, better prepared nurses with creative executive skills are needed to develop and coordinate high-quality, productive nursing systems. As the educational infrastructure for practice in the 21st century, attention must be given to preparing professional nurses to work in a variety of settings, including primary care, long-term care, and community care and with underserved populations in rural and inner city areas.

COMPETENCY AND RELICENSURE

If a clear identification of nursing services is really important under managed care, perhaps an analysis of nursing jobs will become as mandatory as continuing education is in many states. Some questions to be answered in such analysis include: What is the work of nursing? What should it be? Who should be doing which parts of the work? What will be the competencies of the workers? How will the nurse workers maintain competency according to their level of expertise?

Most states have health occupation legislation covering nursing practice and licensure provisions that specifically address professional nursing. In the state of Michigan, for example, the practice of nursing is defined as "the systematic application of substantial specialized knowledge and skill derived from the biological, physical, and behavioral sciences, to the care, treatment, counsel, and health teaching of individuals who are experiencing changes in the normal health processes or who require assistance in the maintenance of health and the prevention or management of illness, injury, or disability" (State of Michigan Public Health Code, 1997). The RN engages in the practice of nursing; the practice of licensed practical nursing is considered a subfield of the practice of nursing performed only under the supervision of an RN, physician, or dentist. Incompetence means a departure from or failure to conform to minimal standards of acceptable and prevailing practice for the health profession, whether or not actual injury to an individual occurs.

Although the laws in most states clearly describe the differences in levels of competency between registered and practical nurses, controversy continues to rage about substitution of LPNs for RNs. Inevitably, nursing must come to grips with the idea of a standard education for a professional activity. Although "BSN or equivalent" is frequently used to state a position requirement, no personnel department would ever argue for an MD equivalent as the minimum requirement for a physician's appointment.

Over the years, nursing has evolved from the services of a trained nurse who learned skills at the bedside to those of a profession with standards of education and practice and recognized accountability to the public. Credentialing at graduation from accredited institutions suggests that minimal criteria with respect to faculty, facilities, and program have been met. Nurse executives set the standards for who will do what in nursing in their settings. They need to consider the basic educational and experiential competency of the participants, among other factors, before deciding on a particular organizational structure or practice pattern (McClure, 1990).

Fragmented, irrelevant discussions prevail nationwide concerning competencies for RNs (Aiken, 1995). It is important that nurses be competent in their assigned roles. However, these assigned roles cannot be determined in educational settings away from the work environment. The technological revolution has created a situation in which education is far behind practice. Nurse executives are the professionals in the best position to see the needs of the patients and the organization.

The LPN role is a dependent role. For minimal-level competency in today's dynamic health care system, the LPN should be prepared at the associate degree level. RNs should be prepared at the baccalaureate level and should have studied supervision and management. As nurse executives conduct job and nursing staff analyses, they need to have competent nurses and nurse assistants to develop practice patterns designed for quality, cost-effective care delivery.

It is no longer acceptable to deny the legal accountability of the professional nurse by creating such titles as primary or team leader or modular nurse. Prospective payment legislation demands a quantification of nursing services.

The first unknown to be defined in the question is *nurse*. The nurse executive has the best key to solving the following:

$$n + \text{practice pattern} = \text{quality care}$$

The practice pattern is easy to identify once a clear decision has been made about n (nurse).

Nurse executives must create practice environments that address the best use of nurses, associate degree through doctorate. Nursing practice patterns based on the creation of new titles without attention to the competence of the participants lack credibility. Institutional licensure is greatly feared as the antithesis of independent professional licensure. If nurses do not assume responsibility for practice as defined in most state practice acts, it may be only a matter of time before institutional licensure takes over as a method of competency maintenance for relicensure.

TRADITIONAL PRACTICE PATTERNS

During the past three decades, an extensive literature has developed on the subject of nursing practice patterns, reflecting the importance of the use of nursing personnel in providing care in hospital settings. Nurses were "assigned" to work rather than considered as participants in a practice pattern. One type of assignment pattern focused on specialization and division of labor, or functional nursing. This type of assignment pattern evolved in response to political and economic factors that demanded a redistribution of RNs during World War II and included the creation of new nursing personnel categories such as LPN and the nurses' aide. Functional nursing focused on getting the greatest amount of task work done at the least cost in time and training. This pattern was accomplished by assigning specific tasks—categorized or ordered according to degree of difficulty and importance to patient well-being—to nursing personnel with corresponding skill levels. The use of multiple personnel to provide elements of a patients' care requires a level of coordination and decision-making best handled within a formal unit structure with a well-defined hierarchy.

Following the focus on specific technical excellence as the basis of assignment patterns, was an emphasis on integrating nursing personnel of varying skill levels into a democratic, close-knit team. Team nursing represents another way of adjusting care to the influx of auxiliary workers and was created to improve patient care by using the diverse skills of team members under the close guidance of RNs. This pattern shifted much of the authority for making nursing decisions to a lower level in the nursing hierarchy: the RN team leader who assumes responsibility for care given by other team members.

One recent pattern to develop places the responsibility for nursing care management within the direct caregiver. Primary nursing requires that the RN's activities change from care manager-personnel organizer to care manager-care implementer.

Nurse aide activities are refocused away from direct contact with the patient and toward equipment and supplies. The services of the LPN are not used in this pattern or fall somewhere on a continuum from direct patient care to direct assistance to the RN. Decisions in the care process are usually made by a single caregiver and are facilitated through horizontal consultation with peers, rather than with line authority. Primary nursing has been the basic nursing practice pattern used in community health nursing.

Each practice pattern has had its day of popularity, and no one best way has emerged for all settings. Indeed, within the same pattern, there is no clear description of nursing responsibility. Within the primary nursing pattern, the time duration in which a primary nurse plans and gives care to a patient might span hospital admission to discharge or be limited to a patients' length of stay on a particular nursing unit. Within a given day, primary nurse responsibility for care management may vary from 8 to 24 hours. In team nursing, the team leader might carefully match patient needs to team member skills so that each patient must cope with only a limited number of personnel, or the team leader could functionally assign tasks within the team itself, with less concern for the number of personnel rendering direct care to an individual patient. In functional nursing, the picture of variation is less clear, for few U.S. nursing departments now identify with this structure. Yet one can recognize this structure in hospitals, where there are separate positions for activities such as discharge planning, patient education, parenteral infusion, and so on.

REDESIGNING NURSING PRACTICE PATTERNS

Work redesign can be exciting with positive outcomes for patient care. There is a great opportunity for maximizing human potential, if nurses are full partners in the workplace and work redesign (Koch & Esmon, 1998). Work redesigners find that the unit culture or established way of doing things exists only to support departments, units or facility. The process of work redesign calls for a break in traditions and routines and puts the patient first. Drucker (1991) notes that the paradigm shift today to a focus on the consumer rather than employees is creating a key impetus for changing the way we do business in health care. A demanding, better educated consumer affects our view of productivity and how to achieve high productivity with intelligent consumers will be a challenge for health care organizations well into the 21st century. Every organization will have to build in the management of change and continuous task simplification. According to Drucker (1992), managers must learn to ask regularly, if we did not do this already, would we do it now.

Task simplification is one of the key elements in any work redesign. It is necessary to look closely at how and by whom tasks required for patient care are done. There are advantages to compressing several jobs into one if it does not take three people to do them. A relatively little discussed idea in work redesign is the issue of patient responsibility in care. Yet Slack (1997) notes that the largest most neglected health care resource today is the patient. Most people can self-manage common important medical problems if they have the clinical information to do so. Slack further notes the excellent response he has had with patients doing their own computerized health assessment. He has found that patients are very interested in the process and provide more accurate information than that acquired only by a health professional.

The purpose of the nursing practice (formerly assignment) patterns study at the University of Michigan was to develop useful tools for nurses in management and clinical practice who are faced with nursing practice pattern decisions. The project included (1) development of instruments to measure nursing practice patterns, patient characteristics, nursing resources, and organizational support; and (2) the publication of a nursing practice user's manual (Beckman & Simms, 1992; Munson, Beckman, Clinton, Kever, & Simms, 1980).

Nursing resources were defined in terms of selected variables, all of which have relevance for care assignment and quality care. Table 19.1 identifies and explains the various nursing resource components, ranging from staff mix and preparation to commitment, stability, availability, and special training. This conceptualization provides a broad perspective on the components of a nursing resource configuration. Consistent with the ANA position on work redesign, nurses participate at every step of the process.

This demonstration project collected data in four hospitals. Preliminary work was essential to the quality of the project and included:

1. Development of a conceptual framework within which the definition of the elements of a nursing pattern could be developed.
2. Literature review of about 270 items selected for their potential contributions to an understanding of the linkage between patient characteristics, nursing resources, and organizational support and appropriate nursing practice patterns.
3. Development of connective propositions from the literature review that could translate the data into appropriate recommendations for a unit's nursing practice pattern.
4. Development of the instruments.

In developing the essential instruments, the study group found it useful to go beyond the traditional nursing practice patterns (functional, team, or primary) and to think of three major dimensions in any nurse utilization pattern: patient characteristics, nursing resources, and organizational support. More recent work by Simms and Erbin-Roesemann (1992) has yielded a fourth major dimension, that of work characteristics and work excitement.

Conceptual Framework

Practice patterns on any patient unit may be seen as a link between problems, as presented by different patient populations, and purpose, as expressed by

Table 19.1 Nursing Resources Variables

Variable	Range	Definitions and Explanation

Mix by shift ratio
   Day
   Evening
   Night
	Ratio	Five-week average count of RNs/LPNs/aides per shift transformed into a standardized ratio

RN/staff ratio
   Day
   Evening
   Night
	Ratio	Five-week average count of RNs/other staff per shift transformed into a standardized ratio

RN/patient ratio	Ratio	Average number of patients per RN over a five-week period by shifts
Part-time/full-time ratio	Ratio	Five-week average of part-time to full-time nursing personnel, all shifts transformed into a standardized ratio
Staff stability: Turnover	0–100%	Proportion of staff replaced each year, separately for RN, LPN, aides
Absenteeism	0–12%	Proportion of staff absent each day, separately for RN, LPN, aides
Staffing instability	0–100%	The proportion of unit staff who change their unit or shift each day; shown for RN, LPN, and aides separately for the day shift
Staff availability	No range	An index of the labor market availability of different categories of nursing personnel
Preparation ratio	Ratio	The ratio of Master's + BSN, to DIP (diploma) + associate's degree (AD), to LPN + aide in the total nursing staff on the unit
Experience ratio	Ratio	The average number of years of experience on the unit for Master's + BSN, to DIP + AD, to LPN + aide
Special training	No range	An estimate of the extent of special training, separately by RN, LPN, and aides, in five skill areas relevant to practice pattern decisions
Staff development resources	No range	A descriptive statement based on responses to questions about staff development

From Beckman, J. S., & Simms, L. M. (1992). *A guide to redesigning nursing practice patterns.* Ann Arbor, MI: Health Administration Press, Foundation of the American College of Healthcare Executives. Copyright 1992 by Health Administration Press. Adapted by permission.

professional standards and purposes of the organization. Figure 19.1 shows the framework within which the definition of the elements of a nursing practice pattern were developed. Four quality attributes identified in the earlier Munson et al. research were used as the basis for the conceptual framework: comprehensiveness, accountability, continuity, and coordination. Instruments were developed to measure the influencing factors of patient characteristics, nursing resources, and organizational support.

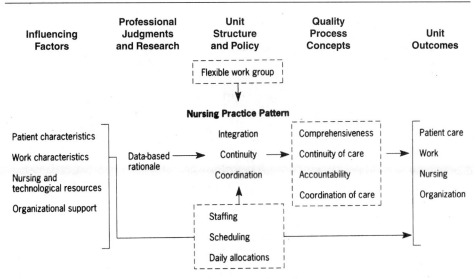

Figure 19.1 Nursing practice pattern conceptual framework. From Beckman, J. S., & Simms, L. M. (1992). *A guide to redesigning nursing practice patterns.* Ann Arbor, MI: Health Administration Press. Foundation of the American College of Healthcare Executives. Copyright 1992 by Health Administration Press. Adapted by permission.

Within the nursing process, two basic activities are recognized: caregiving and care planning, or management. Care management includes assessment of patient requirements for nursing care, formulation of nursing diagnoses, stating outcomes of care and nursing interventions, and evaluation. Caregiving refers only to the implementation of nursing interventions. Table 19.2 highlights the four central elements of a nursing practice pattern.

These elements vary across practice patterns. Care management integration (CMI) would be relatively high in a functional practice pattern and in a primary nursing pattern where one person plans. In a team practice pattern in which the team changes sides of the hall every week, care management continuity (CMC) would be lower. Nursing care integration (NCI) would be high in most primary nursing patterns, lower in team, and lowest in functional, with the greatest number of care givers.

Additional integration, continuity, and coordination variables were conceptualized to complete the profile. Note in Table 19.3 the elements of integration, care management, continuity across settings, and the coordination elements of care-cure, patient services, and intershift coordination.

By collecting specific data on patient, work, nursing, and organizational characteristics, a nursing unit can determine the type of practice pattern actually in use. It is also possible to look at patient characteristics and consider which elements of the nursing practice pattern are most closely related to the needs of the patients. For example, a patient with high psychosocial support needs may benefit

*Table 19.2 Nursing Practice Patterns Concepts and Variables:
Definitions and Relationships*

Concept	Structure Variable
Comprehensive care Nursing care is complete and inclusive; all aspects are well integrated on each shift for each patient	*Integration* The degree to which nursing care of a patient is unified or divided on each shift, measured by the number of personnel managing care, giving care, or both
Continuity of care/Accountability Nursing care over time is consistent over shifts, unit stay, and agency stay The obligation for meeting total nursing care needs resides with an identifiable nurse	*Continuity* The degree to which the patient's care and care management are continuous or shifted among nursing personnel during unit and agency stay
Coordination of care The management of all patients care activities meets patient needs	*Coordination* The person, method, and/or medium used to plan and organize a patient's care within a shift, across shifts, and between nurses and medical staff, patient services

Note: Both concepts and variables are defined and measured from the perspective of the individual patient. These concepts and variables are adapted from Munson, Beckman, Clinton, Kever, and Simms (1980). The concepts were from original work by Dr. Barbara Horn and describe the nursing ideals or goals being sought. The structure variables describe the elements of the nursing unit practice pattern structure that relate to achievement of the concepts. These operationally defined variables are measurable and may vary over time and across units. It is important to note that achievement of the concepts is possible with various levels of the related variables, depending on influencing factors and related adjustments of other practice pattern variables. From Beckman, J. S., & Simms, L. M. (1992). *A guide to redesigning nursing practice patterns.* Ann Arbor, MI: Health Administration Press. Foundation of the American College of Healthcare Executives. Copyright 1992 by Health Administration Press. Adapted by permission.

tremendously from a high level of nursing care integration, that is, care provided by a single person. In contrast, the patient with multiple and complex care requirements may benefit from the care of several specialists.

Based on nursing resources, it is also possible for a unit to consider whether it is appropriate to move toward greater CMI, a different level of CMC, or a different type of intershift coordination. In summary, the elements of a nursing practice pattern can be prioritized in order of importance according to the availability and competence of the nursing resources.

A great advantage in using this approach is the opportunity to look for the weak and strong points in organizational support. For example, it is difficult to have high levels of CMC when nurse staffing or scheduling systems provide a constant rotation of the nursing staff within a hospital. Scheduling and staffing policy are intricately related to nursing practice pattern decisions.

Table 19.3 Elements of Nursing Practice Patterns

Variable	Abbreviation	Basis for Variable Definition
Nursing care integration	NCI	The proportion of total care given by the person providing the most care
Care management integration	CMI	The number of persons managing the care process at a given time
Plan-do integration	PDI	The proportion of caregivers also involved in the planning of care
Nursing care continuity	NCC	The average number of caregivers for a patient over a 7-day period
Care management continuity	CMC	The average number of care planners for a patient over a 7-day period
Care management continuity across settings (transfer)	CMCt	Whether a care planner is responsible for a patient before or after patient's stay on the unit
Nursing coordination	NC	An index that records the most common pattern of on-unit coordination of nursing care activities for a patient; method, level, and model of care delivery are indicated
Intershift coordination	ISC	An index that records the medium of communication by which intershift coordination is achieved; level and method are also indicated
Medical services coordination	MSC	Two indices that record the most common pattern of the nurse's direct involvement, and the proactiveness* of that involvement, in coordinating other inputs to the patient's care requirements from physicians (MSC) and from other professionals (PSC); the level and medium for coordination are included
Patient services coordination	PSC	

*Proactive: taking the initiative in coordination activities; for example, contacting other personnel, making referrals, problem-solving. Reactive: not initiating; a passive or simply cooperative response to coordination initiatives from others. From Beckman, J. S., & Simms, L. M. (1992). *A guide to redesigning nursing practice patterns.* Ann Arbor, MI: Health Administration Press. Foundation of the American College of Healthcare Executives. Copyright 1992 by Health Administration Press. Adapted by permission.

The findings in the Michigan studies suggest a better way to look at practice patterns. The identification of the key elements of the nursing practice pattern lead to the development of data collection instruments specific to four variables: patient characteristics, work characteristics, nursing resources, and organizational support. The new study further demonstrates that this type of information can be quantified and displayed in a format that can be used to defend an existing pattern or a change to a new pattern. This research has had several implications. By providing an effective way to acquire a database, the nurse executive can better evaluate high-cost practice patterns, can select a particular component for concentrated study, or can more logically make comparisons across units. This study further suggests the need to view staff satisfaction and RN/LPN ratios as important aspects of nursing resources.

THE FLEXIBLE WORK GROUP

The flexible work group model is based on the idea of assembling a patient care team according to the needs of patients. In this model, the housekeeper is a member of the work group. The patient and family members may also be members of the work group. The model combines the best of functional, team, and primary or case management ideas and allows the creation of work groups that can expand or decrease in size, depending on patients' needs. The flexible work group is defined as a patient-centered care team that is capable of responding or reforming when the nature of the work changes. Leadership is fluid and responsive to changing patient needs.

Reforming is a process of continuing engagement and disengagement in flexible work group patterns that facilitate the most favorable pattern of care for the patient. As the patient is regarded as an integral member of the work group as well as the focus or purpose of the work group's existence, in a flexible model, direction and decision-making about required work may be a naturally occurring right of the patient or, for that matter, of any other member. Leadership is fluid or free in movement for action. It accrues from the best mix of a flexible team member's skills with the dominant needs of the patient with movement toward recovery or maintenance or promotion of health.

Where ill health is in irreversible progression, then a flexible work group team marries the location, the source, and the provision of care to the optimal comfort (physical, emotional, social, and spiritual) of the patient. The team's existence is validated only by the purpose for which it is formed. Central to that purpose is the planning of care in the realities of that purpose, the individual in need within the family, and all the constellation of variables in a particular lifespace (Idour, 1990).

The flexible work group may also reflect cultural diversity. Cultural diversity is an untapped resource in meeting client needs. To facilitate care planning, client culture can be matched with at least one work group member who is from the same culture (Henkle & Kennerly, 1990).

ENERGIZING RESPONSIBILITIES OF THE NURSE EXECUTIVE

If nursing productivity is low, several avenues of study may be needed to determine the reasons, so that corrective actions may be taken. If study shows that much of nurses' time is spent in nonnursing areas, administration must also determine if it would be cost effective to hire other categories of personnel to assume the nonnursing duties, thus decreasing the number of nurses, or to maintain a percentage of nonnursing tasks in each nurse's assignment. If all nonnursing tasks were taken away from nurses (i.e., if all of them could be identified), the need for nurses could conceivably be decreased by a sizable amount.

The nurse executive must weigh the need for professional judgment in nonnursing tasks and in relating them to patient care. Many categories of nonnurses can be trained to perform tasks, but only the professional nurse has the knowledge and experience to put the nonnursing tasks into the context of total patient care. Instead of being concerned with giving away tasks, the nurse executive may explore ways of eliminating tasks, spreading them more equitably across the nursing staff, or assigning them to personnel under the control of nursing.

The central objective of nursing administration is to maximize the use of human resources toward the achievement of maximum production. There is no automatic way to enhance worker motivation, the key factor influencing productivity and quality of performance. If nurse executives are to energize and create motivating environments, they must understand motivation theories as discussed earlier in this chapter.

There is no such thing as an unmotivated person. All people are motivated. It is a challenge for nurse executives to speculate about why people behave as they do. Goals are accomplished through people and by people. Roles and positions do not interact; people interact, and they do so within their perceptual fields.

The work of nursing is accomplished through the human element. As nurses move up the administrative ladder, there is less need to function at the technical level, but the administrator must never lose sight of the technical demands that must be met. Current nursing practice is highly technical, in keeping with modern times. Although the human body has not changed, the nature of treatments has changed as society has become increasingly computerized and mechanized.

Job enrichment can increase the potential for work satisfaction and help administrators attract and keep a high-quality nursing staff. Although job enrichment can be viewed as part of the energizing function, it must be remembered that not all nurses want enriched jobs: jobs that are high in skill variety, task identity, task significance, autonomy, and feedback. At different times and in different years, individual nurses vary in growth needs and in their interest in their jobs.

In their pioneering research, Hackman and Oldham (1975) identified five core job dimensions that could contribute to job satisfaction in nursing. These are useful for the nurse executive in identifying jobs that have low motivating potential:

1. Skill variety: the degree to which job challenges the individual
2. Task identity: the degree to which the task provides for the completion of a job
3. Task significance: the degree to which the job has an impact on the lives of others
4. Autonomy: the degree to which the job gives the nurse freedom to act independently and use personal discretion

5. Feedback: the degree to which the job provides the nurse with information on job performance

In more recent research, Erbin-Roesemann and Simms (1997) advanced the concept of work excitement as a separate concept, differing from job satisfaction. Their research confirmed the significance of work locus of control, work arrangements, unit culture, and opportunities for learning at work in creating empowering environments.

Sorrentino, Nalli, and Schriesheim (1992) examined the effect of head nurse (unit nurse executive) behaviors on job satisfaction and performance among staff nurses. Using a sample of 103 RNs, the results show significant correlations between unit head nurse behavior and job satisfaction and performance. The findings also suggest the importance of unit nurse executive responsibility in moderating the effects of job anxiety, unit size, and support. Head nurse direction without support had a negative impact on performance.

To energize one's staff is to know what those employees do, not to be expert in their jobs, but to know and understand their work. The executive should walk around the health care setting and stop and observe what individual nurses and patients are doing. This practice conveys to the employee not only that he or she has worth as an individual but also that the particular job or position has worth. This practice also serves as a tracking method for identifying points at which work can be changed. Recognition of the human element is of utmost importance in energizing the division of nursing staff.

Technical and Professional Roles

Does it matter whether technical and professional roles are clarified? Yes, it does matter, not because one role is better than the other, but because they are both important to the quality of patient care and nurses' work lives. Failure to use professional nurses according to their education and expertise is the first great evil in the health care world. Expecting too much of technically prepared nurses is the second greatest malady. There is no nursing shortage today, just a shortage in our thinking about utilization of nursing resources.

SUMMARY

The nurse executive should support the competency of nurses by building on the educational preparation appropriate for their roles and by using practice patterns selected through data-based decisions. Such an approach to using nursing resources differs from that found in traditional nursing texts. The availability of nursing personnel, coupled with organizational and patient characteristics, should dictate nursing practice patterns. Selection of any model without considering these variables is usually a contributing factor in dissatisfaction and high nurse turnover. This chapter has examined the concepts of human potential and motivation as important components of mobilizing nursing resources. Inner-directed individuals are essential for high-performing teams and a productive work force.

STUDY QUESTIONS

1. Define human potential and discuss its relationship to high-performing work teams.
2. What are the symptoms of low productivity?
3. Trace the history of motivation studies starting with the work of Maslow and ending with current theorists such as Senge and Vaill.
4. Describe the factors that influence motivation and describe how motivation theories can be used by nurse executives to energize work groups.
5. The practice pattern redesign model in this chapter is a participatory model that includes all members of the health team. How do you see this model operationalized in your work/clinical setting?
6. Financial status is routinely monitored in organizations today. To what extent would you see outcomes monitored in the same manner?
7. Discuss the implications of differentiating the roles and performance expectations for professional and technical nurses.
8. Anticipating work redesign in your area of practice, identify five tasks that could be performed in a different way and with fewer people. What knowledge skills and equipment are important in your selection?

REFERENCES

Adams, J. D. (1998). *Transforming work* (2nd ed.). Alexandria, VA: Miles River Press.

Aiken, L. H. (1995). Transformation of the nursing workforce. *Nursing Outlook, 43*(5), 201–209.

American Nurses Association. (1996). *ANA position statement on restructuring, work redesign and the job and career security of registered nurses.* Washington DC: American Nurses Publishing.

Beckman, J. S., & Simms, L. M. (1992). *A guide to redesigning nursing practice patterns.* Ann Arbor, MI: Health Administration Press.

Deci, E. L. (1975). *Intrinsic motivation.* New York: Plenum Press.

Drucker, P. F. (1991). The new productivity challenge. *Harvard Business Review, 69*(6), 69–79.

Drucker, P. F. (1992). The new society of organizations. *Harvard Business Review, 70*(5), 95–104.

Erbin-Roesemann, M. A., & Simms, L. M. (1997). Work locus of control: The intrinsic factor behind empowerment and work excitement. *Nursing Economic$, 15*(4), 183–190.

Goertzen, I. E. (1991). *Differentiating nursing practice into the twenty-first century.* Washington, DC: American Academy of Nursing.

Hackman, J. R., & Oldham, G. R. (1975). Development of the job diagnostic survey, *Journal of Applied Psychology, 60*(2), 159–170.

Hammer, M., & Champy, J. (1993). *Reengineering the corporation.* New York: Harper Business.

Henkle, J. O., & Kennerly, S. M. (1990). Cultural diversity: A resource in planning and implementing nursing care. *Public Health Nursing, 7*(3), 145–149.

Herzberg, F., Mausner, B., & Snyderman, B. (1959). *The motivation to work.* New York: Wiley.

Idour, M. (1990). Personal communication from visiting scholar from Massey University, New Zealand.

Koch, R. W., & Esmon, D. (1998). Work redesign: Rethinking resource utilization. In S. A. Price, M. W. Koch & S. Bassett (Eds.), *Health care resource management.* St. Louis: Mosby.

Maslow, A. H. (1962). *Toward a psychology of being.* New York: Wiley.

McClelland, D. (1961). *The achieving society.* New York: Van Nostrand.

McClure, M. L. (1990) Introduction. In I. E. Goertzen (Ed.), *Differentiating nursing practice into the twenty-first century.* Washington, DC: American Academy of Nursing.

Munson, F. C., Beckman, J. S., Clinton, J., Kever, C., & Simms, L. M. (1980). *Nursing assignment patterns.* Ann Arbor, MI: Health Administration Press.

McClusky, H. Y. (1974). Education for aging: The scope of the field and perspectives for the future. In S. M. Grabowski & W. D. Mason (Eds.), *Education for the aging.* Syracuse, NY: ERIC Clearinghouse.

Noer, D. M. (1993). *Healing the wounds.* San Francisco: Jossey-Bass.

Pfoutz, S. K., Simms, L. M., & Price, S. A. (1987). Teaching and learning; Essential components of the nurse executive role. *Image, 19*(3), 138–141.

Robbins, S., & Coulter, M. (1996). *Management* (5th ed.). Englewood Cliffs, NJ: Prentice-Hall.

Senge, P. M. (1990). *The fifth discipline.* New York: Doubleday.

Simms, L. M. (1991). The professional practice of nursing administration: Integrated nursing practice, *Journal of Nursing Administration, 21*(5), 37–46.

Simms, L. M., & Erbin-Roesemann, M. A. (1992). Work characteristics questionnaire. In J. S. Beckman & L. M. Simms (Eds.), *A guide to redesigning nursing practice patterns* (Chap. IV). Ann Arbor, MI: Health Administration Press.

Skinner, B. F. (1953). *Science and human behavior.* New York: Macmillan.

Slack, W. V. (1997). *Cybermedicine.* San Francisco: Jossey-Bass.

Sorrentino, E. A., Nalli, A., & Schriesheim, C. (1992). The effect of head nurse behaviors on nurse job satisfaction and performance. *Hospital and Health Services Administration, 37*(1), 103–113.

State of Michigan Public Health Code. (1997). Article 15, Occupations Part 172, Nursing.

Vaill, P. B. (1982). The purposing of high performing systems. *Organizational Dynamics, 11*(2), 23–39.

CHAPTER

~ 20 ~

Mentorship and Networking

Catherine Buchanan

If you want one year of prosperity, grow grain.
If you want ten years of prosperity, grow trees.
If you want one hundred years of prosperity, grow people.

(Ancient Chinese Proverb)

Chapter Highlights

- The role of mentors and sponsors
- What is a mentor?
- Mentors and mentor relationships
- Barriers for career advancement for women
- Benefits of mentoring for the mentor and the protégé
- Becoming a mentor

Nurse executives now recognize mentors and networking in the development of a successful career. This is particularly true of nurses who occupy middle management positions in health care organizations. A powerful and influential person within an organization acting as a mentor or sponsor can make a crucial difference in providing visibility, credibility, and acceptance. The purpose of this chapter is to present the nature, characteristics, and consequences of mentorship and networking and their application to nursing administrative practice. Both male and female nurses will benefit from this discussion.

In their study of nurse executives Price, Simms, and Pfoutz (1987) substantiated the presence of influential persons in the professional and personal lives of their respondents. The value of role modeling, teaching, and encouragement surfaced as descriptions of career advancement assistance. Vance (1997) stresses that the sustained involvement of support persons, such as mentors, in the life and career path of every human being is a necessity.

THE ROLE OF MENTORS AND SPONSORS

Mentorship has received increased attention as an important element in career development. It has been especially popularized in business literature as the means to a successful climb up the corporate ladder (Cook, 1980; Hennig & Jardim, 1977a; Kanter, 1977; Levinson et al., 1978; Lundig, Clements, & Perkins, 1978; Roche, 1979; Shapiro, Haseltine, & Row, 1978; Warihay, 1980). Men, women are told, hold the key to success in their chosen occupations and professions because they are competitive, politically wise, and help each other via the "old boy's network." Further, if women are to succeed, they must be socialized into this network. This "tuning-in" process for both men and women is accomplished with the assistance of mentors, or sponsors.

Researchers interested in organizational behavior have identified the mentor phenomenon. The distinguishing function of the mentor is to access power and influence for the protégé. Kanter (1977) describes an informal pattern of selection observed in her study of a complex business organization. Individuals in the fast lane were affiliated with sponsors who served as influential and powerful conduits for their protégés. Men and women who moved up without sponsorship were often stalled at some point in their career and denied admission to the inner circles of upwardly mobile elites. Sponsors not only prepare their protégés for upward mobility but also influence how they are received by those in higher echelons.

What Is a Mentor?

The term "sponsor" reached popularity in the 1960s and early 1970s. Today, the commonly accepted term is "mentor." "Sponsor," "mentor," and "role model" are often used interchangeably, but most would agree that mentoring is reserved for a relationship that is more special, intense, and enduring than that implied by modeling (Levinson et al., 1978).

It has been suggested that role modeling is not effective in helping acquire reputations of influence and power. The strategies used by those who have achieved success may not be relevant to succeeding generations. Searching for the role model who encompasses all the attributes associated with success is discouraged. Instead, a combination of models may be more appropriate. This provides novices an opportunity to choose the traits they wish to emulate while rejecting others.

A patron system that embraces a continuum of support is proposed by Shapiro, Haseltine, and Rowe (1978). Mentor and peer pals are the two end points, with sponsor and guide as internal positions on the continuum. Mentor is the most intense and paternalistic relationship on the continuum. Social selection, ascription, and trust are characteristics of this relationship. Next is the sponsor relationship, defined as supportive but not powerful in terms of career advancement. This relationship tends to be encouraging, corroborating, and confidence building in nature. Guides, the next position on the continuum, function to steer individuals. They often provide helpful information about the system, pitfalls to avoid, and standard norms of behavior. Guides are usually administrative assistants or executive secretaries. They also function as gatekeepers who control access to the elite in an organization. Last on the continuum is the relationship between peers: peer pals. Peers share information of mutual interest, serve as a sounding board for one another, support one another, and generally develop relationships that help one another grow, progress, and succeed in career endeavors (Figure 20.1).

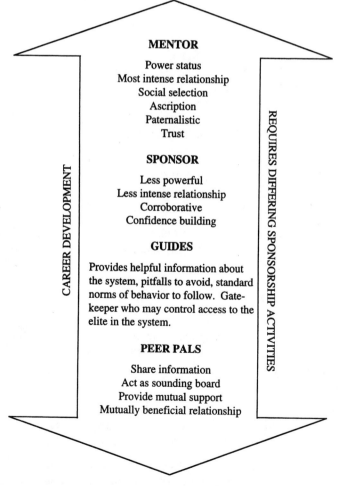

Figure 20.1 Continuum of career development support.

Dalton, Thompson, and Price (1977) advance a model of career organization consisting of four stages: apprentice, colleague, mentor, and sponsor. The apprentice stage is a dependent relationship that involves learning experiences. The collegial stage supports independence. The mentor is involved in helping the apprentice. The sponsor is an individual involved in the direction of an organization through policy formulation and the promotion of key people.

Yoder's (1990) concept analysis of mentoring reveals a more traditional version that she based on Bowen's (1985) definition:

> Mentoring occurs when a senior person (the mentor) in terms of age and experience undertakes to provide information, advice and emotional support for a junior person (the protege) in a relationship lasting over an extended period of time and marked by substantial emotional commitment by both parties. If the opportunity presents itself, the mentor also uses both formal and informal forms of influence to further the career of the protege. (Yoder, 1990, p. 31)

According to Yoder (1990), role modeling, sponsorship, precepting, peer strategizing, as well as being one's own mentor should not be used interchangeably with the mentoring process. The emphasis in this analysis focused on the intensity of the relationship, psychosocial and personal commitment to the relationship by both parties, and the protracted period of time both persons are loyal to the process as being the hallmark of the concept of mentorship.

Characteristics of Mentors and Mentor Relationships

Typically, mentors are highly placed in an organization. They are usually associated with the most powerful and influential people. Frequently they are men, simply because women are not in the higher management echelons in most organizations. Sometimes a mentor has more than one protégé within the organization.

Levinson et al. (1978) describes the relationship between mentor and protégé as a love relationship, intense, not sexual. It often occurs naturally and spontaneously. The experience is described as similar to falling in love in that it cannot be arranged or mandated. Many protégés describe their mentors as father figures, wise, loyal, trustworthy, and protective.

A comparison can be made between mentoring and Erickson's (1963) generativity stage of development. Human beings reach a stage in their development that requires them to give others the benefit of their life's experiences. It is the process of passing from one generation to another the values, standards, and norms of the former generation.

Ideally, a similar process occurs between mentor and protégé. Mentor passes to protégé values and standards that maintain continuity and stability of leadership within the organization. The mentor prepares the next generation of leaders.

Blackburn, Chapman, and Cameron (1981) describe this grooming process as cloning. The mentor fashions the protégé in his or her own image and likeness.

This style of grooming occurs in the preparation of scientists. The novice scientists mimics the master in ways that benefit the continuity of scientific excellence. It is often through the eminence of the mentor that the work of the protégé is recognized.

Zuckerman's (1977) study of the Nobel laureates provides evidence of the valuable link between bright young scientists and their eminent sponsors. The socialization of the next generation of prize winners is the unofficial domain of the laureates in science. It is understood that the work of science is passed from one generation to the next. It is accepted that a laureate will guide and promote the successful achievements of the next generation of Nobel prize winners.

Gray and Gray (1994) created a new mentoring paradigm based on the fact the old paradigm produced a happenstance approach to mentoring. The old paradigm has a cloning effect that falls short in preparing the protégé for the rapidly changing competitive world of today's business climate. The new mentoring model encourages the protégé's diversity, creativity, ideas, and initiative. These characteristics are used through the authority of the mentor to empower the protégé. Today's protégé comes to the workplace better educated and with varied life and work experiences.

Gray's Mentor-Protégé Relationship Model has four mentoring styles based on today's protégé's needs to be equipped and empowered. Mentors can use these four styles flexibly. The four mentoring styles are:

Style 1: Informational Mentoring Style
- Mentor uses one-way communication to impart information to protégé.

Style 2: Guiding Mentoring Style
- Mentor guides a two-way communication with protégé

Style 3: Collaborative Mentoring Style
- Mentor and protégé mutually exchange ideas with no one dominating.

Style 4: Confirming Mentoring Style
- Mentor acknowledges and confirms feelings and ideas expressed by protégé.

Goal = Successful Protégé
- Protégé becomes consciously competent—aware of what to do and can do it (Figure 20.2).

In addition, use of this model requires training in which the mentor-protégé partners are carefully selected, matched, and trained to facilitate the development of a good relationship. This relationship depends on commitment instead of "special chemistry." Gray's model requires recognition by an organization that mentor-protégé pairing is beneficial in the recruitment and retention of the next generation of leaders.

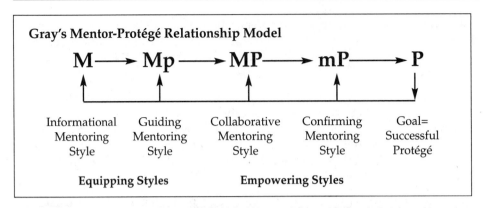

Figure 20.2 Gray's Mentor-Protégé Relationship Model. From Gray, W. A., & Gray, M. M. (1994). *Developing mentor-protégé relationships: A mentor-protégé workbook* (p. 5). Sidney, British Columbia, Canada: The Mentoring Institute. Copyright 1994 by the Mentoring Institute. Reprinted with permission.

BARRIERS FOR CAREER ADVANCEMENT FOR WOMEN

Without question, women entering fields and professions that are traditionally male dominated are encouraged to enter under the aegis of a mentor. Wynter and Soloman (1989) coined the barrier preventing women from moving up the career ladder to top level executive positions as the "glass ceiling." This subtle barrier often stalls women in middle management positions. They are able to view the next level but are unable to break the glass ceiling in order to advance their career.

Lubin (1996) reports on a study done by Catalyst, a nonprofit research group in New York, who recently surveyed 461 senior female managers and 325 male chief executives at the largest companies in the United States. The focus of the study was to look at women above the glass ceiling. Although 44% of the managerial women polled report to the chief executive officer (CEO) or an executive just one level below, more than 60% are in staff support positions such as in human resources and public relations. There were differences in the perceptions of managerial women and their bosses over the extent of women's recent progress. Approximately half the CEOs reported that during the past 5 years opportunities for women to advance to senior leadership in their companies have "greatly improved," compared with only 23% of the female executives. The majority of the women surveyed blamed male stereotyping of women and women's exclusion from informal communication networks, whereas CEOs predominantly cited women's lack of line or general management experience and their scarcity in the executive pipeline. Carole St. Mark stated that the more young women "get experience in line jobs early in their careers, the better the pipeline will be—and the greater the percentage that will get to the top."

The female executives polled by Catalyst often were the first of their gender to reach senior management. They attributed their breakthroughs to consistently exceeding performance expectations. These women stated they outperformed male colleagues by toiling long workdays that stretched from reading reports at 4 AM through business meetings at night. It is interesting to note that few female senior managers stated their advancement resulted from having influential mentors or from corporate strategies designed to assist women, such as affirmative action policies and flexible work hours. The findings suggest that despite women's progress up the management ladder, female chief executives will remain rare in corporate America for years to come.

Women need mentors at two crucial points in their lives: during the early stages of career development and during the final thrust to the top (Holcomb, 1980). The majority of nurses who remain at the practice level and work in hospitals need different sponsorship activities. These nurses need ongoing access to career guidance and informal informational counseling about the hospital system (Campbell-Heider, 1986).

Studies of women in top level management positions indicate that they had help from a mentor, usually a male boss (Hennig & Jardim, 1977b). In contrast, women who failed to establish upwardly mobile career patterns were without sponsors and other support relationships (Kanter, 1977). There are, however, some important considerations for women who engage in mentor-protégé relationships with men.

Cross-gender mentoring—as exists between a male mentor and a female protégé—is discouraged by some authorities (Levinson et al., 1978). Stereotyping is cited as one barrier that influences the relationship negatively. It is believed that commonly held attitudes about women may interfere with the effectiveness of the mentor: "she is bright but not committed," "she is too pretty to be committed to a career," "she will get married, get pregnant, and leave."

Another barrier involves the perception of peers and colleagues. Men and women fear being linked to illicit relationships in the workplace. Mentor-protégé affiliations can fall victim to the faulty perceptions of others, resulting in severe damage to reputation and careers. Organizations can remedy this potential threat by a willingness to recognize the mentor-protégé relationship as a positive and sound force in the preparation of leadership skills. This in turn is beneficial to the organization. Generation continuity and homogeneity of leadership is the prized objective of most organizations (Darling, 1985a; Lundig, Clements, & Perkins, 1970).

The final barrier in cross-gender mentoring is the fear of the mentor-marital triad. The intensity of the relationship can be disruptive when marital partners are not clear about the intent and purpose of the protégé's relationship to the mentor. Working late, an occasional trip out of town, and the importance of the mentor in the professional life of the protégé are all potential problems in the triad.

It is by virtue of its intensity and focus that the mentor-protégé affiliation is the best method for grooming future leaders; by its very nature, mentoring can be both valued and feared. Unless mentoring, especially cross-gender mentoring, is a legitimate structure within an organization, both men and women are reluctant to risk its hazards. Despite the risks, however, cross-gender mentoring has been successful. Women have reported enormous benefit from their work with male mentors (Cameron & Blackburn, 1981; Hennig & Jardim, 1977b).

Murray et al. (1998) interviewed 45 nurse executives in urban and rural locales in the United States. A major objective of the study was to assess the perceptions of influential colleagues, other than the current employer, regarding the leadership roles of the nurse executives with whom they had previously worked. The typical influential colleague identified by most of the nurse executives was a married man with a master's degree in hospital or business administration who had extensive administrative experience. The authors' state that "influential colleagues who are in position to define NEs [nurse executives] roles, mentor them, give them greater support for personal achievement, and otherwise support NEs in their leadership responsibilities can play a major role in helping them to become more effective leaders" (p. 23). These colleagues can create opportunities for nurse executives that will involve them in key decision-making and suggest ways to improve their skills.

Vance (1997) implies that to be successful as mentors and protégés, various qualities are required. A good leader-mentor should be:

- Generous with his or her time and energy—mentoring is going above and beyond the usual commitment.
- Self-confident—members cannot be oppressed and self-absorbed.
- A wise expert—competency and experience provide security in sharing one's knowledge.
- Open to mutual growth—mentors must be respectful of their own and others' need for lifelong learning and development (p. 207).

MENTORING NURSES

The barriers and attitudes concerning the role of women in the workplace are concentrated in nursing. In addition to overcoming the barriers created by cross-gender mentoring already mentioned, nurses must overcome the stereotype attributed to their profession. The attitude that nurses should be content with traditional nursing roles and leave the task of comprehensive health and fiscal planning and management to those best suited—namely, hospital administrators and physicians—is a major barrier. This perception, commonly held by men in health care management, is often shared by nurses (Puetz, 1983).

Another common attitude is that nurses are educated to provide service. They are not expected to provide meaningful management direction for an institution. The nursing profession itself is ambivalent about nurse executive roles in health care organizations. This ambivalence is manifested by confusion about the best arrangement of clinical and management components in graduate programs preparing nurse executives. Nursing staff in health care settings are not supportive of nurse executives who cannot demonstrate clinical practice skills, but they also expect the executive to possess the necessary skills to access power and credibility in the higher echelons of management within the institution.

These attitudes constitute a barrier that thwarts the desire and progress of the nurse executive who is capable of assuming greater responsibility and career diversity. Although same-gender mentoring is advocated for both men and women and would seem to alleviate the problems and attitudes inherent in cross-gender mentor-protégé relationships, the dilemma posed by the employment of too few women in the upper echelons of management is a reality. Women, and especially nurses, are often stalled in middle-management positions because they lack visibility and opportunities for the men who are in power to see them behave effectively.

WOMEN MENTORING WOMEN

Women often are not supportive of each other's efforts in the workplace. Darling (1985b) refers to any negative mentor relationship as toxic. She categorizes these toxic mentor behaviors as avoiders, dumpers, and destroyer/criticizers. Antidotes to a toxic situation include identifying the nature and source of the relationship as well as any past unrelated experiences that are being attributed to the situation, understanding the mentor's current situation and needs so that exceptions can be applied, and finally balancing the relationship with other support networks if getting out of the relationship is not an option.

Most mentor-mentee rifts occur when the mentor has a position of authority over the mentee (Darling, 1985c). Conversely, this similar configuration in the relationship is necessary to promote the credibility and visibility of the one being mentored.

Research has shown that there is another side to the issue of women supporting each other. Warihay (1980) has found that the support giver and the support receiver have different perceptions of the amount of support given. Those in the upper echelons always report giving more than their junior colleagues report receiving. Such perceptions are troublesome, especially in situations in which there are few women at the top levels of management and many in the lower echelons. These perceptions inhibit women in top management from facilitating the career development of other women.

How men in nursing are affected by cross-gender and same-gender mentor-protégé affiliations is not precisely known. There is a paucity of data addressing the issue of male nursing careers and their mentorship experiences. Until the number of men in nursing increases substantially, nursing will continue to be identified as a profession of women. It is important to assume, however, that men in nursing administration are confronted with similar obstacles with respect to cross-gender mentor-protégé relationships. Same-gender mentor-protégé affiliations may be more favorable for the career promotion of men in nursing management, given the tendency of men in senior management ranks to support their junior counterparts.

BENEFITS OF MENTORING FOR THE MENTOR AND THE PROTÉGÉ

Benefits for the protégé include recognition, encouragement, and an opportunity to establish a confidential sounding board. Increased morale and productivity are often related benefits. Honest criticism, informal feedback, nonjudgmental guidance, and an insistence by the mentor that the only performance is the best performance are vital to leadership growth. Knowing that one is being groomed for leadership by a recognized mentor is an experience that has no equal. The nurse executive who demonstrates a power stance beyond his or her expected role needs the support and direction of a recognized mentor who can smooth the way and access power and influence. The nurse executive's credibility and reputation require facilitation by another who is accepted and respected within the organization.

Benefits for the mentor include an opportunity to pass on one's values and standards, increasing the satisfaction that comes from helping another develop the attributes of leadership. The potential to discover oneself by helping others is not a new or different idea. The relationship can help the mentor fulfill professional responsibilities as a supervisor who is interested in those in the lower ranks. It also provides the mentor-manager a support system for policies and activities affecting people in the lower ranks of the organization with whom the protégé may have daily contact. Within the context of nursing administration, there exists for the mentor a nurse executive protégé who can execute a smoother, more cooperative management triad among nursing and support staff, nursing management, and agency administration. The perceived dichotomy between administration and service, which tends to polarize administrators and practitioners, can be ameliorated through the joint efforts of the mentor and the protégé. Such depolarization, in turn, benefits the organization.

CHOOSING MENTORSHIP

It is advisable for upwardly mobile men and women to seek a mentor. Several may be needed at various junctures in a career to serve as information conduits, provide support, and assist in developing leadership behaviors. The following questions and statements are intended to assist the nurse executive in assessing his or her need and desire for sponsorship in career development (Hall & Sandler, 1983). The questions can be altered to adapt to a particular institution or management level. They are not intended to be comprehensive; rather, their purpose is to stimulate a career-planning mode of thought:

1. What circumstances and situations within your organization are best suited for increasing your visibility?
2. What attitudes and behaviors are rewarded by your supervisors in your organization?
3. What are the organization's formal and informal criteria for promotion and salary adjustment beyond the nursing director level of management?
4. Who are the decision-makers involved in your advancement in the organization?

5. Who speaks for you at board meetings and policy planning sessions when you are not invited or are unable to attend?
6. Who can nominate you for promotions, prizes, awards, or important committee assignments or simply indicate you are the best person to get a certain job done?
7. Who defends you when ideas and people come together in conflicting patterns? Who makes certain you are heard even when you voice unpopular or controversial ideas (someone to steady the boat you have just rocked)?
8. How is "inside information" disseminated, policy created, approval for successful change projects achieved, and important decisions regarding staffing, budget, salary, and so on made?
9. Who are the powerful and important people in your organization and who has their ear?
10. Does your organization's structure support the role changes and extensions with respect to nurses and other professionals?

Being able to answer these questions in some detail provides the framework for a decision with respect to one's need for a mentor.

CHOOSING A MENTOR

Selecting a mentor can be a challenge. One should begin by determining career needs and goals. The following characteristics can assist in determining the quality of your mentor choices:

- Good leadership skills
- A professional demeanor
- A track record of advancement
- The ability to empower those around her or him
- Respect peers
- Patience
- Motivation to teach and guide others
- A well developed network of professional contacts
- Excellent problem solving skills
- The ability to inspire others
- A realistic vision of nursing (Laino-Curran, 1995, pp. 78–79)

The list of characteristics should signal that the person possessing these attributes is in demand and has time constraints. However, a good mentor will have time to meet and discuss career goals and progression, conflicts and obstacles in the professional life of the protégé. In turn, with advice is the responsibility to listen and bear the discomfort inherent in career growth activities, relationships and decisions.

It is equally important for the protégé to keep the mentor informed. Providing the mentor with invitations to professional activities in which the protégé has participated or has received accolades are important ways to stay in touch. Being a part of a protégé's professional life gives a mentor that special link "that unbroken line of leadership, of mentor-protégé, that extends into the future" (Kelly, 1987, p. 59).

BECOMING A MENTOR

In deciding whether to become a mentor, one must consider what one can offer a protégé. Equally important is a consideration of the benefits one can derive from a mentoring relationship. What one can offer a protégé has a great deal to do with the allocation of one's time and energy.

The mentor may begin by providing the protégé visibility at meetings, business luncheons, and preparation and feedback sessions in conjunction with presentations and projects initiated by the protégé. Many men and women appreciate a mentor's assistance with appropriate dress, hairstyle, and body language. The management of career, marriage, and childbearing is a crucial area of conflict for women, and learning to juggle these competing responsibilities necessitates a support system, preferably from those with similar experiences. A mentor could provide knowledgeable assistance with such problems. Thus, mentoring is lending one's personal help to a talented person. Ultimately, the mentor must be willing to put his or her reputation on the line for the protégé's sake (Moore, 1982). J. D. Watson remarked, from the perspective of a young scientist, "It is extraordinarily important that you have a . . . patron because there'll be times when you are bound to strike it bad and you'll need somebody to convince people that you are not irresponsible" (Zuckerman, 1977, pp. 134–135).

The critical shortage of qualified, competent professional nurse managers in the higher echelons of health care administration suggests the need for the early identification of leadership talent and the sponsorship of the talent by other talented and respected nurses. In this era of rapidly changing health care demands, nurses must be trained to assume leadership roles. The time required to prepare competent leadership must be shortened and addressed as a professional responsibility. The talents of our current leaders must not be lost.

Dunham-Taylor, Fisher, and Kinion (1993) surveyed 85 hospital nurse executives as to whether there were particular experiences, events or persons that influenced their leadership style. These executives were identified by colleagues as "excellent" leaders. Only 17 stated that no experience, event, or person had influenced their leadership style and that their leadership abilities were inherent. All others described experiences, events, and persons that did influence their leadership style. One-third of the nurse executives stated they had a mentor, often more than one. They were the executive's superiors, directors of vice presidents of nursing chief operating officers, CEOs, or professors in graduate school. These persons recognized "diamonds in the rough" and assisted executives' development by delegating the work to them and then critiquing the work, teaching management techniques or ways to view the political scene realistically, and giving them opportunities. These executives were sometimes promoted to higher positions. These mentors reinforced that the nurse executives were good individuals who had a great deal to offer, could excel in their chosen field, and had leadership potential.

MENTORING ATTITUDES AND BEHAVIOR

Mentors must reconcile the differing perceptions inherent in the roles of mentor and protégé by making explicit the extent to which they can and will offer guidance concerning personal and professional issues. Some authorities suggest that the signing of a contract by both parties in agreement to the terms of the mentorship relationship ensures clarity of purpose and direction (Hart, 1980). Whether the relationship is formal or informal, it is important to know its parameters and constraints ahead of time.

The mentor must provide feedback to the protégé as a function of the mentorship relationship. Such feedback should be framed in an objective context that presents praise and criticism as specifically as possible. The mentor should be prepared to stand by the protégé. The professional stature of the fledgling leader must be protected. At times, the mentor may give the protégé an added degree of credibility and growth advantage by letting others know the protégé speaks for the mentor. For example, the protégé can replace the mentor's contributions at meetings, presentations, and conferences.

Fagan and Fagan (1983) in their research discovered a strong link between job satisfaction and mentoring. They recommended that nurse executives encourage both informal mentoring and formal mentor programs to improve professional development within their organization.

As much as possible, the nurse executive-mentor should include other nurses in both professional and informal activities. Inviting a novice manager to a luncheon session with senior management people is an effective way to advertise the mentor's investment in the protégé. Mentoring need only consist of informing a junior colleague of available resources and being willing to support his or her professional endeavors. This support may consist of advice about job advancement, strategies, or an opportunity to rehearse the presentation of a project to a group of influential leaders in the organization.

The mentor must socialize the protégé into a competitive environment. Female nurses, like many women, are not prepared for this dimension of the workplace. In a sense, nurses are similar to the Nobel laureate who described his need for a sponsor to compete in the institution of science: "I knew the technique . . . I had a lot of knowledge. I had the words, the libretto, but not the music. What was missing was an opportunity to work with men of high quality" (Zuckerman, 1977, p. 123).

Nurses are firmly grounded in their knowledge of nursing care, but they are not equally schooled in the effective discharge of this function in a competitive environment. To establish successful career patterns, nurse executives need to increase their sphere of influence, project credibility, be accepted as important contributors to the policy formulation of their institutions, and be treated as equals with other influential people in the system. Career advances in an organization require the socializing influence of a sponsor. The central purpose of mentoring is to provide the protégé with a competitive advantage so that ability can be transformed into effective leadership skills. For some, mentoring may not be possible, advantageous, or desirable. Whatever the nature of the support, however, we will need someone with whom we can share our hopes and career aspirations, a person who will promote our ideas and our best work and place us in a competitive sphere in which we can prove our abilities and worth. Mentors are in a real sense a necessary ingredient of self-actualization in the workplace. Maestro and pianist, master and artist, and rabbi and student have been paired throughout history so that the very best could give to the best in an effort to preserve the continuity of excellence. Although mentors are not a substitute for competence, commitment, ability, and hard work, these things alone, unfortunately, do not bring the success and reputation that women and men of ability deserve in the workplace.

Holloran's (1993) study investigated mentoring and what is known about its prevalence and application in the nursing service setting. The study sample consisted of 274 female nurse executives from medical center teaching hospitals in the United States. Mentor was defined as a more experienced career role model who guides, coaches, and advises the less seasoned person. "A primary mentor is a person who embodies those qualities of the mentor combined with an intense commitment and a strong belief in the potential strengths and talents of the protégé. A secondary mentor is the 'role model' or 'preceptor' who embodies the qualities of the mentor without demonstrating the emotional intensity and strong beliefs found in the primary mentor." The survey instrument, Mentoring in Nursing Service: A Survey of Nursing Service Executives, consisted of 28 forced-choice questions and four critical incident questions.

The majority of the nurse executives (71%) indicated they had had a mentor, only less than a third (29%) stated they had not. They did not have a mentor because "no one with expertise was available to serve as a mentor" and even though individuals with the talent and qualifications to be mentors existed, the mentor relationship did not develop. Eighty-eight percent of the respondents indicated that their most significant mentor was a primary mentor and that they felt a moderately high or high degree of commitment and belief from their mentor. Only 42% of the nurse executives stated that their most significant mentor was a secondary mentor, and they felt a moderately high degree of commitment and belief from their mentor. This finding reflects a difference in the levels of mentoring with regard to the degree of commitment perceived by the protégé. If a protégé perceives that the mentor has a commitment to or an investment in the relationship, it implies a deeper level to the relationship. The respondents were requested to comment on the importance of their most significant mentor to career development and career advancement. The executives indicated of the two purposes, the

mentor relationship was the most important for the protégé's career development. There were differences between those nurses who had had a mentor versus
those who had not. In the behavioral clusters beneficial for career advancement,
the two groups agree on only one cluster: encouragement and recognition of potential. This finding supports the idea that if one has never been a protégé, one
will not be a mentor. For example, if one has not experienced mentoring, then
one can only imagine what happens and what is beneficial. This also confirms
that ideas about mentoring from one who has not had a mentor do not coincide
with the perception of those who have one.

Two dominant themes merged from the critical incidents where the nurse executives described two interactions with the most significant mentor. These were:
what occurs when mentoring does work, referred to as the power of belief, and
what happens when mentoring does not work, or the power of control. The mentor fostering growth through encouragement and recognition of the protégé illustrated the power of belief. This infused the protégé with the confidence and inspiration drawn from the sense that, if this more experienced, successful person
believes in the protégé, then she must be worth the investment. The power of
control smothered the creative aspects of the mentor-protégé relationship
through the mentor's overpossessive behavior toward the protégé, rejection of
the protégé, and misuse of power. The themes most frequently presented by the
respondents for the power of belief and power of control follow.

Power of Belief

- Encouragement and recognition of potential. The most common theme was
  the significant positive influence the mentor had in instilling confidence in
  the protégé that she could accomplish her goals.
- Opportunities and responsibilities. Once potential was recognized and encouraged, the next most common theme was the mentor provided opportunities to show what one can do, for example, to be given the responsibility
  of managing a large nursing department.
- Inspiration and being a role model. Most of the comments conveyed the
  genuine admiration and gratitude the nurse executives felt for their mentor.
  Respondents spoke of the influence of their mentors, which was deep, pervasive, and lifelong.
- Help with career moves. This theme illustrated ways in which mentors
  made dramatic gestures to promote their protégé.

Power of Control

- Overpossessive behavior toward the protégé. Some felt that their mentors
  were overbearing, promoted overdependence, and did not let the protégé
  make her own decisions.
- Rejection of the protégé. The protégé offered the mentor help in a personal
  matter and later the relationship was never the same. The protégé asked for

help and it was denied, and the protégé expected help in the form of a rec-
ommendation for a new position and it was denied.
- Misuse of power. The patterns that emerged were that the mentor asserted
  her will without apparent concern for others, and the mentor caused the
  protégé to feel used and transgressed the professional boundaries of deco-
  rum. (pp. 51–52)

This study supports the finding that mentoring is a developmental process that
assists with career development and career advancement goals of young professionals. Mentoring involves a process of teaching and learning with a heavy dose
of caring added through the process. Holloran emphasizes that nursing aspects
of mentoring played an insignificant part of the total experience of the nurse executives surveyed, but they must be acknowledged in an effort to promote them.
The respondents confirmed that mentoring is a professional helping relationship
whether there is an emotional investment in or commitment to the development
of the protégé. It is definitely not a casual relationship. Mentoring is an effective
means of preparing for leadership succession. Nurse managers as well as other
administrators should explore opportunities to recognize and develop younger
professional nurses in order to begin their development and advancement
process.

ACADEMIC NURSE ADMINISTRATORS

White (1988), Taylor (1992), and Madison (1994) investigated the presence of
mentor-protégé relationships in the career patterns of nurses in academe. The outcome was inconclusive in terms of research and publication assistance provided
by mentors as compared to productivity by nonmentored nurses. Very few of the
mentored nurses received collaborative or publication co-authoring, grant writing, or paper presentation assistance from their mentors. Instead, mentors were
cited for their esteem and confidence-building relationships with their protégés.

In Taylor's study, the majority of the respondents reported no publications were
generated during their protégé relationship with a mentor, and few reported one
publication while working with a mentor. However, there was a significant difference between the mentored and nonmentored groups in the number of publications. The mean number of publications for the mentored group was significantly greater than for the nonmentored group.

There is a paucity of data in the literature regarding the differential in age of the
protégé as older than the mentor. This variable is usually not addressed by the
investigator perhaps because the number of cohorts in the group is too small to
make inferences.

As more and more women and men change career direction in their lifetime, the
need for skilled assistance may call for a different model of mentor-protégé relationships. This is particularly apparent for women who enter nursing after they
have achieved early developmental goals. Self-esteem issues that are important

to the young fledgling also play an important role for the older career-bound adult who may need assistance at various career stages. Taylor (1992) alluded to the assigned mentor model. The group of nurses in academe reporting this experience was relatively small as compared to the process where they select their own mentor. This reflects a need to investigate the method of assignment and its impact on productivity and career progression.

The purpose of mentoring is achievement. The affiliative socialization needs inherent in women may be counter to the mentor-protégé selection based on "chemistry" in a female-dominated setting as academic nursing. Nurses in these investigations reviewed prized the affiliative needs provided by mentors rather than the achievement needs. Men tend to fare better because their career development issues are oriented toward achievement and results.

If nursing is to compete and earn a distinguished place in academe, methods of intellectual passage from one generation to another must be devised lest the accomplishments of today's nurse scientists will not be realized in the next generation.

THEORY OF NETWORKING

In addition to researching mentor affiliations as a strategy of promoting career advancement and opportunities, social scientists have investigated the phenomenon of networking. Data indicate that inclusion in a profession is associated with career success. A measurement of the degree of inclusion in one's profession is, in turn, associated with networking activities (Buchanan, 1984). Networking provides the visibility and means to disseminate one's ability, talents, and professional support to others. A network is the totality of all the units connected by a certain type of relationship and is constructed by finding the ties between all the members within a bounded system. Further, networks develop basically from two types of relationships: *(1)* family and close friends and *(2)* professional and other infrequent contacts.

The common networking bond between family and close friends is a similarity of beliefs, values, attitudes, and social origins. Support and information exchange characterize the bond between professionals and other social contacts. Family and close friends are strong ties that exert a substantial influence on the behavior of those in the network. Communication patterns tend to be predictable, uniform, and repetitive. Members of such networks are usually few and, thus, have limited access to a wide variety of information sources.

Professional and social contacts are considered weak ties. Relationships within such a network structure exercise less influence on the behavior of members than do strong ties. Because communication patterns are less predictable, more varied, and not repetitive, weak ties provide greater opportunity for the communication of original and expert information. This pattern of communication and its potential for unlimited sources of information is the rationale for the strength of weak ties in facilitating career progress. Thus, the weak-tie theory supports the notion that mobilizing a large weak-tie network enables one to gain access to individuals, groups, and systems for the purpose of achieving occupational, professional, personal, and social goals.

Men and Women and Networking Behavior

Kleiman (1980) considers networks "a step beyond role models and mentors, a necessary next step for women if they want to achieve their professional and career goals" (p. 6). Increasingly, women are turning to other women in an effort to gain professional visibility, exchange information, identify job opportunities, reduce isolationism for women in token positions, support one another in professional growth endeavors, and provide emotional reinforcement. However, networking is a relatively new experience for women. What men achieve quite naturally in their contacts and support of each other is not as commonplace for women.

Patricia Wyskocil observes that "men bond naturally and network instinctively" (Kleiman, 1980, p. 8). Josefowitz (1980) suggests that "just as men relax in a very special way when alone with their own sex group, women too have a special bonding that occurs when they are together without men" (p. 101). It is equally important for men and women to network together in a mixed-gender support group, according to Josefowitz.

The discomfort a woman may feel entering a male-dominated group is identical to that of a man entering an all-female group. However, an effort must be made by both men and women to gain admission to networks within their organizational workplace and professional systems. Not only is work-oriented gossip shared at network meetings—which occur over lunch, after work, or on weekends—but so is important inside information. Through networking, alliances are developed, connections made, and concerns aired. Although it may not be easy to gain entry to certain networks or to subdue feelings of discomfort as a new member in some groups, the nurse executive must seek access to the most influential networks in the health care organization.

Nurses, in particular, encounter difficulty moving out of their sphere of comfort. This is in part due to the traditional separation of the nurse and the physician socially and professionally within health care settings and the lack of assertiveness that continues to be part of the subservient role of traditional nursing service.

Particularly relevant to nurse executives is the contention of Warihay (1980) that in some organizations where few women enjoy the career benefits of upper management, developing a new women's network may be premature. The women in need of support may far outnumber those available to give it. In addition, limiting sources of support to women would tend to narrow career mobility. Thus, any man or woman in one's organization who will be an ally and is supportive of women and men and their achievement perspective warrants inclusion in a network.

Professional Networking

The importance of networking in achieving professional goals has been demonstrated in academe (Buchanan, 1984; Cameron & Blackburn, 1981). Data indicate that a linkage exists among career success, inclusion in one's profession, and networking activities. Successful nurse academicians report that involvement in professional networks is critical in establishing successful career patterns.

Nursing colleagues occupying prestigious positions as journal referees, publishers, grant reviewers, and officers of professional nursing organizations and groups are invaluable sources of professional support for the nurse academician. Networking among academicians is a time-honored institution. Crane (1972) calls such unstructured arrangements "invisible colleges." The dissemination of knowledge is the underlying purpose of such networks. Academicians network about their interests, projects, successes, and each other. These contacts form a valuable link among colleagues within the community of scholars.

Nurse executives must provide similar access to each other as well as senior and junior managers within the health care system. Puetz (1983) and O'Connor (1982) provide a comprehensive overview of the art of networking. They discuss attitudes, skills, and behaviors pertinent to the development of a network culture in nursing. These authors emphasize the necessity of supportive activity between professionals. Using the experience and understanding of others can reduce feelings of isolation and promote self-esteem when career progress is stalled or discouraged by others in an organization.

Networking requires a commitment based on professional competence, reliability, and credibility. O'Connor (1982) aptly points out that "networks provide suggestions, direction, guidance, and support, not solutions" (p. 40). Clarity and honesty based on what one can offer another or what one needs from others is vital to successful networking. In addition, incorporating cross-gender and varied professional representation in one's networking systems will greatly enhance and expand the likelihood of achieving professional goals.

Nurse executives have opportunities to network within their local, state, and national spheres of influence in nursing. This can be accomplished through professional organizations and groups or simply by making contact with others in the professional nurse and health care management community. One reason nurses are rarely invited to debate or report important health issues—as are physicians and other health care specialists—is that they lack professional networking skills. Nurses can also establish important weak ties across professions. For example, they can network with journalists concerning women's health issues, the problems of aging, or clarifying the media-imposed image of professional nursing.

When one needs the assistance and support of others, others often feel the same way. When individuals come together with mutual interests and concerns, a network is created. It is unnecessary to endure self-imposed isolation from peers and colleagues.

SUMMARY

Varying degrees of assistance are identified as positive forces in the development of a satisfying career. Mentorship is one aspect of the patron system of support that nurses are encouraged to adopt. Nurse executives are vulnerable to the barriers women in the workplace encounter as they attempt to move into the higher echelons of power and influence within health care organizations. Evidence supports the view that the assistance of a respected, influential person can be a critical factor in promoting successful career endeavors.

Some people mistakenly believe informal mentoring is superior to formally arranged mentoring. There is no proof that any one form is superior to the other. An intelligent view of both approaches is to concede that they are different for several very good reasons. As humans we need different approaches to mentoring (Gray & Gray, 1994).

Until greater numbers of nurses achieve positions of authority in health care organizations, they must support each other and recognize the need for cross-gender mentor-protégé affiliations. In addition to sponsorship, nurse in leadership positions contact their peers and colleagues through networks. There are data to support the link between networking, inclusion in a profession, and career satisfaction and success. The individual must determine the most effective support system for promoting his or her professional stature and achieving successful
career development.

STUDY QUESTIONS

1. Critically analyze the advantages and disadvantages of mentor-protégé relationships in a health care setting.
2. Develop a role description of the nurse executive as a mentor and as a protégé.
3. Identify various individuals within a health care setting who would be most appropriate to mentor a nurse executive.
4. Evaluate the mentoring strengths and weaknesses of each potential mentor identified in question 3.
5. What are the barriers for career advancement for women?
6. What is the nurse executive's role in creating and legitimating a positive environment for mentoring and networking?
7. Draw up a contract between mentor and protégé explicating the terms of the relationship and the responsibilities of each.
8. Critically evaluate the place of role modeling on the support continuum as it relates to the nurse executive.

9. Cite the paradoxical nature inherent in cross-gender mentor-protégé relationships.

10. Formulate a definition of mentoring applicable to the nurse executive's career advancement.

11. Explain the theory supporting the career advantage of participating in networks.

12. Describe how you as a nurse executive would implement Gray's Mentoring-Protégé Relationship Model. Specify the behaviors you would use in each of the four styles.

REFERENCES

Blackburn, R. T., Chapman, D. W., & Cameron, S. M. (1981). Cloning in academe. *Research in Higher Education, 15*(4), 315–327.

Bowen, D. (1985). Were men meant to mentor women? *Training and Developmental Journal, 39*(1), 30–34.

Buchanan, C. (1984). *An investigation and analysis of the prevalence and effects of sponsorship in the academic career development of nurses.* Unpublished doctoral dissertation, University of Michigan, Ann Arbor.

Cameron, S. M., & Blackburn, R. T. (1981). Sponsorship and academic career success. *Journal of Higher Education, 52*(4), 369–377.

Campbell-Heider, N. (1986). Do nurses need mentors? *Image, 18*(3), 110–113.

Cook, M. (1980). Is the mentor relationship primarily a male experience? *Personal Administrator, 24*(11), 82–84, 86.

Crane, D. (1972). *Invisible colleges.* Chicago: University of Chicago Press.

Dalton, G. W., Thompson, P., & Price, R. L. (1977). The four stages of professional careers: A new look at performance by professionals. *Organizational Dynamics, 6*(1), 19–42.

Darling, L. W. (1985a). Becoming a mentoring manager. *Journal of Nursing Administration, 15*(6), 43–44

Darling, L. W. (1985b). What to do about toxic mentors. *Journal of Nursing Administration, 15*(5), 43–44.

Darling, L. W. (1985c). Endings in mentor relationships. *Journal of Nursing Administration, 15*(11), 38–39.

Dunham-Taylor, J., Fisher, E., & Kinion, E. (1993). Experiences, events, people: Do they influence the leadership style of nurse executives? *Journal of Nursing Administration, 23*(7/8), 30–34.

Erickson, E. H. (1963). *Childhood and society* (2nd ed.). New York: Norton.

Fagan, M. M., & Fagan, P. D. (1983). Mentoring among nurses. *Nursing Outlook, 4*(2), 80–82.

Gray, W. A., & Gray, M. M. (1994). *Developing mentor-protégé relationships: A mentor-protégé workbook.* Sidney, British Columbia, Canada: The Mentoring Institute.

Hall, R. M., & Sandler, B. R. (1983). *Academic mentoring for women students and faculty: A new look at an old way to get ahead.* Washington, DC: Association of American Colleges.

Halloran, S. (1993). Mentoring: The experience of nursing service executives. *Journal of Nursing Administration, 23*(2), 49–54.

Halsey, S. (1978). *Role theory: Perspectives for health care professionals.* New York: Appleton-Century-Crofts.

Hart, L. B. (1980). *Moving up and leadership.* New York: AMACOM.

Hennig, M., & Jardim, A. (1977a). Women executives in the old-boy network. *Psychology Today, 10*(8), 76–81.

Hennig, M., & Jardim, A. (1977b). *The managerial woman.* Garden City, NJ: Doubleday.

Holcomb, R. (1980). Mentors and the successful woman. *Across the Board, 17*(2), 13–18.

Josefowitz, N. (1980). *Paths to power.* Reading, MA: Addison-Wesley.

Kanter, R. M. (1977). *Men and women of the corporation.* New York: Basic Books.

Kelly, L. S. (1987). To touch tomorrow. *Nursing Outlook, 35*(2), 59.

Kleiman, C. (1980). *Women's networks.* New York: Ballantine.

Laino-Curran, D. (1995). Choosing your mentor. *Nursing/95, 25*(7), 78–79.

Levinson, D. J., Darrow, C. N., Klein, E. B., Levinson, M. H., & McKee, B. (1978). *The seasons of a man's life.* New York: Knopf.

Lubin, J. S. (1996). Women at top still are distant from CEO jobs. *The Wall Street Journal,* CCLXXVII (41), B 1.

Lundig, F. J., Clements, G. R., & Perkins, D. S. (1978). Everyone who makes it has a mentor. *Harvard Business Review, 56*(4), 89–101.

Madison, J. (1994). The value of mentoring in leadership: A descriptive study. *Nursing Forum, 29*(4), 16–23.

Moore, K. M. (1982). The role of mentors in developing leaders for academe. *Educational Record, 63*(1), 22–28.

Murray, B., Fosbinder, D., Parsons, R., Dalley, K., Gustafson, G., & Vorderer, L. (1998). Nurse executives' leadership roles: Perceptions of incumbents and influential colleagues. *Journal of Nursing Administration, 28*(6), 17–24.

O'Connor, A. B. (1982). Ingredients for successful networking. *Journal of Nursing Administration, 12*(12), 36–40.

Price, S. A., Simms, L. M., & Pfoutz, S. K. (1987). Career advancement of nurse executives: Planned or accidental? *Nursing Outlook, 34*(8), 236–238.

Puertz, B. E. (1983). *Networking for nurses.* Rockville, MD: Aspen Systems.

Roche, G. (1979). Much ado about mentors. *Harvard Business Review, 57*(1), 14–16, 20, 24–28.

Shapiro, E. C., Haseltine, F. P., & Rowe, M. P. (1978). Moving up: Role models, mentors, and the "patron system." *Sloan Management Review, 20*(2), 51–58.

Taylor, L. J. (1992). A survey of mentoring relationships in academe. *Journal of Professional Nursing, 8*(1), 45–55.

Vance, C. (1997). Mentoring—The nursing leader and mentor's perspective. In C. A. Anderson (Ed.), *Nursing student to nursing leader: The critical path to leadership development.* Albany, NY: Delmar.

Warihay, P. (1980). The climb to the top: Is the network the route for women? *Personnel Administrator, 54*(4), 55–60.

White, J. F. (1988). The perceived role of mentoring in the career development and success of academic nurse-administrators. *Journal of Professional Nursing, 4*(3), 178–185.

Wynter, L. E., & Soloman, J. A. (1989, November). A new push to break the glass ceiling. *The Wall Street Journal,* pp. B1–B2.

Yoder, L. (1990). Mentoring: A concept analysis. *Nursing Administration Quarterly, 15*(1), 9–19.

Zuckerman, G. (1977). *Scientific elite: Nobel laureates in the United States.* New York: The Free Press.

PART
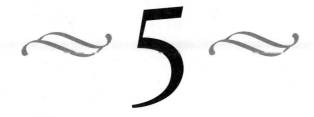
5
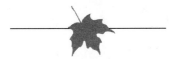

Building and Discovering Resources

CHAPTER

~ 21 ~

Building Effective Work Groups

Sandra R. Byers

Any good coach in the sports field knows that it's a lot easier to build a winning team with skilled and motivated players. (Wellins, Byham, & Wilson, 1991, p. 143)

Chapter Highlights

- Work context
- Hospital context
- The effective unit workplace
- Unit nursing work
- Nursing work within a team
- Unit ethos

Building effective nursing work groups in various settings requires knowledge and skill with planning, coordinating, delegating, and dealing with conflict at the individual, team, and system levels. The need for effective teamwork is self-evident, and the problems of coordination and cooperation require a sophisticated understanding and assessment of teams and groups. Interdisciplinary health care team management requires knowledge of the dynamics of different practice patterns and effective strategies for managing teams, task forces, and task-directed groups. The nursing work group is seen as selected individuals authorized to perform nursing care in an identified location and are working together to accomplish clinical outcomes with a client. This chapter presents an approach to study work groups and workplace environments to plan and build effective work groups.

Planning is a conceptual activity and may be defined as predetermining a carefully detailed course of action that will enable the organization, unit, or individual to achieve specific objectives or goals. Planning requires the ability to think, to analyze data, to envision alternatives, and to make decisions. Planning is essentially a decision-making process and the steps are similar to those of the nursing process. They include assessment of the system or subsystem, including goals and objectives; assessment of present strengths and weaknesses; establishment of assumption and *prediction* of what will influence activities; determination of alternative courses of action; identification of priorities; and selection of a course of action.

Coordination may be described as organizing the work of nursing care within each shift, between shifts, and between nurses and other health professionals throughout the health care delivery system. Delegation is a complementary function of direction. Effective delegation implies that a nurse shares a segment of responsibility, delegates a specific segment of corresponding authority, and demands accountability. Conflict is an inherent part of all organizations, units, and work groups. Within a health care organization, conflict may result from divergence of opinion, incompatibility, transmission of erroneous information, or competition for scarce resources. Although frequently viewed as a negative manifestation of human interaction, conflict in work groups can have positive aspects. The redesign of work groups can be used as a tool for developing shared values and building effective and flexible work groups thus minimizing negative conflict outcomes (Beckman & Simms, 1992).

WORK CONTEXT

Nurses are employed in diverse settings: hospitals, community agencies, long-term care, private practice, physician offices, faith communities and ambulatory clinics, which have an impact on the design of work groups. This diversity has resulted in a variety of employee-employer-consumer contracts that frame the different degrees of independence, accountability, authority, and types of services provided by the nurse and the corresponding work group members. In addition, these contracts, formal or informal, assume the underlying understanding every professional has with clients to provide competent and appropriate service and to be compensated for these services. For example, the nurse in the community-based environment frequently delegates physical care and many basic treatments to family members that in the hospital environment are carried out by the employed staff. Medications are given by family members in the home and some records are kept by family members.

In the hospital setting, it is assumed that the majority of all care must be performed by employees. In contrast, the work group in the home environment has quite different levels of responsibilities, independence, and accountability. In long-term care settings, both the work group's care plans and actual care place more emphasis on the chronic nature of the patient's disease and the physical, social, and emotional needs of the patient over time. Therefore, the work group members may be more consistent as the patient's progress and needs change less dramatically.

In the hospital, although "total patient" is the framework for developing the patient's plan of care, the acute needs of the patient change quickly and take precedence. Team members change frequently as a result of the increased intensity of care required by patients, decreased hospital lengths of stay, and the increased use of assistive personnel to decrease costs. The hospital workforce is changing as other workers are being substituted for the RN (Aiken, Gwyther, & Friese, 1995, p. 2). This creates work environments in which work relationships are not easily maintained and many are broken.

As care is being provided in increasingly different settings and with financial restraints attached to care decisions and potential outcomes, "the complexity and acuity of care needs in the emerging system will require the health professional to be able to work effectively as a team member in organized settings that emphasize the integration of care" (Pew Health Professions Commission, 1995, p. 4). Ann Rowe (1998) has developed a workshop for the self-management of multidisciplinary primary health care teams. The workshop incorporates the theory and research on teamwork and adult learning principles and focuses on values, trust building, and the equality of all to encourage interaction and risk taking. As work environments continue to change, additional study on the effectiveness of teams and work groups will be important.

The Hospital Context

Nursing work groups are affected by factors such as the organization of the hospital and its larger system, costs of health services, and nurse characteristics. One way to understand work groups in any environment is to examine these factors.

Hospitals are large complex organizations frequently within multilevel delivery systems or corporations. They are usually bureaucracies characterized by rules, a division of labor, a hierarchy of authority, specialists, line and staff positions, a separately designated administrative staff, and high tech record-keeping. However, many hospitals are moving away from this bureaucratic "silo-type" structure to a learning organization structure characterized by an integrated approach to organizational effectiveness, systems orientation, horizontal communications, and professional growth and empowerment (Jones, 1997, p. 146). This trend has led to the fact that "health professionals must be prepared to practice in settings that are more intensively managed and integrated" (Pew Health Professions Commission, 1995, p. 34).

The cost of hospital services is increasingly emphasized. Singleton and Nail (1984) explained hospital structure, organization, and relationships from a financial perspective. In "big business," usually the consumer is clearly the purchaser and payer of service. In the hospital, the consumer is the patient who must be admitted for the purchase and receipt of services ordered by the physician and usually paid for by a third party. The physician is not a formal partner in the business enterprise but is responsible for ordering the product of care for the patient. Nurses and others employed by the hospital are responsible for implementing the care prescribed and the care within their practice domain. The payers, usually government agencies, private insurers, or health plans, have a great deal to say about the amount of payment for the health care and the conditions under which the care is provided (Singleton and Nail, 1984). Therefore, the quantity and the quality of the services provided to patients is influenced and monitored by another body outside the hospital environment. This kind of control creates a complex environment for hospitals trying to adjust numbers of personnel and programs to fit with revenue resources. Singleton's analysis supports why the current payment for health care services is becoming increasingly complex. As the system moves to more managed care, discounted contracts, and capitation guidelines (Donaho & Kohles, 1996, p. 49), the ability to control revenue for more than a year has decreased. Consequently, the hospital control has shifted to decreasing hospital resource utilization.

Hospitals are known for employing a large number of professional nurses in proportion to other professionals. Currently, approximately 2 million nurses work in hospitals and are assigned to work on a specific clinical unit or cluster of units. It is estimated that by the year 2020, the 26% of employed nurses over the age of 50 is likely to double and 90% of nurses in hospitals will be under 29 years of age (Thornhill, 1994). Professionals tend to have loyalties to their professional association outside the hospital. They have a mission that is based on their commitment to society not the organization.

The work of nurses is embedded in the structural and role relationships within their practice environment. Aiken (1983) suggested six fundamental tensions between hospitals, physicians, and nurses that continue with few exceptions: *(1)* Nurses' sphere of authority has not changed since World War II even though nurses are now in command of much of the available clinical expertise to care for the seriously ill and make judgments about appropriate use. *(2)* Physicians work fewer hours and are available less for consultation (in the hospital). The authority of the nurse to act in the absence of the physician has not been redefined. *(3)* Nurses have not been recognized for their new level of clinical decision-making with the increase in older and more seriously ill patients. *(4)* There is an increase in medical subspecialties, resulting in numerous physicians involved in a patient's care, fragmentation of care, and the potential of costly and dangerous duplication or omission of services. The role of the nurse to synthesize and monitor multiple diagnostic and treatment regimens has not been recognized. *(5)* Nurses are the coordinators of all the support services involved with the care and safety of a patient, yet they have no authority to deploy or redirect these services to carry out the responsibilities. *(6)* Nurses, mostly women who are now looking at many professional career options, do not find working conditions in hospitals professionally satisfying. These six tensions, which Aiken terms incompatibilities, suggest that nurses' lack recognition and status within the hospital. They may also indicate the need for the nursing profession to communicate to others about what nurses can and do accomplish.

A 5-year program Strengthening Hospital Nursing, concentrated on new work and role designs for nursing in more than 60 grantee hospitals in 6 different health care systems, and 12 individual organizations. Work sampling techniques and in-depth role analysis provided the data to assist in the redesign of the patient care delivery in the hospitals. Four principles were the thread among the hospital sites that guided their efforts in their redesign efforts: *(1)* the number of caregivers providing care to the patient must be limited to increase both continuity and patient satisfaction, *(2)* those doing the work should be included in the redesign, *(3)* the needs of the patients and employees should drive the redesign and not the departmental roles or the bottom line, and *(4)* technology, reimbursement, and demographics must be considered (Donaho & Kohles, 1996, pp. 52–54). The specific outcomes of each site or system were different but were in concert with the program objectives; to develop innovative systems to strengthen patient care through collaborative efforts of all providers, to create work environments that optimally use human resources and improve care in a cost-effective manner, and to establish service delivery patterns that promote provider satisfaction.

The Unit Context

Whereas the clinical unit in community care is the home, the clinical unit in most hospitals is defined by a designated physical space and labeled according to a type of medical specialty. With hospital restructuring, sister units or like-units are identified for staffing flexibility and work efficiency. Patients admitted for care are placed in private or semiprivate rooms. Hospital employees and nonhospital employees come and go on the unit, depending on their assigned responsibilities. Physical structure, organizational structure, management, culture, and work-related variables have constituted the study of the clinical unit.

The workplace of the nurse has received national attention from The American Academy of Nursing in its Task Force on Nursing Practice in Hospitals report, *Magnet Hospitals, Attraction and Retention of Professional Nurses* (American Academy of Nursing, 1983) and the *Secretary's Commission on Nursing Final Report* (USDHHS, 1988). Hospitals that were judged to have outstanding records of nurse recruitment and retention were then labeled "magnet hospitals." This report has been used extensively by nurse executives in trying to correct their own nurse recruitment and retention problems.

The *Magnet Hospital* report identified positive work environment characteristics and encouraged hospitals to design programs incorporating them. They are *(1)* a visible, accessible, and participatory administration; *(2)* knowledgeable and strong leaders who support their work and care about their working conditions;

(3) a collaborative organizational structure with mutual goal setting; *(4)* staffing patterns that recognize the need for adequate quantity, quality, and mix of expertise of staff; *(5)* personnel programs and policies with flexible work schedules, competitive salaries, and benefits; *(6)* active recruitment and retention programs; and *(7)* professional practice support and a drive for quality with models of delivery that support nurse autonomy, constructive feedback on the quality of care, and knowledgeable nursing care consultants available. Nurses in these hospitals, identified for their outstanding recruitment and retention programs, are recognized for their contributions to the total care of the patient and family and are consulted by physicians. Professional development is supported and includes strong orientation programs, inservice, and continuing education, formal education, and career development. *Magnet hospital* chief nurse executives continue to identify distinguishing traits: control of staff nurses over their practice, autonomy and accountability of staff nurses in their nursing practice, and support and recognition of the nurse as caregiver (Credentialing News, 1998, p. 4).

THE EFFECTIVE UNIT WORKPLACE

The Secretary's Commission on Nursing Report (USDHHS, 1988) contained 8 of 16 recommendations addressing reorganization of the workplace. Briefly, these recommendations are *(1)* health care delivery should preserve nurses' time for direct patient care by providing adequate staffing levels for clinical and nonclinical support services; *(2)* innovative staffing patterns should use nurses' different levels of education, competence, and experience; *(3)* automated information systems and other new labor-saving technologies should be developed; *(4)* methods for costing, budgeting, and tracking nursing resource use should be developed; *(5)* involvement of nurses at all policy- and decision-making levels must occur; *(6)* the decision-making level of the nurse in cooperation with medicine should be recognized; *(7)* positive and accurate images of nurses' work should be promoted; and *(8)* the effects of nurse compensation, staffing patterns, decision-making authority, and career development on nurse supply and demand and health care cost and quality should be researched.

The third report of the Pew Health Professions Commission recommends that nursing have a single title for each level of nursing preparation and service and "distinguish between the practice responsibilities of these different levels of nursing, focusing associate preparation on the entry level hospital setting and nursing home practice, baccalaureate on the hospital based care management and community based practice, and masters degree for specialty practice in the hospital and independent practice as a primary care provider." (1995, p. vi).

Nurse retention is used as an indicator of the hospital's and unit's status. Alexander (1988) studied voluntary turnover rate of 1,726 registered nurses and licensed vocational nurses on 146 units within 17 hospitals. The dependent variable, voluntary turnover rate, was correlated with four unit organizational variables: "staff integration," defined as the ratio of RNs assigned to the unit to total patient care staff assigned to unit, extent of RN rotation and among shifts, and ratio of full-time staff to all unit staff; "centralization," defined as RN influence in unit-related decisions and decision-making authority of the head nurse; "communication/coordination," defined as the frequency of contact and communication among nurses during the shift, frequency of patient care conferences, and explicitness of unit policies and procedures; and "evaluation," defined as perceived accuracy of head nurse performance evaluation and the number of patients care hours performed by head nurse per week.

Results indicated four organizational categories significantly related to turnover: salience of evaluation, frequency of patient care conferences, shift rotation, and RN ratio. A positive correlation was found with shift rotations and a negative correlation with the RN ratio suggesting, "A collegial group of professional workers and some degree of organizational stability may be necessary to achieve organizational integration and consequently to reduce turnover" (Alexander, 1988, p. 69). He also contended that where there is formal communication, instrumental communication or informal communication occurs and positively influences turnover. For example, planned meetings and conferences, as patient care conferences, increase the opportunities for staff socialization and positively influences retention. Fair and accurate evaluations legitimize the RN role and, thus, reduce the conflict and alienation that may result in turnover.

Butler and Parsons (1989), Pooyan, Eberhardt, and Szigeti (1990), and Weisman, Alexander, and Chase (1981) studied nurse retention. Butler and Parsons focused on 212 nurses' perceptions of environmental factors, finding inadequate salary, lack of control over scheduling and patient care load, lack of recognition for clinical excellence, and lack of managerial support influencing satisfaction and retention. Pooyan et al. (1990) surveyed 1,250 nurses at three private hospitals, examining the relative contributions of work-related and demographic variables to turnover intention. Demographic variables of age, occupational tenure, education, and marital status did not contribute to nursing job changes in ways not accounted for by work-related variables. The results of Pooyan et al. were consistent with those of Weisman et al. (1981) in suggesting turnover-related variables that can be potentially controlled by management. These variables are satisfaction with promotion, pay, and supervisor, together with three work environment variables: role ambiguity, participation opportunity (e.g., how much "say" the nurses perceived they had in making job-related decisions regarding how to do one's job, the sequence/speed of work, and division of work responsibility as well as the amount of work), and performance constraints (shortage of nursing staff, unavailability of medical equipment/supplies, lab delays, too much paper work, and not having sufficient instructions). Satisfaction with promotion and perceived performance constraints were the first and second most significant predictors of turnover.

Williams (1988) reviewed the literature on hospital and unit design, spatial environment, sound, color, thermal conditions, and weather. These variables have had limited attention from researchers and appear to influence work and environment.

UNIT NURSING WORK

Nursing work has been studied extensively and described in a variety of ways by categorized activities, by physical skills required, by identified "hidden work," by "quality" nursing care characteristics, and by the philosophical and cultural foundations of nursing care.

Yocom (1987) studied practice patterns of over 4,500 newly licensed nurses who responded to questions about nursing activities and client needs. The activity statements were worded in terms of what the nurse does rather than how, how well, or why the nurse performs the activity. The practice domain of the nurse was based on clinical practice area and education program attended. Nurses in medical/surgical clinical units scored high in performing routine nursing measures, monitoring clients at risk, preparing clients for procedures, and controlling pain. They scored low in meeting acute emotional/behavioral needs; staff development, management, and collaboration; and quality assurance and safety. Nurses were very low in categories specific to a setting such as parenting skills associated with teaching new mothers and fathers how to care for a new infant or the administration and teaching of immunizations with pediatric patients' parents. The middle group of categories for the medical/surgical nurses was protecting clients, planning/managing client care, helping clients to cope with stress, assisting clients with needs related to mobility, assisting clients with self-care, meeting acute physical needs, supporting client's family, and ensuring safety during intrusive procedures. The study found work setting (e.g., obstetric, pediatrics, or rehabilitation inpatient units) and type of clients (whether young or old) influenced the frequency of the activities.

A time/task survey was conducted by The Hay Group in over 850 hospitals about nurses working on medical-surgical units ("Misuse of RNs," 1989). They found 26 percent of RN's time on average is spent in "professional nursing": physical assessments, care and treatments, monitoring patients' conditions, planning and documenting care. In a typical shift, 22% of the time was spent with support functions: patient education, family contacts, nursing communications, and coordination. The largest amount of time, 52% was spent in housekeeping details, answering phones, and ordering supplies ("Misuse of RNs," 1989). The investigators reported the reason these nurses stayed or left an institution was based on reasons directly and indirectly related to environment, job, and perceived opportunity for personal and professional growth (Figure 21.1).

Nursing work has been described using words such as "knowing," "caring," "intuitive," the "essence of nursing," or "hidden work" in contrast to the activities/task approach previously presented. Styles (1990) described good nursing care from the patient's perspective and suggested clients should know who is in charge of their personal care and what the plan of care will be. The knowl-

Support Functions 22%   Professional Nursing 26%

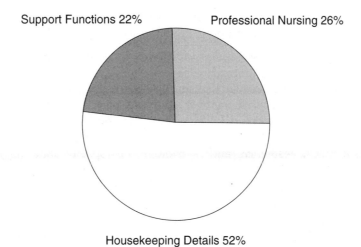

Housekeeping Details 52%

Figure 21.1 Misuse of RNs.

edgeable and technically competent nurse distinguishes between what is nice and what is necessary for client's care and not only cares about the assigned clients but also cares for them. The nurse should be organized and attend to priorities, serve as patient advocate, and allow the patient as much control as possible. The nurse works with others to ensure the treatment progresses as planned and to minimize complications in preparation for discharge and recovery.

Wolf (1989) points out much of nursing work is hidden, thus decreasing societal status and perceived value. She studied a medical unit in a large urban hospital, investigating four "nursing rituals": postmortem care, medication administration, medical aseptic practices, and change of shift report. Wolf observed that nurses pass on their nursing and patient care knowledge chiefly by word of mouth and by demonstration. Nursing in her opinion has both sacred and profane components and described it in terms of unseen work and dirty work. The unseen tasks are common sense and caring work, system maintenance and safety work, interpersonal work, comforting work, privacy work (e.g., collection of private information and personal hygiene needs), sacred work (i.e., moral and ethical problems), and cognitive work. The dirty work is body work and death work. She believes nursing work should be made visible and not taken for granted.

The work of Reverby (1987) in *Ordered to Care* depicts nursing as a form of labor shaped by the obligation to care in a society that does not value or know how to evaluate caring. This obligation has resulted in it being described as "women's work," a "duty" encumbered with societal and ideological constraints and difficulties. She views nurses, historically, as individuals from different classes, with heterogeneous experiences and beliefs. This creates a unity and a language problem as efforts are made to mobilize the group toward professional goals. Caring is not only a subjective construct but it is work. Reverby (1987) challenges nursing via political endeavors, educational and practice clarification, and technological advancement to create the conditions under which caring is valued.

The work of Noddings (1984), Gilligan (1982), and Belenky, Clinchy, Goldberger, and Tarule (1986) can contribute to nurses' awareness and understanding of the complexity of work relationships by considering how the female orientation may affect those relationships. This literature sheds a positive perspective on the capabilities and strengths of women, which would be helpful for nurses to understand as they struggle for identity and a stronger image. Noddings (1984) explored caring from an ethical, aesthetical, and psychological perspective. She suggests one meaning of caring as the charge "to protect, maintain or be concerned about the welfare of something or someone" (p. 9). Gilligan (1982) suggests that women are raised and socialized with an ethic of care, of thinking in terms of the concrete other. Belenky et al. (1986) describe five ways women view reality and define truth, knowledge and authority. Women "know" by using intuition, personal meanings, and self-understanding. They connect with ideas and they seek understanding rather than control over ideas or proof that something is so.

In the work cited above, the individual is the focus of study and not a work group or team. However, with reengineering of nursing work, there is the growing trend to examine the next level of nursing care delivery. Rowland and Rowland (1997) discuss teams as a way to deliver general health care and not just for emergency care situations. Blancett and Flarey (1995) recognize teams as the fundamental work unit with cohesive, interdependent individuals with a shared sense of purpose. Client care is recognized as a product of multiple disciplines.

NURSING WORK WITHIN A TEAM

A basic understanding of who and what is "the team" is fundamental to effective team work. Platt says a "team requires (a) a group of two or more people, (b) a shared sense of purpose or purposes among the group members, and (c) interactions among the members that make them able to accomplish more than each would be able to accomplish working individually toward the shared purpose" (1994, p. 4).

With unit and work restructuring, using professionally advanced care teams (Kohles et al., 1995, p. 118), teamnets or empowered teams (Lipnack & Stamps, 1993, p. 310), the dynamic "bubble" team design (Hamilton, 1993, p. 40), patient care management systems in a holographic organization (Shortell et al., 1993, pp. 23, 25), or interdisciplinary, patient-focused care (Hansen, 1995, p. 11), nursing work focuses on competencies such as consensus decision-making, systems thinking, open communication, relationship building, and interactive processes (Donaho & Kohles, 1996, p. 258).

New team configurations in the different practice environments may have different guidelines. However, "the goal is not just to put together multifunctional and multinational teams, but to create in every employee an eclectic set of perspectives, a set of interchangeable lenses" (Hamel & Prahalad, 1994, p. 96). Competencies, defined as "a bundle of skills and technologies rather than a single discrete skill or technology" are the basis for "competing for the future" (Hamel & Prahalad, 1994, p. 202). With these new team configurations and worker expectations, the five management tasks required are: "*(1)* identifying existing core competencies; *(2)* establishing a core competence acquisition agenda; *(3)* building core competencies; *(4)* deploying core competencies; and *(5)* protecting and defending core competence leadership" (Hamel & Prahalad, 1994, p. 224).

Team building is an essential leadership competency and according to Schaffner and Bermingham, ". . . Is a method of participative management that encourages staff commitment to the unit and the organization" (1993, p. 80). Specific steps are used to assist in the team building process and assess team functioning. The team or work group culture is an important ingredient when facilitating team building. The culture reflects group values and affects group effectiveness, patterns of behavior, and group tasks (Taft, 1997, pp. 47–48). "Group culture is closely related to group identity or self concept. A group that knows what it stands for and where it wants to go is in a better position to move forward than a group that lacks an identity and is aimless" (Coeling, 1997, p. 203).

The strengthening hospital nursing program identified many "lessons learned" that affect team development and the change process, including: *(1)* educational time should be designed for people at all levels of the organization, *(2)* a common language should be established and used throughout the institution, *(3)* individual accountability should shift to team accountability creating a collective "we" for achieving the desired outcome, and *(4)* everyone's competencies should be understood and the unique talents of each person recognized (Kohles et al., 1995, p. 258).

UNIT ETHOS

Byers (1990) explored a hospital's unit ethos, defined as the norms and expectations characteristic of individuals within their work context, by studying 15 staff nurses. They completed questionnaires adapted from Quinn (1988) based on his Competing Values Model, described later. This model appeared meaningful in understanding the complex and competing dynamics on a hospital unit. Underlying beliefs and values are critical to the change process and this model helps to reflect those. In addition, nurses who are in the environment, performing the work, are the experts in judging the effectiveness of that work and in redesigning their work to meet patient care needs. A deeper awareness about how nurses understand their world of work and the norms and expectations in that world might contribute to new organizational models for nursing care delivery and impact retention. An assessment of unit ethos as perceived by the nurse and the work group, may reveal tensions with aspects of organization life such as relationships with hospital administration, physicians, and nurse peers, disillusionment with the work, and inadequate information and communication systems.

Quinn (1988) was concerned about how experts think about effective organizations and tried to understand underlying assumptions causing the behavior. In Quinn's research about organizations, describing effective organizations led to longer and different lists of criteria, based on each organization. The outcome was the competing values framework, which acknowledges organizations as dynamic and confronted with change, ambiguity and contradictions (Figure 21.2). The model, briefly described, has intersecting horizontal and vertical axes, which create four quadrants. The vertical axis ranges from flexibility to control and the horizontal axis ranges from an internal to an external focus. Each quadrant represents one of the four major schools of organization theory: human relations, open systems, rational goal, and the internal process model. Each model has specific characteristics and is in polar contrast to the opposite corner, hence, the notion of competing values.

The model allows the organization to be explored from the perspective that these polar tensions exist in organizations and are not mutually exclusive. The human

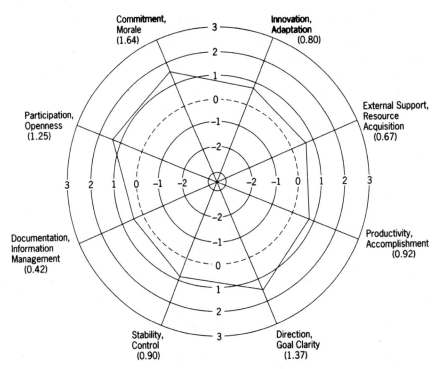

Figure 21.2 The competing values model: organizational effectiveness profile of a nursing unit. The average scores (in parentheses) of the 15 nurses are plotted for the eight organizational components. From Quinn, R. E. (1988). *Beyond rational management.* San Francisco: Jossey-Bass. Copyright 1988 by Jossey-Bass. Reprinted by permission.

relations model stresses internal focus, with criteria as cohesion and morale, and values human resources training, whereas it is in contrast to the external oriented rational goal model that values output, productivity, and efficiency with planning and goal setting. Organizations want and need both ways of functioning, and they are not mutually exclusive. In the same way, the open systems model provides an external orientation, values expansion and adaptation, readiness, growth, competition, and resource acquisition. Its polar opposite, an internal orientation, is the internal process model that values continuity and consolidation with stability and control, information management, and communication. "The model can be used to diagnose and intervene in actual organizations" (Quinn, 1988, p. 50). The information can provide a realistic base for progressive change or adaptation in nurses' work.

The Organizational Effectiveness Questionnaire (Quinn, 1988) places the characteristics in eight groups, which in Byers' study (1990), was used to gain insights into the unit expectations that influence nurses' beliefs about their practice. For example, the average nurse score for participation and openness is 1.25 (in parentheses, Figure 21.2). This particular work group appeared effective and scored highest in commitment to work, positive morale, a clear idea of goals and direction, and participation and openness. The low score was in documentation and information management. The nurses did not value these activities, which might impact a transition to computerization. Nurses who have these same values would probably remain on this unit and find this unit best for them. This type of information can be applied when designing nurses' work, in types of unit work group assignments, in recruitment and retention, and in any planned change.

SUMMARY

The workplace of most nurses is a physical unit that is frequently a closed subsystem of a larger hospital and houses a variety of workers and clients. The units are staffed by nurses who want adequate working conditions, rewards, and benefits, typical of most other workers in our society. The interactions between the mix of workers are complex relationships influenced by the expectations of each other and the way in which the work groups are organized. Nurses are torn between professional allegiance and allegiance to the organization as they continually change and reposition themselves in the organization. The degree to which most hospitals have become individual specialty units, triggered by the increase in complex technology and the specialized nursing care that is required, has influenced the structure of the organization in terms of the need for increased communications and integration.

Nursing studies that explore the effect of unit structure and the kind of integration and communication required at all levels in the organization continue to be essential. The Competing Values Model (Quinn, 1988) offers a way to study the work group and workplace environment. The information currently available on nurses' work and employment conditions suggested by the Byers' study described in this chapter can assist nurses in improving nursing services to patients in all settings. Using Quinn's effective work groups approach can stimulate new care delivery models and promote the delivery of effective and efficient patient-centered nursing care.

STUDY QUESTIONS

1. Compare and contrast work group characteristics between two practice settings, i.e., hospital and home or a congregation of faith and a physician's office.
2. What is the impact of managed care on work group effectiveness?
3. How does an effective work group or team improve morale, job satisfaction, and client care?
4. What are the positive and negative work incentives for a nurse as a multidisciplinary team member?
5. Why are teams important in the current health care system?
6. Apply the eight dimensions of the competing values model to a work group or team that you have been in. What dimensions are similar and what are different?

REFERENCES

Aiken, L. H. (1983). Nurses. In D. Mechanic (Ed.), *Handbook of Health, Health Care and the Health Professions* (pp. 407–431). New York: Free Press.

Aiken, L. H., Gwyther, M. E., & Friese, C. R. (1995, January–March). The Registered Nurse Workforce: Infrastructure for health care reform. *Statistical Bulletin*, pp. 2–10.

Alexander, J. A. (1988). The effects of patient care unit organization on nursing turnover. *Health Care Management Review, 13*(2), 61–72.

American Academy of Nursing Task Force on Nursing Practice in Hospitals. (1983). *Magnet hospitals. Attraction and retention of professional nurses.* Kansas City, MO: American Nurses Association.

Beckman, J. S., & Simms, L. M. (1992). *A guide to redesigning nursing practice patterns.* Ann Arbor, MI: Health Administration Press.

Belenky, M. F., Clinchy, B. M., Goldberger, N. R., & Tarule, J. M. (1986). *Women's ways of knowing.* New York: Basic Books.

Blancett, S., & Flarey, D. (1995). *Reengineering nursing and health care.* Gaithersburg, MD: Aspen.

Butler, J., & Parsons, R. J. (1989). Hospital perceptions of job satisfaction. *Nursing Management, 20*(8), 45–48.

Byers, S. R. (1990). *Relationships among staff nurses' beliefs, nursing practice and unit ethos.* Unpublished dissertation, The Ohio State University, Columbus.

Coeling, H. V. (1997). Organizational subcultures: Where the rubber meets the road. In S. R. Byers (Ed.). *The executive nurse: Leadership for new health care transitions* (pp. 184–206). Albany, NY: Delmar.

Credentialing News. (1998, Spring). Magnet facilities share keys to success in Atlanta. 1(2), 4.

Donaho, B. A., & Kohles, M. K. (1996). *Celebrating the journey: A final report, strengthening hospital nursing: A program to improve patient care.* St. Petersburg, FL: Robert Wood Johnson Foundation and The Pew Charitable Trusts.

Gilligan, C. (1982). *In a different voice.* Cambridge, MA: Harvard University Press.

Hansen, H. E. (1995). A model for collegiality among staff nurses in acute care. *Journal of Nursing Administration, 25*(12), 11–20.

Hamel, G., & Prahalad, C. K. (1994). *Competing for the future.* Boston: Harvard Business School Press.

Hamilton, J. (1993, January 5). Toppling the power of the pyramid, Team-based restructuring for TQM, patient-centered care. *Hospitals,* pp. 38–41.

Jones, L. (1997). Developing a learning organization. In S. R. Byers (Ed.). *The executive nurse: Leadership for new health care transitions* (pp. 134–151). Albany, NY: Delmar.

Kohles, M. K., Baker, W. G. Jr., & Donaho, B. A. (1995). *Transformational leadership. Renewing fundamental values and achieving new relationships in health care.* Chicago: American Hospital Publishing.

Lipnack, J. & Stamps, J. (1993). *The teamnet factor.* Essex Junction, VT: Oliver Wight Publications.

Misuse of RNs spurs shortage, says new study: "Only 26% of time is spent in professional care." (1989). *American Journal of Nursing, 89,* 1223, 1231.

Noddings, N. (1984). *Caring. A feminine approach to ethics and moral education.* Berkeley: University of California Press.

Pew Health Professions Commission. (1995). *Critical challenges: Revitalizing the health professions for the twenty-first century. The Third Report of The Pew Health Professions Commission.* San Francisco: UCSF Center for the Health Professions.

Platt, L. J. (1994). Why bother with teams? An overview. In R. Casto & M. C. Julia (Eds.). *Interprofessional care and collaborative practice* (pp. 3–9). Pacific Grove, CA: Brooks/Cole Publishing.

Pooyan, A., Eberhardt, B. J., & Szigeti, E. (1990). Work related variables and turnover intention among registered nurses. *Nursing and Health Care, 11*(5), 255–258.

Quinn, R. E. (1988). *Beyond rational management.* San Francisco, CA: Jossey-Bass.

Reverby, S. M. (1987). *Ordered to care. The dilemma of American nursing, 1850–1945.* Cambridge: Cambridge University Press.

Rowe, A. (1998). Self-management in Primary Care. *Nursing Times, 94*(29), 60–62.

Rowland, H., & Rowland, B. (Eds.). (1997). *Nursing administration handbook* (4th ed.). Gaithersburg, MD: Aspen.

Schaffner, J. W., & Bermingham, M. (1993). *Creating and maintaining a high-performance team. Nursing leadership, preparing for the 21st* century (pp. 52–92). Chicago: American Organization of Nurse Executives, AHA, American Hospital Publishing.

Shortell, S. M., Anderson, D. A., Gillies, R. R., Mitchell, J. B., & Morgan, K. L. (1993, March–April). The holographic organization. *Healthcare Forum Journal,* pp. 19–26.

Singleton, E. K., & Nail, F. C. (1984). Autonomy in nursing. *Nurse Forum, 21*(3), 123–130.

Styles, M. M. (1990). Ten ways to know . . . , *Nursing and Health Care, 11*(6), 283.

Taft, S. (1997). Paradoxical challenge: Preserve and transform the organizational culture. In S. R. Byers (Ed.). *The executive nurse: Leadership for new health care transitions* (pp. 45–82). Albany, NY: Delmar.

Thornhill, S. K. A., (1994). Hospital clinical advancement programs: Comparing perceptions of nurse participants and nonparticipants. *Health Care Supervisor, 13*(1), 16–25.

U.S. Department of Health and Human Services (USDHHS). Office of the Secretary. (1988). *Secretary's Commission on Nursing, Final Report, Volume 1.* Washington, DC.

Weisman, C., Alexander, C., & Chase, G. (1981). Determinants of hospital staff nurse turnover. *Medical Care, 19*(4), 431–443.

Wellins, R. S., Byham, W. C., & Wilson, J. M. (1991). *Empowered teams.* San Francisco: Jossey-Bass.

Wolf, Z. R. (1989). Uncovering the hidden work of nursing. *Nursing and Health Care, 10*(8), 463–467.

Yocom, C. J. (1987). Practice patterns of newly licensed registered nurses: Results of a job analysis study. *Journal of Professional Nursing, 3*(4), 199–206.

CHAPTER

22

Personal and Group Empowerment

Lillian M. Simms

If management wants employees to take more responsibility for their own destiny, it must encourage the development of internal commitment.

(Argyris, 1998, p. 100)

Chapter Highlights

- Visioning
- Group learning through action research
- Perceptions of work
- Work excitement
- Empowerment and effective practice
- Action learning through action research
- Identifying work penetration points from unit data

The President of the United States cannot alone change the health care system. The Director of Nursing can no longer single-handedly make everything work efficiently and effectively. Tomorrow's leadership must see its prime duty as the empowerment of other people (Simms & Calarco, 1998). The most vital requirements for a leader will be those of self-knowledge and inner balance, and a leader's major attribute will be to facilitate the empowerment of colleagues to be their own leaders. They will facilitate the person in the group who takes the initiative and becomes the point of entry of an idea. They will not squelch ideas, although they may differ in points of view.

The emergence of the phenomenon of transformation is provided a rare opportunity for leaders in nursing. Transformation provides a scenario for a new way of interacting, a new way of problem-solving, and a means for developing a shared vision among health professionals in various settings. The seeds for transformation are in every organization awaiting a cultural climate that will encourage, support, and cultivate them. The essence of transformation is a "metanoic" shift and the realization of personal empowerment that comes from a group with a common vision (Adams, 1998). In metanoic organizations, people do not assume they are powerless and they believe deeply in the power of the individual to assume control of destiny. A growing number of organizations are developing prototypes for a metanoic model with five primary dimensions forming the basis of organizational philosophy:

1. A deep sense of vision
2. Alignment around that vision
3. Empowering people
4. Structural integrity
5. The balance of reason and intuition

How to go about doing this is not so easy. The purpose of this chapter is to discuss the meaning of personal and group empowerment, including an approach to building one's constellation of empowerment through individual assessment, visioning, and continuous learning. Those who wait for someone to hand them power will never know they have it. Power must be recognized from within.

EMPOWERMENT

The key to empowerment is self-development and appreciation of others. Kinsman (1998) speaks of self-development in the truest sense—intellectually, bodily, emotionally, and spiritually. Self-empowered leaders are "focalizers," those who focus the energies of the people in their areas. Focalizers, says Kinsman (1998), help to make decisions in a group but on the basis of input from everyone in the group. Lang (1988, p. 6) defines empowerment as "unleashing—to release from or as from a leash; to set free to pursue; to let loose; to give official power; to enable."

Personal and group empowerment are realized through personal mastery and continuous learning (Senge, 1990; Simms & Calarco, 1998). The ability to focus on future dreams and goals is a cornerstone. One ought to have a purpose for living, and it ought to make a difference that one has lived. Work flows fluidly in enterprises when personal, group, and organizational visions are shared. Personal empowerment can be developed in many ways. One approach is to foster the idea of a continuously developing "dream plan." Figure 22.1 provides a mental model for personal empowerment. It is a picture of components of thoughts and ideas

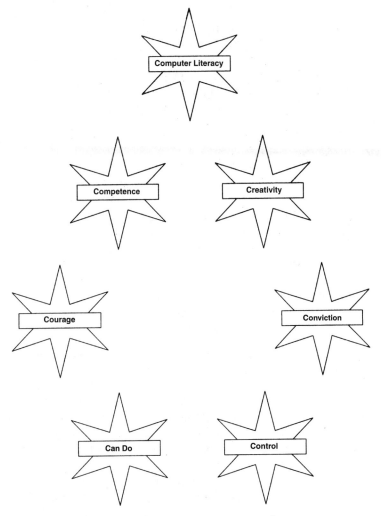

Figure 22.1 The personal empowerment constellation.

that can convey a positive view of the world. Your constellation may be somewhat different and your picture of each star in the constellation may be at a different level of development.

Kornbluh, Pipan, and Schurman (1987) defined empowerment learning as unlimited energy in an organization. Human learning is considered an organizational asset, and in transformed organizations, human learning and problem-solving abilities are viewed as vitally important resources in empowering people—a continuous source of energy. Participation in transformation is seen as a process, not a goal. A zero-sum conception of power in command and control organizations assumes that power is a finite commodity in which some may gain only if others lose. A radically different approach is proposed—a "non-zero sum model" of power in which the total amount of power is always expanding. Based on creation of a learning environment, workers are empowered to use their intellectual abilities to individual and organizational advantage. In this model, every worker counts and every worker exerts control over performance and quality of work and life variables. In transformed metanoic health care organizations, the goal is patient-centered and it is everyone's responsibility to participate in building and advancing a shared vision.

VISIONING

Bennis and Nanus (1985) were among the first to discover that one of the outstanding characteristics of exemplary leaders is the ability to foster organizational learning. Individual visioning unfolds to become a common vision. The group's vision is not the vision of the most articulate or dominant individual but, rather, a distinct entity generated by the group and groups in an organization. Bennis and Nanus (1985) speak of the management of attention through vision. Kinsman (1998) speaks of vision as "powerful to the extent that it expresses one's underlying purpose." Members of high-performing systems have pictures in their heads that are strikingly congruent, drawing people together toward a common reality (Noer, 1993; Ritscher, 1998).

Senge (1990) describes business and other human endeavors as systems, bound by invisible factors of interrelated actions that may take years to fully understand their effects on each other. Each organizational member is part of that lacework (or cobweb) and it is difficult to see the whole system as we tend to focus on isolated snapshots of the system. Personal mastery according to Senge (1990) is the discipline of continually clarifying and deepening one's personal vision, focusing energies, developing patience, and seeing reality objectively. Personal mastery is the essential cornerstone of the learning organization. Because few organizations encourage the growth of their people, there is a pervasive sense of powerlessness in individuals and groups. Resource dependency theory should be advanced to resource discovery theories.

Personal learning and organizational learning are intertwined in building shared visions. Personal mastery begins with understanding the self and the ability to work with our internal mental models. The earlier chapter on making sense of organizations described the organizational window with a variety of images or window panes with differing perceptions of the organization. Building shared vision involves unearthing pictures of the future that form a mission and philosophy that is believed and shared by its members. Group learning is vital to shared vision because work groups or teams are the fundamental learning unit in modern organizations.

If you want to change the world, there is no time like the present. Lang (1988, p. 11) envisions a world in which we as nurses:

- Encourage an entrepreneurial revolution in nursing
- Encourage true competition in the solution of health care problems
- Experiment with nursing corporations and partnerships and nurse-managed centers
- Decrease physician resistance (to nursing practice)
- Increase malpractice and professional liability coverage options for nurses
- Encourage incentives for resolution of dependency, maintenance of health status, and peaceful deaths

As authors of this book, we envision a world in which professional nurses practice independently and collaboratively in the delivery of health care; a world in which nursing has its own recognized and credible technology of knowledge, skills, and equipment and is not totally dependent on other disciplines for energy and innovation.

Figure 22.2 provides a simple approach to nurturing personal empowerment. Imagine the untapped resources discovered in work environments where every-

---

EMPOWERING THYSELF

PART I. Curriculum Vitae
    Name
    Address
    Phone and fax numbers
    Current position
    Academic history including school; degree; specialty; year of graduation
    Professional experience
    Research activities
    Management activities
    Publications
    Professional papers presented
    Honors and awards
    Professional organizations
    Community service
    Other
PART II. Career Plan/Personal Vision
    Important life missions to date—e.g., early years; high school; college; work; etc.
    Personal support system—e.g., people; pets; places; etc.
    Personal learning style
    Strengths/weaknesses
    Dreams for the future
    Ideas in process
    Future life milestones/career points
    Lifelong learning schedule to achieve career points (include projected time schedule) What do you need to learn to achieve career points?
    Fit with current organizational vision (mission and philosophy)

Figure 22.2 Developing self-assessment and personal visioning skills.

one learns self-assessment through the generation of a resumé or curriculum vitae. We have resource abundance in this country. We simply do not recognize it. Personal visioning can be learned through regularly appending one's curriculum vitae with a personal vision or career plan that simply sets out where you have been, where you want to go, and where you fit in your current organizational vision. It is an example of one's lifelong learning plan.

PERSONAL AND GROUP POWER

Power is difficult to define without bringing up images of coercion and domination. Meade (1995) describes empowerment as the process of thinking and behaving as if one has power or control over significant aspects of one's life and work. Nurses must begin to understand power and empowerment to succeed in achieving their professional and organizational goals. Gorman and Clark (1986) defined nursing power as the nurse's ability to do, to achieve nursing objectives. This definition recognized that nursing power does not mean total control over patient care but rather collaboration with other health professionals. Kanter (1977) described organizational power as:

> the ability to get things done, to mobilize resources, to get and use whatever it is that a person needs for the goals he or she is attempting to meet. In this way, a monopoly on power means that only a very few have the capacity, and they prevent the majority of others from being able to act effectively. Thus the total amount of power—the total system effectiveness—is restricted, even though some people seem to have a great deal of it. However, when more people are empowered—that is, allowed to have control over the conditions that make their actions possible—then more is accomplished, more gets done. (p. 166)

GROUP LEARNING THROUGH ACTION RESEARCH

Participatory research offers a strategy for group learning that is consistent with the assumptions of people-centered development (Brown, 1985). It encourages inquiry that focuses on local problems and pragmatic concerns that are reality based. Innovations developed by participants and researchers can catalyze developmental changes. Resultant cooperative relations can combine outside resources with local resources, bringing in commitment to learning new options and energy and skills for solving problems. Interaction with outside researchers links local participants with previously unexplored sources of information and outside alliances that can be sources of political and economic empowerment.

The action-research approach depends on participants learning and working together in unit assessment and planning for redesign. The key characteristics of participatory action research (Israel, Schurman, & House, 1989) are:

- Participation of employees in most aspects of the research and actions; research process is not dependent on theoretical interpretation of the researchers.
- Cooperation of managers, employees, and researchers in a joint process

- A colearning process in which clinical managers, researchers, and employees develop an understanding of the situation under study
- System development in which participants develop the competencies to engage in the process of diagnosing and analyzing problems, planning, implementing, and evaluating changes, such as redesigning work or introducing technology
- An empowering process in which participant organization members gain increased influence and control over their work lives

Participatory action research provides a legitimate model for creating the learning environment essential for this research design. Brown (1985) made a strong case for using people-centered development and participatory research as a means to maximize human resource development. Participatory action research asks adults to be interdependent participants and colearners rather than dependent and researcher controlled. The researchers learn skills for general problem-solving, such as managing meetings, getting information, organizing work, or planning activities. The control of learning in participatory action research can seldom be predicted or planned in detail across projects and is participant-learner dependent rather than research-teacher controlled. Participatory research is a way to promote people-centered development in various systems that encourage local empowerment. This is especially relevant as we work to transform nursing work environments and pave the way for patient-centered care delivery systems.

Examples of successful action research studies have been described in the labor and occupational studies literature. A substantial amount of data exist in Scandinavian documents, wherein the holistic conception of the work environment is considered paramount. Important American studies have been conducted by Deutsch (1988, 1989) in his investigations of workplace democracy and worker health resulting in the postulation of a learning activation process described in Figure 22.3. Kornbluh, Pipan, and Schurman (1987) reported positive findings on empowerment learning and control in workplaces in industry. Schurman and Israel (Schurman, 1989) have a highly credible record in involving workers as researchers and using action research methods in the study of occupational stress. Employee-based and union-initiated efforts to improve the work environment have worked well in various work organizations as well as hospitals.

DIFFERENT PERCEPTIONS OF WORK

Empowerment, personal or group, is related to feelings about work. Studies related to retention and turnover abound in the nursing literature and, in general, have had a negative impact on changing nursing work environments (Simms, Erbin-Roesemann, Darga, & Coeling, 1990). The lack of agreement on the meaning of work in the literature has resulted in a variety of definitions among theoreticians. Work is believed to be different than job with job satisfaction used to refer to affective attitudes or orientations on the part of individuals toward jobs

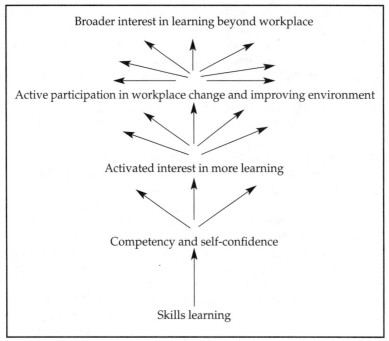

Figure 22.3 Learning activation process.

(Blegen & Mueller, 1987). Work is something individuals and society take very seriously, although authors disagree on the meaning of work.

Schurman (1989) believes that the meaning of work is complex, which is central to the notion that work has a different meaning for every individual, allowing for work to be identified as something other than satisfaction and excitement. Work is viewed as a central human activity in which mind and body unite in actions that not only provide sustenance for the life process, but also generate objects, material and ideational, which have meaning and value to both *self* and others. Attempts to link meaning of work to the organization of work, however, is weak in the literature. Instead, meaning of work is generally associated with job satisfaction, with the former regarded as a reflection of the latter. Sandelands (1988) makes the rare distinction between affect about the work (i.e., meaningfulness of work) and attitudes about the work (i.e., job satisfaction), which he argues are relevant to designing work organizations. Csikszentmihalyi (1990) described positive work experiences when people are in "flow," linking psychic energy with optimal goal achievement and the work experience (see Chapter 6).

Authors of work-enrichment studies often fail to include in their assumptions the meaning of work to the individual. It is likely for individuals to view work as paid employment and not wish to have their jobs enriched. This may be because they have higher level needs met by other forms of work outside their jobs. Fein (1977) concluded that the need for fulfillment from one's job applies only to those workers who choose to find it in their employment. He contends that the vast majority of workers seek fulfillment outside their jobs. In addition, Hackman and Lawler (1971) found that employees with higher order needs satisfied, performed better and were more positive than those without the higher need satisfaction.

The meaning of work has also been examined on intrinsic and extrinsic dimensions by the classic work theorists. Fein (1977) stated that the intrinsic nature of the work performed is not the main cause of the difference between satisfied and dissatisfied workers. Workers' dissatisfaction with their jobs is due less to the nature of work than to other factors such as pay, freedom, and nonwork-related problems. Hackman (1977) disagreed with this conclusion, in that society as a whole has achieved substantial increases in economic benefits; therefore, people today want jobs that provide intrinsic work satisfaction. Trist (1981) identified the intrinsic characteristics of the job as variety and challenge, continuous learning, discretion or autonomy, recognition and support, and meaningful social contribution. The extrinsic characteristics were identified as fair and adequate pay, job security, benefits, safety, and health. These are consistent with the hygiene factors described in earlier work by Herzberg, Mausner, and Snyderman (1959).

JOB SATISFACTION

Hackman (1977) described his basic job characteristics model of work motivation in terms of five core job dimensions. These dimensions create three critical psychological states that, in turn, lead to beneficial personal and work outcomes. Skill variety, task identity, task significance, autonomy, and feedback from the job were noted, with the first three contributing most to a job's meaningfulness. Psychological states include experienced meaningfulness of the work, experienced responsibility for outcomes of the work, and knowledge of the actual results of the work activities. Four outcomes are affected by the level of generated motivation, including high internal work motivation, high "growth" satisfaction, high general job satisfaction, and high work effectiveness.

Mueller and McCloskey (1990) have continued to seek to identify the rewards that keep nurses on the job through the development and validation of an instrument to measure job satisfaction. The McCloskey/Mueller/Satisfaction Scale (MMSS) has acceptable reliability and construct validity and may be used to measure satisfaction with extrinsic rewards, scheduling, family/work balance, co-workers, interaction, professional opportunities, praise/recognition, and control/responsibility. The work is clearly limited to job satisfaction and does not address the more global construct of work.

The organization of people's work may be a major determinant in shaping their health and well-being outside of work. Drawing on years of research on job redesign and work, Karasek and Theorell (1990) attempt to bridge the gap between medical science, psychology, sociology, industrial engineering, and economics to present an approach to the redesign of work organizations to make them more psychologically humane. The authors present a laudable perspective on integrating worker health analysis and job redesign. Citing weaknesses in Quality of Work Life research, the authors further propose job redesign strategies that will promote health-related job change. They further support studies of physiologic changes among workers as part of any work intervention program. In a study designed to improve competence of patients and personnel, physiologic monitoring and educational programs resulted in improvement in patient clinical outcomes and worker health and safety. Important factors in creating an excellent work environment include worker health and safety.

WORK EXCITEMENT

Recent work by the Simms Practice Excitement Project (PEP) team on work excitement has yielded a tool to measure work characteristics and work excitement. To test the model for work excitement, a self-administered fixed-alternatives questionnaire with previously generated key items was used to collect data on 268 nurses' perception of exciting aspects of work and level of excitement about work. Construct validity was obtained using cluster and factor analysis. Cronbach's alpha used to assess internal consistency of the three main questions concerning interest, excitement, and frustration with work yielded reliability coefficients ranging from .85 to .94. Based on these validation studies, work excitement was conceptualized as "personal enthusiasm and interest in work evidenced by creativity, receptivity to learning, and ability to see opportunity in everyday situations." Multiple regression analysis supported five factors as significant predictors of work excitement: growth and development (learning), work arrangements, variety of experiences, working conditions, and change (Table 22.1).

The factor identified as growth and development or learning comprised the variables: taking on challenging problems and projects and solving or accomplishing them and seeing and participating in the growth and development of other nurses. This factor was positively related to work excitement, indicating that the more opportunities for growth and development and learning, the greater the level of work excitement. The second significant factor of work arrangements

Table 22.1 Predictors of Work Excitement

Factor	Component Variables
Growth and development/learning	Taking on new projects and challenging problems; participating in the growth and development of other nurses
Work arrangements	Staffing patterns; time for work accomplishment; optimal communication
Variety	Opportunities available for learning at work; variety in work experiences
Working conditions	Staffing schedules; work hours; money
Change	Pace; variation in patient acuity levels; unpredictable crises
Work locus of control	Perception of personal control of work life

consists of the variables of inappropriate and understaffing, issues of time and getting work finished, and communication problems among nurses, physicians, and other nursing personnel. It is negatively related to work excitement, indicating that the higher the level of frustration with work arrangements, the lower the level of work excitement.

The third important factor, variety, consists of the variables of variety of experiences and availability of learning opportunities. The positive correlation suggests that the more variety and opportunity for learning in the work environment, the higher the level of work excitement. The fourth significant factor was that of working conditions; it comprised the variables of convenient hours, schedules, and money. This factor is negatively related to work excitement, thus indicating that the more frustrated one feels about working conditions, the less work excitement one has.

Finally, the factor of change was a significant predictor of work excitement. This factor contains the variables of fast pace, variety of activities, high-acuity patients, and unpredictable, crisis situations. It is positively related to work excitement, indicating that the more change that occurs in the work environment, the higher the level of work excitement. In other unreported graduate student projects, level of knowledge, working with high technology in critical care settings, and computer use have been found to be significantly related to work excitement. Internal locus of control was the most recent focus of research and was found to be positively related to work excitement, suggesting a link with empowerment (Erbin-Roesemann & Simms, 1997). A theory of work excitement is still in process.

The conceptual framework (Figure 22.4) guiding the research is permeated with opportunities for learning for caregivers and recipients. For example, self-care and the use of assistive technology can be learned and can make a tremendous difference in discharge readiness. Learning new behaviors on the part of caregivers can and should result in continuing clinical competence and other changes in behavior, such as acceptance of assistive technology and the ability to work in flexible groups.

Mastery of the major elements in any unit work or practice pattern redesign will include learning and using the structural concepts of patient characteristics, nursing resources, work group culture characteristics, and work characteristics (Beckman & Simms, 1992); the process components of an action plan; and clinical and workplace outcomes. The concept of work excitement, postulated in terms of person and work environment factors, is considered the catalyst for process and practice outcomes. The latest validation studies have reconfirmed the concept of work excitement (Figure 22.5).

EMPOWERMENT AND EFFECTIVE PRACTICE

In-service management training sessions can function as organizational rituals that maintain the status quo. Hirschhorn (1988) argues that managers and workers

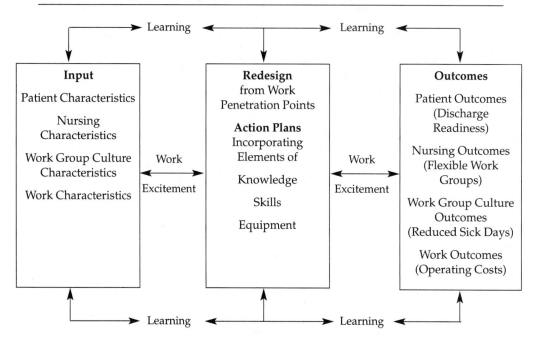

Figure 22.4 Conceptual framework for participatory nursing work redesign.

must enact sophisticated boundaries that help people to acknowledge the claims of outside stakeholders while protecting the coherence of the work group. By failing to do so, they may retreat from role, task, and organizational boundaries, thus creating a more irrational workplace than that found in an industrial milieu. The social defenses at work frequently create a distorted relationship between the group and its wider environment of customers, clients, and competitors. The "outside" is scapegoated or devalued in some way to preserve the "inside." A group dominated by its own social defenses retreats from the boundary it shares with its environment into its collective fantasies and delusions. Group development occurs when group members stop scapegoating others, when they cease using each other or outsiders to manage their shared anxieties. In so doing, they come close to confronting their primary task (Hirschhorn, 1988). In actual practice, this is difficult to do.

However, Gorman and Clark (1986) suggest that group empowerment is possible. During a 3-year period, the Nursing Knowledge Project conducted by Gorman and Clark (1986) examined how nurses applied their clinical knowledge and skills in the practice setting, identified barriers to nursing practice, and evaluated a series of training activities designed to increase nurses' power in practice settings. Four empowerment strategies emerged from their research (summarized as follows):

The practice of analytic nursing: nurses must routinely apply the same analytical skills that enable them to develop a patient's nursing care plan to the interpersonal and organizational problems they encounter daily in the hospital.

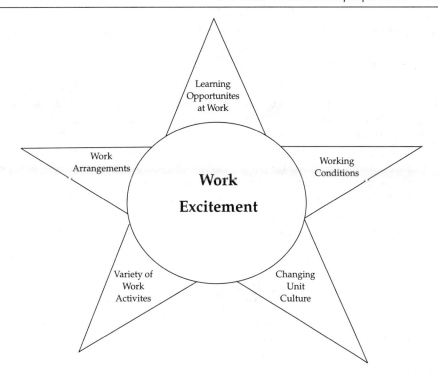

Figure 22.5 Work excitement conceptual model.

Engagement of nurses in change activities: nurses must plan and implement needed change in practice settings.

Strengthening collegiality: nurses must call on the support of their nursing colleagues and the extensive experience of other nurses for counsel and advice in the application of clinical knowledge and skills.

Extending administrative sponsorship: staff nurses must be provided the organizational know-how and support of administrative nurses in efforts to improve patient care. Through sponsorship, more senior nurses guide less experienced nurses to resolve difficult practice problems and link them to needed organizational resources.

Group learning was then encouraged through role-centered case analyses of reality-based unit case studies. The activities of the nurses became highly relevant and extraordinary and visible. In the training program, nurses working in heterogeneous groups, representing various parts of each collaborating hospital, acted as teams and selected common problems to address. The training program, therefore, included both educational and structural solutions for the problems of powerlessness experienced by nurses in the hospital setting. Educationally, the program was designed to empower the participating nurses by teaching them the analytic and interpersonal skills they needed to develop and implement plans for change. Structurally, it established new lines of communication between staff nurses and nurse executives, linking the nurses to needed resources and giving the nurses more control over working conditions.

The implementation of interdisciplinary groups centers on a nucleus of nurses, physicians, and health care executives who appreciate the concept of collaborative work (Simms, Dalston, & Roberts, 1984). The core team should be bright, highly motivated, and closely linked with the recognized organizational leadership, both formal and informal. The core group educates, influences, provides role models, and demonstrates precepts through seminars, quality reviews, persuasion, contribution to the literature, and involvement in solving direct patient care problems. This core group is, above all, persistent, accomplishing what is achievable now, awaiting improved conditions, and then moving forward again. Action learning has been described as team learning by Senge (1990) and as group learning by Svensson (1991). In either case, participants learn from each other and work as a unified team.

AN EXAMPLE OF ACTION LEARNING THROUGH ACTION RESEARCH

Shared purpose/vision must be concerned with active movement from purpose to results. Support for action learning requires an organizational climate conducive to learning new knowledge and skills. One approach to action learning is through action research. In the ongoing Simms, Coeling, and Price redesign research, the researchers meet with unit staff and explain the overall process. Each unit serves as its own control group. The rationale for conducting periodic unit assessment to determine the effectiveness of current practice patterns and quality of patient care needs early discussion. The importance of data for decision-making about changes in practice patterns becomes a natural follow-up of unit discussions. It is important to establish that unit staff will participate in data interpretation and decision-making. Ground rules for maintaining respect for all group members and their opinions will be developed. Organizational mission, unit philosophy, conceptual elements of any practice pattern, flexible work groups, and quality care will be used as discussion themes at each site to lay the groundwork for introduction of assessment instruments.

The entire unit staff becomes part of the process, even though a task force of three to five people may be responsible for collection of data and completing the analysis. This task force includes staff nurses as well as the unit nurse executive. In fact, several task forces can conduct various parts of the unit assessment so that most or all staff members are involved in some way. Thus, unit-based participatory action research teams consisting of unit nurses and researchers will be established at each site and will be selected from volunteers who reflect the different unit skill mix. It will be noted that research teams will be flexible and will change over time so that all interested nurses can become intimately involved with the action research process. The following teams are the work groups, depending on the size of overall staff and different interests of the unit nurses and researchers:

Team A: Initial data collection team

Team B: Work penetration points identification team

Team C: Intervention planning team focused on discharge readiness

Team D: Action planning team

Team E: Follow-up data collection team

Team F: Data analyses and recommendations for future direction

Following introduction of the project and related activities to unit staff, patients will be verbally introduced to the project by a research team member on admission to the unit. The patient consent form will be used to guide the introduction so that all patients will receive consistent information. Patients will be asked to sign the consent form at the time of introduction to the study and will be given the discharge readiness questionnaire at discharge, to be returned in 1 week to the principal investigator.

Unit preparation, collection of baseline data on input and outcome variables, and identification of work penetration points related to discharge readiness will occur over a period of 6 months with data collection from unit staff nurses and nurse managers at all selected hospital sites. In all cases, it is anticipated that the team efforts will not encompass more than 2 months of work.

In sum, the procedure includes the following steps:

1. Unit discussion of mission, philosophy, conceptual elements of any practice pattern, flexible clinical work groups, and clinical outcomes. Technology will be discussed as will knowledge, skills, and equipment, the basic elements of any action plan.
2. Selection of unit task forces and introduction of study to patients
3. Baseline unit data will be collected on:
   - Current patient, nursing, unit work group culture, and work characteristics.
   - Prevailing levels of discharge readiness among patients
   - Prevailing practice pattern (work group membership and arrangements)
   - Prevailing levels of work excitement among unit nurses
   - Prevailing levels of work-related injuries and sick days among unit nurses
   - Prevailing unit operating cost
4. Group discussion of resultant data
5. Development of action plan based on identified work penetration points
6. Implementation of the action plan
7. Follow-up evaluation of input and output variables

IDENTIFYING WORK PENETRATION POINTS FROM UNIT DATA

The process continues with the identification of work penetration points identified from collected data. Resultant baseline data are combined for clinical and systems variances that indicate unit-based work penetration points. Clinical variances are searched for and identified in the patient characteristics and discharge readiness data; systems variances are located in the work, unit culture, nursing resources, and unit nurse executive data. Unit data will be entered into a database using spreadsheet software for easy and quick analysis. In this manner, unit nurses learn how to enter data, analyze data from group generated research questions, and interpret spreadsheets.

Descriptive statistics are used to identify the key patient, nursing, work group culture, and work characteristics requiring immediate attention. The unit research teams generate a summary report describing their units and listing work penetration points that are of primary interest. Prioritizing work penetration points is essential, and the participatory action research teams can decide to address less urgent points at a later time. Some pretest units have identified learning needs related to inadequate knowledge for high-acuity patient care, lack of computer skills, and lack of freedom to leave the unit as immediate concerns. Other pretest units have identified other work penetration points.

For example, cultural analysis of one unit revealed a norm of frequently calling in sick, to the point of abusing the sick-time policy. A comparison of the preferred behaviors with current behaviors indicated the nurses wanted to be able to make patients more comfortable and to spend more time understanding patients' feelings. The work penetration point of altering attendance patterns was identified. The unit nurse executive (head nurse) worked with the staff to help them see that if there were fewer call-ins, they would have a more abundant and stable staff that, in turn, would provide more opportunities to spend time talking with patients and making them comfortable. As a result of this discussion, the staff made a conscious group effort to stop misusing sick time.

Cultural analysis of another unit revealed that it was not expected that nurses offer to help each other. Rather each worked alone to complete the work assigned to them. As budget cuts necessitated staff lay-offs and nurses had to work harder, the unit nurse executive noted a pattern of increased sick days related to back injuries attributed to nurses lifting and moving patients alone without help. A comparison of the preferred behaviors with current behaviors indicated the nurses wanted others to offer to help them more. The work penetration point of altering expectations related to helping each other was identified. Nurses were encouraged to make themselves more aware of their fellow nurses' work load and to take the initiative to offer to help them.

Cultural analysis of a third unit revealed a bimodal norm for attending inservices, attending college, discussing new ideas, and achieving clinical advancement. In other words, on this unit, some nurses valued these behaviors and other nurses rejected them. A new head nurse assigned to the unit noted how these divergent behaviors frequently led to conflict on the unit. She identified the work penetration point of increasing commitment to continued learning. She made her norm of continuous improvement known to the unit. Within a matter of months, those nurses who did not value learning had resigned and the unit was becoming a stable, productive unit.

In sum, following the identification of work penetration points from unit assessment, unit staff determine an action plan for intervention and introduction of redesign of work, work groups, and/or practice patterns based on what they have learned through participation in the action research project. Work groups on the participating units then proceed to implement their individualized action plans with unit-designed interventions (Table 22.2).

PARTICIPATORY ACTION PLANNING FROM ACTION LEARNING

Group-generated action plans are developed, considering collected baseline data, resultant work penetration points, and appropriate technologies (knowledge, skills, and equipment) to design interventions that can yield clinical and systems outcomes. Given knowledge of patient, nursing, culture, and work characteristics, the unit staffs consider the nature of the work to be done and the nursing and technological resources desirable and available to accomplish the work with

Table 22.2 Work Penetration Points (WPPS) and Potential Action Plans

WPPS	Potential Action Plans
Documentation, care plans and discharge planning	Eliminate duplicative assessments, care plans and charting; computerize clinical records
Excessive non-nursing duties	Hire unit clerk with master's preparation in management
High acuity patients with multiple care problems	Improve unit approaches to care through research utilization, new learning and consultation with clinical specialists
Time consuming routine patient care	Optimize use of nursing assistants—invite patient/family participation in care
Inefficient transfer of patients	Initiate development of better people movers; add a rehabilitation engineer to team
Too many patients; no breaks	Conduct time analysis and determine which tasks can be done differently or not at all
Fatigue from being on feet all day	Make ergonomic changes; install exercise bicycles at work for staff use; investigate issues related to improper shoes
Demanding families	Increase family participation in planning care
Negative attitudes among staff	Redesign work groups; eliminate non-essential tasks
Repetitive teaching	Improve use of audiovisual media for individual and group teaching

the best advantage to patients. Consideration in developing the action plan is given to: What pieces of work can or should be done together or by one person? The work should not be characterized only in terms of tasks or time, but also as processes and activities. What work can be delegated to other people or technology? What work should be a patient/family responsibility? What work should be done differently? What work should not be done at all? *In other words, what knowledge, skills, and equipment are needed to redesign the unit work?*

SUMMARY

Group empowerment emerges from personal empowerment, and personal empowerment is related to a sense of purpose and excitement about one's work. One's personal constellation of empowerment can be developed and fine tuned through systematically practicing visioning and self-development. One of the very best self-assessment tools is the simple resumé or curriculum vitae. The individual is the master of one's own life and the curriculum vitae is the history of one's professional life. To add the component of a lifespan career plan promotes the practice setting for envisioning who you may become and where you plan to be over the next 50 years. Visioning skills are practiced frequently in childhood—they need to be continually honed in adulthood and in the later years. If you are envisioning collaborative initiatives, then learning activities must be planned to develop the skill and knowledge necessary for professional collaboration. Group empowerment emanates from group visioning and futuring and, ultimately, is measured in terms of performance and productivity.

STUDY QUESTIONS

1. What is empowerment and how do you differentiate between personal and group empowerment?
2. How does internal locus of control influence empowerment and work excitement?
3. Describe and give examples of opportunities for group learning in your work setting.
4. Why is it important to have participatory activities for group learning to occur?
5. Consider your work setting and identify three examples of work that no longer needs to be done.
6. Review your updated curriculum vitae and identify areas where further personal development is needed.
7. Attend a symphony concert or basketball game and determine how action learning principles are in force.

REFERENCES

Adams, J. D. (1998). *Transforming work.* Alexandria, VA: Miles River Press.
Argyris, C. (1998). Empowerment: The emperor's new clothes. *Harvard Business Review, 76*(3), 98–105.

Beckman, J. S., & Simms, L. M. (1992). *Redesigning nursing practice patterns.* Ann Arbor, MI: Health Administration Press.

Bennis, W., & Nanus, B. (1985). *Leaders: The strategies of taking charge.* New York: Harper & Row.

Blegen, M., & Mueller, C. (1987). Nurses' job satisfaction: A longitudinal analysis. *Research in Nursing and Health, 10,* 227–237.

Brown, L. D. (1985). People-centered development and participatory research. *Harvard Education Review, 55*(1), 69–75.

Csikszentmihalyi, M. (1990). *Flow—the psychology of optimal experience.* New York: Harper & Row.

Deutsch, S. (1988). Workplace democracy and worker health: Strategies for intervention. *International Journal of Health Services, 18,* 647–658. Also reprinted (1991). In J. Johnson & G. Johansson (Eds.), *The psychosocial work environment: Work organization, democratization and health.* Amityville, NY: Baywood.

Deutsch, S. (1989). Worker learning in the context of changing technology and work environment. In H. Leymann & H. Kornbluh (Eds.), *Socialization and learning at work* (pp. 237–255). Brookfield, VT: Gower.

Erbin-Roesemann, M. A., & Simms, L. M. (1997). Work locus of control: The intrinsic factor behind empowerment and work excitement. *Nursing Economic$, 15*(4), 183–190.

Fein, M. (1977). Job enrichment: A reevaluation. In J. R. Hackman, E. E. Lawler, & L. W. Porter (Eds.), *Perspectives on behavior in organization* (pp. 269–281). New York: McGraw-Hill.

Gorman, S., & Clark N. (1986). Power and effective nursing practice. *Nursing Outlook, 34*(3), 129–134.

Hackman, J. R. (1977). The design of work in the 1980s. In J. R. Hackman, E. E. Lawler, & L. W. Porter (Eds.), *Perspectives on behavior organizations* (pp. 458–473). New York: McGraw-Hill.

Hackman, J. R., & Lawler, E. E. (1971). Employer reactions to job characteristics. *Journal of Applied Psychology Monograph, 55,* 259–286.

Herzberg, R., Mausner, B., & Snyderman, B. (1959). *The motivation to work.* New York: Wiley.

Hirschhorn, L. (1988). Psychodynamics of the workplace. In L. Hirschhorn (Ed.), *The workplace within* (pp. 1–15). Cambridge, MA: MIT Press.

Israel, B. A., Schurman, S. J., & House, J. S. (1989). Action research on occupational stress: Involving workers as researchers. *International Journal of Health Services, 19,* 135–155.

Kanter, R. M. (1977). *Men and women of the corporation.* New York: Basic Books.

Karasek, R., & Theorell, T. (1990). *Healthy work.* New York: Basic Books.

Kinsman, F. (1998). Leadership from alongside. In J. Adams (Ed.), *Transforming leadership.* Alexandria, VA: Miles River Press.

Kornbluh, H., Pipan, R., & Schurman, S. J. (1987). Empowerment learning and control in workplaces: A curricular view. *Zeitschrift Fur Sozialisationsforschung Und Erziehungssoziologie (ZSE) J. Jahrgang/Heft 7*(4), 253–268.

Lang, N. (1988). Empower the nurse: A time for renewal. In *Nursing Practice in the 21st Century* (pp. 5–16). Kansas City, MO: American Nurses Foundation.

Meade, R. L. (1995). *How to empower an organization: Unleash the latent power of your workforce from goals to action.* Minneapolis: Lakewood.

Mueller, C. W., & McCloskey, J. C. (1990). Nurses' job satisfaction: A proposed measure. *Nursing Research, 39*(2), 113–117.

Noer, D. M. (1993). *Healing the wounds.* San Francisco: Jossey-Bass.

Ritscher, J. A. (1998). Spiritual leadership. In J. D. Adams (Ed.), *Transforming leadership.* Alexandria, VA: Miles River Press.

Sandelands, L. E. (1988). The concept of work feeling. *Journal for the Theory of Social Behaviour, 18*(4), 437–457.

Schurman, S. J. (1989). Reuniting labour and learning: A holistic theory of work. In H. Leymann & H. Kornbluh (Eds.), *Socialization and learning at work* (pp. 42–68). Brookfield, VT: Gower.

Senge, P. M. (1990). *The fifth discipline: The art and practice of the learning organization.* New York: Doubleday.

Simms, L. M., Dalston, J. W., & Roberts, P. W. (1984). Collaborative practice: Myth or reality. *Hospital and Health Services Administration, 2*(6), 36–48.

Simms, L. M., Erbin-Roesemann, M., Darga, A., & Coeling, H. (1990). Breaking the burnout barrier: Resurrecting work excitement in nursing. *Nursing Economic$, 8*(3), 177–186.

Simms, L. M., & Calarco, M. M. (1998). Maximizing people potential in empowered environments. In S. A. Price, M. W. Koch, & S. Bassett (Eds.), *Health care resource management.* St. Louis: Mosby.

Svensson, L. (1991). A democratic strategy for organizational change. In J. V. Johnson & G. Johansson (Eds.), *The psychosocial work environment: Work organization, democratization and health.* Amityville, NY: Baywood.

Trist, E. (1981). The sociotechnical perspective. In A. H. Van de Ven & W. F. Joyce (Eds.), *Perspective on organization design and behavior* (pp. 19–75). New York: Wiley-Interscience.

CHAPTER

23

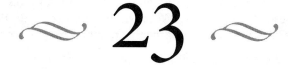

Creating and Managing
Fiscal Resources

Mary G. Nash

To be an executive is to face the reality that resources are limited and choices must be made as to what will be produced and how it will be produced. (Author)

Chapter Highlights

- The operating cycle
- Financial and managerial accounting
- Assets, liabilities, revenues, and expenses
- Revenue centers and cost centers
- Reimbursement methods
- Budgeting and monitoring results
- Resource management system

To be a manager or administrator is to face the reality that resources are limited and choices must be made as to what will be produced and how it will be produced. Implicit in the task of managing fiscal resources is that managers and administrators are held accountable for the resources that are entrusted to them and they are expected to make the most appropriate use of resources. This suggests that they will strive to use resources in a way that is both efficient and effective.

411

Efficiency is the ratio of input to output, and the number that is produced by this computation is only meaningful relative to some standard of comparison with which it can be compared; someone must decide what that standard will be. Whereas efficiency refers to the relative productivity of a resource, the quest for effectiveness raises a different issue: What will be produced with the resources that are available? Again, human judgment is required to make the decision.

It should become clear that managing fiscal resources has both a technical and a policy component. This chapter is largely concerned with the technical component, which is presented in terms of accounting principles, reimbursement rules, budgeting, and management reporting. The policy component is concerned with values and judgments regarding the organization's goals as well as the strategies and structures that are chosen to implement them. How will the work of the organization be divided into operating units and how will the overall effort be coordinated? The technical component takes place within the policy environment, at times shaping that environment and at other times being limited by it.

A complete explication of the complexities of health care financial management is beyond the scope of this chapter. The intention here, instead, is to provide a framework for managing fiscal resources. The center of this framework is the operating cycle supplemented by specific areas that are likely to be most relevant to nurse executives. When you finish this chapter you should have a greater understanding of *(1)* the basic operating cycle of an organization, *(2)* selected accounting and fiscal management concepts that form the basis of many fiscal management routines and decisions, *(3)* reimbursement systems and how they shape and constrain internal management processes, *(4)* budgeting and variance analysis processes, and *(5)* the importance of developing a resource management system.

THE OPERATING CYCLE

A basic accounting concept is that an organization is a "going concern"; that is, it intends to continue to operate for an indefinite period of time. As a going concern, we assume that an organization has an overall mission that defines the nature of its activities. The long-term survival of an organization depends on the ability to create and sustain several operating cycles. By this we mean the ability to:

1. Translate the organization's mission into operating goals and objectives
2. Assess the demand for services it intends to provide
3. Transform or convert resources into a patient care product or service and deliver that service in a method that satisfies patients
4. Realize an amount from the "sale" of those services that is adequate to replenish resources that were used up in the process, thus allowing the cycle to repeat itself

Figure 23.1 depicts an operating cycle.

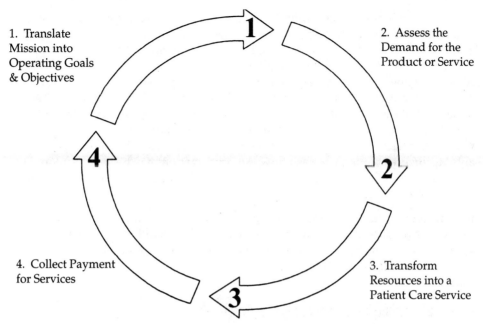

1. Translate Mission into Operating Goals & Objectives

2. Assess the Demand for the Product or Service

4. Collect Payment for Services

3. Transform Resources into a Patient Care Service

Figure 23.1 Operating cycle. Copyright UAB Hospital, University of Alabama, Birmingham. Reprinted with permission.

The translation of an organization's mission into concrete goals is a function of the strategic planning process. Key considerations in the strategic plan are *(1)* how well it reflects the realities of the external environment and *(2)* how it seeks to respond to that environment.

A second feature of the cycle, demand for services, depends on the health status of the community and how health status is recognized and translated into demand, a topic that is beyond the scope of this chapter. The strategic planning process should help to define the type of demand that is to be met to determine what services will be provided. Once this has been agreed to, the budgeting process is used to forecast demand and to determine the appropriate mix of resources necessary to meet that demand. One thing we do know about demand is that in recent years, changes in reimbursement have made health care more competitive; that is, the demand for services is much more sensitive to the prices charged. The section on reimbursement elaborates on this topic.

Nurse executives are most directly involved and therefore should be most influential in the process steps of transforming resources and delivering services. Their decisions along with other departments will determine the ultimate cost of services and the pricing structure. In the absence of philanthropy or other sources of revenue, charges for services must reflect underlying costs if the organization is to recover enough resources to enable it to continue to do business.

The final step in the process, collecting payment for services, is generally not within the purview of nurse executives. However, the success of this activity has a significant influence on cash flow and overall availability of resources to the organization. We will not spend time on this area except to note that the inability to collect revenue on a timely basis may result in an increased cost burden of uncompensated care and interest expense. If the organization must borrow money to pay its bills until the patients pay their bills, it will have less flexibility in operating existing programs or initiating new ones. Some parts of the organization will be charged with reducing the "number of days revenue in accounts receivable" to ensure an adequate cash flow. An organization may be successful in delivering services in a cost-efficient manner but it will not survive if it is not able to collect for services on a timely basis.

Understanding the basic concept of the operating cycle is fundamental to any manager who must function within it or who wishes to influence the process. This section concludes with a discussion of accounting terms and concepts. Those who are comfortable with these concepts already may wish to go on to the next section.

Financial Accounting and Managerial Accounting

The purpose of the **financial accounting** system, simply stated, is to keep track of resources and to make periodic reports summarizing financial transactions. This system has as its goal meeting the internal needs of top management in assessing the overall position of the organization or the reporting requirements of external agencies such as bondholders, other major creditors, or major purchasers.

Managerial accounting builds off the same information collected for financial accounting purposes, but its goal is to provide information that is aggregated at different levels of the organization. A management accounting system should allow individual managers to focus on the activities that affect their areas of responsibility. Standards for financial accounting reports are often defined by external agencies and may be industry specific to ensure comparability. On the other hand, managerial accounting formats are usually internally determined by the needs of the managers and administrators. The capability of the financial information system and the degree to which those who design the information systems understand the needs of line managers and administrators are important factors in the overall utility of the management accounting system.

Assets, Liabilities, Revenues, and Expenses

An **asset** is an item that has value to the organization because of its potential to satisfy a demand. Assets are categorized by their "liquidity," that is, how quickly they can be converted to cash in the even that cash or cash equivalent resources are needed to remain in business. Buildings and equipment, also referred to as "fixed assets," are the least liquid because they are usually specialized for a particular provider and are the most difficult to convert to cash without losing some of their book value.

Liabilities represent debts or amounts owed. They arise because most organizations do not operate on a cash basis; that is, they may delay payment to vendors beyond the usual payment period allowed or they may borrow money for short periods of time to meet current obligations, such as buying supplies or paying salaries. They may borrow for longer periods of time to acquire equipment or buildings. The concept of assets and liabilities allows an entity to record as assets the cost of resources to which they have legal title, even if they are not fully paid for; liabilities represent amounts owed on an asset such as the balance of a mortgage. The difference between total assets and total liabilities is referred to as "net worth." Net worth increases either because assets appreciate in value or because they were used to produce revenue that exceeds the value of the asset that was consumed in its production. Those concerned with the performance of an organization will be interested in evaluating assets, liabilities, and net worth at a particular point, as well as from period to period, to determine whether the changes in these items represent an improvement or deterioration in financial condition. A situation where liabilities exceed assets, that is, a negative net worth, may mean that creditors will be less willing to provide resources to the organization without some additional assurance that they will recover their investment. They may do so only if the organization is willing to pay a premium, such as a higher interest rate or cash in advance. Both approaches add to the cost of doing business and, based on price, make it more difficult to compete.

Revenue refers to the amounts recognized from the sale of a product or service. In health care, the term "sale" is not generally used to refer to the delivery of professional services. **Gross revenue** is the price that is charged for the item. Note that the recording of revenue in the accounting records is a separate process from the actual recording of the cash that is ultimately received. The difference between these two numbers provides useful information for management that would otherwise be lost if we measured revenue in terms of cash received. The difference between gross revenue and cash received may be due to discounts negotiated with purchasers or uncompensated care, which itself may have a variety of sources. The causes of the amounts "written off" should be evaluated to determine whether they are justified because these items reduce available cash.

Expenses are recognized as the value of assets are used up or consumed to produce services or products. For example, as supplies are taken from inventory for use in patient care, they are recognized in the accounting records as expenses. Accounting for the expenses associated with wages and salaries is slightly different. Human resources are not generally recorded as assets on the books. Once an individual is hired and is performing the work of the organization, two accounting transactions occur simultaneously: a liability for wages is incurred during a pay period and the asset that is technically being purchased in increments of payroll hours is recognized as an expense without ever appearing on the books as an asset.

Recognizing the expense associated with the use of buildings and equipment, which have useful lives of several years, is accomplished by the concept of depreciation or amortization. **Depreciation** reflects the gradual deterioration of a fixed asset and allows the organization to recognize its costs gradually over the life of the asset. A simple example is one in which a $10,000,000 piece of equipment with a 10-year life represents a "straight line" depreciation expense of $1,000,000 per year that must be recognized as a cost and included in the prices charged for services. Depreciation may be accelerated in some cases, allowing the cost to be recovered faster. To reduce the need to borrow money and incur interest expense when equipment and buildings need to be replaced, some organizations will **"fund depreciation."** This means that the price charged for a service reflects depreciation expense, and cash realized from the revenue that is generated is set aside to be used to replace the item when it becomes fully depreciated.

Revenue Centers and Cost Centers

Patient billing is frequently based on a "fee-for-service" system; that is, a separate charge is made for each item of professional or ancillary service to the patient. A revenue center is any item that makes a charge for service. For example, separate charges will usually be made for laboratory tests, pharmacy items, operating room use, and respiratory therapy services. These departments are distinguished from "cost centers," which do not issue a separate charge for their services. In the past, increases in costs or expansions in services in these departments were justified by the ability to increase prices. These include, for example, housekeeping, maintenance, dietary, and registration. The cost of these services must be allocated to the revenue-producing departments so that they can be reflected in and recovered through the pricing structure. Is nursing service a revenue center? Generally, not unless the service is billed as a separate item; instead, its cost is included under charges for "routine services," which includes a variety of costs.

The issue of revenue centers and cost centers may become less important if the fee-for-service method of reimbursement is replaced by a single charge for each admission to the hospital or each visit to an outpatient clinic, regardless of services performed. One major payer, Medicare, has already implemented this approach for inpatients. If this method were implemented for all payers, there would be little reason to allocate overhead costs to the traditional revenue-producing departments. All departments would then need to focus on improving internal efficiency. Institution-wide incentives would exist to decrease rather than expand procedures.

The Fiscal Year

Simply recording transactions, as is done by the financial accounting system, will have little meaning unless a time period is specified. A fiscal year is a 12-month period for which transactions are summarized. It does not necessarily need to coincide with a calendar year. Although a business may intend to be in operation indefinitely, establishing a fiscal year reporting period allows owners or trustees to make an assessment of its effectiveness and financial performance at regular intervals. As previously noted, in many cases, annual financial statements are more than a convenience and may be required by external parties. Although not legally required to do so, many organizations break the year down further into quarterly or monthly reporting periods so that results of operations can be assessed and corrective action can be taken on a more timely basis.

Accrual Accounting

Establishment of a fiscal reporting period requires that, for accounting purposes, we behave as if the business were "closed out" at the end of the period. Every attempt is made to reflect all revenue that has been generated as of the end of the period, even though, in fact, it may not actually be recorded until a later time. For example, if revenue from a patient bill is not recorded until the patient is discharged, revenue would not be recorded in the proper period. Accrual accounting requires that the records be adjusted to reflect revenue "as if" the patient had been discharged at the end of the reporting period. The same procedures apply to recording expenses. All significant expenses must be estimated for the period in which they occur, even though the paper work may not be available until sometime after the year end. This means that the organization "holds the books open" until all these expenses can be documented or reasonably estimated. A good example of an accrued expense, also referred to as a liability, is payroll expense. Quite often, the date of payment does not fall neatly at the end of a fiscal period. The portion of the payroll paid after the end of the period that applies to the prior period is accrued into the period where it was actually incurred. Accruing revenues and expenses into the proper fiscal period allows for "matching" of revenues and expenses in the period to which they apply. This adjustment is important if performance is to be compared from period to period.

REIMBURSEMENT METHODS

In the 1990s, health care administrators at all levels felt besieged to reduce costs after years of an expansion that far exceeded the rate of growth in the rest of the economy. Budgets have become more stringent. Practices long established for the organization and delivery of patient care are now being challenged by those who pay the bills. A brief review of the old reimbursement rules is important in understanding how to adapt to the new.

An important feature of health care reimbursement is that most patients are not usually directly responsible for paying the cost of health care. Major third-party payers have assumed this responsibility. These include:

- Medicare, a federal program for patients 65 and over and for individuals who are disabled
- Medicaid, a program financed jointly by the state and federal government for patients who meet tests of low-income levels; eligibility and types of services provided often vary by state.
- A number of commercial insurance companies provide coverage for various

services to individuals either through their employment, as fringe benefits, or as individual policy holders.

- Blue Cross (for hospital service)/Blue Shield (for physician services) provides "group" coverage, generally through an employment relationship as a fringe benefit. Blue Cross is distinguished from commercial insurers because it contracts with individual hospitals that agree to treat patients at reimbursement rates and rules agreed to in advance.

Today's health care reimbursement landscape is diverse and constantly changing at the national and regional levels. Depending on the area of the country in which you live there are differences in reimbursement plans. Regardless of geographical location, the majority of the changes in health care delivery are driven by the increase in managed care penetration.

Whenever an industry is affected by global economic changes it can expect the core businesses to feel a significant impact. The health care industry is no exception. An economic strategy to deal with the escalation of health care expenditures has been the development of managed care systems that emphasize reductions in cost and services.

The impact of managed care has been a major factor in the redesign of the health care delivery system. These new systems have swept the nation as health care providers, such as hospitals and home health care agencies, restructure in response to the changing reimbursement structures. It is expected that managed care systems, such as prepaid group practice plans (capitation), preferred provider organizations (PPOs), provider service organizations (PSOs), integrated service networks (ISNs), independent practice associations (IPAs), and health maintenance organizations (HMOs), will continue to proliferate. More than 100 million people currently are enrolled in managed care programs in the United States (Winslow, 1996).

Wagner (1996) describes the most frequent health care reimbursement structures by the following categories:

- Prospective payment systems
- Per diem
- Managed indemnity
- Capitation

Prospective Payment System

Prospective payment systems are primarily represented by the Medicare program. Medicare's current system of acute care reimbursement was implemented in the early 1980s. This system provides hospitals a preset payment amount for patients based on their discharge diagnoses or diagnostic related group (DRG). Under this system, hospitals that are able to manage their patients' cost below the preset amount are allowed to retain the balance. However, if the cost for the care of these patients exceeds the preset amounts, hospitals must absorb the additional costs incurred. This system has led to dramatic decreases in hospital lengths of stay and increased utilization of postacute care alternatives such as home care, long-term care, and most recently subacute care.

Although this system of payment was initiated by the Health Care Finance Administration (HCFA), it did not take long for other third-party payers to adopt DRG-like systems for reimbursement. Although there are variations in the prospective payment systems for each sector of health care, the basic financial incentive for hospitals remains increased volume and decreased patient days.

Per Diem

The per diem reimbursement structure is used primarily by HMOs. The payers reimburse an acute care facility based on a set rate per day rather than on charges. Reimbursement may vary by service (e.g., medical-surgical, obstetrics, mental health, and intensive care) or can be uniformly applied regardless of intensity of services. For example, with hospitalization, an HMO will adopt utilization management and case management strategies to ensure that the patients are appropriately admitted, that their continued stay is based on the need for clinical services, and that those services are provided in a timely manner. Although they generally pay for each inpatient day, many insurers manage those inpatient days by not paying for any inactivity where the patient no longer meets their clinical criteria.

Indemnity Plans

Managed indemnity plans, sometimes referred to as managed fee-for-service, are usually based on the costs incurred by the health care provider. Basically, the payers reimburse the provider for some percentage of the billed charges. The perceived success of HMOs and other types of managed care organizations is in the control of the utilization and cost of health services. This control has prompted the development of managed overlays that can be combined with traditional indemnity insurance, service plan insurance, or self-insurance. Managed care overlays provide cost control for insured plans while retaining the individuals' freedom of choice of provider and coverage for out-of-plan services.

Historically, indemnity plans paid the hospital the charges billed based on a predetermined agreement. In recent years, these plans have attempted to manage their risk by adding management strategies such as utilization management and case management, once found only in HMOs.

Capitation

The term capitation is the last form of reimbursement to be discussed. *Capitation* is a set amount of money received or paid out. It is based on individual membership rather than on services delivered and usually is expressed in per member per month (PMPM) units.

This fairly new type of reimbursement methodology has had a significant impact on the delivery of health care. Some of these changes have been positive, some not so positive. For example, in the previously described reimbursement strategies, the hospital's financial incentive was volume of admissions and decreased length of stay. In the world of capitation, the financial incentive is to decrease volume of admissions. On the other hand, the entire budgetary process for most acute care hospitals is based on volume and patient days. An increase in admissions and patient days, for all other reimbursement structures, yields an increase in revenue.

In capitation, there continues to be an incentive to decrease length of stay, although the prevention of an admission becomes the primary concern for acute care providers. Under these circumstances, the line between the incentives for the provider and the health plan become blurred and providers begin to act more like health plans as they work to manage their financial risk.

When health care providers are paid a preset amount for the provision of care for their patients, the focus begins to be on maintaining wellness and keeping patients out of the high cost center acute care facilities. To accomplish that end, many health delivery systems focus their attention, and their health care dollars, on prevention and alternatives to the acute care providers such as home care, adult day care, subacute care, and so on. This allows the providers a financial incentive to creatively develop programs that increase quality of care and quality of life outcomes for patient populations as well as fostering goodwill within the community.

Today, the fastest growing capitated enrollment is with the population eligible for Medicare. In 1985, in an effort to curb spending in the Medicare program, HCFA developed Medicare risk programs. In these programs, the HMOs receive a percentage of the actuarial estimate of what it would have typically reimbursed a health care provider or practitioner for coverage of services. HMOs, in turn, contract with providers and pay a PMPM fee. In 1991, only 2.2% of all Medicare beneficiaries were enrolled in managed care plans. In 1998, the number has increased to 13% and is projected to nearly triple, to 35%, by the year 2007 (Health Care Financing Administration, 1997). These increases present special challenges for care delivery systems as they provide health and wellness as well as disease management strategies for elderly populations with multiple chronic illnesses.

In summary, reimbursement structures are constantly changing as insurers, whether government or private, strive to curtail the increasing cost of health care. The leadership challenge will be to ensure the best clinical outcomes while providing value to patients. As responsible health care leaders it is necessary to not only be fiscally responsible but to also be aware of how these health care reimbursement structures affect patients. Health care leaders must continue to manage globally while remaining focused on the needs of individuals.

BUDGETING AND MONITORING RESULTS

This section provides a generalized overview of the budgeting process. Finkler (1996) describes several types of budgets. The budgets covered in this section include the operating, program/product line, capital, and cash types.

A budget is a plan that provides a formal document of what the organization hopes to accomplish and it assists managers in accomplishing the goals and objectives. The budgeting process in any organization will depend on the mission, structure, and culture of an organization, as much as it will depend on formalized mechanical steps involved in budget preparation and use. Given the uniqueness of each institution's budget process, the following section is intended to focus more on budget concepts than on step-by-step mechanics.

Definition and Use of Budgets

A budget is a plan for identifying expected resource expenditures as well as sources of funding or revenue. This plan becomes a formalized document that represents management's intentions and expectations. The budget is used in planning, monitoring, motivating, and communicating expectations (Finkler, 1996).

Planning

Preparation of a budget forces the organization to plan for the future. Forecasting future resource needs allows an organization to respond by anticipating changes rather than reacting to them. A well-prepared budget facilitates the managers' ability to accomplish stated goals within their departments. Careful budgeting also provides an opportunity for a manager to maximize judgment and leadership skills in assisting the organization to accomplish its mission.

Monitoring and Motivation

The budget serves an important role in monitoring the use of resources and in measuring a manager's performance as it relates to the effectiveness of the planning process. The budget can also serve as a motivating tool for managers. However, for the budget to be an effective motivational tool there must be some type of reward for those managers who exceed expectations in planning and monitoring resources. To provide an incentive for gaining additional knowledge in the budgeting process, many organizations are providing a monetary reward to managers who have mastered these skills.

Communication

Another purpose of a budget is to serve as a coordination and communication vehicle within an organization. For example, individuals must work collectively to understand how their department objectives work on behalf of the entire organization. If the hospital finance officer, the medical staff, and the nurse executive are not communicating patient care needs relative to either increases in volume or changes in technology then there will be a lack of coordination and effective budget planning. The process of budget preparation brings information together in a structured method and informs staff of what is needed and expected. Again, the budget provides a target and plan for managers and staff to achieve goals and objectives.

Operating Budgets

The operating budget is a day-to-day management tool and usually covers a period of 1 year. This budget includes the revenues expected from payer sources and the expenses associated with providing services.

Program/Product Line Budgets

The program/product line budgets are special budgeting methods for analyzing and evaluating specific areas. For example, a large ambulatory clinic may have a need for laboratory service for a large number of specialty clinics. A program budget, in this case, would focus on all the costs and benefits associated with laboratory services. In the case of a product line the same principal applies. For example, a center that is trying to focus on the maintenance or development of an oncology product line would focus on all the costs and benefits of all the oncology-related services within the organization or system.

Unlike an operating budget or capital budget that focuses on the coming year, these budgets combine detailed information and long range planning for one specific program/product line. They examine all components of a budget rather than simply looking at the merits of the incremental costs of this year compared with last year. This is especially helpful when a cost accounting system is in place that assists the organization in understanding the profit and loss associated with a program or service.

Capital Budgets

The capital budget is associated with replacement or addition of buildings and equipment. Costs associated with capital budgets are referred to as capital expenditures and generally have a lifetime of more than 1 year. In addition, most organizations have a minimum cost requirement that may range from $500 to $700 for an item to be included in the capital budget.

Because capital expenditures frequently concern large amounts of money, they require careful analysis. The starting point in the capital budgeting process is the generation of proposed investments. Proposals may be direct or indirect to a particular manager. For example, a direct proposal may include the renovation of several patient care rooms on a nursing unit. An indirect proposal might include the purchase of a piece of equipment by another department that assists in decreasing nursing time for a patient care procedure.

After proposals are generated the next step is the evaluation process. This process will require significant collection of data that can be used to justify the proposed financial, patient, or organization benefits. The data analysis should identify the amount of cash that will be spent or received each year over the life of the investment and the financial return to the organization. The analysis may also assist in verifying how patients will benefit from technology enhancements. Organizations can also identify how the data will demonstrate an increase in volume or revenue.

Cash Budgets

The cash budget forecasts the sources and uses of cash and is the lifeline of any organization. The survival of any entity depends on the ability to maintain an adequate supply of cash to meet monetary obligations. Examples of expenses that are paid frequently are employee salaries. These are typically paid at least monthly or biweekly as opposed to revenue collection, which may take several months. Without careful management of cash an organization, even one that appears to be growing in volume, can go bankrupt.

It is important to keep in mind the interrelationship of these budgets; however, we will focus here on the operating budget because this is where nurse executives' knowledge of the patient care process should be most valuable.

RESOURCE MANAGEMENT SYSTEM

Hospitals today are complex organizations that are faced with the challenge of balancing shrinking reimbursement levels with the requirement to deliver quality customer-focused patient care. Nursing services must ensure that the care delivered is appropriate to the patient's need and that the nursing care is scientifically based and technologically sound. In such an environment, the development of comprehensive resource management system (RMS) is imperative to the formulation of a timely response to ever-changing service demands and variable financial reimbursement packages. In a highly regulated environment, an RMS not only meets the requirements of external accrediting agencies but also responds to internal budget constraints and service demand.

A comprehensive RMS complies with the performance standards of the Joint Commission on Accreditation of Healthcare Organizations, the professional standards of the American Nurses Association, and individual state regulations. Consumer expectations must be addressed given the major impact that nursing care has on patient and family attitudes toward a particular health care organization, their services and employees. In addition, the quality of nursing care and patient satisfaction with nursing care is frequently used to market an organization to a broad spectrum of consumers.

Definition/Outcomes of a Resource Management System

An RMS is a structured approach to the dynamic process of identifying and allocating resources in the most effective and efficient manner (Nash, Kuklunski, Sparks, & Knipher, 1998). Integral to the success of a RMS is the accountability for, monitoring of, and benchmarking of resource consumption. Successful management of the demand and supply of all resources requires a perspective targeted to conserving resources.

To develop a comprehensive methodology for the deployment of nursing services, the nurse executive must be able to budget appropriately and provide for the resource requirement of patients in a variety of settings. As a result, methods to measure patient needs, case mix, or acuity are important for financial and quality assessment. The following section describes the benefits and principles of an RMS. The example is focused on an acute care setting but the philosophy and methods can be applied to a variety of settings.

A comprehensive RMS will define nursing resources required by isolating the unit of service as well as intensity of service as measured by patient acuity. The development of the RMS will generally occur in phases and may include assessment, development, implementation, and outcome measurement. The following briefly describes the various phases.

Assessment activities include, but are not limited to, reviewing historical trends related to patient acuity and census, unit activity and staffing patterns; identifying the potential impact of advances in clinical programs and their associated technology; and gathering data on the educational and experiential level of the staff. In addition, the unit size, location, and geographical layout as well as the care delivery model often influence nursing resource utilization.

Development of the RMS entails establishing unit-based nursing care hours in light of internal and external benchmarking activities and staffing and scheduling modification. Interviewing the staff and nurse managers for their input on the development of the system usually identifies related concerns and offers an additional opportunity for clarification of the purpose of the RMS. The integration of the staffing approach with the existing patient care delivery model based don the information gathered during the assessment phase further supports the development phases of the process.

The *implementation* phase of a comprehensive RMS involves the modification of the unit-based budget to meet the identified patient care needs. Clear, concise communication and ongoing educational sessions are a must to keep nurse managers, administrators, and physicians on target to meet the financial objectives of the system. Written reports of data such as operating statistics and productivity indices guide variance analysis and the monitoring of nursing hours and cost per day.

MODEL OF A RESOURCE MANAGEMENT SYSTEM

A systems approach to resource management is a productivity concept and involves identifying system inputs, system throughputs, and system outputs, which are discussed further in Chapter 24. The resources an organization takes in from the environment are called *system inputs* and include resources such as the average daily census, type of service, and method of patient classification. *Throughputs* are the organizational resources used to produce or monitor system outputs. System throughputs might include variable staffing plans, benchmarking data, or productivity reports. Throughputs moderate the process of environmental inputs becoming *organizational outputs*. The organization outputs of patients, staff, and physician satisfaction are often the result of the successful transformation of personnel inputs into the perception of quality organizational outcomes (i.e., output), as shown in Figure 23.2.

After an organization determines the level and type of services it will provide, the nurse executive and managers must be actively involved in leading the process to determine nursing resource needs. With the development of an RMS that focuses on a consistent approach to organizational staffing, scheduling, policies, and procedures, it is possible to predict for and deliver the "right people, to the right place at the right time." A comprehensive patient-driven system approach is necessary in today's health care environment if we are going to consistently delivery quality, cost-effective patient care.

Benefits of a Resource Management System

Regardless of the method chosen, the impact of developing an efficient RMS can result in several important benefits as identified by Cavouras and McKinley (1998):

- Cost-effective flexible budget planning
- Increased productivity

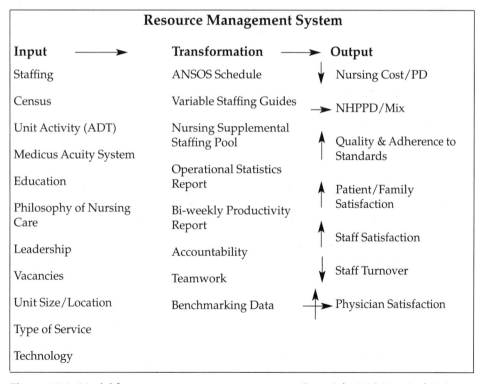

Figure 23.2 Model for resource management system. Copyright UAB Hospital, University of Alabama, Birmingham. Reprinted with permission

- Establishment of criteria for recruitment
- Establishment of criteria for development of staffing patterns
- Establishment of criteria for performance appraisal

The most important implication for nursing leaders, generally, is the establishment of an objective, quantitative base from which to manage a unit/department. Once an RMS is developed and justified, basic planning of budget and program activities may begin, and daily activities can be managed at optimal cost effectiveness and quality, regardless of census fluctuations.

Principles of Resource Management

Every resource management system will be developed to meet the unique needs of the organization. Regardless of the differences in each organization, Cavouras and McKinley (1998) describe the basic principles of an RMS as:

- Patient care cannot be postponed.
- Experienced staff must be available at all times.
- Collaboration is essential.
- Employees are valued.
- Staff prefer not to be reassigned from home unit.
- Costs must continue to be stable or decrease.
- Staff need on less desirable shifts has increased.
- Degree of centralization and decentralization must be operationally clear.
- Comparative data are required for learning and change.
- Census will continue to decrease and be erratic.
- Increased staff flexibility is necessary and desirable.

Nursing Unit of Service: Care Hours Per Day

Determination of a unit of service will depend on the type of setting in which nursing care will be delivered. For example, in an acute care hospital, activities for nursing units are based on the patient days as well as on the hours of care required for that patient population. In an outpatient setting, the unit of service might be measured by number and time needed by visit or procedure.

The ability to accurately determine core staffing needs per patient day is essential to the success of an RMS. Core staff are the number of full-time equivalent employees (FTEs) required to deliver a schedule that provides sufficient staff to meet the patient care needs identified by the nursing care hours per patient day (NHPPD). Finkler (1992) defines the FTE as the standardization of all hours worked based on scheduled formula of 8 hours per day, 5 days per week for 52 weeks. Several points should be considered when identifying the number of FTEs required to meet the desired nursing care hours per patient day: patient care units have a discoverable pattern of staffing needs; the scope and duration of the variations in the demand for nursing care hours are measurable; and the core staffing level must be clearly stated for each clinical business unit.

Figure 23.3 identifies the demand for care at various patient census levels in relation to a core staffing pattern. This schematic illustrates the relationship between unit staffing levels and patient census. Core staffing meets the care demand for the average daily or *certain* census. Core staffing usually also includes the ability to meet the most frequent or *probable* level of care activities based on patient census data. Depending on the organization's overall ability to flex up in *possibly* high or *peak* census times, core staffing might have to be adjusted upward. Determining the most frequent daily patient census along with the scope and duration of patient care demands is important to the identification of the variance in census-specific staffing needs. Although core staffing requirements can focus on the average daily census, the most frequent census should be used to determine core staffing on units where the ability to flex up is limited by personnel or time constraints. If a unit cannot easily respond to a fluctuating census with the necessary additional personnel resources and the unit is not financially prepared to staff at the level of the most frequent census, an organizational response to the need should be developed. The centralized RMS strives to provide personnel resources to those patient care areas that cannot meet their own episodic and short-term demand for an increase in core staffing. Therefore, the financial goals of a centralized RMS are to stabilize the unit's resource response at each census level, to be cost predictive (by using nonpremium pay strategies), and to keep revenue and expenses relatively stable through census-sensitive fluctuations in patient care demand and service variation.

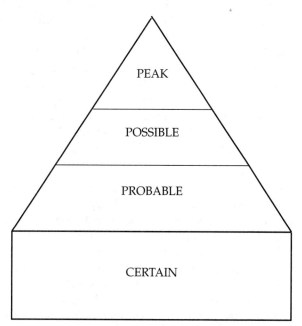

Figure 23.3 Patient care demand pattern schematic. Copyright Lawrenz Consulting. Reprinted with permission.

When any member of the core staff is absent and using nonproductive time off (e.g., vacation, education, sick time) their hours must be replaced to deliver a consistent level of care. In most hospital operating budgets dollars are provided to pay for benefit time. These are the necessary productive hours needed to maintain a consistent level of care. Usually an average of 12% of the total salary budget is used as a proxy for determining the benefit budget for an individual cost center. Historical use patterns are also helpful in determining the desired nonproductive percentage. This percentage may vary based on such things as the number of experienced staff or leave of absences.

The dollars available in each cost center budget to replace paid nonproductive time are usually accrued each payroll based on a formula that considers each employee's allotted vacation and holiday time. The estimated amounts are usually based on historical averages. Some operating budgets also account for expense associated with the replacement staff for leave of absences.

If an organization is methodical in identifying dollars to cover deficit demand, there will be no need for extra resource dollars during the budget year unless volume exceeds budget projections. It is important that each cost center manager be involved in the development of the resource budget and be accountable for the monitoring of the budget according to the aforementioned parameters. Figure 23.4 is an example of a format that could be used to assist managers in tracing resource/expense data.

An important activity for an individual cost center is the ability to monitor expenses. Reports that compare actual resource use to budgeted resource allocation support the financial monitoring activity. Management tools, such as the biweekly operating summary seen in Figure 23.5 include information on dollars, FTEs, and hours per patient day. The biweekly operating summary also provides nurse managers with the necessary unit activity and census data such as budgeted and actual patient days for the pay period. The financial data reported in the summary addresses productive and nonproductive hours as well as direct and indirect costs. The biweekly operating summary assists both the cost center manager and administrative staff in the review of unit performance and variance monitoring.

Another financial management tool that assists nurse managers to understand the reasons for variances in staffing needs and their related costs is the operating statistics report (Figure 23.6). This report focuses on patient day statistics such as weekday versus weekend census and unit activity levels such as the number of daily admissions, discharges and transfers. In addition, the operating statistics report details variance by unit, FTEs, overtime, skill mix, the use of staff from the nursing resource pool, and education and orientation costs. This report along with the biweekly operating summary provides the nurse manager with the data needed to identify the cause(s) of the most budget variances and the information to either justify or correct them, as appropriate.

OPERATING STATISTICS

UNIT	NM	RN	LPN	NA/PCA	PCT/DCT	US	USS/UH	OTHERS	Education FTEs	Dollars	$$/PD	Orientation FTEs	Dollars	SS/PD	Orientation Acct Usage FTEs	Dollars
6911—5NE	0.0	1.8	1.8	1.3	0.0	1.0	0.0	0.0	0.0	16	0.17	0.0	0	0.00	0.0	0
6915—4E/4W	1.0	3.6	0.0	0.0	1.5	0.7	1.0	0.0	0.0	45	0.14	0.0	0	0.00	0.0	0
6928—SCN	0.0	0.7	0.0	0.0	0.6	1.1	0.0	0.0	0.0	26	0.18	0.0	0	0.00	0.0	0
6942—CCU	0.0	3.5	0.0	1.7	0.0	1.0	0.0	0.0	0.2	101	0.58	0.2	194	1.11	1.1	1,536
6943—HTICU	0.0	6.7	0.0	2.8	0.0	1.1	0.0	1.0	0.0	112	0.46	0.0	0	0.00	1.6	2,407
6953—CICU	0.0	10.0	0.0	0.0	3.6	0.0	0.0	0.0	0.0	36	0.26	0.0	0	0.00	0.2	124
6971—CCN	0.0	2.0	0.0	0.0	2.6	1.5	0.0	1.0	0.0	76	0.14	0.0	0	0.00	1.4	1,750
6973—RNICU	1.0	8.1	0.0	0.0	2.6	0.8	1.0	5.1	0.0	86	0.26	0.0	0	0.00	2.6	3,309
6974—CVN	0.0	3.5	0.0	0.2	0.0	0.0	0.0	0.0	0.0	0	0.00	0.0	0	0.00	0.0	0
7401—6S	0.0	2.8	0.0	0.0	2.2	1.1	2.8	0.0	1.2	83	0.24	1.2	1,783	5.27	0.4	737
7408—5N	1.0	9.3	0.0	0.0	2.0	0.9	1.0	0.0	0.5	18	0.07	0.5	635	2.62	0.0	0
7422—8C GYN	0.0	0.5	0.0	0.0	0.0	0.4	0.0	0.0	0.0	1	0.01	0.0	0	0.00	0.0	0
Totals & Avgs	3.0	52.5	1.8	6.0	15.1	9.6	5.8	7.1	1.9	598	0.22	1.9	2,611	0.97	7.3	9,863

Figure 23.4 Operating statistics; vacancies/orientation information. Copyright UAB Hospital, University of Alabama, Birmingham. Reprinted with permission.

OPERATING SUMMARY (Productive Sections and Volume)

UNIT	Prod $$		Prod FTEs		Prod HPPD		VOLUME			
	Bud $/PD	Act $/PD	Flex Bud TAR	ACT FTEs	BUD	ACT	Bud Pt Days	Act Pt Days	Bud ADC	Act ADC
6911—5NE	159.3	189.1	14.0	11.7	11.6	9.9	112	94	8.0	6.7
6915—4E/4W	143.7	119.9	39.2	34.7	9.9	8.4	280	329	20.0	23.5
6928—SCN	158.8	141.1	19.3	15.4	11.3	8.7	112	142	8.0	10.1
6942—CCU	298.1	389.6	41.8	46.9	19.2	21.5	189	174	13.5	12.4
6943—HTICU	270.7	275.4	48.7	49.2	15.9	16.1	266	245	19.0	17.5
6949—ICVU	206.0	242.9	17.3	16.5	14.1	13.6	114	97	10.4	8.8
6953—CICU	393.7	430.3	40.6	41.3	23.0	23.5	196	141	14.0	10.1
6971—CCN	166.9	156.3	71.9	63.1	11.0	9.3	392	542	28.0	38.7
6973—RNICU	369.9	275.6	87.3	64.3	22.3	15.7	263	327	18.8	23.4
6974—CVN	226.2	410.7	4.2	4.8	18.1	23.9	42	16	3.0	2.7
7401—6S	179.9	181.5	54.5	54.2	12.9	12.8	371	338	26.5	24.1
7405—5S	148.0	177.0	31.2	27.0	11.7	10.2	224	212	16.0	15.1
7408—5N	192.2	162.5	37.9	31.4	12.9	10.4	217	242	15.5	17.3
7422—8C GYN	226.0	236.9	18.6	17.7	14.8	14.1	102	100	7.3	7.1
Tot & Averages	222.8	213.4	526.4	478.2	14.6	12.8	2,879	2,999	207.9	217.6

Figure 23.5 Operating summary (productive sections and volume. Copyright UAB Hospital, University of Alabama, Birmingham. Reprinted with permission.

OPERATING STATISTICS

<table>
<tr><th></th><th colspan="7">PATIENT STATISTICS</th></tr>
<tr><th></th><th></th><th></th><th></th><th></th><th colspan="2">Average Census</th><th></th></tr>
<tr><th>UNIT</th><th>ADT Index</th><th>LOS</th><th>Effective Daily Census</th><th>Avg. Midnight Census</th><th>Weekday</th><th>Weekend</th><th>Average Acuity</th></tr>
<tr><td>6911—5NE</td><td>108.5%</td><td>2.2</td><td>6.7</td><td>6.7</td><td>7.6</td><td>4.5</td><td>1.67</td></tr>
<tr><td>6915—4E/4W</td><td>79.6%</td><td>2.7</td><td>23.3</td><td>23.5</td><td>24.8</td><td>20.3</td><td>1.09</td></tr>
<tr><td>6928—SCN</td><td>153.5%</td><td>1.4</td><td>10.4</td><td>10.1</td><td>10.5</td><td>9.3</td><td>1.24</td></tr>
<tr><td>6942—CCU</td><td>58.0%</td><td>3.9</td><td>13.0</td><td>12.4</td><td>12.7</td><td>11.8</td><td>2.78</td></tr>
<tr><td>6943—HTICU</td><td>26.1%</td><td>11.7</td><td>16.6</td><td>17.5</td><td>17.7</td><td>17.0</td><td>2.29</td></tr>
<tr><td>6953—CICU</td><td>61.0%</td><td>141.0</td><td>7.3</td><td>10.1</td><td>11.3</td><td>7.0</td><td>2.96</td></tr>
<tr><td>6971—CCN</td><td>20.7%</td><td>28.5</td><td>36.4</td><td>38.7</td><td>38.7</td><td>38.8</td><td>1.39</td></tr>
<tr><td>6973—RNICU</td><td>35.8%</td><td>29.7</td><td>20.1</td><td>23.4</td><td>23.4</td><td>23.3</td><td>2.61</td></tr>
<tr><td>6974—CVN</td><td>112.5%</td><td>2.3</td><td>2.6</td><td>2.7</td><td>2.8</td><td>2.5</td><td>1.86</td></tr>
<tr><td>7401—6S</td><td>82.5%</td><td>2.7</td><td>24.8</td><td>24.1</td><td>24.3</td><td>23.8</td><td>1.49</td></tr>
<tr><td>7408—5N</td><td>52.1%</td><td>4.5</td><td>16.7</td><td>17.3</td><td>17.4</td><td>17.0</td><td>1.10</td></tr>
<tr><td>7422—8C GYN</td><td>77.0%</td><td>2.8</td><td>6.7</td><td>7.1</td><td>7.8</td><td>5.5</td><td>1.23</td></tr>
<tr><td>Totals & Avgs</td><td>58.1%</td><td>4.6</td><td>184.5</td><td>193.7</td><td>199.0</td><td>180.5</td><td>1.81</td></tr>
</table>

Figure 23.6 Operating statistics (patient statistics). Copyright UAB Hospital, University of Alabama, Birmingham. Reprinted with permission.

There are no national groups or professional associations that solely monitor the supply and demand of nursing resources and against those data our institution could benchmark nursing hours/skill mix. However, institutions frequently compare data with each other.

Most benchmarking data are owned by proprietary companies with a national client base. Comparative data from the Medicus System, which measures patient acuity, can be used to compare and contrast differences in patient's hourly nursing care needs across other contracted organizations.

Patient Acuity Systems

In addition to salary cost information, it is important to measure whether the patients on a nursing unit differ in terms of patient acuity levels. Acuity is a general measure of how sick a patient is and identifies the potential needs related to nursing resources. There are several approaches to developing a classification system. Some organizations work with experts to build their own systems. The most frequent approach is the purchase of an already available system from a national firm. One example of a system used in many hospitals across the country is the Medicus Patient Classification System. Medicus assists in measuring the intensity of nursing resources required per patient. Acuity systems, in general, are useful in providing data for categorizing patient care needs and in projecting appropriate utilization of nursing personnel (Medicus, 1991). In utilizing Medicus, the RN is responsible for assessing acuity level at least once in a 24-hour day. This is done by choosing indicators such as level of consciousness, bed rest, complex intake and output, and oxygen therapy. Each indicator present is assigned a point value and the points assigned to each indicator yield a total score for each patient. Classifications are based on the total number of assigned points and range from a type I with 0 to 24 points up to a maximum of 181 points for a type VI patient, with type VI being the most acutely ill patient.

The above information is generated to determine the unit workload index and patient acuity. Although typically not used to determine staffing patterns shift to shift, these data do assist in determining trends. The workload index is a weighted census of the patient population and calculated by the daily classification score and number of patients in each category, yielding an overall patient mix. The workload index is determined by multiplying the number of patients in each category by the numerical weighing factor specific to each category and summarizing to produce a total. By using the workload index, it is possible to internally compare units with different patient populations. The workload index divided by the census gives the average daily acuity. The average daily acuity is a single measure describing the overall mix of patients on the unit. For example, the average acuity of 2.3 indicates that the average patient mix on a unit is a type IV patient.

Patient Satisfaction

One of the most pressing issues for hospital executive management teams, in today's competitive managed care marketplace, is to provide the right amount of staff, at the right time, at the right place, and for the right number of nursing hours in the least costly manner. Both nursing resource management and patient satisfaction are linked at the point of service. Patients' judgments of nursing care depend on positive perceptions of the patient care experience (Cavouras & McKinley, 1997).

Decreased length of stay has further compressed the patient care experience and blurred nursing resource consumption needs. The most recent Lawrenz Consulting (1997) survey of 104 hospitals nationwide shows length of stay continuing to decrease, particularly in the intensive care units. At the same time inpatient nursing care staff, as a percentage of total hospital staff, have remained the same or decreased. These trends suggest that the need for stabilization of patients with intensive nursing care before discharge has increased. The management of patients' complex nursing needs continues to be an important variable in the success of an organization in relation to resource management and patient satisfaction.

The patient care experience in the hospital setting becomes the ultimate test of whether the chosen approach to a resource management system is efficient for the institution and effective in providing positive patient care outcomes. To adequately evaluate the effectiveness of a resource management system there should be an assessment of its impact on patient satisfaction. The RMS should include an integration of patient satisfaction findings.

Patient satisfaction is the match between what the patient expects from the care delivery system and what is actually received. Meeting the patient's needs is the most challenging of all the patient satisfaction issues primarily due to the diversity of the population served and the complexity of nursing care required. Figure 23.7 assists nurses in understanding the relationship between hospital care delivery and staffing. Cavouras and McKinley (1997) suggest asking the following questions when evaluating patient staffing and patient satisfaction:

- Did patients and families have access to care, services, and comfort measures when they thought they needed them?
- What were the patients or families ease of doing business with hospital staff?
- Did patients or family members perceive that they were given the information and control to make decisions about their own or family members care?
- What judgment did they have about the quality of care they received?

In summary, each aspect of the RMS can be tested by specific patient satisfaction indicators of best practices. This data-driven method equates findings of the patient satisfaction survey to known aspects of resource management, such as staffing and scheduling patterns, staff mix, service demand patterns, and unit activity monitor (ADT index). All of this data can be unit specific. Asking the right

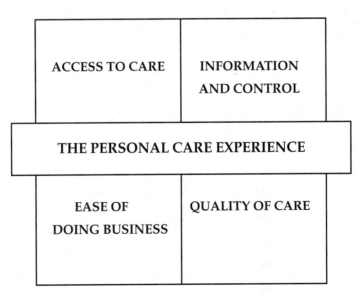

Figure 23.7 Patient satisfaction specifics. Copyright Lawrenz Consulting. Reprinted with permission.

question about patient satisfaction provides critical feedback necessary to enhance the patient care delivery processes.

SUMMARY

Managing fiscal resources implies not only authority over resources but accountability for the productive use of those resources. The task is an integral part of every manager's job. In health care, it is more challenging because of the dramatic changes that have resulted in more stringent reimbursement rules. With fewer slack resources and greater uncertainty in the new competitive environment, managers are called on to manage to "a finer tolerance." This is particularly challenging for nursing services because they provide much of the direct patient care that is the heart of the health care endeavor. To be accountable and responsive to patient needs, nurse executives must have an understanding of both the technical aspects and the larger policy environment where value judgments are made in developing assumptions and standards for the appropriate use of resources. This chapter has attempted to present the technical aspects of reimbursement, budgeting, and resource management in the context of the larger environment. Nurse executives are challenged to keep both the technical and policy aspects in mind as they assume greater roles in managing health care resources.

STUDY QUESTIONS

1. The operating cycle is an important concept. Describe the four basic cycles of an organization's operating cycle.
2. A key consideration for an organization's survival is its strategic plan. Discuss the concepts that assist in the accomplishment of an organization's financial mission through strategic planning.
3. Discuss the differences between financial and managerial accounting.
4. The development of a resource management system includes four phases. Discuss the importance of each phase in planning and coordinating resources.
5. What are the main components of the program budgeting process?

REFERENCES

Cavouras, C., & McKinley, J. (1997). Patient satisfaction. In: *Perspectives on staffing and scheduling.* (Vol. XVI, Number 6). Phoenix, AZ: Lawrenz Consulting.

Cavouras, C., & McKinley, J. (1998). Principles of resource management. In: *Perspectives on staffing and scheduling.* (Vol. XVII, Number 2). Phoenix, AZ: Lawrenz Consulting.

Finkler, S. (1992). *Budgeting concepts for nurse manager.* (2nd ed.). Philadelphia: Sanders.

Finkler, S. (1996). *The complete guide to finance and accounting for non-financial managers.* Englewood Cliffs, NJ: Prentice Hall.

Health Care Financing Administration. (1997). *Health Care Financing Review.* Washington, DC: Congressional Budget Office.

Lawrenz Consulting. (1997). Consultant to UAB Hospital, University of Alabama, Birmingham. Personal Discussion.

Medicus. (1991). *The Medicus patient classification instrument.* Chicago: Author.

Nash, M. G., Kuklinski, S., Sparks, D., & Kniphfer, K. (1998). *Development of a RMS system: An executives summary.* Unpublished manuscript, University of Alabama, Birmingham.

UAB Hospital. (1998). University of Alabama, Birmingham.

Wagner, E. R. (1996). Types of managed care organizations. In: P. R. Kongstzedt (Ed.), *Managed care handbook* (3rd ed., pp. 33–39). Gaithersburg, MD: Aspen.

Winslow, R. (1996, January 30). Health care costs were steady last year. *The Wall Street Journal,* A: 2, 20.

C H A P T E R

24

Computer Information Systems and Productivity Management

Mary L. McHugh

The concept of productivity goes far beyond the idea of gaining greater output and being efficient. (Simms, Price, & Ervin, 1994, p. 340)

Chapter Highlights

- A conceptual framework for productivity concepts
- Computer information system applications in nursing
- Clinical applications
- Efficiency and its relationship to productivity
- Data entry technology
- Care scheduling

Computer information systems are tools to support information handling activities. They can be used to facilitate nursing documentation. More importantly, they can be used to increase the efficiency and quality of nursing care. That is, they can increase nursing productivity in both clinical and administrative domains. Examples of areas that are now or could be computerized can be found in Figure 24.1. Chapter 23 provides several excellent examples of computerized financial reports.

A framework that organizes a variety of concepts concerned with "productivity" is suggested as a logical structure within which to organize and evaluate concepts

Clinical Nursing Practice	Nursing Administration

1. Reduction in clinical errors
2. Clinical care scheduling
3. Clinical consultation
4. Reducing the volume of documentation
5. Making clinical documents more complete and reliable
6. Increasing clinical records' accuracy, precision, and timeliness
7. Quality management
8. Tracing of clinical outocmes
 	
  • Unexpected mortality rates
  • Nosocomical infection rates
  • Functional status changes
 	
9. Analysis of the relationship between care protocols and changes in patient status
	1. Staffing and scheduling
	2. Performance evaluation
	3. Project design, scheduling, and evaluation
	4. Management decision support:
	
	  • System simulation/modeling and analysis of effectiveness/outcomes of management decidsions
	  • Forecasting
	  • Trend analysis
	  • Project evaluation
	
	5. Financial planning and management
	6. Strategic planning
	
	  • Productivity evaluation
	  • Analysis of program costs versus lost opportunity costs for cost comparisons of competing programs
	  • Cost analysis/cost projections

Figure 24.1 Examples of computer applications to enhance nursing productivity.

and propositions pertaining to computer information systems. This chapter will address the concepts of productivity, quality, and efficiency and explore the relationships among productivity, efficiency, and quality of care. It will address the role of computer information systems in the management of nursing productivity.

A CONCEPTUAL FRAMEWORK FOR PRODUCTIVITY CONCEPTS

Productivity is conceptually defined as the ratio of inputs to outputs. Inputs include all the human, time, and material resources used to produce a given unit of output. Inputs are usually converted into equivalent dollar costs, including concepts such as the time value of money as well as direct and indirect costs of producing the unit of output. Therefore, "inputs" are often expressed as "costs." Outputs are defined as the number of units of product "of a specific quality." Mathematically, the relationship is expressed as a ratio (McHugh, 1986a) in the following manner:

$$P = I \div O$$

where P is productivity (an expression of the relationship between invested resources and products of work); I is inputs (invested resources); and O outputs (products of work).

Traditionally, the health care industry has focused on the "number of units" component of the concept "outputs" while sometimes omitting the "quality" component of outputs, simply because service quality is so difficult to quantify. Thus, we have measures of clinical outputs such as "patient days" or "patient visits" and the like. Part of the problem with this approach is that it is insufficient to meet the evolving expectations of consumers and third-party payers. Nobody seeks health care to buy "a patient day" or a "service encounter." Patients seek health care for prevention or discovery of health problems, or to achieve a cure of an actual problem, or to abate the negative impact of a health problem on the quality of their lives. The interests of third-party payers focus on ensuring that the money they spend on care for subscribers is used in ways that actually improve health status not on ineffective or harmful treatments.

Recently, there has been increasing interest in using computer-based tools and improved collaborative models to improve productivity in health care. Staff workload and productivity of nursing and medical staff have been studied (Atkins, 1995; Cohn, Rosborough, & Fernandez, 1997; Kalton et al., 1997; McHugh, 1997; Moreno & Reis-Miranda, 1998; Wulff, Westphal, Shray, & Hunkeler, 1997). Some of these papers have explicitly addressed the importance of maintaining quality while improving efficiency, but others have not. The three studies that focused primarily on efficiency (Atkins, 1995; Kalton et al., 1997; McHugh, 1997) all used computer simulation modeling to examine very different factors related to efficiency in hospitals and clinics and so had quite different findings.

McHugh (1997) studied the effects of three different nurse floating patterns on wage costs and on the extent to which each of the floating patterns produced understaffed and overstaffed shifts. She found that restricting the practice of floating nurses only to the units in which the nurses were competent to practice was equally cost effective to the model that forced nurses to float to any unit in the hospital. This latter model is the one usually promoted by industrial engineers who are not familiar with the high degree of skill specialization in nursing today. Kalton et al. (1997) used computer simulation modeling to attempt to improve the efficiency of a breast care center that tried to provide true, multidisciplinary care to its patients. They found that the computer could help with scheduling so that long waits were reduced, or in some cases, eliminated. Atkins' study (1995) attempted to link performance expectations in a psychiatric treatment program to nonnursing staffing requirements. They used two different models to study the effects of managed care on variables that influence staffing. Their results showed that as mean length of stay (LOS) decreased, reimbursement also decreased while at the same time, cost of care rose because of the increased admissions and discharges.

The Cohn et al. (1997), Moreno and Reis-Miranda (1998), and Wulff et al. (1997) studies all sought to find ways to minimize cost while at the same time maintaining or improving quality of health care. Wulff et al. (1997) sought to use computerized assessment and analysis tools and method to study the process of health care and to find ways to improve the process. Cohn et al. (1997) focused almost exclusively on building an interdisciplinary team at Brigham and Women's Hospital in Boston. Their purpose was to find ways to improve efficiency by using the combined expertise of the medical teams, nursing, perfusionists, and case managers. They found that the collaborative efforts of the group reduced LOS and cost while volume increased and outcomes improved. Finally, Moreno and Reis-Miranda (1998) used a computer-based tool to examine the match between levels of care (patient acuity) and staff availability. They discovered a "large mismatch" between planned and utilized level of care in the intensive care units (ICUs) in Lisbon, Portugal.

Attention has also focused on using principles of ergonomics to improve the safety (and therefore efficiency) of health care providers (Busse & Bridger, 1997; Geraci, 1997; Hendrickson, Kovner, Knickman, & Finkler, 1995; Kovner, Schuchman, & Mallard, 1997; Krall, 1995; McHugh & Schaller, 1997). Unfortunately, with the increasing competitiveness among insurers, the rapidly increasing dominance of managed care in the health care marketplace and the expected move toward fully capitated systems, quality of care has, in some cases, suffered. Increasingly, providers and consumers have begun to fear that profit needs of powerful third-party payers will be met at the expense of safe patient care and availability of services. There is even the possibility that advances in care will be impaired by these changes in health care financing.

All of these changes coexist with a continuing problem—the meaning of quality in health care has not been well defined. Questions such as, "What constitutes essential services and products and should be covered by insurance?" and "What health services and products are discretionary and should not be covered by insurance?" are very difficult to answer and can lead to perceived inequities in the market. For example, witness the public reaction to the introduction of Viagra for male impotence since the government (Medicare and Medicaid) decided (at least in some cases) to pay for this drug to treat male impotence. It has been argued that that is discriminatory against women because those sources will not pay for women's oral contraceptives—clearly drugs used to treat the "problem" of excessive fertility. Purely cosmetic surgery and drugs are usually not covered by health insurance.

The emerging tenor of our clientele (patients and payers) is to demand that we demonstrate (and, of course, document) that patients obtain what they are seeking. In the past, third-party payers and health care managers have defined "what patients are seeking" as the services delivered. Services were generally presumed to be effective in producing desired changes in health status. Thus, health services are equated with desired changes in health status. The United States now stands on the verge of a redefinition of the concept, "what patients are seeking." The new approach abandons the assumption that services are effective and defines "what patients are seeking" in terms of changes in the patient's health status or functional status. This change is so radical as to constitute a major paradigm shift in providers' and consumers' view of health care and reimbursement for health care. It will force health care professionals to stop focusing on the quantity of services and to expend more effort in measuring the quality of outputs (defined as patient outcomes).

It may now be useful to redefine a term used in industry that does not fit with the realities of the health care environment. In industry, "throughput" is used to mean a specific quantity of input, "put through" processing in a specific amount of time to produce outputs. This conceptualization fails in health care because patients, on whom health care actions are performed, can never be defined as inputs or outputs per se. Patients are not used or consumed in the process of producing "health care" and therefore are not inputs. Neither are patients created or produced within the health care system, so the patient cannot be defined properly as an output.

Health care services ought to act on the patient *in the process of care delivery* in such a way as to produce beneficial changes in the patient's health or functional status. In this sense, the concept of health care services is similar to the concept of throughput. There is not a comparable term to "throughput" in health care. However, such a term may be useful to describe services provided or actions performed on patients. Such a conversion of the term "throughput" may be useful for providing a clear discrimination between inputs (materials and labor), the actions of the supplier (health care providers), which would be called throughput, and the effects of those actions on patients, which would be defined as outcomes of services or care (McHugh, 1989a). Agreement is not yet available on the meaning of the term "outputs" in health care, but clearly differentiating among other, less controversial terms will reduce the amount of confusion about how terms are applied in the health care setting.

In this context, services delivered will be described as throughput. The health care industry has often measured throughput and called it output. For example, nursing outputs have often been defined as counts of services such as "number of intravenous (IV) starts" or "number of dressing changes" and the like. In fact, services are a means to an end, not an end in themselves. This is the crucial problem in defining services as output. The conceptual change now emerging in health care involves redefining services as throughput and patient health/functional status changes as outcomes of care. Eventually, outcomes should constitute one component of the concept "outputs" in health care.

As the concepts "services" and "patient outcomes" change in health care, the concept of "quality" in health care must also change. "Quality of care" has been defined as adherence to standards (written or assumed) defining what services to provide, how to provide them (performance standards), and specifications for documenting those services. In other words, "quality of care" has actually been a measure of quality of throughput. As the health care delivery paradigm shifts to a focus on health/functional status outcomes, the measures of "quality of care" most familiar to quality improvement (QI) nurses will no longer suffice. "Quality" will be subsumed under measures of productivity. New measures of productivity in the health care industry need to be developed. The new measures need to specify changes in health status as outputs and to clearly differentiate between services and the effects of those services on patients. The implications of this change are at least as significant to the health care industry as was prospective reimbursement. This change will transform quality assessment from a minor irritation—an activity conducted primarily to meet the requirements of accrediting and regulatory bodies—into a critical element in the financial success of the institution.

It is unlikely that most existing paper chart systems and current work processes in the QI department will be able to support the future requirements of quality measurement and documentation (Oatway, 1987). The volume of data and the content of data required to identify patient outcomes will be such that only a computer-based patient chart will permit the work to be accomplished. Furthermore, the computer chart must be able to be accessed by (or linked to a computer with) programs designed to aggregate data across patients, perform statistical analyses, and facilitate the creation of QI reports. Accordingly, a more detailed consideration of emerging concepts of quality in health care is germane to discussion of the implications of computer information systems for the future of nursing management.

Changing Concepts of Quality in Health Care

Satisfactory measures of productivity are extremely difficult to obtain in nursing and health care (Young & Hayne, 1988), in part because of the difficulty of incorporating quality indicators into productivity measures. Yet, productivity measures that fail to take account of the quality of the output are so seriously flawed as to be nearly barren of meaning. An example from manufacturing may help to illuminate the concept of quality and the contribution of quality to productivity.

> In machine tool manufacturing, industrial engineers often develop precise performance specifications for the product. The performance specifications then dictate objective measures of product performance. In this context, quality outcomes may be dichotomized as either "acceptable performance" or "unacceptable performance." The product is "acceptable" only if it meets *all* of the performance specifications. It is "unacceptable" if it fails to meet *even one* specification. A product that fails to meet specifications cannot be sold, and thus counts as zero when the number of outputs are counted. However, inputs necessary to produce a flawed product are usually the same as those used to produce an acceptable product. Therefore, the rate of rejection (quality problems) increases the number of inputs relative to the number of *counted* outputs.

This example illustrates that quality problems are merely one type of productivity problem. Integral to the concept of quality is the concept "performance standards" for the *output.* Performance standards pertaining to throughput refers to aspects of work similar to aspects of care in nursing QI. These must often be done to ensure that degradation of throughput does not produce flawed outputs. But control of quality of throughput is useful only insofar as it improves the quality of outputs.

In nursing, the concept "quality of care" has traditionally been interpreted to mean adherence to throughput standards. Output standards (patient care outcomes) have been difficult to measure. In fact, for many patient problems, measures of patient care outcomes do not yet exist. It must be most strongly emphasized that the term "patient care outcomes" has changed significantly. It no longer refers to nursing services. That term now refers to objective, measurable changes in patient condition and/or functional status.

The Concept "Efficiency" and Its Relationship to Productivity

Efficiency refers to measures of how fast a particular task or unit of work is accomplished. Efficiency translates into productivity only indirectly. As an example, consider the amount of time an infusion pump can save by eliminating the need to count "drops per minute" when the nurse regulates an IV. If that time saved is spent at the nurses' station in personal conversation with a colleague, no productivity increase is realized. Only if the time saved is used to care for more patients or to deliver better quality care is productivity enhanced (Channon, 1983). The manager must make a conscious effort to use efficiency improvements wisely. Whereas increases in efficiency may or may not be translated into productivity increases, decreased efficiency will almost always damage productivity. This principle can easily be observed by any nurse who must replace an experienced staff nurse with a nurse who is new to the institution. During orientation, the new employee will need to spend significant amounts of time learning where supplies are kept, what numbers to call for lab, pharmacy, dietary, and all the myriad details the experienced nurse will have at her fingertips. Even if the new employee has many years of experience in nursing, the new setting will hamper efficiency for a period of time. That is why most nursing services do not count a new employee as part of the productive staff for a period during orientation. Clearly, although increases in efficiency may not be easily translated into productivity improvement, efficiency decreases will almost automatically translate into productivity decreases.

Efficiency, Human Effort, and Productivity

The second component of the productivity formula involves the number of outputs (per unit of input). When one considers productivity enhancement in terms of increasing the number of outputs, the concept of efficiency is critical. Managers with concerns about their department's productivity may try to increase productivity by increasing the efficiency of people's personal work habits. This approach has two problems. First, efficiency improvements translate to productivity increases only when the time saved through greater efficiency is reinvested in producing more outputs or into decreasing inputs per unit of output. In nursing, this becomes problematic if increased efficiency produces an extra minute here and 3 minutes there. It then becomes difficult to reinvest those saved minutes effectively. Second, unsustained productivity improvements represent a zero percent net change. Individual work habits are notoriously difficult to change, and each individual has a personal comfort work pace. The comfortable work pace can be *temporarily* speeded up. Unfortunately, people cannot sustain a work pace that is uncomfortable for long periods of time, and they are *less* efficient for a time after exhaustion is reached. Thus, the productivity gains during the speeded up period are usually lost during recovery from exhaustion.

This author has noticed confusion about the relationships between efficiency improvements and human performance dynamics among many health care managers. All too often managers try to improve productivity through motivational lectures or threats. Sustained productivity increases are *never* achieved in that manner. Sustained productivity improvements are a product of improved work tools.

Improving Productivity

From these definitions, it is clear that one may increase productivity in two ways. Productivity is enhanced by increasing the number of outputs while holding constant the number of inputs. Alternately, productivity is increased whenever the quality is increased, assuming outputs and inputs are held constant. For sustained productivity improvements to occur, something in the workplace must change to enable the system to produce more or better outputs. History demonstrates that significant, sustained productivity increases have always resulted from application of technological advances in the workplace. Consider the following situation:

> A 2-inch-long nail must be driven into a standard 2″ × 4″ piece of lumber. The carpenter has only his bare hand with which to accomplish the work. How long will it take to pound that nail into the board? If the carpenter is provided with a simple hammer, how long will it take? Finally, how many 2-inch nails can the carpenter drive into a house under construction with an electric nail gun?

Clearly, the carpenter will never get a house built without at least a hammer. The carpenter with a hammer might get the house built in a matter of months, whereas with a nail gun, the house may go up in a matter of weeks or, perhaps, even days! To improve productivity, managers must improve work technology and work processes.

Nurse managers need to avoid unsuccessful strategies and address productivity by seeking out better tools for the work of nurses. In today's resource-constrained environment, it is too costly to add full-time equivalents (FTEs). Expecting people to work harder is an approach that cannot succeed. Nursing administration needs to take leadership in changing the productivity paradigm now in use in the health care industry. For as long as economic resources for health care delivery are constrained, the old paradigm will be unsuccessful. It cannot succeed because it is founded on a false understanding of the nature of work output and it fails to recognize real, measurable limitations of human performance. What is required of nurse managers is a new look at how nursing work is accomplished—and how that work might be completed more efficiently. The key to productivity lies not in the average nurse's character or work ethic. The key paradigm change involves a view of tools as the key to productivity improvement.

Sources of Productivity Improvement

As nurse managers examine their departments for productivity improvement opportunities, two questions can be used to guide the search. First, "Is the work activity under scrutiny a large enough component of the work of the nurse that a significant efficiency gain in this area can be translated into a meaningful productivity increase?" Second, "Does the technology now exist to achieve a significant efficiency improvement?"

When considering the size of the work activity, time studies may be helpful in determining precisely how much nursing time the activity consumes. If, for example, one can achieve a 90% improvement in the efficiency of a nursing activity, but the activity only constitutes 1% of the work day, only 4.3 minutes per nurse have been saved per 8-hour shift. On the other hand, if a 20% improvement in the efficiency of a nurse can be achieved for an activity that constitutes 40% of the nurse's time, 38.4 minutes in an 8-hour shift have been saved. In a unit staffed with five nurses, that savings translates into an extra 3.2 hours available for teaching the patient/family, responding to patient requests, or providing care to one additional patient (assuming 9.6 hours of care per patient day).

When considering availability of technology, it is important to focus on what is available here and now. All too often, investigations into productivity enhancement technology are derailed by speculation about the productivity gains that will be achievable when this or that technology advance becomes available. Such conjecture is interesting and valuable when communicating possible directions for product development to vendors. However, it is not productive in the context of current strategic planning. These two questions will serve as a guide to focus attention on realistic planning and budgeting for productivity enhancement technology investments. Once an investment opportunity is identified, determining the value of the investment is necessary.

Justifying Investments in Productivity Enhancement Technology

To justify investment in an item of technology, the manager needs to determine if the investment will produce a net improvement or decrease in productivity. Justifications have more credibility when they focus on a comparative analysis of the cost versus the value of the technology to the institution. "Value" may focus on return on investment, strategic match, competitive advantage, and management information (Parker, Benson, & Trainor, 1988). For nurse managers, this may translate into FTE reductions or cost avoidance (avoid the need to add FTEs to accomplish new work required by patient condition or by regulation), improvement in quality of care, improved reimbursement, achievement of strategic goals, etc. For cost justifications the manager often needs to obtain items of information such as:

1. Ability to offer new or expanded services with a good reimbursement profile
2. Capacity to offer a service or program desired by customers (that may or may not be available from a competitor)
3. The number of nursing hours saved per month or year by the new tool, including both indirect activity hours and direct activity hours
4. The cost of those nursing hours
5. A full costing of the labor saving technology. The cost analysis will include yearly maintenance costs and the cost of any incidentals such as manufacturer provided support, in-service education, new FTEs required to support the technology, etc. The purchase price must also be adjusted for the time value of money to determine the full cost of the labor saving device.

The adjusted cost of the technology should be divided by the cost of the nursing hours saved. The point at which the dollars saved in nursing hours equals the adjusted dollars spent to purchase and support the item is the "break even" point. All useful life of the technology after that point is "profit." Of course, if the useful life of the technology is less than the time necessary to reach the break even point, productivity is decreased by the purchase rather than increased. (This is true because the inputs invested have increased, whereas outputs have remained constant and the organization has suffered a net loss.)

Nursing Productivity Enhancement Opportunities

Information handling is the most promising area in nursing for successful productivity enhancement projects. It fits all the criteria previously outlined: it constitutes a large portion of the job, and technology to achieve significant gains now exists. The amount of time nurses spend on communications was measured at 35 to 40% during the middle and late 1960s (Jydstrup & Gross, 1966; Richart, 1970). It is obvious that the time spent on information handling has not decreased in the past 20 years. It may have even increased to as much as 45 to 50%. As for the technology, a variety of applications have been developed to support nursing. A careful study of the use of computer information systems in industry reveals that no one industry has information-handling needs like nursing. Nursing has complex and data-intense information-handling and decision support problems. Yet, virtually all of the types of information-handling problems found in nursing have computer solutions in at least one other industry. Therefore, the following propositions are offered for the reader's consideration. Significant and material increases in nursing productivity are needed now. These increases in productivity can be achieved with application of existing computer technology to nursing information-handling functions.

COMPUTER INFORMATION SYSTEM APPLICATIONS IN NURSING

Computer information systems can be used to enhance nursing productivity in two ways. First, they can reduce the amount of time required to complete tasks.

To the extent that the time saved is invested in accomplishing more work, productivity is enhanced because the number of outputs is increased. Practically, this may be exhibited by doing the same work with fewer people (an FTE reduction is achieved without decreasing number or quality of outputs) or by achieving more work outputs from the people now available. Second, computers can be used to increase quality of outputs. It is important to understand that both clinical and administrative productivity can be enhanced with computer information system technology.

Clinical Applications

Today, nurses spend many hours completing flow sheets, care plans, nurses' notes, vital sign graphics, and other records of nursing care. Some of these are in an easy "checklist" or "fill in the blanks" type of flow sheet format. Others continue to require extensive narrative charting. In many care settings, virtually all of this work is done manually. When one considers that performing free-hand narrative charting is similar to having to write a school term paper or concept paper, it can be appreciated how tedious and time consuming much of this paperwork load has become. The primary goal of putting the clinical chart on computers is to reduce the time required to complete these documents.

Computers can help reduce this burden in several ways. Only a few will be described in this chapter. First, there now exists data entry technology that can greatly streamline the process by which a nurse enters patient care information onto the chart. Second, for some types of data, computers can collect, record, analyze and prepare reports automatically. Third, computers can eliminate or dramatically decrease the work involved in transcribing data (e.g., physician orders) and entering data in several formats (e.g., writing the vital signs and then graphing them). Fourth, computers can help the nurse to organize, prioritize, and schedule the many tasks to be performed each shift.

Data Entry Technology

Writing information on paper in narrative format is the least efficient method of data collection available. Once entered, the use of that narrative information is strictly constrained (Nolan, 1973). Paper-based narrative data cannot be located, retrieved, or analyzed efficiently—even during the care episode that occasioned the narrative note. Costly human time must be invested to convert that narrative information into data that can be aggregated across many patients and analyzed in some fashion. Once stored in medical records, narrative information is effectively lost because of the large amount of time needed to retrieve and search the entire chart for that one note.

Technology exists to permit data to be entered into a computer with minimal or no typing. This technology may consist of application of informatics techniques or of computer technology (machines and programs) or both. Informatics techniques involve redesigning the chart to permit the majority of data to be entered in numeric format. These formats usually consist of checklists, numbers in a structured format (e.g., vital signs), or graphical data representations.

Checklists may be the most common format for assessment data. Data such as cardiac sounds, lung sounds, skin condition, cardiac rhythms, and the like have a limited number of possible descriptors. These descriptors are presented on the screen as a list and the nurse selects from the list. For example, from normal sinus rhythm to asystole there are 23 commonly described cardiac rhythms. Much time can be saved with a system in which the nurse merely needs to check one of the rhythms instead of writing out a rhythm such as "wandering atrial pacemaker." The checklist format for charting will also help to eliminate the problem of unapproved abbreviations that many health care organizations must address.

Structured number formats and graphical representations of data are informatics methods found in nearly all nursing flow sheets. Structured number formats have proved useful in ICU flow sheets and in other settings where routine care or assessments must be performed and documented in a repetitive manner. Graphics are less commonly applied. Most settings use a vital signs graphics form, but this is by no means the only application of graphics for representing assessment findings. For example, pupil size is often graphically represented in neurologic trauma settings. Some units that specialize in care of the patient with respiratory problems may document adventitious sounds on a drawing of the lungs on the flow sheet. These techniques may be applied to either paper- or computer-based charts, but combined with computerized data entry technology, they offer their greatest power and economy.

A variety of data entry technologies are now available for use in clinical areas. Available today are the light pen, the mouse or track ball, touch screens, and of course, the keyboard and number pad. There are also hand-held terminals, modems for remote access to the computer, and computer networks that permit a direct link to a distant computer.

Light pens function by either detecting light from the screen or by flashing a light onto a point on the screen. With a checklist or graphic, the nurse places the light pen over the part of the screen to be marked and clicks a button to register "enter." Documenting the average admission assessment with its many checklists and graphics could be made many times faster with light pen entry. With a touch screen the nurse uses a finger to "mark" the correct place on the screen to enter data. A mouse or track ball has a sensor in a movable ball structure. As the mouse or the ball on a track ball is moved, the computer senses the direction change and changes the location of the screen cursor in response. A button on the mouse or track ball serves as an "enter" key.

For data in checklist or graphic format the light pen, mouse, or track ball can be used with a high degree of efficiency. Numeric data can also be selected from a "menu" of numbers with these technologies. However, they require a permanent terminal. Very few settings now have point-of-care clinical computers. Until bedside computers become standard, other data entry methods will be required.

The goal of efficiency is not furthered by increasing the amount of transcribing required in the clinical setting. Paper charts can easily be carried to the bedside. A 70-pound computer cannot. However, it is possible to acquire pocket-sized terminals (similar to a calculator) on which assessment data can be entered. The pocket terminal can be plugged into the main computer for electronic data transfer. In this way, the nurse will not find a need to write down care notes on a piece of scrap paper for later data entry into the computer or paper record. The point here is that there will be problems encountered in converting paper charts to computer information systems. Implementing a computer could be a serious mistake if it forces people to continue their current paperwork load and add computer data entry to the process. It is important to consider tool solutions for these problems rather than FTE solutions when developing a computerized patient record system.

Automatic Data Collection

In some settings, machines are now being used to monitor physical parameters. The monitors in ICUs are now called physiologic monitors instead of heart monitors because they monitor so many different physiologic variables. All of the monitors sold today are based on computer technology, and most (if not all) are designed to permit the monitored data to be stored, trended, and transferred electronically to another computer. Some of the other machines that use computer chips are IV pumps, syringe infusion pumps, ventilators, oximetry, and so forth. Most of these have some capability for transferring data.

These can improve efficiency in two ways. First, they can record the data so that the nurse does not have to enter the data in any format. Second, they can, independently or through data transfer to another computer, perform automatic trending and graphing of the data. In this way, they permit the nurse to avoid some transcribing of data from one part of the record (flow sheet or narrative notes) to another (the graphical record). It may also be that in some cases, they can substitute for manually performed nursing assessment tasks.

For example, if an arterial line is present, the physiologic monitor computer can be programmed to automatically measure and record mean arterial pressure readings and to graph the waveforms. The nurse may not need to take any blood pressure readings but only to validate the accuracy of the machine's measures at the beginning of a shift. For a patient who requires extremely close blood pressure monitoring (e.g., every 5 minutes), this can save the nurse up to 90 minutes of work during an 8-hour shift.

Once data are in a computer, programs can be written to perform operations on that data—assuming the computer was designed to permit the data to be used in a variety of ways (Martin, 1976). Computers can be programmed to select a subset of the data for each of many patients. It can store the subset in a new file. Programs can be used to access the data in the new file and perform statistical manipulations and analysis on the data. Some programs will take raw data or analysis results and format them into a final report. All these activities can be performed manually. Manual data manipulation, however, is tedious, error prone, and so time consuming that by the time the report is prepared, it may be obsolete. Properly designed computer systems can be programmed to perform all these tasks in a matter of seconds or minutes.

Efficiencies from Reduction in Transcription Time

Nurses transcribe large amounts of information from one place to another. Part of noting physician orders is usually accompanied by copying the order onto a medication ticket, Kardex, PT schedule, lab requisition, and so forth. People make errors when copying information from one place to another. Children often play the game "telephone" in which one child originates a message and whispers to the next child, who repeats the message to another, and so on until the message at last returns to the originator. As the length and complexity of the "message" increases, the final story is increasingly garbled. Transcribing activities are merely a written and abbreviated form of the telephone game. We ought to expect a certain rate of change with transcribed orders. Yet, nurses always seem surprised when an order is miscopied or omitted entirely. The surprise—not to mention the harsh condemnation of the nurse involved—is inappropriate. A system that relies on human beings to copy large volumes of written materials from one data site to another is a badly designed system.

In industry, there are many examples of computers transcribing important messages to large numbers of different individuals and sites. Computer transmittal is virtually error free. The few errors that do occur in computer data transmission are usually identified by the computer itself as it checks the data for errors. The efficiencies obtained from computer transcription will be augmented by the reduction in time required to complete and investigate incident reports for transcription errors.

Care Scheduling

Nursing care today is more intense, complex, and detailed than at any time in history. Current trends suggest that the situation will worsen. It is also known that the average person usually can retain only about seven items of information in short-term memory. (Most people can remember a number they looked up in the telephone book long enough to dial it. If an area code needs to be added, however, most people need to write the number down. A telephone number without the area code is seven digits.) Nurses today have far more than seven items of information to keep in short-term memory. Most have developed their own informal techniques to allow them to function. Yet, many care omissions still happen.

Perhaps a new paradigm is needed. The care system we now have *requires* nurses to function beyond normal human performance limits. Instead of increasing FTEs or, worse, blaming and punishing people for less than super performance, we should redesign the system. Existing manual systems offer few memory supports and little or no assistance with scheduling care tasks to the individual nurse. Nurses generally are responsible for a group of patients. The care must be planned so that each patient's requirements are met in a timely fashion. Essentially, nurses schedule care tasks, and scheduling is a cognitive activity.

The cognitive work involved in scheduling is iterative and hierarchical. That is, priorities are determined for each care item and for each patient. Some are bound by time limits such as medications. Others may be scheduled according to unit routine or the nurse's convenience. Once priorities are determined, they are listed on the schedule (whether that be a paper or mental schedule). As higher priority care items are scheduled, lower priority items are left on the unscheduled list. Each review of the unscheduled item list and the partially completed schedule is a cycle or iteration. Computers can iterate rapidly and endlessly. If properly programmed, a computer will produce a work schedule much faster (and thus more efficiently) than a human being could. Furthermore, computers can instantly revise the schedule if a new patient is admitted or new orders written. Preparing or revising a care schedule can be tedious and stressful. That kind of stress often reduces efficiency. A computer scheduler can enhance efficiency by saving time and by reducing the stress factor associated with scheduling tasks.

Clinical Care Quality Improvement

Many of the facilities that promote efficiency can also serve to improve patient outcomes by improving the quality of nursing care. The computer can do this in three ways. First, it can be programmed to reduce or eliminate many errors. Second, it can make expert clinical consultation instantly available to the nurse as care is delivered. Third, it can permit a level of analysis of outcomes of care that is far beyond what can be accomplished with paper charts. Nurses will be able to empirically demonstrate the effects of nursing care on patient health status and functioning. That information will enable nurses to exert more control over changes in practice patterns through the ability to demonstrate the benefits of nursing care protocols.

Performance Limitations and Error Reduction

Previously, it was argued that the current environment requires nurses to function at levels that are beyond normal performance limits. Limits may be absolute or relative. For example, no person can start 500 IVs in an 8-hour shift. Even if the patients were all lined up and all supplies at the ready, a nurse would have to average no more than 57 seconds per IV. That limit is absolute. However, a nurse could start 90 IVs in an 8-hour shift if all the conditions were right, the patients were all lined up, and nobody had difficult-to-access veins. In that case, an average of 5 minutes per IV would be possible. Even under the best conditions, however, nobody could sustain that average forever.

The point is that people can sometimes perform extraordinary feats. Nobody can perform extraordinarily all the time. A system that requires people to function at peak performance at all times is a source of error. The current care environment is so complex and busy and offers so few supports to human memory and cognition that it predisposes to clinical error. Most people do the best they can with the resources they have. Very few nurses are deliberately sloppy or careless. No system can protect against the occasional error. But when we see incident reports averaging more than one or two serious errors a week per unit and notice that even our best nurses are making more errors than expected, we should begin to question the system instead of the quality of the people. Quality cannot be consistently maintained with a seriously flawed care delivery system.

To the extent the computer information system can serve to reduce clinical errors, it will improve quality of care. A medication system provides one example of how a computer can improve care quality. Medication errors can be virtually eliminated by means of a program designed to permit physicians to enter directly their medication orders. It is possible to program the computer to calculate automatically the proper dose range for the patient's body weight and to warn the doctor of a potential dosage error while the order is being entered. The computer can also check the on-line PDR listing for that drug against the patient's medical diagnoses (or clinical problem list) and warn of a possible incorrect drug or of drug interactions or allergies. Furthermore, incorrect routes or methods of administration can be brought to the physician's attention before a clinical error is made. The computer can be programmed to expect the medication to be charted by a certain time and to warn the nurse about the omission in time to give the drug. If a nurse attempted to enter the wrong dose, the computer could instantly detect and report the error. If an incorrect dose was actually administered, early discovery might permit immediate action to protect the patient from harm. If the error was merely a typographical error, the nurse would have the opportunity to correct the error on the screen before it was permanently recorded in the patient's chart.

Medication errors are only one type of clinical problem that can be alleviated by computer technology. Other situations include activities that require math calculations or need to be performed at specific times. For example, computers can automatically calculate data derived from monitored variables. Therefore, a pulse pressure that is widening in a head trauma patient can be detected and alarmed by a computer attached to the blood pressure monitor. Many errors in documentation could be avoided if computer charts were programmed to recognize the range of correct values and alarm on values that were out of range (e.g., a BP recorded as 60/120). Wrong chart notes would still occur, but would be less frequent if the record itself could detect care not ordered or inconsistent with certain types of expectations. For example, a dressing change charted on a patient who had no wounds or a PAP test recorded on a male patient should not pass unchallenged.

Clinical Consultation

The computer can serve to support the clinical knowledge base and decision processes of nurses (Ozbolt, Schultz, Swain, & Abraham, 1985). A few systems have been developed to support the clinical judgment of physicians. These systems work by offering advice or by guiding the thinking and decision processes of the clinician (Brennan & McHugh, 1988). These systems help to improve the quality of clinical judgments by ensuring that all the important information that should be considered is, in fact, taken into account (McHugh, 1986b).

A system that provides a draft care plan derived from the initial nursing assessment is another form of clinical consultation. Ideally, the system should guide and support patient assessment and planning of care (McHugh, 1989b; Zielstorff, McHugh, & Clinton, 1988). Although a nurse might overlook or forget a low-priority nursing diagnosis in a multiproblem patient, the computer will not.

Clinical decision support could be of immense value. For the first time in history, a basic level competency in assessment and nursing diagnosis could be defined and maintained. Even very inexperienced nurses would be unlikely to miss important clinical phenomena. The computer would present not only the data, but also a basic level of interpretation of the clinical meaning and importance of the data.

Equally important, the nurse could use the computer as a clinical learning tool. It could be asked to show the nurse the information it used to determine its nursing diagnosis or its care-planning strategy. The computer could be queried by the nurse about its decision process and the decision rules it used to draw its conclusions. Thus, nurses could use the computer to learn new facts and also to improve their own critical thinking and clinical judgment skills.

Improving Clinical Practice

Clinical practice is only partially based on evidence of its efficacy. Advancements in the science of nursing are hampered by the expense of research and by the amount of time such research requires. Data collection and preparing data for computer entry usually consumes 70 to 80% of all research costs. It is frustrating for a researcher to realize that most of the data needed for a particular study have been collected and stored in the paper chart but, because of the expense, cannot be retrieved. Despite the great expense of collecting data anew, it is often still less expensive than data retrieval from paper charts. Thus, the paper chart often acts as more of an impediment to quality improvement than an asset. A properly designed computer-based patient record could provide enormous opportunity to examine, analyze, and evaluate nursing care protocols and activities across many hundreds or thousands of patients.

If the capacity to evaluate the effects of nursing care on hundreds or thousands of patients were available, changes in practice could be more easily based on sound evidence of the benefits of those changes. Programs could be developed to flag and track unexpected deaths, prolonged lengths of stay, nosocomial infection rates, unusually good patient outcomes, and the like. This information could be linked with the nursing care provided. Commonalities or special differences in these special cases could be evaluated for the need to change practice. If one approach is found to be more highly associated with successful patient outcomes than another, nurses could discover this fact and then change practice to increase success rates. Conversely, care that is ineffective or even deleterious could be identified and abandoned in favor of successful care approaches. The problem now is that we are unable to use the data in our own nursing records to discover and document the effects of our work.

As health care looks more toward changes in patient health status as the most important indicators of care quality, it will become increasingly important for nurses to link nursing practices to patient outcomes. Every blood pressure test, bed bath, dressing change, and patient education session costs money. Some studies have documented the benefits of particular nursing care protocols. However, too much of our care is now based on unit routines or unproven ideas about what will benefit the patient. In the future, we will need to justify nursing care expense with far more credible evidence of the benefits to patients of that care. Until and unless nursing care is documented in a system that permits rapid and inexpensive retrieval, aggregation, and analysis of that data, nursing will be unprepared to respond to the demands of third-party payers and regulatory bodies for proof of the quality and effectiveness of our care.

Applications for Nursing Service Administration

In these challenging times, it is increasingly important for nursing care delivery systems to be well managed. All of the principles pertaining to quality, efficiency, and productivity addressed in the context of clinical nursing apply equally to the practice of nursing administration. In some ways, it may be even more important for administrators to examine their practice than for staff. Nursing service administrators must make critical decisions about the fate of their employees and the direction nursing care will take in their institutions. Poor decisions may lead to poor patient care, loss of staff, and ultimately, perhaps, even failure of the entire institution.

Quality of Management Decisions

The body of information needed by nurse managers to make good decisions has increased dramatically in the past 20 years. They have always needed a good foundation in the realities of clinical practice, people management skills, project management skills, and good skills in resource management. None of those skills are obsolete. However, today, managers must also have a good working knowledge of third-party payer trends, financial analysis, public relations, requirements of accrediting bodies and regulatory agencies, and a myriad of other facets of the health care industry and its political and social environment.

Increasingly, more pieces of information, more complex information, and the dynamics of interrelationships among disparate items of information need to be understood and analyzed if good management decisions are to be made.

Meanwhile, the situation of health care is highly volatile. Almost no one has the time to spend manually collecting, aggregating, and analyzing large volumes of data—even if they have the economic resources to invest in those activities. All too often, these problems force managers to make decisions with faulty and insufficient information. Such decisions may work out well enough if the manager is lucky. Many health care organizations are at risk, however, and poor decisions may threaten their survival.

Computer information systems can be used to improve the quality of management by permitting managers to acquire and *use* more information in their decision-making processes. In this way, they improve the quality of their decisions.

Consider trying to make a decision about choosing between devoting resources to adding four birthing rooms in obstetrics or adding two new operating rooms to surgery. What factors might influence the decision if the only information related to the hospital management team was that both the obstetricians and the surgeons wanted their respective expansions very badly? One suspects that personal relationships with the physicians might influence the decision, or the clinical preference of the decision-maker might take precedence. Obviously, the decision has only a 50% chance of being the right decision with this paucity of information. Most managers would identify at least five or six more items of information they would need to make a good decision. Critical items of information might include:

1. Information about which program was currently providing the most profit
2. Community birth rates and the trend upward or downward in births in the service area
3. The number of women in their childbearing years and population trends in females in the service area
4. The amount of elective surgery that currently must be delayed due to insufficient operating rooms
5. Cost projections for each expansion project
6. Any anticipated loss of surgeons or anesthesiologists because of retirement or relocation and the hospital's potential for replacing those losses
7. Information about the plans of competing hospitals in the service area

The answers to any *one* of these questions might have a strong influence on management's decision. If managers have answers to *all* of these questions, they would have a more complete picture of the hospital, its resources, and its environment than any part of the answers could offer. No one aspect of the problem would be likely to create a distorted image of the situation and, thus, have a disproportionate influence on the final choices of the management team. Full information decreases the probability that a wrong choice will be selected.

Unfortunately, the quality of most management decisions can only be evaluated retrospectively. However, some computer-decision support technology exists to permit managers to evaluate in advance the problem outcomes of some types of decisions. These types of applications are called management-decision support systems.

Currently available management-decision support tools include computer simulations, forecasting and trend analysis programs, statistical analysis programs, and financial planning programs. Computer simulations are procedural models. They express dynamic relationships in a system by means of precise symbols and directions about how those symbols remain static or move about in relation to each other. For example, a model of a unit and its access to nursing staff in relation to changing workloads has been developed for the purpose of examining costs and staffing adequacy of a variety of nurse staffing patterns (McHugh, 1988).

Nurse executives must perform financial analysis and make projections about changes in skill mix, clinical specialty requirements, and a host of other problems in which past experience can offer a guide to future performance. Computer programs can be used to support the quality of decisions involving these issues. Specifically, financial planning, forecasting, statistical analysis, and trend analysis programs can be used to improve predictions of changes in the internal and external environment. They can also be used to link these predicted changes to possible outcomes of selected managerial decisions. The computer's predictions of outcomes of decisions can be used as early warning of a need to make adjustments in strategic plans.

Nursing service administrators may want to investigate the value of these types of decision support tools in their own practice. To the extent that nursing service administrators make use of all available resources to support assessment, planning, and evaluation in their management practice, they will be better managers. They will make better quality decisions, and their institutions will have a better chance to survive the stresses of this rapidly changing health care environment.

Efficiency in Nursing Administration

Computer information systems can be used for a wide variety of applications to increase the efficiency of administration. A variety of tasks that must be performed by the nursing service administration require significant amounts of number processing or other data manipulation. Patient classification systems, staffing and scheduling systems, budgeting, and the like are data intensive and data manipulation intensive. Computers can greatly speed up the processing and reduce errors of manual handling.

In this area, conversion from manual processes to computer processing may well permit reduction in FTEs. However, it is more common to find that managers seek computers to avoid increasing secretarial FTEs when their people are simply overwhelmed. On the other hand, they may realize that information that would be extremely useful can be obtained only with the processing power of a computer. Some types of computer programs that have been developed to improve managerial efficiency are patient acuity classification systems, staff scheduling systems, project planning and scheduling applications, budget development and control systems, and programs to support strategic planning efforts. These programs require substantial amounts of information about the current operations of the organization (e.g., average census, workload amount and stability, number of staff, staff mix, among others). These types of programs provide new information by performing analysis on the data about the experience. The value of all of these programs is constrained by the availability of data about the operations of the organization.

Perhaps the greatest danger facing administrators' ability to avail themselves of computer-decision support technology is the dearth and poor quality of information they can retrieve from their own operations. The clinical record contains the source data on the operations of any clinical agency. Few industries would allow their operations data to be lost to illegible, inaccessible paper records. Yet, that is exactly how many hospitals treat their clinical operations data. Consider how rapidly your hospital could obtain precise answers to the following questions:

1. How many CCU patients overflowed into SICU last month? Does that number represent our usual experience?
2. How many patients who were at risk for decubitus ulcers actually experienced some degree of skin breakdown?
3. Does the current nursing workload in terms of number and acuity of patients per nursing FTE match the nursing care we had planned to deliver when we prepared the budget?

Many hospitals can quickly answer the third question. Those data are found in an automated patient classification system, if the hospital has such a system. The first question can also be answered fairly quickly. Someone must retrieve the SICU log and make a judgment about every patient listed as to whether or not the patient should have been placed in CCU. A precise answer may never be available, but a good estimate should be obtained in 1 or 2 weeks.

The second question may be a problem. Most hospitals have no practical way to identify patients at risk of complications. Actual complications are usually only available if tracked in a QI study. Yet, answers to the second question relate directly to the effects of the nursing care on patients. The only way that such data can be made available economically is through implementation of the computer-based patient chart. Even then, the desired functionality will be achievable only if the computer-based chart meets the criteria for such systems as described in the ANA publication, *Computer Design Criteria for Systems that Support the Nursing Process.*

SUMMARY

Computer information systems are primarily useful in the context of productivity enhancement. They help achieve productivity gains by increasing the efficiency or quality of work. In both the clinical and administrative arenas, the amount and complexity of information required for success has grown to such proportions that manual data and information processes no longer suffice. Good decisions are not made in the absence of relevant information. Nurse managers and clinicians need rapid and economical access to an ever-increasing volume and variety of information if their decisions are to lead to clinical and institutional successes. However, computer technology now exists to greatly enhance the power of nurses to improve their performance and the benefits of nursing care. The seeds of future success should be planted now with vendors and other members of the health care delivery team. Vendors must be informed of our needs and the expectations of our computing systems. Other members of the health care delivery team should collaborate with nurses and vendors on the design and implementation of powerful new clinical information systems. The effort will be worthwhile because the benefits of clinical and administrative computing will accrue to all of us—patients, clinicians, and administrators.

STUDY QUESTIONS

1. Define productivity and discuss the factors that influence it.
2. What recent developments have provided the impetus to measure and increase nursing productivity?
3. Review the questions raised in the above section and prepare answers for your work setting.
4. How will computer information systems improve productivity and quality across settings?

REFERENCES

Atkins, R. (1995). A computer-based model for analyzing staffing needs of psychiatric treatment programs. *Psychiatric Services, 46*(12), 1272–1278.

Brennan, P., & McHugh, M. (1988). Clinical decision-making and computer support. *Applied Nursing Research, 1*(2), 89–93.

Busse, M., & Bridger, B. (1997). Cost benefits of ergonomic intervention in a hospital: A preliminary study using Oxenburgh's productivity model. *Curationis, 20*(3), 54–58.

Channon, B. (1983). Dispelling productivity myths. *Hospitals, 57*(19), 103–119.

Cohn, L., Rosborough, D., & Fernandez, J. (1997). Reducing costs and length of stay and improving efficiency and quality of care in cardiac surgery. *Annals of Thoracic Surgery, 64*(6-Suppl), S58–60; discussion S80–82.

Geraci, E. (1997). Computers in home care. Application of change theory. *Computers in Nursing, 15*(4), 199–203.

Hendrickson, G., Kovner, C., Knickman, J., & Finkler, S. (1995). Implementation of a variety of computerized bedside nursing information systems in 17 New Jersey hospitals. *Computers in Nursing, 13*(3), 96–102.

Jydstrup, R. A., & Gross, M. J. (1966). Cost of information handling in hospitals. *Health Services Research, 1*(3), 235–261.

Kalton, A., Singh, M., August, D. Parin, C., & Othman, E. (1997). Using simulation to improve the operational efficiency of a multi-disciplinary clinic. *Journal of Social Health Systems, 5*(3), 43–62.

Kovner, C., Schuchman, L., & Mallard, C. (1997). The application of pen-based computer technology to home health care. *Computers in Nursing, 15*(5), 237–244.

Krall, M. (1995). Acceptance and performance by clinicians using an ambulatory electronic medical record in an HMO. *Proceedings of the 19th Annual Symposium on Computer Applications in Medical Care,* pp. 708–711. Silver Spring, MD: IEEE Computer Society.

Martin, J. (1976). *Principles of data-base management.* Englewood Cliffs, NJ: Prentice-Hall.

McHugh, M. (1986a). Increasing productivity through computer communications. *Dimensions of Critical Care Nursing, 5*(5), 284–302.

McHugh, M. (1986b). Information access: A basis for strategic planning and control of operations. *Nursing Administration Quarterly, 10*(1), 10–20.

McHugh, M. (1988, May). Comparison of four hospital nurse staffing patterns for wage costs and staffing adequacy using computer simulation. *Dissertation Abstracts International, 48*(11), 3250-B. B-The Sciences and Engineering. (University Microfilms International Order No. DA8801370)

McHugh, M. (1989a). Productivity measurement in nursing. *Applied Nursing Research, 2*(2), 99–102.

McHugh, M. (1989b). Computer support for the nursing process. *Health Matrix, 7*(1), 57–60.

McHugh, M. (1997). Cost effectiveness of clustered versus unclustered unit transfers of nursing staff. *Nursing Economic$, 15*(6), 294–300.

McHugh, M., & Schaller, P. (1997). Ergonomic nursing workstation design to prevent cumulative trauma disorders. *Computers in Nursing, 15*(5), 245–254.

Moreno, R., & Reis-Miranda, D. (1998). Nursing staff in intensive care in Europe: The mismatch between planning and practice. *Chest, 113*(3), 752–758.

Nolan, R. (1973). Computer data bases: The future is now. *Harvard Business Review, 51*(5), 98–114.

Oatway, D. (1987). The future of computer applications for nursing quality assurance. *Journal of Nursing Quality Assurance, 1*(4), 61–71.

Ozbolt, J., Schultz, S., Swain, M., & Abraham, I. (1985). A proposed expert system for nursing practice. *Journal of Medical Systems, 9,* 57–68.

Parker, M., Benson, R., & Trainor, H. (1988). *Information economics: Linking business performance to information technology.* Englewood Cliffs, NJ: Prentice-Hall.

Richart, R. (1970). Evaluation of a medical data system. *Computers in Biomedical Research, 3*(5), 415–425.

Simms, L. M., Price, S. A., & Ervin, N. E. (1994). *The professional practice of nursing administration,* (2nd ed.). Albany, NY: Delmar.

Wulff, K., Westphal, J., Shray, S., & Hunkeler, E. (1997). Using automated continual performance assessment to improve health care. *MD Computing, 4*(1), 24–30, 32–35.

Young, L., & Hayne, A. (1988). *Nursing administration: From concepts to practice.* Philadelphia: Saunders.

Zielstorff, R., McHugh, M., & Clinton, J. (1988). *Computer design criteria for systems that support the nursing process.* Kansas City, MO: American Nurses Association.

CHAPTER

25

Nurse Staffing and Scheduling

Yvonne Marie Abdoo

The development of nurse staffing systems arose from the concern of nurse executives that there are not enough personnel to provide necessary nursing care. (Author)

Chapter Highlights

- The evolution of nurse staffing systems
- Patient classification as a component of staffing systems
- The development of staffing systems
- Work measurement in nursing
- Scheduling and workweek patterns for nursing personnel
- Current and next generation nurse staffing systems

One of the most critical issues confronting nurse executives today is nurse staffing. Staffing policies and needs affect the nursing department budget, staff productivity, quality of care provided to clients, nursing staff morale, and even nurse retention. At the same time nurse staffing requirements are affected by overall hospital policies and by nearly every other department in the organization, including admitting, lab, x-ray, dietary, and the like. Thus, it is essential that nursing administrators thoroughly understand the components and issues in nurse staffing. This chapter provides a history of staffing systems, reviews classic research, and proposes alternatives for the future.

Nurse staffing is a term often used but subject to a variety of interpretations. For purposes of this discussion, *nurse staffing* is a broad area composed of three main components: planning, scheduling, and allocation. Planning encompasses determination of the number of nursing personnel needed over a long-term period. The scheduling component entails assigning nursing staff for specific time periods by shift, based on patient care needs. Allocation of nursing staff involves staffing assignments or readjustments on a daily or shift basis.

A great wealth of information has been written in the realm of nurse staffing, but the articles tend to recount personal experiences and to describe trial-and-error rather than scientific approaches. Aydelotte (1973) asserts that:

> Nurse staffing methodology should be an orderly systematic process, based upon sound rationale, applied to determine the number and kind of nursing personnel required to provide nursing care of a predetermined standard to a group of patients in a particular setting. The end result is prediction of the kind and number of staff required to give care to patients. This prediction of the number and kinds of personnel to give patients nursing care 24 hours a day, 7 days a week . . . is no small task. The aim is to provide, at reasonable cost to the general public the agency serves, a standard of nursing care acceptable to its clientele and the nursing staff serving it. (p. 3)

The planning or staffing methodology phase should be based on quantifiable, measurable data. This systematic nurse staffing determination must include the following variables: *(1)* an assessment of patient care needs (patient classification), *(2)* an assessment of required nursing time to meet patient needs (nursing work load determination), and *(3)* an algorithm that uses the first two variables. Average occupancy and seasonal fluctuations in the occupancy rate are also helpful supplemental variables.

Deviation from the intuitive approach to a systematic research approach can be achieved only after those involved in nurse staffing decisions thoroughly understand the history of nurse staffing, its trends, its complexity, and its needs.

THE EVOLUTION OF NURSE STAFFING SYSTEMS

Nurse staffing systems have evolved since early 1960, when Connor (1961) published a research report, based on his earlier doctoral dissertation, on the utilization of nursing staff. A major result of Connor's work was the development of a three-category patient classification tool in which a hospital's medical and surgical inpatients are identified by the unit's head nurse as category I, self-care; category II, partial or intermediate care; or category III, intensive or total care. Guidelines describing the typical characteristics of a patient in a particular category were developed for the head nurse to use in categorizing patients.

An average nursing time for each patient category was determined through work measurement studies, and each of the average times was significantly different from each other when tested statistically. A staffing algorithm using a patient care index (I) was developed:

$$I = 0.5N_1 + 1.0N_2 + 2.5N_3$$

where *I* is the patient care index, *N* is the number of patients in each category; the constants represent the amount of direct care in hours, and the subscripts represent the specific clarification level (Connor, 1961).

Connor noted even in 1960 the effect of the variation of patient needs on the nursing workload. The nursing workload varied only slightly if the number and distribution of patients by classification were constant. "On the other hand," noted Connor, "if the number of each class of patients is also variable, we may expect wide variation in total daily demand on staff. It is, therefore, important to determine how the classes of patients vary within the census, for this, in conjunction with the average times required, would permit the estimation of variation in nursing staff requirements for a single ward or in the hospital" (Connor, Flagle, Hsieh, Preston, & Singer, 1961, p. 33).

The Commission for Administrative Services in Hospitals (CASH) (Des Ormeaux, 1977) adapted the work of Connor and his colleagues (1961) from the Johns Hopkins University using additional systems analysis and other industrial engineering techniques to prepare a staffing manual to assist hospitals in determining their own nurse staffing requirements. The components of the staffing system include: *(1)* a three-level patient classification tool (self-care, partial care, and total care); *(2)* standard time allowance for the performance of each nursing procedure or task; *(3)* census data (the number of admissions, discharges, transfers, and occupied beds); and *(4)* the number and types of personnel employed on a nursing unit (Figure 25.1). The following reports, as summarized by Aydelotte (1973), could then be generated:

- Actual staffing plan (as it is in operation)
- Recommended staffing plan
- Report of accumulated hours, giving the amount of time for each worker and each task
- Work distribution sampling
- Recommendations for redistribution of the procedure (the work)

Other staffing systems (Center for Hospital Management Engineering, 1978; Cochran & Derr, 1975; Georgette, 1970; McCormick, Roche, & Steinwacks, 1973; Minetti & Hutchinson, 1975) developed during the 1960s and early 1970s for specific hospitals adapted the work of Connor (1961) to fit a particular institution's specific needs. Although a modification of the classification tool might occur—for example, expanding the tool from three patient category types to four or five types with descriptive criteria—the basic methodology remained the same. The average amount of nursing care time needed was calculated from the patient classification input and converted to the average number of nursing staff needed to provide nursing care. The variances of the average nursing care time and nursing staff were not determined.

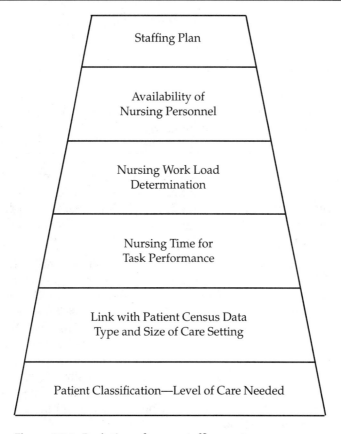

Figure 25.1 Evolution of nurse staffing systems.

PATIENT CLASSIFICATION AS A COMPONENT OF NURSE STAFFING SYSTEMS

The component of traditional nurse staffing systems essential to all facets of the total system is patient classification. *Classification* may be defined as the ordering or arrangement of objects or properties conceptually, physically, or in both ways. This process has long been used in many fields and is evidenced by various taxonomies that have been developed in most sciences.

According to Sokal (1974), taxonomy is the theoretical study of classification, including its bases, principles, procedures, and rules. Taxonomy actually includes two phases: classification and identification. Identification encompasses assigning previously unidentified objects or concepts to the proper or correct class according to an established classification system. Thus, taxonomy is the science of how to classify and identify.

The major purpose of classification is to describe the structure or relationship of the constituent objects to each other and to similar objects and to simplify these relationships in such a way that general statements can be made about classes of objects (Sokal, 1974), which should facilitate the understanding of users. Another goal of a classification system is ease of manipulation or retrieval of information, because complex relationships are often simplified by a classification schema. Classification systems also facilitate economy of memory by summarizing information about relationships and attaching a specified label.

Patient Classification Tools

Since 1960, patient classification tools have been developed to categorize or group patients according to their prospective nursing care requirements for a specified period of time. Because the health needs—and, as a result, the nursing needs—vary from patient to patient, tools have been developed to predict the nursing time required based on the identified patient needs at a given time. According to Giovannetti (1978), the "concept of patient classification entails the categorization or grouping of patients according to some assessment of their nursing care requirements over a specified period of time" (p. 3). The main purpose of these early patient classification tools or instruments was to predict nurse staffing needs on a shift to shift basis.

Determining and agreeing on assessment criteria are not simple feats, however, because there are several ways of viewing patients' requirements for nursing care. A major issue that must first be resolved is whether the assessment categories should focus on health maintenance, illness problems, or degree of independence in meeting one's own health or illness needs. Abdellah and Levine (1965) discussed the concept of patient classification as an area of interest for nurse researchers. Patient classification was defined as a scaling scheme in which the underlying continuum can be conceptualized as expressing a quantitative statement of a patient's requirements for nursing services. These may range from no requirements at all—representing a condition of maximum self-help ability—to the other extreme, total requirements for nursing services—representing a condition of minimum self-help ability. One may also visualize the continuum as levels of wellness. The degree or amount of nursing care required by the patient is not necessarily positively correlated with the level of wellness; one cannot say that the less well the patient, the more nursing care he or she will require. For example, a terminally ill patient may require fewer nursing services than a person with a fractured leg (moderate level of illness).

The early patient classification systems documented in the literature (Connor et al., 1961; Chagnon et al., 1978; Meyer, 1978a, 1978b; Norby & Freund, 1977; Norby, Freund, & Wagner, 1977) are based on defining the patient's physical needs during hospitalization and tend to exclude psychosocial and long-range health maintenance and sustenance needs. Various nursing models have evolved since 1970—for example, those of Kinlein, Orem, Rogers, and Roy—that do not view the patient according to an illness or disease state, as in the traditional medical model, but, rather, look at the whole person, including the person's health maintenance and promotion needs and relationship to the total environment. Since the advent of these conceptual frameworks, patient classification criteria based solely on physical needs have been criticized by nurses.

Thus, establishing the viewpoint for a patient classification system is not simple. Since 1970, the issue has been compounded by the expanding and changing role of nursing, lack of nursing research on the topic, and reexamination of the patient's health illness status. A perusal of the published patient classification schemes indicates that the majority have been developed for adult populations in acute care settings and focus on determining the degree of patient dependency on nursing personnel to meet the patient's basic needs.

Once the viewpoint for the development of the patient classification system (PCS) has been decided, problems with generics and semantics can arise. Common categorization schema of many PCSs currently in existence use three or four general groupings, for example, self-care, partial care, and total care; or minimal care, standard care, intensive care, and critical care. The terms by themselves, however, are not self-explanatory or mutually exclusive. What is the distinction between the intensive and critical care categories used in a particular patient tool? It is imperative that clear, detailed explanations describe the various classification groupings so that any existing ambiguity might be minimized.

It is important to realize that patients in a particular classification are not necessarily identical but, rather, possess many similarities related to the defined classification characteristics. Nor are the given classes mutually exclusive, though some authorities believe this is desirable. According to Giovannetti (1978), "each class should be mutually exclusive—classes should not overlap. However, it has already been shown that some overlapping is usually *unavoidable* because of variations in viewpoint which must be accommodated" (p. 9).

Sokal (1974), on the other hand, points out that classifications need not be hierarchic, and the clusters may overlap (intersect). "From studies in a variety of fields, the representation of taxonomic structure as overlapping clusters or as ordinations appears far preferable to mutual exclusivity. By ordination, we mean projection of the operational taxonomic units (OTUs) in a space of fewer dimensions than the original number of descriptors. When tested by any of several measures of distortion, ordinations in as few as two or three dimensions frequently represent the original similarity matrices considerably more faithfully than do dendrograms" (Sokal, 1974, p. 1121).

There have been a wide variety of patient classification instruments in use in hospitals throughout the United States, especially once the Joint Commission on the Accreditation of Healthcare Organizations (JCAHO) (1993) mandated that every area must have a process to determine the level of care required by patients being served in that specific area, and that the method used has interrater reliability and face validity. It is sometimes facetiously remarked that there are as many different tools as there are hospitals. The tools vary in format and length. Patient classification schemes have several common characteristics:

1. Categories are used that describe patient characteristics or critical indicators of a patient's nursing care requirements that might encompass any or all of the following, as mentioned by Aydelotte (1973):
   - 1.1. Capabilities of the patient to care for himself or herself
   - 1.2. Special characteristics of the patient related to sensory deprivation
   - 1.3. Acuity of illness
   - 1.4. Requirements for specific nursing activities
   - 1.5. Skill level of personnel required in the care
   - 1.6. Patient's geographical placement or status in the hospital system

2. Most schemes include class designations ranging in number from three to nine, with descriptive statements regarding patient characteristics for each level. Examples of labels assigned to classes are self-care, partial care, and complete care; or I (minimum care), II (average care), III (more than average care), and IV (maximum care). The patient is then categorized as either a I, II, III, or IV based on the most characteristics the patient exhibits.

3. Physiologic dimensions of nursing care are definitely designated, whereas psychosocial, religious, and cultural behavioral needs or requirements are generally not considered.

4. Most systems define nursing care times that can be assigned to activities in the appropriate class or category designation.

5. Many patient classification schemes have not been tested for validity and reliability.

In examining a patient classification tool, one should critically analyze whether it recognizes professional nursing activities other than technical tasks. Connor's work in 1960 (Connor, 1961), the first published work in this area, emphasizes technical, or task, components of nursing care. But Connor's classification must be considered in the context of what nurses did at that particular time in nursing history. An increasing number of tools now are designating emotional support needs and teaching needs. But if emotional support and teaching needs are checked off for every patient without any way to differentiate the amount of teaching and emotional support needed to determine the nursing time required, then teaching and emotional support could actually be considered mathematical constants and could be built into the time allowances for the particular classification levels.

One should also realize that a complex patient classification tool may not be any more accurate or reliable in determining the number of nursing staff needed than a simple system. The necessity of reading lengthy directions may lead to utter frustration and increase the number of mistakes made while trying to follow the directions. The amount of time required to complete the classification tool must also be considered. Important goals for a patient classification instrument are *(1)* internal consistency, or a high interrater reliability; *(2)* simplicity of use; and *(3)* minimal time and cost for the users.

Abdoo (1987) demonstrated that it is difficult to quantitatively support the 90% agreement level for a patient classification instrument, which is usually recommended in the literature (Giovannetti, 1985). The desirable level indicative of achieving interrater reliability depends on the type of patient classification instrument used and should be based on the number of disagreements that can be tolerated before a difference in patient care demand (and the resulting nurse staffing requirements) occurs. On certain days when the percent agreement dropped below 90% in certain classification categories, a significant difference in nursing staff occurred while at other times a significant difference did not occur ($p = .10$). It appears that orientation may be the more important item to attain agreement. The patient care demand requirements increase for each orientation level (with the specific classification instrument used in this study), because there is an inference that if a patient is not oriented to time, place, and person, then he or she will require more nursing assistance. The major factors that contributed to the lack of agreement between raters were incomplete or incorrect information and differences in professional judgments (Abdoo, 1987).

It is important to note that most patient classification tools have been developed for acute medical-surgical patient populations prior to changes in reimbursement practices for inpatient care, redesigned care delivery systems such as "patient-focused care" and other models that use cross-trained workers or lesser skilled workers than RNs in an effort to contain inpatient hospitalization costs, and the expansion in skilled care, home care, and outpatient services. Changes have occurred in the distribution of patient acuity and length of stay (LOS) has decreased. It is also important to note that most of these patient classification systems are not necessarily generalizable to critical care, psychiatric (Eklof & Qu, 1986; Forchuk, 1996), maternity (Killeen, 1986), community health, pediatric patients, ambulatory care or outpatient services (Hoffman & Wakefield, 1986; Johnson, 1989; Karr & Fisher, 1997), home care (Saba, 1992), skilled care, long-term care, and other community settings (Martin & Scheet, 1992). Although modifications of acute care patient classification tools have been made for both skilled and long-term care settings, the frequency (daily versus weekly versus biweekly, etc.) of classifying patients needs to be carefully evaluated as well as the associated nursing care demand times for each classification level.

Noyes (1994) reinforces the importance of achieving interrater reliability and face validity to meet both JCAHO requirements and also regain credibility with the institution's nursing staff and the financial officer in a changing health care market.

> The credibility of PCS [patient classification system] slipped because we (CNEs) and the nursing staff learned that point values could be 'tweaked' to reduce or expand staffing levels requirements. This was true for the projected numbers of nurses required to meet the demand levels and in skill mix. Skill mix was decided on arbitrarily. Patients were getting 'more acute' because of shortening length of stay, and work loads were changing. Financial constraints were an ever increasing reality. (p. 7)

THE DEVELOPMENT OF STAFFING SYSTEMS

During the 1970s, several commercial staffing systems were introduced that have gained popularity. The Medicus system (Freund & Mauksch, 1975; Norby & Freund, 1977; Norby et al., 1977) uses a computer-read classification tool with weights assigned to each of approximately 25 classification indicators. An algorithm utilizing the sum of the weights for the inpatient census and coefficients obtained from regression analysis from previous work determines the number of nursing personnel needed to provide the care. Although the classification tool was computer-read using Scan-tron sheets, the original system did not operate in real time. Some hospitals have the nursing staff classify the patients on-line (directly on the computer screen), whereas other institutions batch the classification sheets and obtain monthly reports for budgeting purposes.

From the work of Poland, English, Thornton, and Owens—the PETO group—evolved the GRASP (Grace-Reynolds Application Study of PETO) nurse staffing system (Clark & Diggs, 1971; Meyer, 1978a, 1978b). The patient care units (PCUs) used are obtained from the patient classification tool for inpatients, and PCUs for incoming admissions are also estimated. New admissions are assigned a bed on a nursing unit with the lowest PCU count to achieve an even distribution or workload among the nursing units. The system, although initially not designed to run on computers, now has a computerized version available .

Chagnon, Audette, Lebrun, and Tilquin (1978) developed a patient classification tool listing 129 possible nursing interventions, each having an estimated weighting for a 24-hour period. The number of staff needed (*P*) is determined using the following equation:

$$P = \frac{(S + TUP)}{360}$$

where *P* is the number of staff needed for a particular shift, *S* is the patient care time, *TUP* are the tasks performed unrelated to individual patient care time, and 360 is the amount of productive time available by a staff member, with time for breaks, meetings, and so on subtracted from the total paid work time (Chagnon et al., 1978). The census form, which includes the number of patients on the unit and their classification, is completed before each shift and submitted to the nursing office to facilitate decisions to balance supply and demand of nursing staff.

It is interesting to note that the published staffing systems derive the number of nursing personnel needed to provide care but do not quantitatively deal with the variance in the number of nursing hours needed. In most cases, the unit is staffed at the mean, and the variance in nursing time demand around the mean is not calculated. Although Connor (1961) discussed how variation in patient needs affects the nursing workload, the GRASP system attempts to reduce the variation in nursing workload by admitting the patient to a bed where there is available nursing time; no attempt has been made to estimate the variance.

Hancock, Segal, Rostafinski, Abdoo, DeRosa, and Conway (1981) have developed a computer-aided nurse staffing system that operates in real time and considers the variation within nurse staffing requirements. The system uses a patient classification schema adapted from Trivedi (1975, 1976) using the ambulation, bathing, feeding, and orientation categories with three possible levels—1, 2, 3,—as the initial indicators of nursing care requirements. This schema results in 3^4, or 81, possible basic classification configurations, each with its own mean nursing time and variance in nursing time to reflect the nursing workload of medical patients, and another 81 means and variances for surgical patients. Intravenous therapy, catheter care, dressing care, and isolation are included in a special procedures section, because these activities reflect a high amount of nursing time.

The development of nurse staffing systems arose from the concern of most nursing departments that there are enough personnel to provide the necessary nursing care. But does the fact that actual staff equals or exceeds recommended staff mean that patients receive the necessary nursing care? Unfortunately, this cannot be concluded for several reasons. It is important to realize that inexperienced personnel, improper skill mix of nursing staff, lack of productivity, inadequate support services, and unpredicted patient crises affect the accuracy of the predicted number of nursing staff. Overstaffing does not ensure that the patients receive more attention or prevents adverse patient outcomes. McCloskey (1998) found after collecting data on six identified adverse patient outcomes (medication errors, patient falls, urinary and respiratory tract infections, skin breakdown, patient complaints, and mortality) for one fiscal year from a large university hospital, that as the "RN proportion of care rose to an 87.5% level, it related to a lower incidence of negative outcomes; however, when the RN proportion of care went beyond that level, the adverse outcome rates also increased" (p. 199). Ongoing and retrospective audits are necessary to evaluate the nursing care services provided and resulting adverse patient outcomes such as patient falls, medication errors, and skin breakdown.

WORK MEASUREMENT IN NURSING

The determination of the amount of nursing time required by each patient for every shift is an essential but by no means simple component of a staffing methodology. Nursing has relied primarily on industrial engineers and engineering work measurement techniques to quantify nursing actions, but there are often problems with the values obtained. For example, many of the allocated time values for patient care deal only with technical tasks. Abdoo (1987) delineates factors that contribute to difficulties in conducting work measurement studies to quantify nursing time:

1. The industrial engineer or nonnurse observer does not recognize the assessment, evaluation, and psychosocial aspects of the nurse-patient contact, and the nurse often does not convey these components of professional nursing practice to the industrial engineer, due to the nurse's unfamiliarity with work measurement techniques.

2. It is often difficult to differentiate between the start and completion of a nursing activity. For example, while giving a patient a bath, the nurse interacts with the patient. How much of the time spent with the patient should be allocated to the technical task of bathing and how much to assessment and interaction?

3. Although often referred to as time-study or efficiency experts, industrial engineers cannot easily measure the time spent in assessment and interaction. Measurement of repetitious, technical tasks can readily be done, but determination of times involving professional judgment and skills is much more difficult.

4. There is a lack of uniformity in the methods used by nursing personnel in performing technical procedures.

5. The procedure often is not completed from start to finish without some type of interruption (e.g., physician, another patient, nursing staff, or visitor asking for information).

Hudson's dissertation, summarized in Aydelotte (1973), presents:

> criteria that support the classification of nursing work as nonrepetitive. He also examines questions relating to variations in task prediction time, to procedure development, and to the incentive problem. Hudson found it difficult to encourage individuals to complete task assignments within the time predicted for their accomplishment. He concluded that a task's time variation was due not only to the individuality of the patient and his condition but also to the individuality of the nurse, the concept of nursing practice, and the preconceived notion of how to perform it. Adherence to a present plan or procedure was not seen by nursing personnel as either essential or desirable. The work sequence and pace were set by other kinds of priorities. (p. 27)

Improvement and refinements in determination of nursing activity times can only occur if the nurse has a basic understanding of work measurement principles so that effective collaboration with industrial engineers will occur. Four basic work measurement techniques have been used in nursing studies to determine the time involved in nursing activities (Williams, 1977):

1. Time study and task frequency
2. Work sampling of nurse activity
3. Continuous observation of nurses performing activities
4. Self-reporting of nurse activity.

Lindner (1989) discusses methods-time measurement (MTM), which was developed in the 1940s for industrial applications, and how a newer method, methods time measurement-universal analyzing system (MTM-UAS) can be used to break down nursing activities into small elements. "In order to develop a time standard for any task, it is necessary only to combine the small elements in the order necessary to complete the task. The order, or sequencing, in which these elements are combined is referred to as the "method" for the activity. . . . By adding the time required for each small activity, total time for the process can be determined . . ." (p. 46).

Difficulties encountered by nursing in using industrial-based work measurement methods to measure nursing practice are:

1. Many of the allotted time values deal with technical tasks because the industrial engineer or observer does not recognize the assessment, evaluation, and psychosocial aspects of the nurse-patient contact. Thus, a patient who requires technical tasks could very likely be rated in a higher category than one who requires psychosocial or teaching activities.
2. In developing a PCS, some nursing departments borrow the nursing times from the classification systems of others. It is important to realize that the times for one agency may not be accurate for another because the nursing policies and procedures, unit architecture, experience of the nurse, and methods of implementing the work can vary from agency to agency.
3. Many systems use the mean time for a task without any consideration of the variance. Abdoo, Hancock, Luttman, and Rostafinski (1979) have found that nursing tasks often vary widely with who performs the activity and the method used. For example, report time on one studied unit ranged from 15 to 90 minutes, with a mean of 30 minutes.
4. The educational and experience background of the observee is often not considered, nor is a differentiation made among the levels of RN, LPN, and nurse assistant or aide.
5. Times obtained by nurses self-recording the nursing actions they performed may not be accurate because it is difficult to accurately perform and simultaneously time the work as one is actually doing it. But if observers had been used, observer bias could also occur. The observers would need to be trained in time studying nursing activities and tested for interrater reliability.
6. Most studies do not consider:

   - The appropriateness of the nursing intervention occurring at the time of intervention
   - The staffing situation at the time of the study (over-, under-, or satisfactorily staffed)
   - The type of nursing care delivery model such as primary, functional, modular, team nursing with skilled nursing staff such as RNs, LPNs or RNs, or LPNs with other cross-trained workers that was in effect.

At present, there is a lack of research dealing with these issues to support what differentiation should be made.

In summary, determination of accurate nursing activity times is very complex but extremely important, because it, along with a reliable and valid PCS, should serve as the foundation for the determination of the number of nursing staff required.

SCHEDULING AND WORKWEEK PATTERNS FOR NURSING PERSONNEL

Once the long-range determination of the average or minimum number of nursing personnel needed to supply daily patient needs has been made, the personnel scheduling can begin. At first glance, scheduling seems to be an easy task of marking on and off days on scheduling sheets. In reality, however, effective scheduling is a science as well as an art. The most overwhelming problem is the interrelatedness between the staffing determination and the scheduling function, because the weekend and holiday-off policies have a direct impact on the necessary number of budgeted nursing positions to provide daily coverage. For example, if the policy is every other weekend off and a minimum of four nurses are needed daily on the day shift, then additional nursing positions are needed to provide the necessary personnel on weekends and required days off. Weekend staffing policies also have direct impact on the nursing budget because the number of extra personnel needed will vary with the number of weekends off in a given scheduling period. Other institutional policies, such as handling of overtime, shift rotation, and number of different shifts that can be worked in a week, also affect scheduling.

Various scheduling systems have been published and deserve consideration: cyclic, supplemental, block, and computerized. There does not appear to be much difference between cyclic and block scheduling, except that the assignment pattern of the former repeats itself in cycles. One advantage of the cyclic method is that the staff can determine their schedule far in advance if the system is strictly adhered to. Requests for certain days off can also be eliminated, because the nursing personnel would be responsible for switching their days off with someone else. Both cyclic and block scheduling lend themselves easily to computerized scheduling.

The practice of float, or supplemental, scheduling has been used intermittently. At one time, float nursing pools were common in hospitals, but they were eliminated as nursing departments were forced to cut their budgets. The pendulum seems to have swung in the opposite direction with "dial-a-nurse," or agency nursing, coming into the picture. Many of these nursing agencies are businesses owned and managed by nurses to provide contract staffing. Although many nursing service departments initially used these contractual services, some nursing departments decided it would be more cost effective to create or reinstitute their own float pool to supplement daily nursing needs. A number of factors must be considered for a successful float pool: selection of float personnel, job satisfaction, in-service education, method of unit assignment, support system, and other factors. The utilization of float nurses to supplement regular unit staffing is a viable, cost-effective option when used properly.

Computerized nurse scheduling was originally conceived as the cure-all for the monotony of nurse scheduling, as well as a cost-effective solution to scheduling problems. A nurse or staffing clerk would no longer be needed to do the technical task of scheduling personnel. Cyclic scheduling lends itself naturally to computerization because, after defining the constraints, the algorithm repeats itself. But manual staffing systems that honor employee requests for days off, require shift rotation, have a nursing shortage, or have high personnel turnover are not as amenable to computer programming. Warner (1976) described his methodology for more flexible staffing options with a mainframe computer; it was based on building in a large number of assumptions and definitions in the computer program algorithm. Warner's system initially appeared successful but still required human handwork afterward to fine-tune the schedule. For example, on Tuesday, there may be only four nurses assigned (the defined minimum number needed) yet on Wednesday, seven nurses might be assigned to the same unit. Warner later converted this mainframe computerized scheduling system to work on the personal computer. The computer algorithm was refined to better allocate the nursing staff, and this personal computer operated system is being marketed as ANSOS (Warner, Keller, & Martel, 1991).

With the decreasing cost and at the same time improved performance of personal computers, other computerized scheduling systems such as the Interactive Scheduler developed by Medicus in the late 1980s (Jelinek & Kavois, 1992) and artificial intelligence-based software systems such as NURSPREF (Applied Interactive Management Corporation, 1987) and NURSE-HELP (Chen & Yeung, 1993) have evolved and are being used in acute care settings. Cost savings are difficult to determine with computerized scheduling systems because one must consider the hardware, software, and associated personnel costs to set up and maintain the system. Some have tried to cost justify the purchase, installation, and maintenance of a scheduling system because the number of full-time equivalent (FTE) personnel needed later to maintain the system will decrease. One must still plan on having the equivalent of one FTE to work with the individual head nurses or unit personnel to implement and maintain the system for about a 400-bed institution. When staff vacancies are minimal, a good staffing clerk can produce a good schedule as efficiently as can a computer. When staff vacancies are high, a computer cannot replace the human judgment necessary to adjust the nursing resources to provide inadequate staffing coverage.

Innovative practices from industry regarding the length of the workday have also affected nursing. Debate continues over 8-hour, 10-hour, and 12-hour workdays, as well as 1-week-on, 1-week-off patterns. The 10-hour workday has been found to work best in areas where continuous 24-hour coverage is not essential. If 24-hour coverage is required, then a mechanism must exist to provide an additional 4 hours of coverage. Two advantages of the 10-hour workday are extra days off in the workweek and decreased transportation-related expenses. Potential child care difficulties, fatigue, and handling of call-ins are some of the disadvantages. In addition, workers may not be used in the best manner when overlapping shifts occur, which can result in extra staffing for a 2-hour period.

Twelve-hour shifts easily provide the necessary 24-hour coverage. Advantages are similar to those of the 10-hour day, whereas the disadvantages could be more severe, for example, the employees may notice more fatigue, and staff may not be able to work overtime to cover a call-in.

Although compressed workweeks have been gaining popularity in nursing settings, more research is needed regarding employee fatigue, employee productivity, cost effectiveness, and fatigue-produced errors. Each method must be examined regarding:

1. Adaptability to institutional personnel and payroll policies and procedures
2. Impact on nonnursing departments
3. Willingness of the nursing staff to work nontraditional hours
4. Cost savings, if any, not only to the employer, but also to the employee (for example 4-day workweeks eliminate 1 day's worth of driving)
5. Present overtime worked by nursing staff on 8-hour workdays

Because these five considerations can vary from institution to institution, one ideal workday length for every agency may not exist. There may not even be unanimous consensus for all units within one institution.

Shift rotation is another important component of nurse scheduling. The preferred trend has been to hire staff for each of the shifts, but because there is often difficulty finding enough personnel to work afternoons and midnights, the day-shift personnel must often rotate. Felton (1975) has written an interesting report concerning her findings related to the effects of shift rotation on physiologic body rhythms:

> The temperature and potassium levels did not return to the before-night rotation levels even 10 days post night duty. . . . In addition to averaging one and a quarter hours less sleep during the day when subjects worked at night, five factors were related to a higher disruption of the quality of their sleep and restfulness: (1) trouble staying asleep, (2) trouble sleeping because of noise or environmental temperature, (3) fatigue, (4) difficulty switching from night to day shift, and (5) requiring a week to adjust bowel habits after night duty. One factor was related to lower disruption: satisfaction with the regular work schedule. (Felton, 1975, pp. 18–19)

Interestingly, there are no further published studies regarding the effects of shift rotation on nursing staff 20 years later. More studies regarding shift rotation of nurses and circadian rhythms, as well as comparisons of the physiologic effects among day-to-night, day-to-afternoon, and afternoon-to-night rotating shifts are needed. One implication thus far is that it is better for a regular day-shift employee to work several consecutive night shifts rather than to work a day-night-off, day-night-off type of rotation.

The issue of centralization adds another dimension to the scheduling and staffing issue. Proponents of decentralization feel that this approach conveys an interest in the individual needs of the employee, while the employee may feel he or she is only a number when dealing with a centralized scheduling office. A centralized scheduling office can usually provide a better balanced schedule in terms of personnel for each shift, whereas a decentralized system may have difficulty providing adequate coverage on certain shifts, especially if the unit is totally responsible to provide its own personnel. An important question arises as to which type of scheduling is more cost effective and which is better able to use the needed nursing staff, based on nursing resource demand. According to Sitompul and Randhawa (1990), "nursing salaries make up the largest single element in hospital costs. Thus, effective scheduling of nursing personnel is important in controlling health-care costs" (p. 62).

CURRENT AND NEXT GENERATION NURSE STAFFING SYSTEMS

The development of patient classification, nurse staffing, and nurse scheduling systems was summarized in the previous sections. Questions arise as to whether current systems meet the needs of nursing service departments, and where these systems should be going to meet future needs in a competitive, dynamic health care environment that emphasizes decreasing health care costs. Changes in nursing care delivery have been implemented to react to decreased LOS and the increasing demand to remain competitive and reduce the costs of inpatient and community-based services. Advances in computer technology, diagnosis-related groups (DRGs) and the adoption of a prospective payment system, managed care, increasing emphasis on productivity, patient outcomes, cost-effective nursing care delivery, changing nursing care delivery models, and total quality management

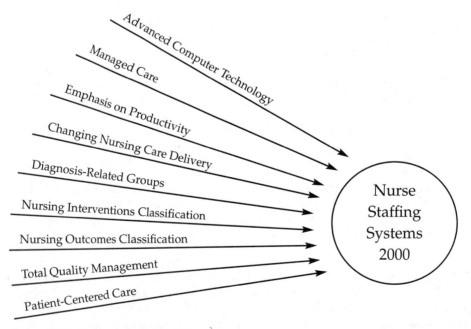

Figure 25.2 Next generation staffing systems.

are factors that have had and will continue to have great impact on the current utilization and future development of nursing staffing systems (Figure 25.2).

Computerized patient classification, staffing, and scheduling systems have become more common as the personal computers have become increasingly powerful and there is less need to have these systems run on hospital mainframe computers. Giovannetti (1990) discusses a second-generation patient classification system, ARIC (allocation, resource identification and costing), incorporating innovative design features made possible with recent software advances. This system provides unit-specific classification information and ongoing reliability and validity monitoring capabilities. DeGroot (1994a) offers another approach to conceptualize and evaluate current methods of PCS-related staffing, and describes a new method of PCS-related staffing with implementation strategies (1994b).

If one critically looks at the current systems in place, one sees that they tend to be fragmented systems developed for a very specific purpose, rather than separate pieces that can easily interface with other specialized systems to result in a completely integrated, (closed feedback loop) system. The patient classification tool was originally developed to classify patients, which then, in turn can be used to predict demand for nursing care time. That information, however, does not typically interrelate with the purchased computerized scheduling package, unless the daily patient classification summary data for a nursing unit is manually reentered into the scheduling system.

The question also arises as to whether a patient classification tool is actually needed if computerized nursing care plans can be developed with associated nursing care times as part of the computerized clinical nursing information system, which then allows the amount of nursing care time required by each patient to be calculated. It is the opinion of this author that this is the direction that patient classification and nurse staffing systems should be taking, rather than trying to develop a patient classification instrument that will satisfy both the nursing staff and nurse managers. As automated or computerized nurse charting becomes more available, then the nursing care that the patient needed can be compared to the documented nursing care that the patient received. Budd and Propotnik (1989) describe a patient classification system driven by computerized nursing notes developed at LDS Hospital, that determines appropriate staffing and also bills patients directly for nursing services.

Daily patient acuity information, the resulting nursing staff predicted necessary to deliver patient care, and the actual staffing with the computed variance in predicted number of staff needed versus actual can be used by nurse managers for decision-making and budget forecasting and in quality assurance programs. The predicted number of staff should be compared with actual staffing on a daily, weekly, and monthly basis. Information aggregated by day of the week can help allocate nursing staff during scheduling. For example, if a surgical unit consistently shows less staff needed than usually provided on Tuesday, the scheduler may be able to adjust future schedules accordingly.

The relationship between patient classification (acuity), DRGs, case mix models, schemas for classifying nursing interventions and outcomes such as the Nursing Interventions Classification (NIC), and Nursing Outcomes Classification (NOC), as well as the feasibility of determining nursing care costs, based on nursing care provided, are being studied in a number of institutions. The major problems have been that the patient classification data, if computerized, has been typically stored as aggregate data (summed over the total number of patients) for a specific patient care unit either by day or by each shift, rather than storing each patient's individual classification configuration for every classification occurrence for that patient, and the variety of patient classification tools that are used across institutions. In addition, the Institute of Medicine (1996) discussed the need for research on the impact of changes in health care and nursing care delivery models with the resulting changes in nurse staffing mix on patient outcomes, and recommended the development of "performance and outcome measures sensitive to nursing interventions and care with uniform definitions that are measurable in a uniform manner across all hospitals" (p. 124).

Nursing departments have been forced to seriously examine nursing resource use and in many cases reduce staff in reaction to the increased emphasis on reducing health care costs from third-party payers. "Nurses account for approximately 35–40% of the total budget of the average hospital (Bridel, 1993; Halloran, 1985), making the utilization of the nursing resource perhaps the highest priority to achieve effective and efficient delivery of care " (Campbell, Taylor, & Shuldham, 1997, p. 237). It is very important for nursing not to just react, but to make decisions based on data and ensure that the changes do not endanger the quality of patient care. McCloskey (1998) examined the relationship between medication errors, patient falls, urinary and respiratory tract infections, skin breakdown, patient complaints, and mortality in one large university hospital, and found an inverse relationship between RN hours of care and rates of medication errors, decubiti, and patient complaints. More studies are needed in this area to document the effects on patient care due to substitutions of licensed nursing personnel with unlicensed personnel. Additional research is needed across all nursing care delivery systems (which includes long-term care and community health facilities) not only to determine the quality and cost of nursing care delivered, but also in other indicator areas such as those pointed out by the Institute of Medicine (1996), for example, rates of injury, illness, stress, and turnover of nursing staff, because of these changing workplace demands.

SUMMARY

Nurse staffing has traditionally consisted of several components: planning, scheduling, and allocation. The planning or staffing methodology phase should be based on quantifiable, measurable data. This systematic nurse staffing determination must include the following variables: *(1)* an assessment of required nursing time to meet patient care needs (patient classification), *(2)* an assessment of required nursing time to meet patient needs (nursing workload determination), and *(3)* an algorithm that uses the first two variables.

The predicted number of nursing staff can be used for personnel scheduling, budgeting, and productivity tracking. A variety of scheduling options are currently used by nursing departments: computerized, compress workweek (with 10-hour and 12-hour workdays); cyclic, block, and float, or supplemental; and centralized or decentralized. It is important to realize that what works well in one institution or even one unit may not work well in a different institution or unit. Although many nurse staffing systems have evolved over the past 35 years, external forces such as the change from a retrospective to a prospective payment system, the shift to a managed care environment, and advances in computer technology and information systems allowing management local and remote access to clinical information will continue to affect the development and utilization of future staffing systems. It is critical that those systems used be modified and new systems be developed and implemented when necessary to reflect the changes in the health care environment and delivery system and to evaluate the impact on quality of care in addition to the financial implications.

STUDY QUESTIONS

1. Interview a nurse executive in an acute care, long-term care, or home care facility. Ask how staffing and scheduling patterns are determined. To what extent does patient acuity affect staffing levels?
2. Explore the legal requirements in your state for on-site availability of RNs in various settings for health care delivery. How does your setting meet or deviate from these requirements?
3. Review this chapter and trace the history of the development of staffing and scheduling systems. How will patient-focused care or the substitution of unlicensed personnel for licensed nursing staff alter these staffing patterns? How can one measure the effects of this type of change and the quality of patient care delivered?
4. Discuss reasons why it is difficult to find nursing staff to work in long-term care facilities, and give examples of strategies that nurse managers can use to improve employee retention.

REFERENCES

Abdellah, F. G., & Levine, E. (1965). *Better patient care through nursing research.* New York: Macmillan.

Abdoo, Y. M. (1987). A model for nurse staffing and the impact of inter-rater reliability of patient classification on nurse staffing requirements. (Doctoral dissertation, University of Michigan, 1987) *Dissertation Abstracts International, 48*(2).

Abdoo, Y. M., Hancock, W. M., Luttman, R., & Rostafinski, M. (1979). *Determination of nurse staffing requirements: A case study.* Unpublished doctoral dissertation, report, University of Michigan, Ann Arbor.

Applied Interactive Management Corporation. (1987). *NURSPREF.* Seattle, WA: Author.

Aydelotte, M. K. (1973). *Nurse staffing methodology: A review and critique of selected literature.* (DHEW Publication No. (NIH) 73-433). Washington, DC: US Government Printing Office.

Bridel, J. E. (1993). Why measure workload? *Professional Nurse, 8,* 362–365.

Budd, M. C., & Propotnik, T. (1989). A computerized system for staffing, billing and productivity measurement. *Journal of Nursing Administration, 19*(7), 17–23.

Campbell, T., Taylor, S., Callaghan, S., & Shuldham, C. (1997). Case mix type as a predictor of nursing workload. *Journal of Nursing Management, 5*(4), 237–240.

Center for Hospital Management Engineering. (1978). *Nurse scheduling: An examination of case studies, proceedings of a forum.* Chicago: American Hospital Association.

Chagnon, M., Audette, L. M., Lebrun, L., & Tilquin, C. A. (1978). A patient classification system by level of nursing care requirements. *Nursing Research, 27*(2), 107–113.

Chen, J. G., & Yeung, T. W. (1993). Hybrid expert-system approach to nurse scheduling. *Computers in Nursing, 11*(4), 183–190.

Clark, E. L., & Diggs, W. W. (1971). Quantifying patient care needs. *Hospitals, 45*(18), 96, 98, 100.

Cochran, J., & Derr, D. (1975). Patient acuity system for nurse staffing. *Hospital Progress, 56*(11), 51–54.

Connor, R. J. (1961). A work sampling study of variations in nursing workload. *Hospitals, 35*(9), 40–41.

Connor, R. J., Flagle, C. D., Hsieh, R. K., Preston, R. A., & Singer, S. (1961). Effective use of nursing resources: A research report. *Hospitals, 35*(9), 30–39.

Des Ormeaux, S. P. (1977). Implementation of the CASH patient classification system for staffing determination. *Supervisor Nurse, 8*(4), 29–35.

DeGroot, H. A. (1994a). Patient classification systems and staffing. Part 1, problems and promise. *Journal of Nursing Administration, 24*(9), 43–51.

DeGroot, H. A. (1994b). Patient classification systems and staffing. Part 2, practice and process. *Journal of Nursing Administration, 24*(10), 17–23.

Eklof, M., & Qu, W. H. (1986). Validating a psychiatric patient classification system. *Journal of Nursing Administration, 16*(5), 10–17.

Felton, G. (1975). Body rhythm effects on rotating work shifts. *Journal of Nursing Administration, 5*(3), 16–19.

Forchuk, C. (1996). Workload measurement and psychiatric mental health nursing: Mathematical and philosophical difficulties. *Canadian Journal of Nursing Administration, 9*(3), 67–81.

Freund, L. E., & Mauksch, I. (1975). *Optimal nursing assignments based on difficulty.* (Final Project Report USPHS 1-R18-Hs001391). Washington, DC: US Government Printing Office.

Georgette, J. K. (1970). Staffing by patient classification. *Nursing Clinics of North America, 5*(2), 329–339.

Giovannetti, P. (1978). *Patient classification systems in nursing.* (DHEW Publication No. (HRA) 78-22). Hyattsville, MD: US Government Printing Office.

Giovannetti, P. (1985). DRGs and nursing workload measures. *Computers in Nursing, 3*(2), 88–91.

Giovannetti, P. (1990). A new generation patient classification system. *Journal of Nursing Administration, 20*(5), 33–40.

Halloran, E. J. (1985). Nursing workload, medical diagnosis related groups, and nursing diagnosis. *Research in Nursing and Health, 8,* 421–423.

Hancock, W. M., Segal, D., Rostafinski, M., Abdoo, Y. M., DeRosa, S., & Conway, C. A. (1981). A computer-aided patient classification system where variation within a patient classification is considered. In C. Tilquin (Ed.), *Systems science in health care.* Toronto: Pergamon Press.

Hoffman F., & Wakefield, D. S. (1986). Ambulatory care patient classification. *Journal of Nursing Administration, 16*(4), 23–30.

Jelinek, R. C., & Kavois, J. A. (1992). Nurse staffing and scheduling: Past solutions and future directions. *Journal of the Society for Health Systems, 3*(4), 75–82.

Johnson, J. M. (1989). Quantifying an ambulatory care patient classification instrument. *Journal of Nursing Administration, 19*(11), 36–42.

Joint Commission on the Accreditation of Healthcare Organizations. (1999). *1999 accreditation manual for hospitals volume I standards.* Oakbrook Terrace, IL: Author.

Karr, J., & Fisher, R. (1997). A patient classification system for ambulatory care. *Nursing Management, 28*(9), 27–28.

Killeen, M. B. (1986). A patient classification tool for maternity services. *NLN Publication,* (20-2155), 293–306.

Lindner, C. (1989). Work measurement and nursing time standards. *Nursing Management, 20*(10), 44–48.

Martin, K. S., & Scheet, N. J. (1992). *The Omaha system: applications for community health nursing.* Philadelphia: Saunders.

McCloskey, J. M. (1998). Nurse staffing and patient outcomes. *Nursing Outlook, 46*(5), 199–200.

McCormick, P., Roche, J. M., & Steinwacks, D. M. (1973). Predicting nurse staffing. *Hospitals, 47*(9), 68, 73–77.

Meyer, D. (1978a). *GRASP: A patient information and workload management system.* Morgantown, NC: MCS.

Meyer, D. (1978b). Work load management system ensures stable nurse-patient ratio. *Hospitals, 52*(5), 81–85.

Minetti, R., & Hutchinson, J. (1975). System achieves optimal staffing. *Hospitals, 49*(9), 61–64.

Institute of Medicine. (1996). *Nursing staff in hospitals and nursing homes: Is it adequate?* Washington, DC: National Academy Press.

Norby, R. B., & Freund, L. E. (1977). A model for nurse staffing and organizational analysis. *Nursing Administration Quarterly, 1*(4), 1–13.

Norby, R. B., Freund, L. E., & Wagner, B. A. (1977). A nurse staffing system based upon assignment difficulty. *Journal of Nursing Administration, 7*(9), 2–24.

Noyes, B. (1994). Inter-rater reliability: Regaining credibility with your staff and financial officer while meeting JCAHO standards. *Journal of Nursing Administration, 24*(9), 7–8.

Saba, V. K. (1992). Home health care classification. *Caring, 11,* 58–60.

Sitompul, D., & Randhawa, S. U. (1990). Nurse scheduling models: A state-of-the-art review. *Journal of the Society for Health Systems, 2*(1), 62–72.

Sokal, R. R. (1974). Classification: Purposes, principles, progress, prospects. *Science, 185*(4157), 1115–1123.

Trivedi, V. M. (1976). Daily allocation of nursing resources. In J. R. Griffith, W. M. Hancock, & F. C. Munson (Eds.), *Cost control in hospitals.* Ann Arbor, MI: Health Administration Press.

Trivedi, V. M., & Hancock, W. M. (1975). Measurement of nursing workload using head nurses' perceptions. *Nursing Research, 24*(5), 371–376.

Warner, D. M. (1976). Computer-aided system for nurse scheduling. In J. R. Griffith, W. M. Hancock, & F. C. Munson (Eds.), *Cost control in hospitals.* Ann Arbor, MI: Health Administration Press.

Warner, M., Keller, B. J., & Martel, S. H. (1991). Automated nurse scheduling. *Journal of the Society for Health Systems, 2*(2), 66–80.

Williams, M. A. (1977). Quantification of direct nursing care activities. *Journal of Nursing Administration, 7*(8), 15–18.

PART
6

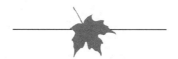

Current and
Emerging Challenges

CHAPTER
26

Impact of Aging on Nursing Practice Patterns

Lillian M. Simms • Naomi E. Ervin

To the matter of increasing capability must be added the aging factor and the nation's apparent unwillingness to address issues of when doing more is appropriate—that is the rationing issue. (Zelman, 1996, p. 40)

Chapter Highlights

- Changing demographics
- Standards of health care
- The frail older people
- Assuming leadership for new practice patterns
- Obstacles to a geriatric emphasis
- Older women: a special need

The rapid growth in the older population in this country is one of the most influential forces shaping the health care delivery system and society as a whole now and well into the next century. Americans over age 65 will increase from 25 million in 1980 to 66 million by 2040 according to projections by the U.S. Bureau of the Census in Projections of the Population of the United States: 1982 to 2050 (Figure 26.1). This represents a surge from 11% to 21% of the total population. These changing demographics are not confined to the older population. Worldwide, the

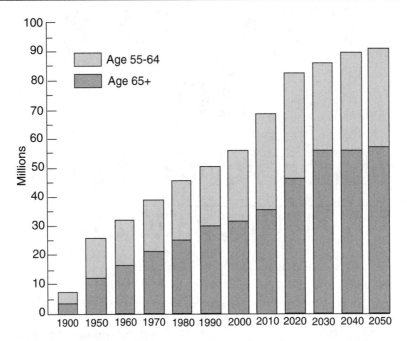

Figure 26.1 Number of persons aged 55 and over by age group, 1900 and 1950 to 2050 (data for 1980–2050 are projections). (From the National Center for Health Statistics.)

number of women is increasing at all age levels (American Academy of Nursing [AAN], 1997). As the global society moves from a situation of high rates of fertility and mortality to low rates, whole populations begin to age. With the decline in infant and childhood mortality rates, the elderly portion of the world's population will continue to increase (Figure 26.2). The question arises as to whether or not this group represents a vast group of untapped human resources or a burgeoning pocket of individuals in the upper age ranges who have the greatest need for social, income maintenance, housing, and health services. History will decide the outcome of this argument, but in the meantime, drastic changes in the thinking of nurse executives must occur.

CHANGING DEMOGRAPHICS

Traditionally, the health care field has been facility driven (Zelman, 1996). However, it is becoming increasingly evident that new programs must be developed with creative solutions that go beyond bricks and mortar if the benefits of longevity are not to bankrupt America and other countries around the world. Some level of clinical integration along a full continuum of care in an organized system must be provided. The majority of older people are active individuals who prefer to live at home in apartments, houses, and mobile homes. Although home health services have mushroomed, a major gap remains in the market for

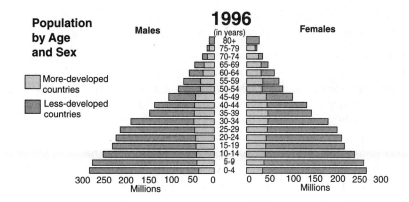

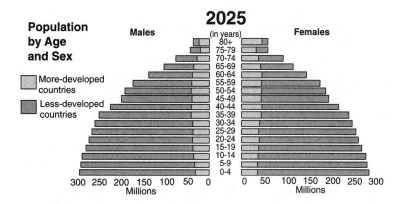

Figure 26.2 The changing global age structure. U.S. Bureau of the Census, International Programs Center, International Data Base.

creative individualized services. A network of services is essential to the provision of a system that will support older people living at home. One of the most important linkages could be ambulatory centers that provide health maintenance information and activities as well as numerous social activities for clients or their families. Another is the nursing home model that serves as a rehabilitation center. Walk-in ambulatory day centers and redesigned nursing homes may serve as the key to liberation of older people in the 21st century. Chapter 8 discusses a variety of relevant community settings.

The application of assistive technology to the problems of older people has had two major effects (Haber, 1986). First, it reduces the costs of care by providing additional help to older people so they can remain independent, and second, it enhances the quality of life. Numerous devices, described in Chapter 32, will minimize the problems of vision, hearing, musculoskeletal disabilities, proprioceptive loss, and the dementias. It is conceivable that many tasks now performed by nursing staff could be assisted by robotics. Nurse executives may wish to analyze critically current and emerging technologies that could not only enhance the quality of life of older people but could greatly affect the nature of nursing care.

The fastest growing group is the old-old, those over 85 years. If the nursing profession is to respond adequately to the growing numbers of older adults, it must intensify its commitment to the special health and health-related problems of older people at every level of administration, education, practice, and research (Rowe & Kahn, 1998). Since 1950, life expectancy in the older ages has increased at an accelerated pace. Most of the increase in life expectancy before 1950 was due to decreasing mortality at the younger ages: growing numbers of people reached old age because of decreased mortality rates in the younger age groups. Since World War II, life expectancy at the older ages has increased at a faster rate than at birth.

It is anticipated that the number of older people will increase even more in the decades ahead. This is not an unreasonable or unwanted speculation when one considers the fact that for humans to travel to and live on other planets, a much longer life span will be required.

For health care professionals, including nurses, the impact of the increased aging population is one of major importance. The use of all health care services increases dramatically with age. Most older people have at least one chronic condition, and older people with multiple chronic diseases are common. The most common chronic condition in old age requiring health care services are arthritis, hypertension, hearing impairment, heart conditions, orthopedic impairment, sinusitis, visual impairments, and diabetes (Belsky, 1988). Therefore, chronic conditions have a serious impact on care needs for those who require services ranging from daily personal care to hospitalization in acute or long-term care facilities.

The use of hospitals and nursing homes increases significantly with old age. The hospitalization rate for people 65 and older is much greater than for younger people (Zelman, 1996). Although most people 65 and older are not hospitalized in any given year, older people will continue to account for an increasing share of total hospital usage.

The nursing home population has also increased remarkably. Although less than 5% of all people over 65 are in nursing homes, this figure increases significantly in the middle-old and old-old groups. Seven of 100 people in the 75 to 84 age group and one out of five in the 85-plus group are in nursing homes (Rowe & Kahn, 1998). Women are likely to be present in larger numbers than men because there are more women in this age bracket. However, worldwide, women tend to be more disabled than men by age 65 and require more health services (Figure 26.3).

The causes of death, and therefore the nature of health care, for old people are markedly different than for young people. Heart disease, stroke, and cancer account for three-fourths of all deaths in the group aged 65 and older.

Thus, the demographic changes in our population project an increasing number of older people as well as an increased need for health care services. The signifi-

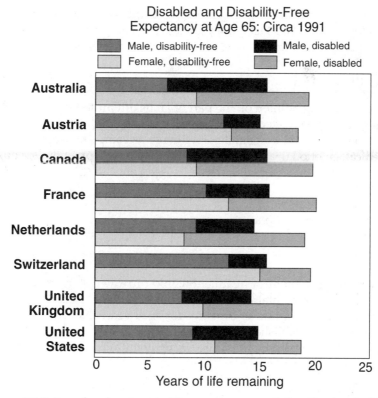

Figure 26.3 Female advantage in life expectancy partially offset by disability. World Health Organization. (1995). *World Health Report 1995.* Geneva, Switzerland.

cance of long-term care—long considered less important than short-term care—will become fully recognized in the next decade. Long-term care encompasses a continuum of interrelated health and social services. It includes both institutional and noninstitutional services and requires coordination of public policies, funding, and case management to provide appropriate services for individuals with changing needs (Zelman, 1996).

The concern for older people in today's health care world is not solely the result of the greatly increased number of them. Changes in federal legislation since the 1930s have contributed much to the economic status of the 65-and-over group. As a result of the Great Depression, the Social Security Act was passed, establishing a retirement income system and a system of federal grants to states to provide financial assistance to the aged (Rowe & Kahn, 1998).

Nurses can expect to deliver care to increasing numbers of older people who can pay for health care either through private insurance or Medicare-Medicaid reimbursement. All facets of care are available, ranging from highly complex technological procedures to wellness-based, self-care, teaching-learning approaches. For most of the old-age group who are not incapacitated by disease, intellectual functioning and the capacity for learning neither cease nor diminish because of chronological age. This fact allows nurses to develop creatively those options for nursing care that uniquely meet the nursing care needs of older people.

STANDARDS OF HEALTH CARE

There is a rapidly growing opinion on the part of all health professionals that older people should not be treated as separate systems, organs, and diseases. Rather, they should be treated by a single practitioner as complete people with individual medical, emotional, and social histories. This single practitioner could provide:

- Accessibility to care
- Competence of the practitioner
- Caring focus
- Affordable care

Translated into reality, this mode of treatment would provide patient-centered care, with an emphasis on maintaining cost-effective, humane services. Older people today pay more out-of-pocket expenses for health care than when Medicare programs were first established. Even though a large percent of the total health care bill is currently paid by Medicare, many items of need are excluded (1995 White House Conference on Aging, 1996).

Much of the inefficiency in care delivery is related to the lack of optimal services geared toward the special needs of older people. Dr. Leslie S. Libow (1982), the medical director at the Jewish Institute for Geriatric Care, Long Island, New York, envisioned the nursing homes as a respected place for treating people. A pioneer in health care, he saw the nursing home as a major center of activity in the nation's health care scene and an extension of the university health sciences campus. Training of undergraduate and graduate students in medicine, nursing, social services, and allied health sciences would involve exposure to geriatric and nursing home patients.

In proposing a framework for a continuum of care for aged people, Libow suggested that aging is the celebration of survival and geriatrics the fruition of the clinician. Increasingly, the nursing home—if not all long-term care facilities—is the place for that celebration and fruition to occur. Libow saw the nursing home image changing from a place in which to die to a respected place for treating people. Libow maintained that there is no respectable science and art of medicine without geriatric medicine and no true geriatric medicine without the nursing home. Many of Libow's ideas have already come to fruition with the development of assisted living complexes and teaching nursing homes.

Therefore, it is conceivable to imagine a full-service geriatric program that involves provision of services across settings from the patient's own home to a skilled nursing home to an acute hospital, and so on. Older people are no more limited to place of care than are younger people. Frequently, the acute care hospital is the point of entrance to the health care system, at which nursing has the greatest opportunity to influence decisions about continuity of care and linkage with other settings. Figure 26.4 presents a model of the type of geriatric health care system first outlined by Libow (1982). A similar systems approach has been proposed by Denson (1992) as the result of tracing older people through the health care system. The nursing home as a rehabilitation site has been vastly underused. Unfortunately, standard hospital rehabilitation programs often reject the very patients who require rehabilitation prior to discharge. Frail older people are a very large part of this group. As hospitals seek to diversify, it becomes essential for nurse executives to design new nursing patterns that will promote continuity of care across various settings. To establish a rehabilitation unit in a nursing home is to depart from the traditional role of the nursing home and offer a setting in which a full interdisciplinary team can excel. Rehabilitation in the United States has traditionally been applied primarily to persons in youth and midlife. The widespread association of aging with infirmity and the assumption that loss of function is normal in advanced age have contributed to denial of essential therapies. Rehabilitation could be embedded in the total care program rather

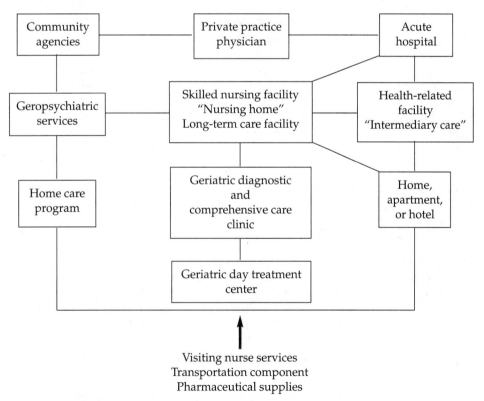

Figure 26.4 The geriatric health care system. From Libow, L. S. (1982). Geriatric medicine and the nursing home. *The Gerontologist, 22*(2), 139. Reprinted by permission.

than an add-on, fee-for-service treatment. Health professionals must recognize that rehabilitation or its lack may be the determining factor in whether an individual will require care from others and what level and duration of continuing care will be required.

Research on aging conducted by Rowe and Kahn (1998) found evidence of the successful influence of exercise, diet changes, and meaningful everyday activities on disease prevention and longevity. Nurse executives could be instrumental in planning behavioral programs that nurture prevention of disease in old age.

THE FRAIL OLDER PEOPLE AND SECONDARY AGING

In the medical world, where a disease-illness orientation is predominant, social-psychological theories of aging are less important than biologic theories. The identification of the causes of the numerous physical and mental afflictions is the goal of research in the biology of aging. The average human life has increased mainly because infectious diseases have succumbed to antibiotics, immunization, and improved sanitation.

Various biologic studies indicate that the cause of aging may not be outside us but within us. Simple descriptions of changes in the physical and mental characteristics of the aged are not sufficient to explain the aging process. A number of investigators have shown that cultured human fibroblasts double only a limited number of times before they deteriorate, lose their capacity to divide, and die. However, they do not think that people age because some of their cells lose the capacity to divide. Rather, they attribute aging to the loss of cell function that occurs before cells reach their limit for division. As cells malfunction, body organs and whole systems are affected and eventually die (Abrams, 1997).

Other investigators attribute senescence to errors in cell operations regulated by DNA. The aging body's increasing susceptibility to disease may be directly related to declining levels of thymosin. The increase in disease in older people occurs during the same period that the thymosin-producing thymus gland shrinks with age. Other biologic theorists espouse the wear-and-tear theory, the lipofuscin theory, the cross-linkage theory, and the immunologic theory (Abrams, 1997).

One cannot help but think that theories of aging that focus on changes in individual cells are not comprehensive enough. Yet the nature of this kind of research and the interest in prolonging life at any cost necessarily affects physicians and nurses and the decisions they make in caring for people. Many doctors and nurses still speak of finding a cure for old age, as if it is a disease rather than part of the life cycle. There always seems to be hope that some medication will be found to block the aging process. The genetic revolution and its impact on aging and disease is discussed in Chapter 34.

In a sense, then, aging presents a negative picture to health professionals. In care settings, the loss of physical functions tends to blur the image of older people as lively, unique individuals. Students in nursing and medical schools must understand the function of all body systems; failure of these systems is viewed as an indication of the decline of the whole person. The MacArthur Foundation Studies of Aging in America (Rowe & Kahn, 1998) have debunked the myths that to be old in America means to be sick and frail. Three key factors have been found to predict mental function in old age: *(1)* regular physical activity, *(2)* strong social support systems, and *(3)* belief in self and ability to cope.

Loss of function in primary aging, aging without disease, occurs at varying levels in all organs and systems. Diseases, however, contribute a secondary aging effect and are the cheif barrier to extended longevity. In primary aging, changes occur in audio-visual, neurologic, cardiovascular, metabolic, renal, and respiratory function (Abrams, 1997). When disease is present, more function is lost and at a faster pace.

Nurse executives are responsible for nursing practice, research, and education as they relate to professional nursing within the institution. Yet, little if any attention is directed toward the care of old people, who now account for more than 25% of all health care costs (Zelman, 1996). The health care system in the United States has two standards of care: one for the aged and one for younger patients. These problems of a double standard are primarily due to failure of the nursing and medical professions to incorporate gerontologic and geriatric knowledge into their educational curricula, research, and clinical practice.

In hospitals, nursing homes, and home care settings, there is a need for health care workers to prevent confusion, minimize dependence, and provide physical care for older patients. Skill in caring for the aged patient can be improved only if someone in a leadership position demands new standards of care. The nurse executive has wide influence throughout the institution and, aside from the physician, is the single person most likely to affect the care of large numbers of patients. Nurse executives can establish the goal of having better prepared nurses by sharing gerontologic knowledge and providing resources with which staff nurses may enhance their skills.

Nurses are in a unique position to influence care of older people. The frail, disabled, and dysfunctional older people are a particularly powerless and voiceless constituency. Burnside (1981) first described the frail older people as those who have reached a great age, over 75, and who have, during their long lives, accumulated multiple disabilities, chronic illnesses, or both. These changes, combined with an aging physiology, put such people at increased risk of physical and psychosocial impairments. The frail older person is under constant stress from within and without and has difficulty maintaining daily living activities. Maintenance of wellness is difficult and illness is frequent. Recognizing the real and potential physical changes in old age, nurse executives face a tremendous challenge in planning patient-centered care that requires recognition of environmental and learning needs.

ASSUMING LEADERSHIP FOR NEW PRACTICE PATTERNS

The basic assumption underlying all rehabilitation, remotivation, and reality-orientation care models is that older adults have the ability to learn new behaviors.

In the words of Howard McClusky (1971), who lived and functioned as a professor until the age of 82:

> In general, then, we are justified in saying that even into the 70s and 80s, and for all we know as long as we live on the functioning side of senility, age per se is no barrier to learning. There is no one at any age, even the most gifted, who is without limitation in learning. Thus limitation per se—age related or otherwise—should not be our criterion for appraising the capacity of older people for education. We can teach an old dog new tricks, for it is never too late to learn. (pp. 12–13)

The lag between nursing knowledge and practice is greater for older people than for any other age group. Few nurses are prepared for geriatric care, and few nurses know that the aging process alone is not a cause of a patient's psychological condition; other causes might be drugs, nutrition, disease, or depression due to grief. The nurse executive has wide influence in an institution and is in a better position than any other person to affect the care of large numbers of patients. For every organization that becomes a center of geriatric expertise, higher expectations of care will be sought in other organizations.

The nurse executive role in nursing homes is at a significant crossroad. The last White House Conference on Aging of the 20th century provided an additional stimulus for the nursing profession to offer leadership in the care of older people. Major emphasis was given to the importance of nursing leadership in health care services. Nurses have already demonstrated leadership in establishing preventive health care services in nontraditional settings with a focus on wellness. Nurses have served as health caregivers, counselors, and client advocates, and it is important now to direct such efforts to promoting health for older adults. Health was recognized at the conference as the chief determinant in improving quality of life for senior citizens and was cited as the first core issue of concern. Ensuring comprehensive health care including long-term care was the primary core issue with the following items identified:

- Promotion and prevention
- Access to quality care
- Continuity of care across settings
- Preservation Medicare/Medicaid
- Research and education (1995 White House Conference on Aging, 1996)

A variety of educational programs can be designed, irrespective of health care setting, that can improve the physical health, mental health, self-esteem, and independence of the aged person. The best mode for restoring psychological health and, indirectly, physical health is through remotivation techniques that encourage patients to use their own past experiences and skills in coping with the present. Prior life experiences, values, and interests can be used by a knowledgeable staff in assisting older adults to greater independence and improved quality of life.

Attention to functional competence and the need to teach staff how to work with older people and change behavior are necessary. Because institutional dependency is related to poor self-concept and low life satisfaction, it is important to investigate altering both behavior and setting to enhance resident autonomy. Nurses have a major role to play in identifying measures that will offset the effects of cognitive, elimination, audiovisual, and mobility problems. Regardless of disease processes, these functional disabilities commonly interfere with activities that could enhance self-esteem and encourage independence. The same principles of care apply in acute, long-term, and home care settings.

Luskin et al. (1998) conducted an exploration of successful aging by reviewing studies of prominent mind-body therapies with particular focus on cardiovascular and musculoskeletal disease as the most disabling conditions for older people. A compelling body of evidence supports the linkage between mind and body and the current distinction between mind and body therapies may no longer be tenable. Hope and spirituality were found to enhance well-being in older individuals and thus influenced adaptation to illness and continued function during chronic illness.

The various studies reviewed by Luskin et al. (1998) suggest that social support may be the predominant influencing factor for mitigating the harmful effects of cardiovascular disease. As a specific form of social support, attendance at church or religious services appears to have a protective effect on the health of older people, having positive effects on both mortality and morbidity rates. In other studies of social support, those who frequently attend church have lower death rates, smoke less, exercise more, and have better social contact than those who rarely or never attend church.

Other studies evaluated the effects of forgiveness training on anger management, cognitive-behavioral therapy, imagery, meditation, music therapy, hypnosis, energy/spiritual healing, yoga, and the martial arts. The implications of this research are multiple. Nursing practice patterns of the future will have to reflect therapies that not only achieve symptom reduction in those with identified diseases but will also have to include teaching behaviors that encourage successful aging. There is compelling need for nursing interventions that will guide prevention of disease and reduction of cost of care for an estimated 70 million people by the year 2030.

OBSTACLES TO A GERIATRIC EMPHASIS

A negative attitude toward older people is frequently cited as the major cause of disinterest in working with older people in any health care setting. Aging may be equated with disease or even death, both having negative connotations in our society. All societies deny death. This is manifested in various ways of ignoring the dying person or carrying on elaborate rituals to keep the dead with the living, as seen, for example, in the practice of keeping cremated ashes in the living room or preserving departed family members in cryogenic vaults. Belief in an afterlife is one of many societal supports, and the clear if unwritten goal in the institutions where most of us will die is to preserve life at any cost. In fact, modern medicine has added more to immortality than have all the theologians and church people in history combined. Physicians seem determined to do almost anything to keep a human system going.

Overcoming negative attitudes is difficult, for they are usually strongly held. In defining programs and goals with a geriatric emphasis, the nurse executive will have to facilitate learning behaviors that will produce positive attitudes. Despite the prevailing belief that old age is synonymous with a decline in creativity, Simonton (1990) proposes that a much more favorable outlook can be gained by reviewing the actual careers of artists and scientists in their later years. The author cites the work of Galileo, Goethe, Bach, Handel, Beethoven, Hawking, and Rosenweig as individuals who refused to let physical handicaps stop them from generating ideas. Creativity in the later years may be dependent on an individual's initial creative potential in earlier life and seems unrelated to age. The potential for late-life creativity has implications for planning health care services and in viewing human resources in care-giving roles. Perhaps every individual patient has untapped creativity and potential for living a meaningful life. It is up to the caregiver to spot this potential and to match nursing therapies with abilities. Depression is a major dysfunction in old age but is one that can be addressed with holistic patient-centered care that recognizes individual goals for creative activities.

Older adults are the biggest users of illness care in U.S. hospitals and nurse executives need to know and understand concerns of older adults. Knowledge of concerns could lead to establishing services that might be offered on an outpatient basis without hospital admission. Older adults comprise 20% of hospital admissions, 40% of inpatient days, and 30% of hospital discharges (Halbur & Freeberg, 1991). Recognizing that comprehensive geriatric programs are needed, Halbur and Freeberg conducted a survey of older adults' concerns in an urban community hospital. Handling changes in life and staying active and involved were high on the list of identified concerns of older people. The results further suggested involvement of older people in planning geriatric programs.

Contrary to popular belief, the economic situation of older people has improved dramatically over the past several years. Older people as a group have impressive financial assets despite areas of deep poverty. Aging of the population and the related requirements for home personal assistance have increased the demand for unskilled home care services, whereas the supply of acceptable quality, paid custodial home care is threatened by the increasingly precarious financial condition of providers (Zelman, 1996). As hospitals seek new markets, the creative nurse executive must attend to the rapidly increasing need for housekeeping services at home in combination with skilled nursing services. A creative nurse executive could design a unique geriatric home care program that links housekeeping services with health care services in a product that has appeal for a large number of clients.

Many older people live in rural areas of our country and many of them suffer from some form of chronic disease (1995 White House Conference on Aging, 1996). Nurse executives, seeking to develop marketable health promotion product lines, may well be interested in recognizing this group as they work to develop a positive geriatric emphasis. The present system of activities by agencies is based on a belief that old people are sick, disabled, and poor and unable to participate independently in society. Those who are actively concerned about the aged can play an active role in shaping the nature of change by devoting more attention to the positive side of aging to balance the past emphasis on dependency, helplessness, deprivation, and cure of disease (Rowe & Kahn, 1998).

OLDER WOMEN: A SPECIAL NEED

Nursing care programs often ignore the special health needs of older people, and, in particular, they may not even recognize the needs of older women. Older women are economically disadvantaged, socially isolated, and negatively stereotyped (AAN Writing Group, 1997). The medical profession takes a different view of men and women experiencing the same medical problems, and it is not uncommon for women to receive tranquilizers that are not appropriate. Ageism and sexism form a double-edged sword. Postmenopausal women have frequently outlived their culturally ascribed usefulness and frequently face additional negative attitudes toward feminine aging. The vast majority of elderly people are older women, and because the care of older people is primarily a nursing task, the opportunities for negative behavior are compounded if nurses do not have a geriatric interest.

Women are less apt to have supportive family groups (AAN Writing Group, 1997). They become widowed before men, and they have fewer remarriage options. It is not socially acceptable for older women in our culture to marry men substantially younger than themselves. Health problems abound in older women, and few doctors seem interested in these problems. "Postmenopausal syndrome" and "senility" frequently cover up a medical diagnosis or lack of it.

The story of poverty in old age is the story of women without job skills and knowledge of financial management. Nursing practice patterns should be designed to address the broader circumstances of women's lives, including sanitation, environmental health, housing, infectious disease surveillance, and control. Programs for community-based health promotion and disease prevention, nutrition supplementation and screening services are essential. According to a special report by the AAN Writing Group for Women's Health (1997), fundamental features of excellent women's health care should include:

- A grounding in an awareness of women's everyday lives
- Reflection of diversity

- Oriented to comprehensive care across the life span
- A wide range of services provided
- Multidisciplinary care providers
- Accessible to all women

Women's health care across the life span should begin in childhood with elements of community care emphasizing prevention of disease and promotion of health.

Nurse executives need to develop new practice pattern models for better delivery of health services to underserved populations of women and children. Access to health care services is strongly related to financial ability to obtain the services. It is estimated that 12 million adult women in the U.S. are uninsured. Their incomes, if any, remain lower than men's and their health insurance packages may be available only through their husband. Nurse executives are in a unique position to transform existing patient education programs to include career planning, counseling, and financial training.

Fitness programs could well include a creative education packet that includes assistance with diverse aspects of daily living including physical, mental, family, and fiscal fitness. Patient-centered practice patterns need to be designed to fit the coming age in which care recipients are part of the planning process for care over the life span. Nurses are uniquely prepared to provide whole family services in a variety of settings. Chapter 8 discusses the wide range of practice settings beyond the hospital including community and rural practice settings, which are especially relevant for family care.

SUMMARY

Responsibility for care of older people as a significant part of the nurse executive's role has not been addressed in most organizations. Most staffing studies focus on high turnover rather than on the potential for nursing leadership in providing quality care for older people. Our society's concept of aging and the attitudes of health professionals and patients influence the development of optimal care programs. Nurse executives should encourage creative approaches to care, ranging from changing attitudes toward older people to designing programs that meet their special needs. They are also in a unique position to support the development of assistive technology for older people. Older women's health is a special need requiring new approaches to health care over the life span.

STUDY QUESTIONS

1. How does the increasing older population relate to nursing administration and practice?
2. Why are population trends considered important aspects of society?

3. People are living longer in the United States today than at any other time in history. Explain how this affects the health care delivery system. Include the effects of Social Security and Medicare-Medicaid.

4. Explain Libow's position on nursing homes, and contrast it with your own concept of nursing homes.

5. Discuss the concepts of primary and secondary aging.

6. Explain the importance of distinguishing the aging process from a disease process and give the major reasons why aging is sometimes considered a disease.

7. Review the demographic charts in this chapter and develop a proposal for a nurse-managed clinic.

8. List the steps essential for nurse executives to provide leadership in stimulating better care for older people.

9. Give reasons why it is vitally important that nursing personnel understand the concepts of geriatrics.

10. What is the most frequently cited reason for disinterest in working with older people? What are some of the others?

11. List some of the special needs of older women.

REFERENCES

Abrams, G. D. (1997). Cellular injury and death. In S. A. Price & L. M. Wilson (Eds.), *Pathophysiology* (5th ed.). St. Louis: Mosby-Year Book.

American Academy of Nursing. (1997). Global migration: The health care implications of immigration and population movements. Proceedings of the American Academy of Nursing 1995 Annual Meeting and Conference, *Health care in times of global transitions*. Washington, DC: Author.

Belsky, J. K. (1988). *Here tomorrow. Making the most of life after fifty*. Baltimore: Johns Hopkins University Press.

Burnside, I. M. (1981). *Nursing and the aged*. New York: McGraw-Hill.

Denson, P. M. (1992). Tracing the elderly through the health care system: An update. *AHCPR Monographs. DHHS, PHS, Agency for Health Care Policy and Research (AHCPR)*. Information and Publications Division, 18-12 Parklawn Building, Rockville, MD.

Haber, P. A. L. (1986). Technology in aging. *The Gerontologist, 26*(4), 350–357.

Halbur, B., & Freeberg, K. (1991). Older and wiser: A hospital-based comprehensive geriatric program. *The Gerontologist, 30*(6), 833–836.

Libow, L. S. (1982). Geriatric medicine and the nursing home: A mechanism for mutual excellence. *The Gerontologist, 22*(2), 134–141.

Luskin, F. M., Newell, K. A., Griffith, M., et al. (1998). A review of mind-body therapies in the treatment of cardiovascular disease. Part 1: Implications for the elderly. *Alternative Therapies, 4*(3), 46–61.

McClusky, H. Y. (1971). *Education*. Background paper for 1971 White House Conference on Aging. Washington, DC: U.S. Government Printing Office.

National Center for Health Statistics. (1996). *Current population reports*. U.S. Bureau of the Census. Washington, DC: U.S. Government Printing Office.

Rowe, J. W., & Kahn, R. L. (1998). *Successful aging.* New York: Pantheon Books.

Simonton, D. K. (1990). Creativity in the later years: Optimistic prospects for achievement. *The Gerontologist, 30*(5), 626–631.

U.S. Bureau of the Census. (1996). International Programs Center, International Data Base.

U.S. Department of Commerce, Economics and Statistics Administration, Bureau of the Census. (1996). *Global aging into the 21st century.* Washington, DC: U.S. Government Printing Office.

1995 White House Conference on Aging. (1996). *The Michigan experience final report.* State of Michigan: Michigan Office of Services to the Aging.

World Health Organization. (1995). *World Health Report 1995.* Geneva, Switzerland: Author.

Writing Group of the 1996 AAN Expert Panel on Women's Health. (1997). Women's health and women's health care: Recommendations of the 1996 AAN expert panel on women's health. *Nursing Outlook, 45*(1), 7–15.

Zelman, W. A. (1996). *The changing health care marketplace.* San Francisco: Jossey-Bass.

CHAPTER
27

Beyond Managed Care: Person-Centered Care

Ingrid A. Deininger • Naomi E. Ervin

The person is a whole being and cannot be separated into segments for diagnosis and cure. (Carson, 1989, p. 8)

Chapter Highlights

* Effects of managed care
* Person-centered care—a holistic model
* Nurse-managed home care
* Individualized hospice care
* A great place to work
* Role of the nurse executive
* Challenges to person-centered care

The advent of managed care has created an unexpected opportunity for professional nurses to expand their clinical and management skills in various primary care and nurse-managed environments. The delivery of health care in the United States was revolutionized in 1973 with the passage of the Health Maintenance Organization (HMO) Act that legitimized HMOs and authorized government funds for implementation. Medicare and Medicaid were born and employers began to offer numerous health care insurance options. Long-term care and primary care became realistic options for care and consumers developed, for the first time in history, an appreciation for health care as a lifetime concept, not entirely related to medical care. The purpose of this chapter is to present a theoretical and practical approach to person-centered home care with special emphasis on hospice care. There are multiple health professionals today, but it is the professional nurse who can best coordinate care for the whole person. Although managed care continues to get mixed ratings, the hue and cry for person-centered care remains a major focus of consumer interest.

EFFECTS OF MANAGED CARE

The health care system has changed substantially over the last decade and will continue to do so in the 21st century. Managed care systems have emerged in response to the HMO legislation. Models for managed care are discussed in Chapter 30. These systems are generally defined as systems that integrate the financing and delivery of appropriate health care services to enrollees by means of one or more of the following elements:

- Arrangements with selected providers to provide a comprehensive set of health care services
- Explicit standards for the selection of health care providers
- Formal programs for ongoing quality improvement and utilization review
- Emphasis on keeping enrollees healthy
- Financial incentives for enrollees to use providers and services associated with the plan (Health Insurance Association of America [HIAA], 1996)

Although physicians initially resisted this change in the way health care business is conducted, opposition has gradually decreased. For the first time, consumers are taking a new look at health care and are becoming knowledgeable participants, not only selecting the type of health insurance plan but working actively with health professionals in planning their care. Nurse practitioners (NPs, a specialized role for nurse executives) are increasingly more involved in primary and family care settings, as well as long-term care settings (Reyes, 1999).

Nurse Practitioners

Nurse practitioners are RNs whose formal education and clinical training extend beyond the basic nursing licensure requirements. An integral part of the managed care system, NPs are frequently case managers whose central role is to obtain and negotiate the most cost-effective service for the patient. NPs are trained to diagnose and recommend treatment for common acute illnesses, disease prevention, management of chronic illnesses, and numerous other primary care and long-term care services. NPs treat the whole person and in general bring a focus on health care prevention and education as well as long-term chronic oversight. Although their contribution is largely to the care of women and children, NPs also provide valuable services for the mushrooming aging population. The age group growing most rapidly is senior citizens 85 years and older who are increasingly requiring long-term care in institutions or at home (HIAA, 1996). Chapter

26 provides a continuum of care model for older people that includes home care, long-term care, and acute care settings. Hospice programs are emerging as unique person-centered, holistic multidisciplinary models that are viable nurse-managed options for many consumers.

PERSON-CENTERED CARE—A HOLISTIC MODEL

Person-centered nursing is based on the assumption that each person is a unique and complex human being comprising biologic, psychological, sociologic, and spiritual components (Lindberg, Hunter, & Kruszewski, 1998). As an open system, the components of the person are constantly changing and interacting. Inherent in this concept is the unifying element of spirit, which is not necessarily religious in nature, but is the inspiring or animating principle that pervades thought, feeling, and action. Thus, professional nurses view the person as a holistic being who is greater than the sum of one's parts with a spiritual component that makes one unique. Figure 27.1 depicts an example of an holistic model.

The philosophy of person-centered, individualized care is based on the belief that the individual is a person with intrinsic worth and dignity, a person who deserves respect. Because patients have worth as persons, their wishes—how they desire to live the remainder of their life, where they want to live, and the manner and place of their dying—are to be respected. The patients' desires dictate the course and manner of the care they receive. Nurses realize that "everything has its season," even death. Death, then, is not an event that occurs in a vacuum, but an inevitable part of the process of living that derives its value and worth from life lived to the fullest and from the person who has lived it.

Spiritual Component

The spiritual component can be an integral part of nursing practice in any care setting. This can range from a personally selected or composed prayer to inspirational

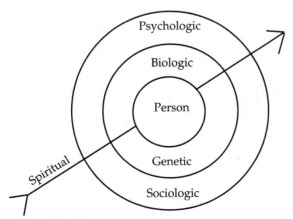

Figure 27.1 Components of a holistic model.

messages or stories created by others. Although nurses may not share the same spiritual orientation as their patients, they can respect another's spiritual beliefs and try to understand them. In home care settings, staff realize that we do not live forever . . . also called *impermanence.* The struggle to accept our mortality is daily experienced. Sogyal Rinpoche (1994) writes:

> One of the chief reasons we have so much anguish and difficulty facing death is that we ignore the truth of impermanence. We so desperately want everything to continue as it is that we have to believe that things will always stay the same. . . . Reflect on this: The realization of impermanence is paradoxically the only thing we can hold onto, perhaps our only lasting possession. . . . It is only when we believe things to be permanent that we shut off this possibility of learning from change. If we shut off this possibility, we become closed, and we become grasping. Grasping is the source of all our problems. Since impermanence to us spells anguish, we grasp on to things desperately, even though all things change. We are terrified of letting go, terrified, in fact, of living at all, since learning to live is learning to let go. And this is the tragedy and the irony, but it brings us the very pain we are seeking to avoid. (p. 43)

It has been well stated by Verna Benner Carson (1989) that the *call to wholeness* reaches each individual in the depth of his or her being. To heed that call is to respond to the invitation to live life fully, with purpose, in wellness, and with the totality of one's personhood. When health and wellness cannot be reached, nurses can understand that the focus of care has to be changed and they will do their best to help patients die in peace and comfort.

NURSE-MANAGED HOME CARE

An organization that provides person-centered care should ideally have the patient/family on top of its organizational chart. Co-author Deininger's Individualized Home Nursing Care (IHNC) agency is an example of a nurse-managed business with the concept of patient-centered care as the organizational vision. The agency is organizationally divided into three businesses: Individualized Home Nursing Care, Inc., Individualized Home Care, Inc., and Individualized Hospice (Figure 27.2). The same Board of Directors is responsible for operating and advising the management of the three component agencies. Seamless care is thus provided by the three agencies: one that provides skilled nursing care and all the therapies, one that provides private, custodial care, and one that provides hospice services.

Deininger believes that accountability to patients and to the consumer public as a whole is essential. Talbot (1995) states, that consumer accountability implies a duty or obligation to clients to provide quality care with predictable outcomes. Knowledge of nursing research is essential for quality care and the nurse executive needs to seek opportunities to work collaboratively and cooperatively with researchers in academic institutions in gathering data and measuring outcomes.

Skilled Nursing Care

Nurses are central in agencies that provide skilled nursing and hospice care. This embodies care provided by an agency that is certified under Medicare/Medicaid/

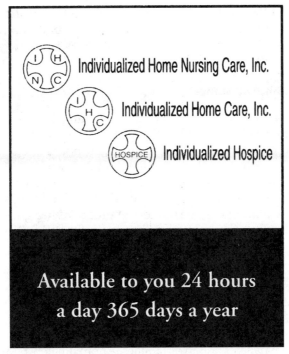

Figure 27.2 Three component agencies of a person-centered care model. Reprinted with permission of Individualized Home Nursing Care, Inc.

Blue Cross and Blue Shield and has contracts with various managed care organizations. Health care organizations must be able to provide hospice and private duty care to reduce fragmentation of care. The nurse executive must have the necessary knowledge and skills to foster teamwork and coordinate the best quality care for the patient. This means that excellent clinical skills in addition to administrative and business skills are needed by the nurse executive.

Expected outcomes include patient/family satisfaction, increased independence of patients (when appropriate), and decreased hospitalization and visits to physicians. As the individual moves from the skilled nursing agency to hospice care, or vice versa, it is essential that the same caregiving staff is retained. Patient and families will experience greater satisfaction from the provision of "seamless care," which is the continuity of care from the same staff. Individual persons benefit from the specialized knowledge and skills of staff members of the interdisciplinary team. Continuity of the same home care staff is essential, which includes the nurse who works collaboratively with the patient's primary physician.

INDIVIDUALIZED HOSPICE CARE

Hospice programs as formally recognized entities have a short history in the United States, but are gaining in recognition and acceptance by the public

(National Hospice Organization, 1997). Hospice care offers an alternative to denial of impending death and related issues. Because the philosophy of hospice is to treat the dying person and the family as a unit, many issues may be addressed within the context of support and caring.

History of the Hospice Movement

Hospice is a concept of care for people who have terminal illnesses and for their families. Care is planned and delivered by an interdisciplinary team that is usually composed of physicians, nurses, social workers, pharmacists, and chaplains. The focus of the care is on pain management, symptom control, and a holistic approach to coordinate care and meet the needs of both the dying patient and the family (Hayslip & Leon, 1992). In a little over 25 years that the hospice concept has existed in the United States, the number of programs has grown from one in 1974 to over 3,000 now serving terminal patients and their families.

Although the concept of hospice care was observed in medieval times in Europe, the United States owes the existence of the current movement to England. St. Christopher's hospice was founded in London by Dr. Cecily Saunders in 1967 (Mor & Masterson-Allen, 1987). In 1974 under the leadership of Florence Wald, Dean of the Yale School of Nursing, the first hospice was opened in New Haven, Connecticut as a home-based service (Baker, 1992). As of 1997, 3,000 hospices served approximately 450,000 patients and their families. Approximately one of every two people who died of cancer in 1997 received hospice services (Mahoney, 1998).

Hospice Care Philosophy

Hospice is a philosophy and an attitude about caring for others. "Hospice emphasizes the quality over quantity of life and the importance of both physical and spiritual contact between people as life draws to a close" (Hayslip & Leon, 1992, p. 2). To achieve this philosophy and demonstrate the attitude of caring, hospice promotes a natural acceptance of death as well as returning personal control and decision-making to the dying patient. In addition, hospice care endeavors to support the dying person in continuing to live until the moment of death.

A second major philosophical component of hospice care is to treat the dying person and the family as a unit of care. Often the dying person and family have difficulty expressing feelings or taking care of unfinished business. Hospice staff are trained to be able to cope with and facilitate the acknowledgement of death and to help the person and family work through their issues. "Energy is directed toward coping and comforting and not toward denial of the problem" (Paradis, 1985, p. 19).

Payment for Hospice Services

Reimbursement for hospice services is now provided by a wide variety of health insurance plans, but this was not always the case. With approval of the Medicare hospice benefit, hospice services became more accessible in many parts of the country.

Medicare Hospice Benefit

The Medicare hospice benefit was mandated as part of the Tax Equity and Fiscal Responsibility Act (TEFRA) of 1982 and went into effect November 1, 1983 with a 3-year sunset provision. Legislation in 1986 made the hospice benefit permanent. Reimbursement of hospice services is allowed to organizations that meet the hospice conditions of participation. The organization must be engaged primarily in delivery of care to the terminally ill and have an interdisciplinary approach. Nursing care, physician services, and drugs/biologicals must be available 24 hours a day. Core services of nursing, physicians, medical social services, and counseling (bereavement, dietary, spiritual, personal, and family) must be provided. Several other conditions of participation are spelled out in the legislation (Hayslip & Leon, 1992; Paradis, 1985).

Under provisions of the Medicare benefit, patients may be voluntarily admitted to a hospice if a physician certifies that the patient has 6 months or less to live. In choosing the hospice benefit, patients waive their rights to other Medicare benefits except for care not related to the terminal illness and for physician care under Part B when the attending physician is not an employee of the hospice program.

A broad range of home care and inpatient services are covered including bereavement counseling for the family within 1 year of the patient's death. In addition to the core services listed above, required covered services include therapies (e.g., physical and speech), homemaker and home health aide services, drugs, supplies, durable medical equipment, inpatient respite care, and nutritional counseling. The involvement of volunteers in administrative or direct patient care roles is also required for participating hospices (Figure 27.3).

Reimbursement to hospices is on a prospective daily rate for each patient based on four levels of care: routine home care, continuous home care, hospice inpatient care, and inpatient respite. Eighty percent of care must be delivered in the home for a hospice program overall. A plan of care must be established by an interdisciplinary team and the attending physician before hospice care is begun. The hospice legislation states that an RN must be designated to coordinate the implementation of the care plan (Hayslip & Leon, 1992).

Private Health Insurance

Establishment of the Medicare hospice benefit created an environment for the major insurance companies to need to respond. By 1983, the 11 major insurance carriers offered some form of hospice coverage (Paradis, 1985). Coverage for hospice services under private health insurance has tended to be extensions of home health benefits, but some plans do offer an explicit hospice benefit. The coverage has been geared more toward the costs of medical services with less emphasis on counseling and bereavement services.

Models of Hospice Care

Four dominant models of hospice care have emerged in the United States:

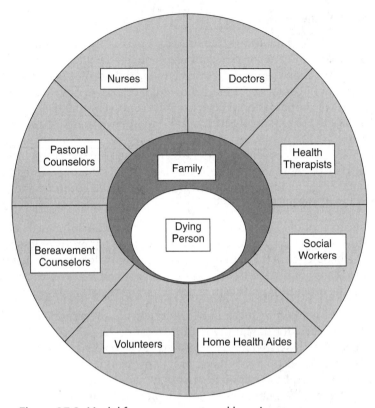

Figure 27.3 Model for person-centered hospice care.

- Home care that is hospital based, nursing home based, or community based (visiting nurse associations or home health care agencies)
- Free-standing autonomous hospice facility
- Separate hospital-based palliative care unit
- Hospital-based subacute unit emphasizing continuum of care (Hayslip & Leon, 1992; Paradis, 1985)

About 40% of hospices provide hospice care exclusively; others are affiliated with home health care agencies, hospitals, or multiple-agency coalitions (Mor, Greer, & Kastenbaum, 1988). One study found that 49% of all hospices were hospital based, 17% were operated by home health care agencies, and 34% were free-standing in the late 1980s (Mor & Masterson-Allen, 1987).

Because of the tremendous changes in health care reimbursement and structure in the last decade, changes may be anticipated in the future for hospice care. Debate partially centers around the role of profit as opposed to maintaining the person-centered focus of hospice care. Traditionally hospice care has been provided regardless of the patient's ability to pay. This tradition faces an uncertain future with the greater penetration of managed care businesses and health care corporations into the health care market.

A GREAT PLACE TO WORK

In addition to a hospice philosophy, Deininger's holistic nursing agency reflects chaos theory first presented by Freedman (1992) and is described in detail in Chapter 3. The nurses working in this organizational structure must be multitalented, enjoy autonomy, and willing to accept challenges daily; they each must be willing to be the patient's advocate and be a leader with excellent critical thinking and public relation skills. They must be willing to learn continuously, be aware of the ever-changing reimbursement issues, have excellent assessment skills and a broad knowledge base, as well as certain high-tech skills. These nurses are an essential part of an interdisciplinary team and they must coordinate care and services with other staff members and be aware which services are reimbursable and which require private pay. As active team members, they recognize how each staff member can contribute to the goals of the agency and become an important part of the care team.

Seamless Care

Seamless care agencies such as IHNC provide counselors within the agency for counseling staff. A built-in support system will foster retention of staff, assist in the recruitment of staff, and enable staff to continue to provide holistic, person-centered, quality care to patients. Initial orientation and ongoing support are imperative to retain loyal and excellent staff. Terminating relationships, especially in hospice care, calls for group and individual support.

Realizing that staff members will react differently to change, they are encouraged to participate in planning the implementation of change as well as give input regarding changes needed. This should include a clearly defined statement of what the change is, why the change is necessary, how the change will be implemented, and how it will affect each staff member. Regularly scheduled staff meetings, written announcements, and individual meetings are essential.

To meet the many needs of care providers and patients, different leadership styles are needed. In IHNC, the nurse manager actively participates in most care conferences, occasionally makes patient visits, and is on call if needed. It is of utmost importance to have excellent communication skills, both verbal and written. Working effectively together as a team requires not only honest communication, but also respect, trust, and appreciation for each other. Leadership skills, including administrative and organizational knowledge and excellent interpersonal and motivational skills, are imperative. Skills are needed to identify the strength of each staff member, allow for weaknesses, and recognize where coaching and developing individual skills may be appropriate.

The IHNC Holistic Approach

Knowledge of complementary therapies, such as massage, therapeutic touch, tai chi, music therapy, guided imagery, visualization, homeopathy, and others is shared with the IHNC staff (Custer, 1989). Several educational programs focused on these therapies. In practice, the efficacy of complementary therapies is recognized and staff have realized that the therapies should not only be used as part of hospice care, but also part of wellness care. Always treating the individual first, and then the disease has been part of the agency's philosophy. One learns to appreciate the uniqueness of each individual and each family situation.

One of the biggest failures in the 20th century Western scientific medicine has been the failure to deal with death and to adequately control the pain and suffering of dying patients (Henkelman & Dalinis, 1998; Loeb, 1999). End-of-life decisions require often deep struggles within our hearts. *Letting go* is a way of life that can be experienced throughout our lifetime. If we have learned to let life go and be flexible, we are better prepared for our decline. If we have been controlling individuals then we tend to be so to the end of our life. If we live life with a sense of a gift and grace then we tend to do so to the very end of life (Dunn, 1994). Life-prolonging procedures, such as cardiopulmonary resuscitation and artificial hydration and nutrition, must be discussed. Useful information for caregivers in long-term and home care settings should include material explaining dehydration and the signs and symptoms of death.

All of the IHNC agency nurses care for acutely, chronically, and terminally ill patients. Incorporating the hospice concept as part of their practice requires additional teaching and support. Watson (1988) writes that when an event occurs between the nurse and the patient, the spirit of both is present in what becomes a caring occasion. The nurse has often limited training and experience in the area of palliative care; therefore, nursing competencies in end-of-life care must be individually addressed. Experienced nurses become the designated mentors. Soon the "trainee" trusts the mentor and is able to share her fears and beliefs. When the nurse is involved with a person at the end of life, the caring and recognition of spiritual needs are the two most important elements defining nursing practice (From, 1995).

Mentoring

The empowerment and care of others through mentoring are important leadership tasks. To truly make the environment such that it is a great place to work, support and mentoring must be part of the daily activities. Mentors guide, model, encourage, and inspire protegés and professional colleagues in both formal and informal environments (Vance, 1999). To mentor the staff means to be there for them, to be in touch with them, to care, to support, to believe in them, to encourage them so that they can do the job, to assist where help is needed, to develop leadership and interpersonal skills, to be willing to share, to be trustworthy and to be knowledgable.

In the hospice/home care arena extra administrative support is needed as staff encounter end-of-life situations. Additional time is often required by the nurse and the social worker to coordinate the necessary resources. This may affect the daily visit schedule of the staff. Administration then needs to empower the scheduler or intake nurse to rearrange the schedule of each staff member. They may require extra time for the care of the patient/family and if needed, some time off for themselves.

ROLE OF THE NURSE EXECUTIVE

The nurse executive in home care agencies must be flexible, overseeing the staff during the day-to-day operation, assist where needed with daily crises, and able to function in different roles, such a home health aide, on-call nurse, field supervisor, and educator. The nurse executive must make sure that the environment is healthy, harmonious, and supportive. The nurse executive must work closely with the business manager to ensure financial stability. Budgets must be developed and accounts need to be reviewed. Weekly meetings with the nurse managers and the business manager are essential.

Benchmarking is of vital importance (Solovy, 1999). How does an agency compare to others in regard to quality of care, patient satisfaction, and staff retention? Statistics are needed to assess if the agency is fulfilling its expectations and living up to its mission. The nurse executive's job is to nurture the shared vision, prepare for the future, plan realistic goals, and see that these goals are implemented and fulfill the stated vision and mission. Building a shared vision is an important part of goal setting and achievement.

Daily awareness of regulatory and legal requirements for nonprofit, tax-exempt, certified health care agencies and hospice is essential and the constant changes need to be monitored. Increased support by management is needed because frequent federal regulatory changes in documentation and nursing practice occur. For example, documentation is becoming increasingly complex, is burdensome, and leads to shorter nurse visits. One has to ask "What can I do to keep the values which are essential to the agency? How can I adapt to the daily changes? What help do I need so that I don't feel helpless and out of control?"

Clinical and Management Skills

In the ever-changing health care arena, the nurse executive must demonstrate multiple skills. These include not only clinical skills, but also business, management, teaching, and research skills. Good negotiating skills and being an advocate for patients are of major importance. One must be able to assess one's knowledge and abilities in each one of these areas. Networking with other nurse executives is imperative. They can be an invaluable resource and assist the nurse executive when consultant help is needed. Developing and cultivating relationships with colleagues in different areas of nursing is essential. To be able to exchange information and knowledge and draw on each other's expertise are needed for survival.

Support is especially needed when nurses are involved with hospice patients with complex problems. Although they have been trained in palliative care, the fear of hastening a patient's death can be a barrier to providing comfort care to the dying individual. Explaining the double effect of pain relief with the possible side effect of hastening death is imperative (Loeb, 1999). This complex problem can be discussed at the weekly meetings of the interdisciplinary team or with a seasoned palliative care/hospice nurse, or the nurse executive. Support is given as the nurse attains practical knowledge and becomes comfortable to give the best care and greatest comfort to the dying individual.

How can we learn to save time and to be efficient? Time must be used wisely. Agencies cannot afford to do things twice. Doing things right the first time saves time and money. An example is to check annually all paperwork/forms used in the operation of the agency. Check what is being duplicated, that is, what information is gathered more than once. What can be combined? How many individuals handle the information? Are staff using available support systems efficiently (e.g., cellular phones, computers)? Do staff have the necessary tools to be efficient?

Fostering teamwork in often stressful situations is a challenge for the nurse executive who must not swerve from the mission of the agency. Only the collaborative effort of each team member can make the vision and the mission of the agency a reality. The nurse executive cannot face all tasks alone—the vision and the work must be shared. The able nurse executive corrects everyone who says, "I work for you" with "Oh, no you work WITH me." The environment plays a major role in fostering teamwork. Staff appreciate a supportive environment. When many of the personnel have been in the agency for many years, close relationships have formed. IHNC staff members and patients are remembered on their birthdays with a card signed by many.

Administering Hospice Programs

Hospice care provides great opportunities for nursing management as well as for clinical practice. The philosophy of hospice care is generally compatible with the foundations of nursing practice and the caring ethos of the nursing profession. Perhaps more than any other delivery system for nursing care, hospice incorporates the structure and processes to reach the outcomes desired in providing services.

Marketing the service is not always easy because of numerous barriers. Chief among these are the public's perceptions that hospice care is for dying not living, physicians' reluctance to "give up" on patients, and family denial of the terminal state of a family member's illness. Because referral for hospice care must come from the physician, marketing to physicians and their office staff is a key to developing and sustaining a viable hospice program.

Difficulties with determining that a patient has 6 months or less to live is a barrier for physician referral to hospice. Lack of training for physicians in terminal care and accurate prognosis were identified as barriers to hospice referral in one study (Miller, Miller, & Single, 1997). Providing continuing education programs for physicians and health care staff in all health care settings in a community can assist with marketing hospice services as well as improve the quality of care for terminally ill patients who are not referred for hospice care (Brenneis & Bruera, 1998; Hall, Hupe, & Scott, 1998).

Another challenge facing the nurse executive in hospice care is maintaining the balance between person-centered care and meeting the fiscal demands to stay in operation. Although Medicare reimbursement has made revenue generation easier in some respects, not all hospice programs qualify for or choose to become Medicare certified. It is estimated that about 75% of hospices in the United States are certified. On the other hand, one study has suggested that Medicare-certified hospice programs may tend more toward a medical model of palliative care than noncertified programs (Sontag, 1996).

The fiscal challenges are addressed more effectively with thorough knowledge of reimbursement regulations, methods to increase staff productivity, management of drugs and durable medical equipment, inpatient admissions, use of volunteers, and fundraising. The role of the nurse executive in a hospice program integrates to a great extent these knowledge areas with that of the hospice philosophy and clinical management of patient care. Integration of the various knowledge bases allows the nurse executive to provide clinical leadership and program management that are both focused on maintaining the cost effectiveness of hospice services.

CHALLENGES TO PERSON-CENTERED CARE

The biggest issue in home care is reimbursement. The challenge of providing care is to retain the components of quality, holistic care in a most cost-effective manner. The Balanced Budget Act of 1997 indicates that cost-based reimbursement for the Medicare Home Health Benefit program will be drastically changed, and home care agencies will receive less! Nurse executives in all settings face many challenges.

Medicare patient's hospital and nursing home length of stay is shortened. Patients are discharged to home care with continuing acute care needs. There is an improved survival rate for those who have chronic illnesses. The aging population is increasing, and home care needs are on the increase—but who will and can pay? Hospice benefits and end-of-life care do help those who are willing to admit they are terminally ill and do not wish further active treatment. Within the acute home care model, agencies often support a patient/family who is not quite ready to forsake all treatment. Agencies must then provide pre-hospice care, which includes palliative care, pain management, symptom control, and spiritual and psychosocial support.

Fundraising

Fundraising is an integral part of hospice care. The establishment of a patient care fund, with the necessary procedures for its use, is an important part of any seamless home health care agency. Memorial donations and private endowments are the source of such a fund, which enable patients to receive additional care as needed. For example, a family may have been caring around the clock for a family member. The family is in desperate need of relief at night and is unable to pay for private duty care. Patient care funds can be used to provide the necessary assistance. If it is a hospice patient, the agency asks the family to mention the agency in the obituary. Thus memorials assist in replenishing the fund. The terms *marketing* and *fundraising* are often difficult for nurse executives. It is imperative, however, that a nurse executive understand and devote time to both marketing and fundraising. As costs increase and resources decrease, the responsible nurse leader must ensure that agencies are financially secure.

Regulatory Restrictions

Managed care will continue to change. Numerous regulations in documentation changes and restrictions in how we practice nursing must be followed by the nursing staff. Increased management support is imperative. Increased consumerism and increased tension between the purchasers and providers of managed care will ultimately create a different picture. More and better information is demanded by consumers and providers (American Nurses Association, 1998). While continuing to be caring, nurses also must be astute business persons. Nurses must be patient advocates and also control costs. This role may be very difficult at times and cause conflict. Multidisciplinary participation is needed. The nurse will have to develop skills as a negotiator and a change agent to work effectively with the ever-changing health care environment.

Commitment to Quality

Commitment to quality and accountability are at the pulse of any nursing organization. Everyone should be able to articulate the values and beliefs of the organization. Values encompass the abstract of what is right, not only to the public, to other health care organizations but also to insurers (Omery, 1989). Nurses are identified by the values and beliefs they have adopted. This is seen in their daily activities and by their choices and decisions as they practice their profession (Pellegrino, 1990). Effective nurse executives train staff well, provide ongoing in-service education, and recognize work well done.

Nurse executives have to get out of the office and keep in touch with what is happening in the field. Seeing patients and supporting staff assist in keeping staff moving in the same direction, encourage self management, make empowerment a reality, and inspire staff to give quality care. The mission has to be shared by all. Words have to be put into action. Each person in an organization can make a difference. Agency staff must feel appreciated, have a positive attitude, and feel a sense of worth as if the agency also belongs to them. Teamwork and having a caring, positive, and motivational work environment are essential. These are the bases for successful person-centered care and a flexible care delivery structure. Home care is a key component of the health care system today. What the next health care model will be, no one really knows, but person-centered care is here to stay.

SUMMARY

Nurse executives in home care agencies must be knowledgeable about acute, long-term, and home care and must understand business practices, legal aspects, the importance of collegial networking and mentoring. Nurse-managed person-centered care delivery systems offer a viable alternative to profit-centered organizations. Hospice is a philosophy and an attitude about patient-centered caring that emphasizes the quality of life rather than quantity of life. The multidisciplinary approach to palliative care in hospice programs encompasses physical care for the patient as well as spiritual care for both the patient and the family.

It is the dying who teach us and they are often the ones who give us courage and strength. We try to listen to them, to their wishes, to their hopes, and to their fears. Hospice home care is truly the humblest kind of nursing. We strive to alleviate the fear of a painful death, control symptoms as much as possible, and preserve the personal dignity of the individual. We must consider the patient's goals, personal values, and what constitutes his quality of a meaningful life. Only then can we understand the *benefits and harms*—the ethical principle of beneficence.

STUDY QUESTIONS

1. What are the characteristics of a person-centered care model?
2. How does participatory management fit in with a nurse-managed organizational structure?
3. Review Chapter 3 for a description of chaos theory. How does IHNC's organizational structure reflect this theory?
4. What are the models of hospice care?
5. How does the hospice philosophy fit the definition of person-centered care?
6. Describe three challenges for the hospice home care nurse executive.
7. Describe how managed care could assist the development of person-centered care.

REFERENCES

American Nurses Association. (1998). *Managed care: Nursing's blueprint for action.* Washington, DC: ANA Publishing.

Baker, M. (1992). Cost-effective management of the hospital-based hospice program. *Journal of Nursing Administration, 22*(1), 40–45.

Brenneis, C., & Bruera, E. (1998). The interaction between family physicians and palliative care consultants in the delivery of palliative care: Clinical and educational issues. *Journal of Palliative Care, 14*(3), 58–61.

Carson, V. B. (1989). *Spiritual dimensions of nursing practice.* Philadelphia: Saunders.

Custer, G. (1989). Individualized Home Nursing Care, Inc. nonpublished report. Ann Arbor, MI.

Dunn, H. (1994). *Hard choices for loving people* (3rd ed.). Herndon, VA: A & A Publishers.

Freedman, D. (1992). Is management still a science? *Harvard Business Review, 70*(6), 26–38.

From, M. (1995). Utilizing the home setting to teach Watson's theory of human caring. *Nursing Forum, 30,* 5–11.

Hall, P., Hupe, D., & Scott, J. (1998). Palliative care education for community-based family physicians: The development of a program, the evaluation, and its consequences. *Journal of Palliative Care, 14*(3), 69–74.

Hayslip, B., Jr., & Leon, J. (1992). *Hospice care.* Newbury Park, CA: Sage.

Health Insurance Association of America. (1996). *Managed care: Integrating the delivery and financing of health care.* Washington, DC: Author.

Henkelman, W., & Dalinis, P. (1998). A protocol for palliative care measures. *Nursing Management, 29*(1), 40–46.

Lindberg, J. B., Hunter, M. L., & Kruszewski, A. Z. (1998). *Introduction to Nursing.* Philadelphia: Lippincott-Raven.

Loeb, J. L. (1999). Pain management in long-term care. *American Journal of Nursing, 99*(2), 48–52.

Mahoney, J. (1998). An update on efforts by the hospice community and the national hospice organization to improve access to quality hospice care. *The Hospice Journal, 13*(1/2), 139–144.

Miller, K. E., Miller, M. M., & Single, N. (1997). Barriers to hospice care: Family physicians' perceptions. *The Hospice Journal, 12*(4), 29–41.

Mor, V., Greer, D. S., & Kastenbaum, R. (1988). *The hospice experiment.* Baltimore: Johns Hopkins.

Mor, V., & Masterson-Allen, S. (1987). *Hospice care systems: Structure, process, costs, and outcome.* New York: Springer.

National Hospice Organization. (1997). A pathway for patients and families facing terminal illness, Standards and Accreditation Committee.

Omery, A. (1989). Values, moral reasoning and ethics, *Nursing Clinics of North America, 24*(2), 499–507.

Paradis, L. F. (Ed.). (1985). *Hospice handbook: A guide for managers and planners.* Rockville, MD: Aspen.

Pellegrino, E. D. (1990). Values and academic health centers: A commentary and recommendations. In R. E. Bulgers & S. J. Reiser (Eds.), *Integrity in health care institutions* (pp. 167–178). Iowa City, IA. University of Iowa Press.

Reyes, A. (1999, April 12). Nurse practitioners, physician assistants focus of UM study. *The University Record, 54*(27), 6.

Rinpoche, S. (1994). The Tibetan book of living and dying. In H. Dunn (Ed.), *Hard choices for loving people* (3rd ed.). Herndon, VA: A & A Publishers.

Solovy, A. (1999). Benchmarking under managed care. *Hospital & Health Networks, 73*(1), 49–62.

Sontag, M.-A. (1996). A comparison of hospice programs based on Medicare certification status. *The American Journal of Hospice & Palliative Care, 13*(2), 32–41.

Talbot, L. A. (1995). *Principles and practice of nursing research* (pp. 4–5). St. Louis: Mosby-Yearbook.

Vance, C. (1999). Mentoring the nurse leader and mentor's perspective. In C. A. F. Anderson (Ed.), *Nursing student to nursing leader.* Albany, NY: Delmar.

Watson, J. (1988). *Nursing: Human science and human care.* New York: National League for Nursing.

CHAPTER
28

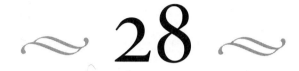

Collective Action—
Labor Relations

Richard W. Redman

Although the right to bargain collectively is a legislated right, it is often viewed with ambivalence when professional employees are involved. (Author)

Chapter Highlights

- Concept of collective bargaining
- Major collective bargaining legislation
- Nursing and collective bargaining
- Process of union recognition
- Contract negotiations and impasse procedures
- Life with a contract

The purpose of this chapter is to discuss protective legislation for employees and employers as it relates to collective bargaining by nurses. The evolution of collective bargaining in the United States, in general industry and in nursing, is explained briefly. The major legal requirements for collective bargaining are examined and their implications for the nurse administrator are discussed.

CONCEPT OF COLLECTIVE BARGAINING

Collective bargaining is often referred to as "bilateral determinism," meaning that two parties, management and a representative group of employees, participate in making decisions that affect the employees in the workplace. This collective or

515

bilateral approach is seen as an alternative to management unilaterally making employee-related decisions. Generally, collective bargaining is viewed as having a close relationship with human resource management. Although they are two distinct programs, they can become related at times; if management does an inadequate job in managing the human resource, they will generally find themselves dealing with a petition by employees to bargain collectively.

The American labor movement has been an important part of U.S. social and economic history. Many feel that American industry owes its present standing in the world marketplace to the labor movement. History supports the fact that prior to the legislated protection of employee rights in the workplace, many employees were exploited and had little say in workplace issues. Unionism generally has played an integral part in balancing out the relationship between management and staff (O'Rourke and Barton, 1981).

Although the right to bargain collectively is a legislated right, it is often viewed with ambivalence when professional employees are involved. The idea of nurses, physicians, or teachers being involved in collective bargaining activities often evokes strong emotional responses, either pro or con. Those who support collective bargaining for professionals take the position that it is the legal right of all employee groups to seek collective representation over those areas protected by legislation: the mandatory bargaining subjects of wages, hours, and other conditions of employment. Furthermore, it is felt that collective bargaining is the only way to maintain control over professional practice. Those who are against professional employee involvement in collective action generally view unionism as a blue collar activity that promotes strikes, that is, is unprofessional.

In nursing, it presents the additional challenge in that both management and staff generally are professional nurses who are colleagues, yet sitting on different sides of an issue. Also, there are issues related to what type of organization is most appropriate to represent nurses in a bargaining situation, for example, an industrial or trade union or a professional organization that deals with and understands nursing practice issues. These issues notwithstanding, it is the legal right of nurses to bargain collectively just as it is the right of other employee groups to do so. Although management in most organizations would undoubtedly prefer to work directly with employees rather than work with a third party, such as a union, it also is a fact that employees are not always given their due work place rights and collective action is the only way to ensure that. Many nurses view collective bargaining as the only way to balance their relationship with management and to enhance their professional status (Wilson, Hamilton, & Murphy, 1990). Regardless of personal views, it is essential for the nurse executive to have a thorough understanding of employee and employer rights as they relate to collective action.

MAJOR COLLECTIVE BARGAINING LEGISLATION

Legislation to protect employee rights in the workplace is essentially a 20th century phenomenon. The initial legislation focused on railroad employees but subsequent legislation covered employees in almost all types of industries. Table 28.1 presents a brief chronology of the major federal legislation that defines the rights of employees and employers with regard to collective bargaining.

The National Labor Relations Act (NLRA), passed in 1935, is the major piece of legislation that began to define the rights of employees to organize and bargain collectively. It has been amended three times. Initially the NLRA covered all health care employees. The 1947 amendments, however, excluded the nonprofit health care industry from the NLRA, because it viewed nonprofit health care organizations as charitable organizations that were not involved in interstate commerce and thereby exempt (Hirsh, 1990).

The 1947 legislation also excluded federal and nonfederal government-controlled hospitals from collective bargaining. Thus, Veteran's Administration facilities and state and local government-controlled hospitals' employees, as well, could not bargain collectively. This effectively closed off the majority of health care employees from the right to unionize.

Gradually, health care employees were granted rights to organize. In 1962, an executive order established the rights of federal health care employees to organize

Table 28.1 Chronology of Major Federal Labor Legislation in the United States

1898	Erdman Act
	First federal legislation to deal with collective bargaining; outlawed discrimination by employers against union activities.
1926	Railway Labor Act
	Established mediation and voluntary arbitration as means to decrease labor/management conflict.
1935	National Labor Relations Act (NLRA)
	Designed to promote greater self-determination for employees through establishing protected rights to organize and bargain collectively; established the National Labor Relations Board to conduct union elections and provide remedy for unfair labor practices; initially covered all industries, including health care; also known as the Wagner Act.
1947	Taft-Hartley Act
	Amended the NLRA; quite restrictive of union activities; established the Federal Mediation and Conciliation Service; specifically excluded nonprofit private and governmental health care organizations.
1959	Landrum-Griffin Act
	Directed at the internal affairs of unions.
1962	Executive Order 10988
	President Kennedy's order that established employees' right to organize in federal hospitals (such as the VA); prohibits strikes in those facilities.
1974	Taft-Hartley Amendments
	Amended the NLRA; permitted non-public, non-profit health care facility employees to bargain collectively; established a series of rules specifically for the health care industry (such as required advance notice for strikes).

but prohibited them from striking if an impasse was reached. In 1974, NLRA amendments established the rights of all health care employees in private not-for-profit facilities to bargain collectively.

The legal arena which covers employees' right to organize in a particular type of health care organization is often referred to as the "patchwork quilt of legislation." Federal employees are covered by the EO 10988; employees in the private not-for-profit sector are covered by the 1974 NLRA Amendments. Employees in other types of health care facilities, for example, a state- or city-owned facility, may be covered by "right-to-work" laws if they exist in a particular state. Thus, the right to organize can vary for nurses from one organization to another within the same locale, depending on the type of facility ownership and whether appropriate legislation exists.

The National Labor Relations Board (NLRB), established by the 1935 NLRA, oversees the conduct of the NLRA. The two major activities of the NLRB are *(1)* determination and certification of bargaining units through regulated election procedures and *(2)* prevention and remedy of unfair labor practices (NLRB, 1978). The NLRB also regulates and interprets the NLRA and its amendments through the establishment and promulgation of rules. One important rule which relates to the number of bargaining units permitted in a health care facility has been monitored and challenged over the past 20 years by both nursing groups and hospital management. This rule pertains to the number of bargaining units that can exist in one facility.

The NLRB has ruled that as many as eight bargaining units are appropriate in a given health care facility. The eight bargaining units that may exist in one facility are:

1. Nurses
2. Physicians
3. Other professionals
4. Technical employees
5. Business office clericals
6. Skilled maintenance employees
7. All other non-professionals
8. Security guards

This is quite different from an earlier NLRB position that assumed only two bargaining units were appropriate: professional employees (which would include RN's) and nonprofessional employees.

Eligible membership is determined by the "community of interest" doctrine that compares job families in terms of economic concerns, degree to which their work is integrated, and the management structures that apply to them. Nursing groups, such as the American Nurses Association (ANA), have been concerned about RN-only units, taking the position that the "community of interest" of nurses is unique and other job families should not be eligible to participate in a nurses' bargaining unit. Hospital management has been concerned about the number of bargaining units that a facility could potentially have to deal with. Their position has been that bargaining with up to eight units in a facility would be too time consuming and increases the potential for disruption of workflow if negotiations break down with any one group (Gullett and Kroll, 1990).

The NLRB ruling on eight bargaining units was contested in court by the American Hospital Association (AHA). The case was eventually argued before the U.S. Supreme Court which upheld the NLRB position (AHA vs. NLRB, 1991). Thus, it appears that the potential for eight bargaining units as well as RN-only units will likely remain in any given facility.

Related to this community of interest issue is the status of individuals designated as supervisors. By law, anyone who is classified as a supervisor is excluded from membership in a bargaining unit. Supervisor is defined by the NLRA as someone who has authority to hire, suspend, lay off, promote, discharge, reward, or discipline an employee (Shepard & Doudera, 1981). Generally, employee positions are reviewed on a case-by-case basis and inconsistencies may be found across different health care organizations. For example, assistant head nurses, clinical nurse specialists, and patient care coordinators may be classified as a supervisor in one organization and as a potential union member in another. It depends on how an organization defines a particular job title in terms of actual supervisory responsibilities.

A recent case examined the role of the charge nurse. Hospital management challenged the eligibility of charge nurses for membership in a collective bargaining unit on the grounds that they function as supervisors (Ketter, 1996). The U.S. Court of Appeals for the Ninth Circuit upheld an NLRB ruling that charge nurses were not supervisors and thus eligible for membership in a collective bargaining unit (Nguyen, 1997; Smith, 1996).

These kinds of challenges can be expected to continue. Many issues in contemporary labor relations are grounded in a 60-year-old industrial relations model. The issues of the rapidly transforming work environment, with self-directed work teams comprised of staff of varied skill mix, will continue to blur the distinctions between workers and supervisors (Cohen, 1995).

NURSING AND COLLECTIVE BARGAINING

Collective bargaining in the health care industry is a relatively new development, with most of the activity taking place in the past 20 years. Most of this activity, especially within nursing, was stimulated by the 1974 NLRA Amendments. Currently, approximately one-third of all RNs are organized in units that represent 20% of all hospitals in the United States (Merker, Blank & Rhodes, 1990).

Major leadership for collective bargaining in nursing has come from the ANA. The ANA established its commitment to representing the professional and economic interests of nurses when it was established in 1896. In 1946, a national economic security program was developed by ANA. In 1949, the ANA filed with the NLRB as a bargaining agent for nurses. Although the ANA is registered as a national labor organization, it does not directly represent nurses for collective bargaining purposes. That role is filled by the state nurses associations that have economic and general welfare programs. Approximately 70% of all unionized nurses are represented by these state associations (Flanagan, 1983). The remainder of organized nurses are represented by other health care unions or general trade and industrial unions that also are involved with health care employees.

Nurses join unions for all the same reasons that any employee group seeks collective bargaining. The major reason is that nurses are dissatisfied with management practices. This dissatisfaction generally relates to inadequate grievance procedures, unsatisfactory wage and fringe benefit packages, inconsistent interpretation of policies by management, and a lack of control over decision-making concerning their work and responsibilities. The general levels of dissatisfaction that nurses evidence are generally the type of catalyst that increases interest in what unions can do to address the contributing factors.

Several factors in the contemporary environment have also contributed to an increased interest in collective bargaining by nurses. Many nurses are looking for an increase in autonomy to go along with the increased responsibility they are assuming. Other professionals such as teachers and, to a lesser degree, physicians are increasing their involvement in collective bargaining and this adds legitimacy for nurses who are interested. The impact of the feminist movement has encouraged women to stand up for their rights (Flanagan, 1983). The literature is replete with nurses' growing discontent over general working conditions. Finally, the continuing problems with the economic status of nursing, especially wage compression, remain a major issue in nursing (Secretary's Commission on Nursing, 1988).

The impact of workplace restructuring and the pressures of managed care in the health care industry also contribute to precedents in collective bargaining contracts. In 1998, a contract between Kaiser Permanente, the nation's largest health maintenance organization, and the California Nurses Association established "quality liaison" nurses who will monitor the quality of patient care at each Kaiser facility. The nurses' union demanded this role in response to the many changes occurring in the practice environment, including downsizing of nursing staff and the introduction of unlicensed assistive personnel. These union-selected nurses will function as independent advocates for patient care standards, staffing levels, and other factors that impact on the quality of care. Given that Kaiser has facilities in 18 states, federal officials view this agreement as a breakthrough in both patient protection and labor-management relations (Sherer, 1998; Kilborn, 1998).

Although economic factors are often cited as a major factor for unionizing, limited data are available on the success rate of unions in addressing economic dissatisfaction. Some generalizations about the effect of unions on wages of hospital employees can be made. Overall, wages have increased at a statistically significant level for unionized hospital employees. The effect on nursing salaries has been smaller (about 6%) than on nonprofessional salaries (about 10%). Another effect to be considered is the "spillover effect," that is, the impact on pay levels in hospitals that are not unionized but compete in the same marketplace for employees with other hospitals which are unionized. Generally, these non-unionized hospitals have to pay higher wages to compete. In addition, the spillover effect can occur within one institution where non-unionized employees benefit from the effects of other employees who are unionized. This effect on wages ranges from 1% to 8% (Wilson, 1985).

Critics of unionization often attribute increased costs in health care to union activities. While limited data exist, it does appear that the impact of unionization on hospital costs has been modest. Less than 10% of the increase in hospital costs in the 1970's was attributable to union activity. Furthermore, it was predicted that the impact during the 1980's and 1990's will be even less (Becker, Sloan, & Steinwald, 1982). In the 1990s, this has continued to be the case.

Overall, it appears that the debate over nursing's involvement in collective bargaining is diminishing. Although that does not negate the debate over appropriateness, it does suggest an increased acceptance and recognition of the legal right of nurses to engage in union activities to address both workplace and professional practice issues.

PROCESS OF UNION RECOGNITION

When a group of employees is interested in forming a bargaining unit, stringent requirements as outlined by the NLRB, must be followed. These legal requirements guide the actions of management, the employees who are potential members of the bargaining unit, and the labor organization that is attempting to represent the employees. Any violation of the legal requirements outlined in the NLRA is designated as an unfair labor practice and punishable by the NLRB, which functions like an administrative court (NLRB, 1978).

The nurse executive must have a good working knowledge of the appropriate legal requirements and must ensure that the entire nursing management team is informed. Generally, when organizing efforts are developing, the senior management team in the facility will work closely with consultants who specialize in responding to union recognition campaigns. These consultants are often referred to as "union busters" by the union representatives (Ballman, 1985). It is important to keep in mind that the employees who are promoting the cause of the union are relying heavily on union staff members and in this regard are working with consultants as well. Several guides exist that offer strategies to both management and the employees interested in forming a bargaining group (see, for example, American Hospital Association, 1991; O'Rourke and Barton, 1981).

The process of union recognition begins with the labor organization filing a petition or a series of union authorization cards signed by a minimum of 30% of the employees in the potential bargaining unit. The NLRB then conducts a hearing to determine the appropriate unit membership based on the "community of interest" doctrine. In addition to a determination of which job families are to be included, the NLRB conducts a review of all job titles and the positions they represent to ensure that any title categorized as a supervisor is excluded from the bargaining unit election.

After the eligible membership for the proposed bargaining unit has been determined, there is a 30-day period which is referred to as a "laboratory environment." During this time, both management and the union will conduct active campaigns, presenting their views and recommendations to the employee group. Both sides are closely regulated by the NLRB. The NLRA is biased toward the union during this time in that the union can essentially promise the employees all types of gains that will be achieved if the union election is successful. Management, on the other hand, can make no promises about what they will do if the union is not voted in. The intent is that management has had the opportunity for those promises prior to the "laboratory" period and now it is too late for quick fixes. Management can, however, hold informational sessions, called captive audience sessions, in which factual information is presented to employees. Employees are required to attend these sessions if scheduled during work time. During this period the union will also be campaigning actively, conducting informational sessions and rallies. Often, other unions in the region will assist with the campaign in support of the labor movement (American Hospital Association, 1991).

At the end of the 30 day period, the NLRB will conduct a secret ballot election. A 51% majority of those voting is required to elect the bargaining unit. If successful, the labor organization is then designated as the exclusive bargaining agent for the employees. If not, no additional elections can be held for a period of 12 months (Hirsh, 1990).

In the past 10 years, there has been a general decrease in the number of elections held in health care organizations, although the percentage of those won by unions has increased during that same time. Most predict there will be an increase in election activity, given the impact of prospective payment, the general financial constraints in the health care industry, and the recent Supreme Court ruling that upholds the NLRB position for bargaining units (Merker, Blank, & Rhodes, 1990; Scott & Simpson, 1989). The trends in the 1990s indicate that election activities have continued to increase gradually.

CONTRACT NEGOTIATION AND IMPASSE PROCEDURES

If the union is recognized by election, then both management and union representatives must bargain in "good faith" to develop a labor contract. The contract covers the mandatory topics outlined in the legislation that applies to that health care facility. The scope of bargaining usually includes wages, hours, and conditions of employment. Any other topic is permissible for bargaining, provided both parties agree to bargain over it.

Over the past 15 years, a new negotiation technique has been used increasingly in collective bargaining situations. The "mutual gains" approach, developed by the Harvard Negotiation Project, has been developed as an alternative to traditional negotiation techniques that often are a test of wills framed within a win/lose paradigm. Mutual gains is a new model that promotes a collaborative labor-management relationship rather than the more typical adversarial relationship. The technique is a structured process in which interests of all parties are discussed and options are generated for all issues. The options are then evaluated using agreed-on criteria and solutions are developed out of the evaluated options (Moore, 1996; Ury, 1991). This mutual gains approach has been used successfully in nursing with demonstrated effectiveness and efficiency (Himali, 1995). Evidence also indicates that it generates better quality decisions that are based on data and evaluated with objective criteria (Ury, 1991).

After the contract is negotiated and agreed to by both parties, the union membership votes to ratify or reject the contract. If ratified, the contract then serves as the legal set of policies that must be adhered to by both parties. Contracts are either 2 or 3 years in length.

Sometimes the negotiation process reaches an impasse where neither side will change its position on a particular contract item. Although a strike is always a potential outcome in impasse situations, generally there are a series of intermediate activities as an attempt to resolve the differences. Some legislation or existing contracts require that unresolvable differences be reported to the Federal Mediation and Conciliation Service (FMCS), which may require mediation before a strike can occur. The FMCS will investigate, conduct hearings in which both sides present their position, and present recommendations that are advisory, not binding. Some contracts may require binding arbitration in which a third party intervenes on unsettled issues. In this situation, an arbitrator holds hearings and makes a binding decision, that is, both parties must accept it.

If an impasse is reached after fact finding and the appropriate legislation permits the union membership to strike, the union generally conducts a vote among its membership. The NLRA requires a 10-day notification of the NLRB before a strike can occur in a health care organization so that necessary arrangements can be made to transfer patients, decrease admissions, and take other appropriate steps to ensure safe patient care.

Two types of strikes are legal: economic strikes and unfair labor practice strikes. An economic strike is called by the union in response to demands made by the employer in terms of wages, hours, or working conditions. In this type of strike, employers cannot discharge workers who are on strike but they can hire either temporary or permanent replacements. The second type of strike is called by the union to protest an unfair labor practice, such as management's bargaining in poor faith. In this type of strike, employees have a legal right to reinstatement and cannot be permanently replaced (Rothman, 1983).

If a strike is to occur, very careful strategic planning is required by the health care facility. The nurse executive assumes a key leadership role in determining patient care management and staffing of those beds that will remain open during the work stoppage. General guidelines are available to assist the facility in planning for a strike (Rothman, 1983).

The overall strike rate in health care facilities is approximately 4%, with the majority of work stoppages occurring over first contracts. The major reasons for strikes are not always economic, although management tends to view them as such. Key issues are often related to overtime hours, weekend duty, grievance management, and overall working conditions, such as degree of employee involvement in decision-making and general communication patterns between management and employees (Imberman, 1989).

Every attempt is made to encourage settlement of a work stoppage, generally by both parties involved as well as the NLRB. On settlement of a work stoppage, careful consideration must be given to reintegration of the employees as they return to work. This planning should take place during the strike, not after it is settled. Consideration is needed by both employees and management as the organization goes through what is best viewed as a healing process. Blaming and personalizing of issues should be avoided and open communication encouraged. The nurse executive plays an important leadership role for the entire organization by creating an environment where both management and staff can work through their feelings of resentment, anger, and betrayal (Rosenthal, 1990).

LIFE WITH A CONTRACT

After a ratified contract is in place, it becomes important for the organization and its members to accept the reality of the union contract. The existence of the contract will present both advantages and disadvantages to both parties. Most important, it standardizes the treatment of all employees and removes ambiguity from management decision-making. The existence of a contract should be viewed as something that will now be used by the organization to move forward and get on with its daily goals.

The contract does not negate the need for a human resource management program. It defines only those areas that have been bargained over and does not address many areas that go beyond the mandatory scope of bargaining. In fact, it would be a mistake for any organization to use the contract as its human resource program.

The nurse executive must ensure that an orientation to the contract is conducted for all members of the nursing management team. It is the management team that will be interpreting the contract on a daily basis through their interaction with bargained-for employees. If they do not have a good understanding of the terms of the contract, they will be generating a lot of grievances for the organization. The managers should also be informed on who to contact if they are not sure how to handle a situation. Periodically, the contract should be reviewed with nurse managers to ensure that they are interpreting the contract with consistency.

Data should be gathered by management throughout the life of the contract in terms of what problems are surfacing that need to be reexamined at contract renewal time. Vague contract language, sources of continual grievances, and areas where the contract is silent all provide important evaluation information for the nurse executive when the next contract is being negotiated.

Living with a negotiated contract does not have to be a difficult experience. Mutual respect and understanding by both parties can provide a solid foundation for collaborative working relationships among management and staff.

SUMMARY

The protective legislation for employers and employees that addresses collective bargaining provides an extremely important body of knowledge for the nurse executive. Often, it is experienced in a crisis situation which is laden with emotions, rather than rational actions. The nurse executive plays a key role in the organization in terms of dealing with employees' concerns and potential collective action. Having a good working knowledge of the rights and responsibilities of both employers and employees in the workplace is essential for the nurse executive. If a collective bargaining contract is in place, it must be integrated into the overall human resource management program that exists within the organization. The nurse executive can assume an important leadership role for the entire organization by creating a working environment wherein the concerns of the employees and the well-being of patients and families are the primary values.

STUDY QUESTIONS

1. Identify the major pieces of Federal legislation designed to protect the rights of employees and employers in the collective bargaining domain.
2. Describe the prevalence of collective bargaining activities in the health care industry in general and nursing in particular.
3. Discuss the legal requirements that must be followed by employees and employers when collective action is undertaken by employee groups.
4. Discuss the advantages and disadvantages of collective bargaining for employees and employers.
5. Explain the relationship between a collective bargaining contract and a human resources management program.

REFERENCES

American Hospital Association v. *NLRB*, S. Ct. 90–97 (1991).
American Hospital Association. (1991). *Collective bargaining units in the health care industry.* Office of Legal Regulatory Affairs. Legal Memorandum, No. 16. Chicago.

Ballman, C. S. (1985). Union busters. *American Journal of Nursing, 85*(9), 963–966.

Becker, E. R., Sloan, F. A., & Steinwald, B. (1982). Union activity in hospitals: Past, present, and future. *Health Care Financing Review, 3*(4), 1–13.

Cohen, D. M., & Wick, E. F. (1995). Healthcare in transition: Labor law impact on nurse-supervisor roles. *Journal of Nursing Administration, 25*(6), 15–18.

Flanagan, L. (1983). *Collective bargaining and the nursing profession.* (Publication No. D72E IM). Kansas City: American Nurses Association.

Gullett, C. R., & Kroll, M. J. (1990). Rule making and the National Labor Relations Board: Implications for the health care industry. *Health Care Management Review, 15*(2), 61–65.

Himali, U. (1995). New bargaining technique protects the role of the RN. *American Nurse, 27*(5), 10.

Hirsh, H. L. (1990). Legal aspects of nursing administration. In J. A. Dienemann (Ed.), *Nursing administration: Strategic perspectives and application* (pp. 29–55). Norwalk, CT: Appleton & Lange.

Imberman, W. (1989). Rx: Strike prevention in hospitals. *Hospital & Health Services Administration, 34*(2), 195–211.

Ketter, J. (1996). The National Labor Relations Act: Tracing the history of nursing empowerment. *American Nurse, 28*(6), 13.

Kilborn, P. (1998, March 26). Nurses get new role in patient protection: Pact with biggest HMO allows care givers to guard standards. *New York Times,* p. A12.

Merker, L. R., Blank, M. A., & Rhodes, R. (1990). *Collective bargaining strategy briefings.* (No. 154902). Chicago: American Hospital Association Center for Nursing.

Moore, C. (1996). *The mediation process: Practical strategies for resolving conflict* (2nd ed.). San Francisco: Jossey-Bass.

National Labor Relations Board (1978). *A guide to basic law and procedures under the National Labor Relations Act.* (No. 031-000-00187-1). Washington, DC: U.S. Government Printing Office.

Nguyen, B. (1997). Long-awaited Providence ruling upholds right of charge nurses to bargain. *American Nurse, 29* (5), 1, 14.

O'Rourke, K. A., & Barton, S. R. (1981). *Nurse power: Unions and the law.* Bowie, MD: Robert J. Brady Co.

Rosenthal, E. A. (1990). Good planning alleviates bad effects of stoppages. *Health Care Strategic Management, 8*(12), 13–15.

Rothman, W. A. (1983). *Strikes in health care organizations.* Owings Mills, MD: National Health Publishing.

Scott, C., & Simpson, J. (1989). Union election activity in the hospital industry. *Health Care Management Review, 14*(4), 21–28.

Shepard, I. M., & Doudera, A. E. (Eds.). (1981). *Health care labor law.* Ann Arbor, MI: AUPHA Press.

Sherer, J. (1998). Kaiser's labor pains. *Hospitals & Health Networks, 72*(6), 30–32.

Smith, M. H. (1996). NLRB v. Health Care & Retirement Corporation of America, Inc.: A challenge for the nursing profession. *Nursing Outlook, 44:*(4), 191–196.

Ury, W. (1991). *Getting past no: Negotiating with difficult people.* New York: Bantam Books.

U.S. Department of Health and Human Services. (1988). *Secretary's commission on nursing.* Final Report. Volume I.

Wilson, C. N. (1985). Unionization in the hospital industry: How are wages affected? *Healthcare Financial Management, 8,* 30–35.

Wilson, C. N., Hamilton, C. L., & Murphy, E. (1990). Union dynamics in nursing. *Journal of Nursing Administration, 20*(2), 35–39.

C H A P T E R

29

Facilities Planning for Diverse Health Care Delivery Settings

Judith A. Bernhardt

Nurse executives have a significant role in the facility planning process because of their clinical experience related to the technical and sophisticated nursing and medical services provided today. (Author)

Chapter Highlights

- Role of nursing in facility planning
- Facility planning and design process
- Physical and functional evaluations
- Construction documents, the bid-award process, and construction
- Postoccupancy evaluation
- Impact of managed care on facility design

The purpose of this chapter is to provide basic knowledge of the process and content of planning the physical environment for health care facilities. Conceptualization of the physical environment has resulted in the recognition that staff functioning and patient recovery are affected by the human organization within health care facilities. Because the delivery of nursing care extends into and depends on all other areas in a health care facility, the importance of effective nursing administration in facility planning cannot be underestimated. This basic facility planning knowledge can be applied to a variety of health care settings.

For any administrator, planning is an essential component of the administrative process and includes the major activities of setting objectives, determining policies and resources, making decisions, and ensuring that the desired outcomes are achieved. Planning is the first conceptual skill required in an administrative role and is the dominant process in the design and construction of health care facilities. A useful way of thinking about planning is to consider both strategic and tactical planning.

Strategic planning encompasses long-range goals and objectives for an organization, whereas tactical planning focuses on goals and objectives in more detail and for a shorter time span. In the health care environment, strategic planning includes such tasks as describing the mission and role, determining the scope of services and the level of care to be provided, and choosing the site location and design concept. Tactical planning includes budgeting, identifying staffing ratios, and determining patient admission and scheduling procedures. The function of facilities planning is to strategically conceptualize and plan how an individual health care environment will function in the future. To plan facilities strategically is to commit to the risk of conceptualizing about the future.

THE ROLE OF NURSING IN FACILITY PLANNING

Nurse executives have a significant role in the facility planning process because of their clinical experience related to the technical and sophisticated nursing and medical services provided today. Nursing accounts for more than 50% of a hospital's payroll, and total payroll constitutes more than 50% of all hospital operating costs. Nursing merits active involvement throughout the planning process to produce management and operating efficiencies. The very nature of nursing's role as nursing service's representative and patient advocate makes it a source of invaluable experience and insight about nursing practice, the flow of materials and people, functional requirements of space, and environmental issues important to nursing staff, patients, families, and other health care providers. All of these elements can be enhanced or hindered by the design of the environment (Price, Koch & Bassett, 1998).

The planning and design of building programs require a decision-making process that involves several levels within an organization. For major building programs, there is usually a director of planning who functions as the representative of hospital administration, a planning committee, special committees with broad and diverse user representation, and the governing board, which retains ultimate authority and responsibility for the entire building program. Smaller building programs and renovation projects may compress these decision-making levels. Nursing has an opportunity to provide input into the organization at the levels where strategic program management and operational planning occur throughout the planning and design process.

The task of strategically planning health facilities is generally accomplished by a planning committee typically composed of representatives from various departments or disciplines. Nursing administration must be represented at this level, where needs and future programs of the organization will be determined. At the same time, nursing can develop its own internal organizational structure to designate the appropriate staff who need to be involved on any special committees to influence the management of the program design and provide educated direction on nursing practice and function. Such organization is important whether the facility planning project is large or small, for the design portion of the process itself demands significant time commitments to the development, review, and approval of final design schemes.

For a large replacement project spanning a number of years, consideration should be given to establishing and assigning a full-time nursing representative to serve as a consultant and a link between the nursing staff and the architect, providing knowledge about the impacts of the physical environment on nursing practice.

Additionally, the facility planning arena introduces nursing to the world of planners, architects, engineers, and health consultants and brings with it techniques and terminology that are relatively new and unfamiliar. The nurse consultant must learn such techniques and terminology through daily interaction with these planning professionals to be able to communicate in planning jargon, anticipate information needed by the architect in each design phase, and evaluate design schemes. Well-prepared and relevant functional spatial requirements for nursing have a good chance of successfully becoming incorporated into the final design.

The following responsibilities are essential to the role of nurse consultant:

1. Coordinate the involvement of nursing in the planning and design decision-making processes.
2. Gather data and prepare documentation to facilitate decision-making.
3. Examine and evaluate innovative design concepts, care delivery organization, and new technology, and make recommendations related to planning objectives.
4. Review program plans and assist in the definition of nursing practice requirements.
5. Act as liaison to interpret terminology and professional concerns between the staff, consultants, and external planning and regulatory approval agencies.
6. Monitor the design and construction for consistency with the original planning concepts.

Because the profession of nursing serves as a practical advocate, a number of patient and family needs can be coordinated by nursing in facility planning. Nursing care is approached from a holistic view that recognizes the physical, spiritual, psychosocial, and developmental needs of patients, with the patient, family, and community central to nursing's concern and program implementation. The design or plan of the health care environment, therefore, should support patient and family needs for a therapeutic milieu (Zelman, 1996).

Nursing can, through experience, sensitize planners and architects to environmental design and behavior as it affects not only staff, but patients and their families as well. The needs of patients and their families basically relate to the degree of control they have over an otherwise stressful environment. Six such needs have been identified:

1. The ability to find one's way between destinations
2. The ability to control what is likely to be seen and heard as a result of space relationships
3. The ability to regulate the amount of interaction with others, visually and acoustically
4. The security and safety of the environment
5. The convenience with which various amenities and destinations can be reached
6. Special needs because of age or physical or mental limitations

Incorporating these needs into design enhances the delivery of quality patient care (Carpman & Grant, 1993).

THE FACILITY PLANNING AND DESIGN PROCESS

Whether in building a new health care facility or accomplishing major additions or alterations to an existing facility, optimal long-term outcomes are achieved when those involved have a basic understanding of the planning process and a concept of design objectives (Hardy & Lammers, 1986; Munn & Saulsbery, 1992). This section describes the process phases and discusses ways in which nursing can positively influence the phases (Figure 29.1).

Mission and Role Study

The first phase of the planning process defines the mission and role for at least 10 years in terms of programs, physical facilities, and general space requirements for departments of all types. Recently, health facilities have employed independent, professional consultants to develop long-range role and program plans. The mission and role study has the dimensions of a community-wide survey and includes such elements as patient origin studies, population projections, utilization trends, length of stay, patient days, average daily census, and bed requirements. The study includes the examination of plans of other health care providers in the area, community characteristics, the effects of legislation, and its primary, secondary, and tertiary care roles on a defined area-wide basis.

At the same time, required health care resources, the role of education and research, and long-range personnel requirements are evaluated. On completion and acceptance of this survey of health care needs and the services to be provided, capital costs and the ability to finance the project must be determined by a financial feasibility study. Effective nursing involvement later in the design

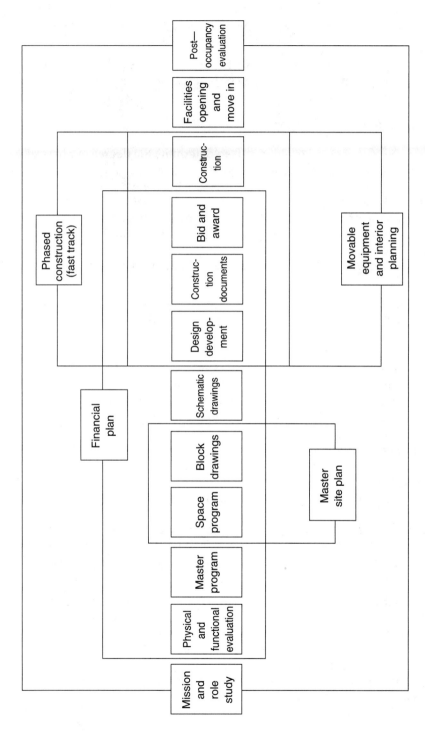

Figure 29.1 The planning and design process continuum. From the Office of Planning, Research, and Development. The University of Michigan Hospitals, Ann Arbor, MI.

process as it relates to types of patients and services to be provided requires that nursing be part of the prior development of long-range goals and be aware of the impetus for the design project (Hardy & Lammers, 1986).

The mission and role study is also necessitated by the high degree of regulation of the health care environment. Nursing may be involved in collecting and analyzing data to convince review agencies of the need for and economics of the project.

Physical and Functional Evaluation

The basic purpose of physical evaluation is to determine the degree of physical obsolescence of existing space, identify major code violations, and project usability in the future. The functional evaluation assesses the ability of space to serve as an efficient work place for personnel and to provide a supportive environment for patients and their families. The methodology used to functionally evaluate spaces compares functional attributes with adopted criteria. *Guidelines for Construction and Equipment of Hospital and Medical Facilities,* The American Institute of Architects 92-42212 and pertinent state rules and regulations serve as the basis for criteria.

In addition to the codes and regulations, a number of functional concepts provide standards for evaluating functional features. The more common concepts include:

1. Viewing the whole facility as a single, efficient system
2. Physical relationships required between departments
3. Room size and shape needed to accommodate function
4. The ability of the facility to expand
5. Space and equipment flexibility
6. The degree of automation
7. Separation of cleaned and soiled zones
8. Privacy accommodations for patients
9. Building circulation patterns (Hardy & Lammers, 1986)

The functional concept of flexibility deserves much emphasis. For health care environments, flexibility is critical in allowing for changing techniques of professional practice, alteration of department layouts to meet those changes, and addition of new departments in the future.

If a major design effort is to be undertaken as a result of the physical and functional evaluation, then usually at this phase of the planning process, a project team is formed, roles of the members are defined, and the decision-making process is clarified. This is when a well thought-out process of designating staff or nursing committees for ongoing involvement in the remainder of the process can also be developed. It is not unreasonable to request that a nurse consultant or several nurses be assigned to the project team on a major renovation or replacement project. For minor projects, a consistent point of contact in nursing can be designated to coordinate and provide input at each major phase in the project.

The importance of this involvement cannot be overemphasized. The quality of the planning and design effort in the remaining phases depends on those assigned to plan in detail and on the architect. Health care facilities are composed of complex relationships, flows of people and supplies, technological requirements, and operational procedures. These relationships necessitate a series of planning and design decisions and compromises to create a project that balances user needs, is aesthetically pleasing, and is of reasonable cost and optimal utility. To achieve these goals, it behooves nursing to be an integral part of the decision-making process and assist in determining which program planning and design compromises minimally affect the functions required to care for patients.

Master Program

The master program phase of planning health care facilities precedes actual design efforts. The master program describes operational concepts and specifies functions in terms of procedures, required equipment, and numbers and categories of space users. The projected number of procedures or tests is based on the number of admissions, patient days, and clinic visits projected in the mission and role study.

Master programming is one of the most important planning activities. The master program is reviewed by external regulatory agencies and becomes the major approved policy document. It serves as a guide for the architect, the manager responsible for construction, administration, and the people who will use the space. This programming effort, once the province of the design architect, is now frequently conducted by planners familiar with health care functions. Titled functional planners usually have a background in hospital management, and many are trained by consulting firms that specialize in both health care programs and facility planning.

A number of nursing-related operational concepts require decisions at this stage (Hardy & Lammers, 1986):

1. Types and mix of patient rooms (single, double, four-bed)
2. Centralized versus decentralized supply processing and material distribution systems
3. Size of nursing units
4. Presence or absence of a nursing station
5. Type of care delivery
6. Degree of automation for processing data
7. Degree of centralization for laboratories and pharmacies.

Clinical factors that drive facilities planning include infection control, accessibility, visibility, traffic patterns, patient privacy, staffing patterns, nursing efficiency, support spaces, storage, communication, acoustical requirements, and technology requirements (Harrell & Swaim, 1993).

It is in this part of the planning process that the nurse executive can make a significant contribution by using designated nursing planning resources to describe and document for the planners the planning objectives and design concepts that are not only required but desired to implement nursing practice in a new setting.

The planning objectives and design concepts can begin with a description of the patient population and the philosophy of delivering patient care within the overall mission and role of the health care facility. Such objectives include but are not limited to the operational concepts previously described.

Once the philosophy of care and the patient population are identified, it is useful to identify the program goals and assumptions for nursing, including definition of terms. An example of a program goal is to maintain a system of decentralized nursing administration. Once all the goals have been listed, with objectives stated for each, the operational and physical space requirements to implement each goal can be identified. Examples of operational and physical space requirements for the goal of decentralized nursing administration are to locate units with similar patient populations in close geographical proximity and to require office space for each head nurse on the unit for which he or she is responsible.

As part of the master program, it is valuable if the documentation of planning objectives and design concepts for nursing itself are stated in a format that all parties can understand. To assist in the description of these objectives and concepts, the nurse consultant, designated nursing personnel, or both should review layouts of nursing areas and systems in other health care facilities. Such a review can be accomplished through carefully documented visits to other health care facilities; reviews of hospital, medical, and design journals; and operational analyses to prepare adequate documentation to support the proposed space requirements. An example of an operational analysis that may need to be performed is to describe and document the rationale for desiring a certain size nursing unit.

Space Program

A space program is a listing of every room or area to which a function is assigned in a proposed construction project. As a direct derivative of the master program, a space program is used to communicate facility needs to the architect and is frequently prepared by a functional planner. The traditional space program lists the type of room required within a unit or department and the quantity, size, and functional requirements of each. The space program should provide the architect with a clear understanding of not only what function is to be performed in the space, but the quantity and type of personnel required for the function, in addition to the equipment and environmental needs. The listing of rooms follows the order of the master program, and rooms are grouped by department, functional entity, or both (Table 29.1).

Table 29.1 Example of a Partial Space Program for a Nursing Unit

Room Type	Functional Requirements	Quantity	Square Feet per Space	Total Square Feet
Family waiting room	Provide seating for 12 people at 15 square feet per person. Should have exterior windows and window to corridor. Close to drinking fountains and phone. Locate two toilets adjacent to but not inside room. Conversational environment. Provide for hanging coats, boots, and so on.	1	180	180
Single-patient room	Bed, access to bed, visitor seating space, patient chair space, exterior window, wardrobe for clothing, adequate circulation at foot of bed for equipment, accommodate flowers, tack board, patient clock.	16	130	2,080
Double-patient room	Same as single. Note: adequate clearance between beds.	8	200	1,600
Patient bathroom	One for each patient room, toilet with bed pan flusher, shower, lavatory, bed pan storage, staff shelf for specimens, patient shelving for toilet articles, wheelchair accessible, night light.	24	40	960
Nursing station	Space for charting, forms, and communication for 6 to 8 people. Counter for computer terminal capability and chart rack. Space for telephone, nurse call, patient locator, tack board, clock, pneumatic tube station. Visual surveillance of corridor. Adjacent to medication station, physician dictation, and conference room. Provide good acoustical attenuation.	1	300	300

Several factors influence the space program phase. Different conclusions about the dimensions and space identified by the functional planner for a room can be arrived at during the actual design by different architects. For example, an intensive care patient care room programmed for a certain size might need a generous width to allow adequate clearance at the foot of the bed during a cardiac arrest. However, the architect might believe that the length dimension is more important for the medical gas outlets and equipment required at the bedside. Thus, one important requirement might be needlessly compromised at the expense of another, equally important functional requirement.

Another factor influencing the space program includes minimum square footage assignments or the amount of space stipulated by most state and federal regulatory agencies for certain functions. Although these minimum requirements must be met for licensure, certain spaces need to be larger to accommodate specific functions; for example, a teaching hospital would require spaces to accommodate students. Finally, construction budgets influence space assignment size. When budgets are restricted, space sizes for rooms are usually at their functional minimum; when budgets are unrestricted, optimal space sizing can be achieved. Nursing can provide assistance in monitoring those essential spaces that may be in danger of becoming dysfunctional under budget constraints (Hardy & Lammers, 1986).

A carefully prepared master program and a well-defined space program can assist in achieving functional rooms and spaces for a health care facility, which enables administration to make many important design-related decisions without repeating the trial-and-error process often encountered in design.

Block Plan Drawings

Block plan drawings represent the beginning of design, the point at which the architect translates the program and space descriptions into simple drawings of blocks of space. Block plans graphically depict a facilities evaluation of necessary functional adjacencies between departments; for example, the emergency room should be located near the intensive care units to minimize travel distance for critically ill patients. The block of space for each department and the departments it relates to are shown along with major corridors and elevators. Alternative ways in which these blocks of space can be designed are then evaluated as to how well they fit in their new location.

At this phase, three-dimensional models are useful for major building programs in demonstrating alternative schemes to assist in the selection of optimum relationships and configurations. Because the nursing unit is the major determinant of the building's shape, the architect first focuses on its location within the building. Nursing can assist the architect by providing criteria on departmental adjacencies important to nursing and on functional requirements that will influence the shape of a nursing area. Criteria of importance include nursing travel distances between spaces and the location of supplies for those spaces.

As block plan drawings are developed, a master site plan is formulated for major building programs. This process encompasses selection of a site, analysis of the site, and development of drawings to visually portray the buildings and uses of all parts of the site. A site plan is the rational selection of a location to accommodate all construction envisioned during a 15- to 20-year future period for a health care facility. The plan reflects vehicle and pedestrian traffic flows, parking, building configurations, placement, organization, and landscape details. With the advancement of technology in health care, provisions for flexibility of site use and expandability of structures is an important part of the facility planning process (Hardy & Lammers, 1986).

The block plan phase is also the stage in the design process at which an evaluation of full-size mock-ups of various fully equipped rooms are of extreme importance. In planning and designing health care facilities, no other adequate substitute exists for seeing spaces in three dimensions. Users of the space can be involved at this point in evaluating function and predicting the operational quality of certain spaces, building materials, equipment, and furnishings. Mock-ups can also be of significant value to administration in introducing a new facility to the community. In fact, mock-ups should be installed permanently in a new facility as an in-service education tool for everyone from health care personnel to maintenance and housekeeping.

As part of the initial design phase, a mock-up program can be undertaken in several steps:

1. The project team and architect can evaluate two-dimensional drawings (sketches or floor plans).
2. Visits can be made to mock-up displays prepared by manufacturers of specific health care equipment.
3. The team can study three-dimensional scale models of specific spaces and participate in evaluating full-scale mock-ups with actual or simulated equipment and furnishings. Full-scale mock-ups can be built in the existing facility or in a nearby building and can be constructed for a small percentage of the overall project budget, particularly if planned from the onset.

A space can be considered a prime candidate for mocking up if:

1. The space recurs frequently in the design.
2. The space is complex and needs to be visualized to understand its functional relationships with people, equipment, and other spaces.
3. A mock-up is the best way to acquire, evaluate, and transmit meaningful user input about the space.
4. The capital and operating costs of the space are great.
5. The space is expensive to renovate after occupancy.

Spaces that might be mocked up include a general and an intensive care patient bedroom, a nursing station, an examination room, and an operating room. If full-scale room mock-ups are not financially feasible for a project, three-dimensional models should be used as a fallback predesign evaluation tool (Rogoff, Couture, & Bernhardt, 1979).

The first step in evaluating full-scale mock-up rooms is to develop performance criteria for how the space is expected to function; for example, there should be adequate space in a two-patient room at the foot of the bed to allow the second bed to be removed during a cardiac arrest without unduly disrupting the arrest procedure. The next step is to determine what tools will be used to evaluate the spaces, for example, questionnaires, interviews, and checklists. Activities that will routinely occur in the space can be role-played or simulated and can be photographed or videotaped to document which aspects of the design function well and which do not. With clear documentation, designers and the project team can address the findings and modify the design accordingly. Performance criteria and evaluation methodologies can also be used to test equipment, material, and furnishings.

Schematic Drawings

In schematic drawings, a detailed version of block plans, the shape of every room is outlined. In addition to showing the corridors shown in the block plans, schematic drawings also reflect mechanical spaces, such as ventilation and pipe shafts and the location of building-support columns, stairs, and doors. All the assumptions about the equipment and furnishings that will be provided in each space must be known during the schematic phase (Figure 29.2).

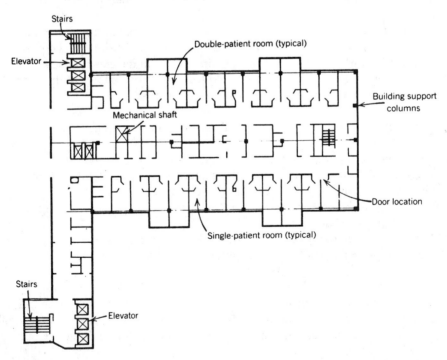

Figure 29.2 Example of schematic drawing of a patient unit. From the Office of Planning, Research, and Development. The University of Michigan Hospitals, Ann Arbor, MI.

With the nursing units' location already established in the design of a new building, the relationship of spaces and flow of staff, patients, and materials within a department is determined during this phase. Nursing can prepare performance criteria for the unit in terms of number of people using the spaces, degree of privacy or openness, visual and acoustical needs, and control and monitoring requirements. If mock-ups are being used, this design information should be incorporated in the mock-ups, along with the criteria for the other spaces, and communicated to the architect.

The nurse consultant, the staff nurses, or both can work with the architect to develop multiple schemes and options for laying out the spaces. Previous research and visits to other facilities can assist them in choosing from a range of options. The clearer the nursing design guidelines, the easier it is to develop alternative schemes and to evaluate the design that best meets original planning objectives.

Although the best time to decide which planning, design, and construction approach to take is before the facility planning and design activities are undertaken, the approach nevertheless must be selected no later than at the completion of schematic drawings. The two types of design and construction approaches are conventional and "fast track." In the conventional approach, construction is not begun until all the design and contractor documents are completed.

In a fast-track approach, construction begins on certain elements of the project while planning and design continues on other elements; for example, the lower portion of the building may be constructed while the nursing units are still being designed in detail. The theoretical advantage of fast tracking is an earlier construction completion date, which saves time and money. For health care facilities, fast tracking can force actions to keep the project on schedule in an industry where decision-making is not always timely (Hardy & Lammers, 1986).

If a fast-track approach is used, the development of goals and objectives by nursing early in the master programming phase is especially crucial to avoid fragmented, reactive design decisions. Schematic drawings may allow some adjustments to the scope of the project, but at their completion, the scope and functional relationships of departments and rooms are usually fixed. Schematic drawings need to be reviewed by the state health department before final approval to be certain they are in compliance with all codes.

Design Development

Once decisions are made regarding functional space locations and basic departmental configurations as reflected in single-line schematic drawings, the architect begins to determine the details of design for each room. The drawing dimensions are more precise for all spaces than in a schematic design.

To determine the detailed design of each room, the project team collects detailed data about the physical requirements of each space. Examples of physical requirements include equipment, characteristics of the materials to be used, lighting types and levels, medical gases, mechanical and electrical systems, nurse call systems, telephone, intercom, and dictation and pneumatic tube systems.

It is not uncommon for rooms, doors, and even corridors to be relocated at this phase as mechanical and structural systems are better understood and evaluated by the engineers. Continued nursing input during this phase is important because design relocations can significantly change how some rooms function. The mock-ups can assist in evaluating these changes as well as to further test detailed room requirements. For example, for the layout of the head wall in patient rooms, the exact height, location, and quantity of gases, outlets, and equipment can be evaluated to determine the impact on efficient patient care delivery and bed placement within a patient room.

During the design development phase, definitive planning occurs for major movable medical equipment, such as dialysis machines and operating room tables. Finalizing the placement of such equipment is necessary to determine the precise room dimensions and the location of plumbing fixtures and electrical outlets. Interior design planning also begins during design development and entails decisions about color, wall and flooring materials, signs, furnishings, artwork, and plants. Input from nursing and from mock-ups or other research can contribute to the creation of a functional and aesthetically pleasing environment (Hardy & Lammers, 1986).

CONSTRUCTION DOCUMENTS, THE BID-AWARD PROCESS, AND CONSTRUCTION

Construction documents consist of the design specifications, working drawings, and conditions for construction that are incorporated into a contract. They represent the decisions throughout the process and specify the dimensions and layout of what will be built. During this phase, the final details are worked out between the architect and the engineers. As problems are identified, design decisions are reevaluated and modified. If significant architectural or functional changes are required in patient care and related spaces, a review by nursing can verify that the changes are acceptable, based on functional goals and objectives.

During the bid-award phase, competitive bids are taken, and contracts are negotiated and awarded before construction commences. Again, changes can occur with respect to materials and equipment. Alternative materials and equipment are listed to increase competition for better prices. Such alternatives must be acceptable to nursing, because the contract will be awarded to the lowest bidder. Many times, substitutions beyond the acceptable alternatives are proposed by contractors and administrators as a way to reduce costs. This fact emphasizes the need for well-documented specifications on how staff expects all items to function. Nursing can provide input to assist in evaluating whether a substitution is appropriate, based on the construction cost, operating cost, depreciation, appearance, and functional requirements.

The most critical task for the project team during the construction phase is to make sure that the construction work proceeds according to the intent of the drawings and specifications and that it is on schedule and stays within budget (Hardy & Lammers, 1986). Contractors who are not aware of the original goals and concepts of the project might attempt to make changes that may directly affect the appearance and functioning of patient care areas, such as changes in the location and type of fixtures. Meetings with the project team and construction site tours can assure continued nursing participation during this phase.

Facilities Opening

During construction and before opening, attention must be turned to both how people will function in the new design and plan the move. A smooth transition from old to new can require a minimum of 1 year or more of advanced planning, depending on the size of the project.

Therefore, there is a need to develop a move-in schedule, write policies and procedures, and orient employees to any new functional concepts and equipment. If this is not done, existing and new employees, because of an incomplete understanding of the new design, may attempt to carry over the current methods of functioning from the old to the new. In all probability, the new space will have been designed to accommodate very different ways of operating (Hardy & Lammers, 1986). Moving into a new wing or a new patient tower is no simpler than moving into a new facility across town because both situations involve the same process.

POSTOCCUPANCY EVALUATION

Postoccupancy evaluations of building and spaces have two major purposes. The first is to provide feedback to functional planners and designers on how well the spaces function based on the original design goals. The second purpose is to gather data that can be applied to future design. The evaluation should be done within the first year after occupancy and consist of an objective assessment using a variety of research methods.

The research methods include gathering quantitative data on the number of users and uses of space and collecting qualitative data, such as data on the attitudes of people using the space and photographs depicting the behavior of the users. If there is consistency with the original design concepts and these concepts are still appropriate, then the design can be considered a success. Learning about what is inconsistent allows for immediate improvements and for information that can contribute to future design (Zimring & Reizenstein, 1981). Nursing has much to gain by being involved in postoccupancy evaluations from the standpoint of enhancing future practice and achieving a therapeutic environment.

THE IMPACT OF MANAGED CARE ON FACILITY DESIGN

The 1990s have seen more change in the way health care is delivered than at any time in the past. These changes include a shift to ambulatory services, the development of ambulatory care centers, and a growth in home health, skilled nursing facilities, and subacute care to name a few. Perhaps the most significant change has been the shift to a capitated reimbursement system as a form of managed care (Health Insurance Association of America, 1996). This shift is the driving force in changing health care delivery from a disease-oriented system to a wellness-oriented system, focusing on prevention and a continuum of care and not just on illness and hospitalization. For the nurse executive, this means changing the way nursing practice is perceived. It means examining the various care delivery processes on an ongoing basis and seeking ways to improve quality while reducing costs (Flarey, 1997).

Primary care delivery is the core of managed care and has become a critical component in the health care system. Its impact on design can be seen in newer facilities that are increasingly providing more comfortable and welcoming spaces with abundant natural light and plants. More attention is being paid to patient preferences and privacy and how staff interact. Facilities have shifted from large scale to smaller scale with an emphasis on convenient access. Centralized and decentralized functions are mixed. Patient education spaces and accessible community rooms are readily available. Spaces and furnishings are flexible and more adaptable to meet the rapidly changing health care environment (Kantrowitz & Associates, Inc., 1993).

Significant design concepts have emerged in the midst of all this change. These concepts affect facility planning and require consideration and evaluation by nurse executives. Additionally, these design concepts have the potential to improve the ability to market to managed care organizations if patient care is improved at a reduction in cost. The major ones include, but are not limited to, cooperative care, patient-focused care, postsurgical recovery centers, the Planetree Model, and ambulatory health campus models.

Cooperative care places an emphasis on patients and their families learning to care for themselves. It requires supportive staff who respond to patients and families in a noninstitutional manner and setting. Patients who qualify for this setting are inpatients who are essentially mobile and have a care partner. The care partner is the key element in this concept and most knowledgeable about the patient. The inpatient environment is residential and comfortable. Patient rooms are designed to look like hotel rooms and the caregiver resides in the same room with the patient (Bacher & Komiske, 1993).

Patient-focused care seeks to restructure traditional hospital operations and reduce the many compartmental nursing units supported by a multitude of centrally dispatched services. This new approach basically cross-trains caregivers to provide a high percentage of the services the patients need with select equipment found in x-ray and the laboratory relocated on the nursing unit. Routine ancillary services are performed for the convenience of patients and doctors, the level of direct care is increased, care is protocol driven, and patients interact with dramatically fewer employees (Lathrop, 1991).

A postsurgical recovery center is an inpatient facility that provides short-term, postsurgical nursing care for many routine elective surgeries performed in an ambulatory setting. The concept is that patients recuperating here receive a personalized form of postoperative nursing care at a reduced cost from what they would incur for similar care in a hospital. There are free-standing and facility-based models, and hospital- and physician-sponsored programs (Steinman & Sexauer, 1990).

The Planetree Model has a philosophy of care with an emphasis on patient choices and a higher level of patient education, self-care, and family care. The design of the environment is intended to soothe and cater to the ill. A health resource center, kitchenette, homelike lounge equipped with a large-screen TV and VCR, an open nurses' station, a carpeted central corridor and a cozy ambiance are some of the major features of this concept. A "care partner" theme is also part of this philosophy as well (Weber, 1992).

The premise of an ambulatory health campus is to provide one-stop shopping for families seeking health care. These campuses are envisioned to become the primary care sites in regionally managed care networks and be on the front line of profitable health care delivery. They are intended to unite diverse ambulatory services such as laser clinics, birthing centers, hospice centers, self-health shops, medical supply outlets, and discount pharmacies among others. A fitness center might coexist with a surgical center on this campus for the health-minded consumer. Design principles include family-centered care, team care, care for the impaired or aged, structural flexibility to respond to change, and enhanced technology systems. Many are now or will be linked to hospitals and the largest ones may include a limited number of inpatient beds, for same-day or short-stay patients (Coile, 1994) (Figure 29.3).

All of these concepts have been driven by the changing forces in health care in this decade and from an examination of how health care is delivered. New or redesigned facilities will have a totally different appearance from the traditional health care design with these innovative approaches to health care delivery.

SUMMARY

Facility planning and design is a process that moves from macroscopic conceptual planning to the more microscopic details of design for renovations or new construction of health care facilities. This process is a complex one with many constraints. Yet nurse executives should not be overwhelmed by the task. The most important people in the process are the administrator and the staff who have the final responsibility for developing and implementing the program and then for using the building or spaces. Therefore, it is critical that the nursing staff be knowledgeable about and actively involved in the planning and design process from beginning to end. Nursing knowledge and involvement can assist in anticipating and solving problems, which will lead to better design of health care facilities for staff and patients in the future.

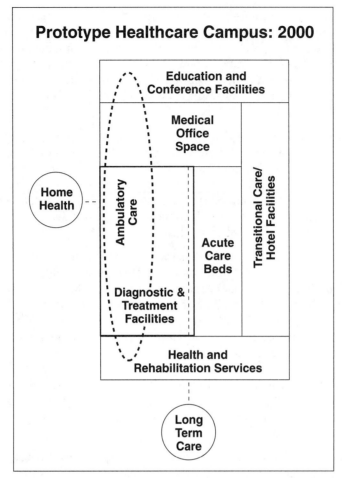

Figure 29.3 Example of an ambulatory health campus. From the refocus of hospitals on ambulatory care systems in the 21st century, exhibit 3. Paper presented at the 1993 International Conference and Exhibition on Health Facility Planning, Design, and Construction, New Orleans, September 14–16, p. 674 by D. Moser, 1993. Reprinted with permission of the American Hospital Association/American Society for Hospital Engineering.

STUDY QUESTIONS

1. What are the major steps of the design and planning process for building any new health care facility?
2. How has managed care influenced facility design in your area?
3. Explain how the Planetree Model for care influences the design of patient environments.

REFERENCES

Bacher, L., & Komiske, B. (1993). *New directions: Cooperative care.* Paper presented at the 1993 International Conference and Exhibition on Health Facility Planning, Design and Construction, New Orleans, September 14–16, 1993, pp. 107–139.

Carpman, J., & Grant, M. (1993). *Design that cares: Planning health facilities for patients and visitors* (2nd ed.). Chicago: American Hospital Publishing, Inc.

Coile, R. (Ed.). (1994). Ambulatory health campus: The "lite" hospital of the future. *Hospital Strategy Report, Newsletter* 6(5), pp. 1–8. Frederick, MD: Aspen.

Flarey, D. (1997). Managed care changing the way we practice, *Journal of Nursing Administration, 27*(7/8), 16–20.

Hardy, O., & Lammers, L. (1986). *Hospitals: The planning and design process* (2nd ed.). Rockville, MD: Aspen Systems Corporation.

Harrell, M., & Swaim, T. (1993). *Maximizing patient welfare in critical care unit design.* Paper presented at the 1993 International Conference and Exhibition on Health Facility Planning, Design and Construction, New Orleans, September 14–16, 1993, pp. 353–369.

Health Insurance Association of America. (1996). *Managed care: Integrating the delivery and financing of health care,* Part A. Washington, DC: Author.

Kantrowitz & Associates, Inc. (1993). *Design evaluation of six primary care facilities for the purpose of informing future design decisions.* The Center for Health Design.

Lathrop, J. (1991, July/August). The patient-focused hospital. *Healthcare Forum Journal,* pp. 17–20.

Moser, D. (1993). *The refocus of hospitals on ambulatory care systems in the 21st century.* Paper presented at the 1993 International Conference and Exhibition on Health Facility Planning Design and Construction, New Orleans, September 14–16, 1993, pp. 670–675.

Munn, E., & Saulsbery, P. (1992). Facility planning—A blueprint for nurse executives, *Journal of Nursing Administration, 22*(1), 13–17.

Price, S. A., Koch, M. W., & Bassett, S. (1998). *Health care resource management.* St. Louis: Mosby.

Rogoff, D., Couture, P., & Bernhardt, J. (1979). *Staff analysis on mock-ups.* Ann Arbor, MI: Office of Planning, Research and Development, the University of Michigan Hospitals.

Steinman, B., & Sexauer, J. (1993). *Hospitals and postsurgical recovery centers: Reinventing hospital-based surgical services.* Paper presented at the 1993 International Conference and Exhibition on Health Facility Planning, Design and Construction, New Orleans, September 14–16, 1993, pp. 341–346.

Weber, D. (1992, September/October). Planetree transplanted. *Healthcare Forum Journal,* pp. 30–37.

Zelman, W. A. (1996). *The changing healthcare marketplace.* San Francisco: Jossey-Bass.

Zimring, C., & Reizenstein, J. (1981). A primer on postoccupancy evaluation, *American Institute of Architects Journal, 70*(13), 52.

CHAPTER

30

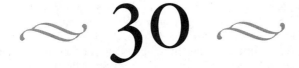

Marketing Nursing and Nursing Services

Sylvia A. Price • Debra Keene

Marketing ... is the whole business seen from the point of view of its final result, that is, from the customer's point of view. (Drucker, 1974, p. 63)

Chapter Highlights

- Marketing
- Marketing management
- Marketing management philosophies
- Nursing market arena
- Market segmentation
- Marketing information and research
- Marketing strategies
- Models of managed care
- Wellness movement

Marketing is a discipline that enables organizations to identify human wants and needs to achieve organizational goals and objectives. Effective marketing is a key factor associated with the survival of health care organizations. An introduction to principles of marketing that will enable nurse executives to integrate these concepts into their nursing administrative practice is the focus of this chapter.

MARKETING

Marketing implies being sensitive to and satisfying individuals' needs and wants through the process of exchange. It involves identifying products that are viewed as capable of satisfying a human want, need, or exchange. Kotler (1994) states that exchange is the core concept of marketing and requires that the following conditions must be satisfied:

- There are at least two parties.
- Each party has something that might be of value to the other party.
- Each party is capable of communication and delivery.
- Each party is free to accept or reject the offer.
- Each party believes it is appropriate or desirable to deal with the other party (p. 9).

If these conditions prevail, there is potential for exchange. Whether exchange occurs depends on whether the two parties can agree on terms of that exchange that will leave both parties better off than before. Exchange is referred to as a value-creating process because exchange normally leaves both parties better off than before the exchange.

A market is a place of potential exchanges or trade. Marketing is working within the context of a market to actualize potential exchanges to satisfy human needs and wants. Coping with exchange processes requires considerable deftness. Organizations must demonstrate expertise in managing exchange processes. They need to attract resources from specific market arenas, change them into useful products, and trade them in other market arenas.

MARKETING MANAGEMENT

Kotler and Scheff (1997) define marketing management as the "analysis, planning, implementation, and control of programs designed to create, build, and maintain beneficial exchange relationships with target audiences for the purpose of achieving marketing objectives. It relies on a disciplined analysis of the needs, wants, perceptions, and preferences of target and intermediary markets as the basis for effective product design, pricing, communication, and distribution" (p. 31). Health care marketing management is defined as "the *process* of understanding the needs and wants of a *target* market. Its purpose is to provide a viewpoint from which to *integrate* the analysis, planning, and implementation and control of the health care delivery system. The output of the health care marketing process is the development of the means to satisfy or facilitate exchange of values between health care providers and the target market(s)" (Cooper, 1994, p. 7).

Marketing management is essentially demand management. The organization apparently forms an idea of a desired level of transactions with a target market. Kotler (1994) states that "marketing management has the task of influencing the level, timing, and composition of demand in a way that will help the organization achieve its objectives" (p. 14). He distinguishes eight different states of demand, each presenting a different marketing challenge:

1. *Negative demand.* A market is in a state of negative demand if a major part of it dislikes the product and may even pay a price to afford it. People often have a negative demand for preventive health care (dental services, mammograms). A manager's task is to analyze the reasons the market dislikes the product, if redesigning a program, lower prices, and more positive promotion can change the market's beliefs and attitudes.

2. *No demand.* Target consumers are disinterested or indifferent to the product. The service may be either unknown or the client is not interested in it. Thus, individuals may not be interested in a well-child clinic, new technology, or surgical procedure. The marketing task is to devise ways to emphasize the benefits of the product with the person's needs and interests.

3. *Latent demand.* Clients may share a strong need that cannot be satisfied by any existing product. Drug treatment centers and crisis rape centers are examples of strong latent demand services that are slowly being used. The marketing task is to determine the size and need of the potential market and develop effective services to satisfy the demand.

4. *Declining demand.* Previous levels of demand are declining. Declining visits to a well-child clinic and decreasing hospital admissions are examples of declining demand. The marketing task is to analyze the causes of the decline and attempt to reverse it through creative remarketing of the service or product.

5. *Irregular demand.* Demand varies and creates inefficiencies in staffing, production, and distribution, such as when hospital operating rooms are overbooked early in the week and underbooked toward the end of the week. The marketing task, referred to as syncromarketing, is to find ways to alter the same pattern in demand through incentives such as flexible pricing or promotion.

6. *Full demand.* This occurs when organizations are pleased with their volume of business. For example, the client is satisfied with the managed health care point-of-service model and is willing to risk inconveniences and still desires it. The marketing task is to maintain the current level of demand, maintain quality, and measure client satisfaction.

7. *Overfull demand.* The demand level is higher than the desired demand. An example would be more patients on a critical care unit than can be safely treated. The marketing task, called demarketing, requires finding ways to reduce the demand by closing nursing units, increasing prices, reducing promotion or service, or referring patients to other units. The aim of demarketing is not to destroy demand but only to reduce its level, temporarily or permanently.

8. *Unwholesome demand.* Products are considered undesirable and attract organized efforts to discourage consumption. Alcohol, hand guns, and cigarettes are examples of undesirable products. The marketing task is to

encourage consumers to give these products up through advertising campaigns, taxes, public service announcements, price increases, and reduced availability.

Marketing challenges health care organizations to be responsive to the motivations of clients or consumers to seek or avoid care: their wants, needs, attitudes, and perceptions of the risks versus the benefits of various services. The influence of such factors as escalating health costs and consumerism has resulted in significant changes in health care delivery. To reduce expenditures, hospitals and community health agencies have responded with incentives to attract more clients. For example, hospitals offer a broad range of services geared to ambulatory care and allied health services (e.g., home care, hospice, home medical equipment). Home health agencies are also expanding their services to meet their clients' needs and desires (e.g., high-tech ventilator support systems, infusion therapy). Prospective reimbursement based on diagnosis-related groups also provides incentives for hospitals to reduce length of stay and procedures and to control expenditures (see Chapter 23).

The advent of wellness and primary care programs is a challenge to hospitals because such programs extend the hospital's traditional role as a provider of inpatient and emergency services. These programs are based on the premise that the consumer or client has a choice as to whether, when, and where to seek health care. In initiating health promotion and primary care programs, hospitals, as well as other community health agencies, must attract clients to the use of such services through the implementation of a marketing approach to health care delivery. Another mechanism to use resources more efficiently is through multihospital systems. These systems have attracted independent hospitals because of the benefit from economies of scale, especially in shared operations such as finance, purchasing, and other services.

MARKETING MANAGEMENT PHILOSOPHIES

Marketing management is the deliberate effort to achieve outcomes with target markets. It is imperative that organizations formulate philosophies to direct their marketing endeavors. Marketing activities should be administered according to a concept of responsible marketing practices. Three alternative concepts can assist organizations in their marketing activity: the product concept, the selling concept, and the marketing concept.

Product Concept

The product concept is a management orientation that assumes the consumers' desire those products that are good and reasonably priced. Such products require minimal marketing strategies to achieve satisfactory sales and profits. In health care, physician, as consumer of the product, will respond favorably to good products (or services) and facilities; therefore, minimal marketing strategies are usually required to ensure sufficient use. Nurse executives and practitioners are also consumers who are seeking new products that will enhance services to their clients. It is important to have nursing's active participation in developing and implementing the organization's marketing plan, which will help ensure the success of an innovative product line.

Consumers are becoming more knowledgeable about health care through such mechanisms as patient education programs and the media. Federal regulations such as the Patient Self-Determination Act are explained to consumers in the news and other educational literature that is available in the health care agency. These mechanisms will enable the consumer to take a more active role in the decision-making process in the health care marketplace. In some cases, consumers actually drive changes in health care practices (e.g., birthing rooms, rooming-in for parents of hospitalized children).

Both profit and not-for-profit organizations can operate according to a product concept. A classic example of the failure of the concept is the demise of the railroad industry, whose management was so convinced it had a superior form of transportation that it underserved its customers. The railroad industry ignored the challenges of the efficient service of the airlines and the trucking industry's capacity to pick up and deliver door to door.

Selling Concept

The selling concept is a management orientation that assumes that users will usually not purchase enough of the organization's products unless they are approached with a considerable selling and promotional venture. The major focus of the concept is obtaining sufficient sales for an organization's products. The concept is based on the assumption that customers will buy again, but even if they do not, a sufficient number of other customers will buy the product. This practice has many disadvantages, particularly when customer satisfaction is secondary to selling the product or service. For example, pharmaceutical sales promotions often engender hopes with unrealistic promises of weight reduction drugs to control obesity without emphasizing the drug's side effects.

Marketing Concept

The marketing concept is a management orientation that accepts the fact that the key task of the organization or system is to ascertain the needs, wants, and values of the target market. The objective is to modify the organization or system so that it delivers the desired level of satisfaction more effectively and efficiently than its competitors.

Drucker (1974) contrasts selling and marketing by emphasizing that "selling and marketing are antithetical rather than synonymous or even complimentary. There will always, one can assume, be need for some selling. But the aim of marketing is to make selling superfluous." He stresses that "the aim of marketing is to know and understand the customer so well that the product or service fits him/her and sells itself. Ideally, marketing should result in a customer who is ready to buy. All that should be needed is to make the product or service available, i.e., logistics rather than salesmanship, and statistical distribution rather than promotion" (pp. 64–65).

To implement a marketing approach, an organization must have a strategic plan of marketing research to determine and attempt to satisfy a defined set of wants of a target group. The enterprise must also recognize that activities related directly or indirectly to the target market must be located under an integrated market control. Cooper (1994) notes that the marketing concept becomes the focus for integrating the efforts of the enterprise. *Consumer satisfaction* is this focus. As health care in the United States departs from horizontal care (hospital-based) toward more vertical care (ambulatory facilities), the consumer or patient will become a more predominant focus. It is this function that helps integrate the previously insulated elements of the organization and emphasizes the necessity for planning from a marketing management perspective.

Implementing the marketing concept starts with ascertaining existing or potential consumer needs, followed by planning a coordinated set of services and programs to serve those needs and wants. The services and programs are aimed at generating consumer satisfaction as the stimulus to satisfying organizational goals.

The initial step in the implementation process is to identify the market, the individuals who might exchange something they have that the organization desires for something they want that the organization possesses. In this process, important attributes of each party are identified. The next step is to divide the market into homogeneous, distinctive groups to cultivate separate strategies for each one. Specific opportunities and high-probability exchanges with various market segments are then identified. The final step is to decide which of those opportunities to target for specific action and what results are desired.

The marketing concept is particularly significant in nursing because nurse executives must be cognizant of the exchange relationships within the context of the health care organization's external and internal environments. The exchange relationships in nursing practice, whether in the hospital or the community setting, are fundamentally unstable because the value of what is exchanged is constantly changing.

NURSING MARKET ARENA

Within the nursing division, the target market arenas are the members of the organization and the client or service populations. Other internal constituents may include the governing board, employees of other departments, physicians, and volunteers. External environments include clients, community, visitors, suppliers, regulators, supporters, professional associations, and colleagues in other organizations.

These exchange relationships are depicted in the following scenario. The nurse executive represents the organization, such as the hospital, home care agency, long-term care facility, in exchanges with the nursing personnel. The nurse executive is the spokesperson for nursing. The agency exchanges benefits, salary, rewards, and accomplishments for the staff nurse's endeavors, allegiance, and support of the organizational goals, whereas the consumers exchange money, approval, and satisfaction for technically competent and humane nursing care to improve their health status.

Nurse executives exchange their services for a position of respect, influence, and a desirable place to practice, whereas the physician exchanges client referrals for a workplace, prestige, influence, and other conveniences. In a hospital setting, physicians are primarily responsible for admitting patients and providing medical care (writing orders for treatment and medications). Nurses perform autonomous nursing activities as well as administer the physician's orders. Client satisfaction is directly related to the attentiveness and competency of the nursing personnel.

MARKET SEGMENTATION

Every market consists of consumers with different needs, preferences, and responses; thus, no one approach will satisfy all consumers. Selecting a target market requires an appraisal of the market opportunities that are available. Each segment of the market requires its own services, marketing strategies, and goals.

For a health care organization, it is imperative to identify whether a distinct group of individuals would or might use a particular service if the need arose. Lovelock (1979) identifies three criteria for the development of meaningful market segments: (1) measurability: it must be possible to obtain information on the specific characteristics of interest; (2) accessibility: management must be able to identify chosen segments within the overall market and effectively focus marketing efforts on those segments; and (3) substantiality: the segments must be large enough or sufficiently important to merit the time and cost of separate attention.

It is difficult to implement market segmentation strategies when the target segment is not clearly identifiable with the population. For example, a health promotion program may be developed to screen potential diabetics, clinics may be established in strategic locations, and a pricing policy determined. However, informing individuals who could benefit from early diagnosis and persuading them to use the services may be difficult.

MARKETING INFORMATION AND RESEARCH

The nurse executive must identify actual and potential markets and institute a two-way flow of communication with all markets to determine the elements that are valued by each segment and what each desires to exchange. Marketing data, such as the needs, wants, and values of the market, must be systematically reviewed and analyzed by the health care organization. When this initial process is completed, strategies are then devised for each segment. To accomplish this, the organization systematically collects and analyzes data from which to make policy regarding consumer preferences in the health care marketplace.

The nurse executive must be intimately involved in forecasting volume and frequency of demands for nursing services, perceptions of clients about the organization and its health care services, and potential demand for new services that are required by the client, physician, and nursing staff. The nurse executive must recognize nursing as a potential revenue-generating service and project the numbers and types of nursing personnel that are needed to meet these demands. Nursing has the potential to be revenue generating with regard to such areas as home care, patient education, midwifery, and rehabilitation.

Marketing Information System

Many health care organizations are analyzing their information needs and developing information systems as a basis for decision-making. Kotler (1994) uses the term *marketing information systems* (MIS), which consists of individuals, equipment, and procedures for gathering, sorting, analyzing, evaluating, and distributing needed, timely, and accurate information to marketing decision-makers.

The MIS subsystems that provide market information are: *(1)* internal records, such as patient records, quality improvement records, patient satisfaction surveys, exit interviews with employees; *(2)* marketing intelligence, which refers to sources and procedures by which marketing managers obtain everyday information about pertinent events in the marketing environment (e.g., nursing journals, newsletters, television, nursing professional organizations); *(3)* marketing research or the systematic design, collection, analysis, and reporting of findings and relevant findings to a specific marketing situation. Many institutions have added a fourth information service, a marketing decision support system (MDDS), to assist marketing managers make better decisions. The model consists of data that are analyzed statistically. The manager can use a program to determine the optimum course of action. Then the manager takes this action, along with other factors that affect the environment and result in new data. Kotler (1994) stresses that new software programs appear to assist marketing managers analyze, plan, and control their operations. These programs provide support for designing marketing research studies, segmenting markets, setting prices, and so on.

Marketing Research Consultants

An important issue is whether an organization should conduct its own research or hire a marketing research consultant. A cost-benefit analysis of using an external consultant versus an organization conducting its own research must be evaluated before a decision is made to hire a consultant. Clarke and Shyavitz (1994) suggest that market research should typically be conducted with the assistance of or by external consultants with expertise in the area of market research. Because such research must be objective, it is important that it be carried out in an unbiased manner. It is difficult for the internal staff of any organization to be objective and unbiased in the way they ask questions of clients; also, confusing market research with promotion activities in an attempt to "sell," or promote, the organization is less likely to occur if market professionals are consulted. These researchers realize that the purpose of market research is for the health care organization to become educated about its market, whereas the purpose of promotion is to educate the market about the health care organization.

Qualitative and Quantitative Research

Market research emphasizes the identification and analysis of information on consumer attitudes, perceptions, opinions, and preferences to devise market strategies. For example, in the health care arena, it is important to analyze consumer reports, after the hospitalization stay, to determine their interest and needs. Qualitative research is a comprehensive analysis of the characteristics and importance of human experience. Qualitative market research emphasizes why consumers like or dislike a product and examines what would change their attitudes and perceptions. Various research techniques are used to identify and evaluate this process. One technique is the focus-group discussion for which a representative group of actual or potential users is brought together. A subject should be introduced by a trained moderator who generates discussion through a few selected "probing" questions. The purpose is to elicit statements regarding the group's preferences concerning the topics under discussion. These statements are analyzed in an attempt to identify the components of the issues that should be explored with quantitative measures such as a telephone or mail survey.

A second qualitative research technique is the individual depth, or one-to-one, interview. This method is appropriate to use, particularly, when topics may be personal or confidential for the person to discuss in a focus-group situation. This technique may take the form of detailed interviews with an individual conducted by a trained interviewer. The decision-making or reasoning of the participants is probed on a one-to-one basis, generally through predominantly open-ended questions. The responses are analyzed to identify and clarify issues rather than to formulate a specific action plan.

Another technique, the nominal group, or Delphi technique, is used when group consensus is desired. A structured format is often used to minimize group interaction and assist the group-reach innovative or judgmental decisions. For example, in a study of nursing shortages, Wandelt, Pierce, and Widdowson (1981) used the nominal group technique at a conference of health care experts. They generated over 150 suggestions for attracting nurses back into the workforce.

Quantitative market research, by contrast, refers to systematic statistical sampling of a target market population. Studies are conducted to identify consumer segments in the health care market so that forecasts can be made about their future behavior. The demographic and behavior profiles of the consumers indicate who comprises the market and who provides services to the segments within it.

Much of the data needed for these studies can be obtained from secondary sources both internal and external to the organization, such as previous similar research studies and discharge or case-mix records. Data may be collected through survey instruments, such as mailed questionnaires and telephone and personal interviews. The data are then analyzed so that patterns of association or relationship among variables can be determined. In the health care market, quantitative research is conducted in an attempt to control segments so that forecasts predict how the target market will behave (Flexner & Berkowitz, 1979). The information obtained from the qualitative and quantitative phases of the research is used to devise marketing program strategies. Criteria for evaluating these programs are also included. For example, program effectiveness is measured in the health care market by analyses of service utilization, revenues and costs, consumer compliance and satisfaction, and health outcomes.

MARKETING STRATEGIES

In the implementation phase of a marketing plan, the organization should translate marketing research information into strategies and tactics. An important element that must be considered when developing market strategies is planning the marketing mix, represented by the four Ps: product (service), place, promotion, and price. Product, as defined previously, is whatever is offered to a market that is viewed as capable of satisfying a human want, need, or exchange. Place, or distribution, refers to how the product is made available to target segments of the market. Promotion is the activities that make the product available to the consumer. Price refers to the amount of money individuals have to pay for the product. The decision regarding the combination of the various elements—which can be combined in several ways and coordinated in a systematic way to reach targets—is an integral component of marketing strategies. Ireland (1979) emphasizes that success in understanding and applying the marketing mix to a given market "lies in developing a thorough understanding of the people in the market so that the right product can be afforded at the right time in the right place supported by the right promotional effort" (p. 258).

Marketing Plan

Hillestad and Berkowitz (1991) describe a six-step market-based approach. The steps include:

1. Setting the mission
2. Performing an external/internal analysis
3. Determining the strategy action match and marketing objectives
4. Developing action strategies
5. Integrating the plan and making revisions
6. Providing appropriate control procedures, feedback, and integration of all plans into a unified effort (p. 54)

Within each step, three types of activities are necessary for success: the process of performing the staff work necessary to support decision-making, actually making decisions, and integrating all units or services to support coordination of efforts. Each step and its constituent parts are diagrammed in relation to these activities (Figure 30.1).

An organization's business plan is also an important component of its strategy formulation. The initial step in a business plan is to formulate a statement of the organization's mission and goals. Following this is the marketing plan. The marketing plan feeds the operations plan, which works into the personnel plan, which then flows into the financial plan. All of these elements are an integral part of the business plan (see Figure 30.1). Refer to the Appendix for examples of nursing businesses.

Marketing plans require internal data along with information on attitudes, opinions, and the external environment of the organization. The marketing orientation requires that nurses must have an impact on decision-making. For example, in an extended health care facility nurse-physician collaboration was identified as the primary goal of the agency. The nurse practitioners and physicians developed and implemented a marketing plan that enabled the organization to achieve its goal of cost-effective, high-quality patient care.

Cost and Pricing

The determination of price in health care organizations is one of the most complex areas of administration. The direct and indirect costs generally related to a specific cost center do not form an accurate indicator of the actual cost of providing and maintaining these services. Pricing practices must be evaluated to make them more equitable and competitive in the marketplace. Health care agencies must develop a pricing structure that reflects the actual cost of providing services. Nurse executives are close to the consumer and capable of evaluating pricing practices. They need to be much more involved in determining product costs.

Kotler (1994) describes a six-step procedure for determining the price of a product. He notes that an organization must decide, in attempting to ascertain a price or pricing policy the objective that it is trying to achieve such as survival, to maximize current profit or sales growth. Second, the organization determines the demand schedule indicating the probable quantity purchased per period at alternative price levels. Third, the organization estimates how its cost varies according to different output levels with varying levels have accumulated production experience. Fourth, the agency examines competitors' prices as a basis for positioning its own price. Fifth, the organization selects one of various pricing methods. The following examples illustrate this concept:

- Markup pricing—to add a standard markup to the product's cost.
- Target-return pricing—determine the price that would yield its target rate of return on investment.

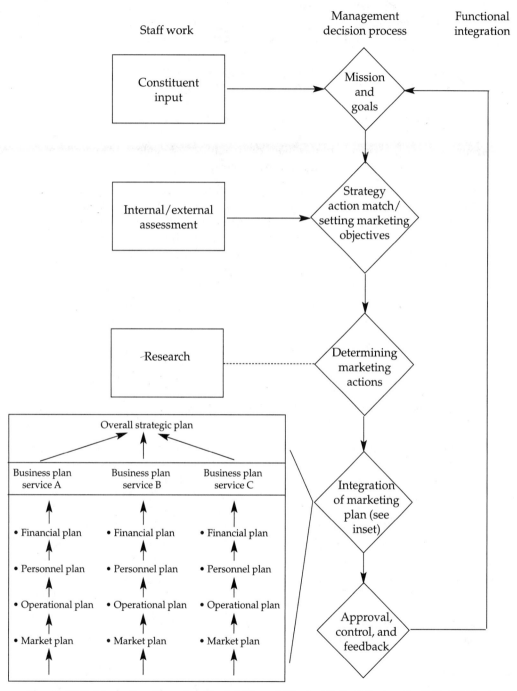

Figure 30.1 Marketing Planning Model. (From Hillestad, S. G., & Berkowitz, E. N. (1991). *Health care marketing plans: From strategy to action.* Gaithersburg, MD: Aspen. Reprinted with permission.

- Perceived value-pricing—based on the product's perceived value. The buyer's perception of value rather than the seller's cost is the key to pricing. The company should price at a level that captures what the buyer thinks the product is worth.
- Value pricing—companies charge a low price for a high-quality product. The price should represent an extraordinary bargain for consumers.

The company determines its final price, communicating it in the most effective psychological way, coordinating it with other marketing-mix elements, and determining if it will gain acceptance with distributors and dealers, the company salesforce, competitors, suppliers, and the government.

Kotler states that when an organization is initiating a price change it must carefully consider customers' and competitors' reactions. These reactions are influenced by the meaning customers' see in the price change, whereas competitors' reactions flow from a specific reaction policy or from a fresh appraisal of each situation. The action is certain to affect buyers, competitors, distributors, and suppliers. The success of such a change depends on how the parties respond and their responses are among the most difficult things to predict. Thus, a contemplated price change implies great risks. A market-oriented pricing system that enables health care agencies to more closely match prices and costs is needed.

Promotion

Promotional activities are a strategic part of a marketing campaign. Prospective clients should be knowledgeable regarding the service or product and its desired attributes. The information disseminated must be based on what consumers should know.

Promotion involves advertising, selling, and public relations. In a health care setting, promotional activities usually include identification of services, for example, educational services. Recruitment of nursing staff is also an example of a promotional activity. Recruiters publicize their agency by distributing promotional brochures, participating in professional meetings, and advertising in professional journals. Patton (1991) stresses that a marketing approach to nurse recruitment "promotes your hospital as a competitively superior place of work for satisfying the needs of nurses (and, consequently, the needs of your hospital for competent, motivated, and stable nursing personnel)" (p. 17). Health care agencies are becoming more aggressive in their advertising efforts. Publications and news releases are most effective when designed within the context of a total hospital marketing plan. In the present health care arena, competition is evident for the attraction of consumers in the marketplace.

Competition

In health care, competition is geared toward demand, which restricts the dollars coming into the health system. The assumption is that consumers are involved in making different choices depending on their particular needs. Some spend dollars to have more services. Through control of costs and prices, providers such as physicians compete for clients. There is bargaining with providers over prices by such groups as business and labor unions. It is assumed that cost containment results through market forces and consumer choice.

Congress has been involved in several pro-competition measures aimed at reducing health care costs. These proposals provide consumers with incentives to decrease unwarranted use of health care and to select the most cost-effective health care plans. The attempt is to reduce the deductions employers can claim for medical benefits, which would encourage them to choose less costly health insurance programs. The proposals also advocate an increase in cost sharing through deductibles and copayments, which would be included in plans for the employed and Medicare and Medicaid recipients. An example of recent legislation is the passage of a provision, contained in the budget bill Public Law 105-33, that will expand Medicare reimbursement at 85% of physician rates for nurse practitioners and clinical nurse specialists to all geographical and clinical settings. As of January 1, 1998, Medicare clients, those with mental disorders, and the disabled will have access to the cost-effective, quality health care provided by advanced practice RNs in both rural and urban areas and in hospital- and community-based health care settings. Also in this spending bill were provisions to reauthorize the Community Nursing Organization (CNO) demonstration project. CNOs are pilot managed care programs administered by nurses who offer Medicare benefits to the elderly in noninstitutional settings. These nurse-managed coordinated care programs have been recognized since they began in 1994 for delivering high-quality, cost-effective patient care.

The American Nurses Association has advocated the importance of nursing's interest in developing competition in the health industry. Nursing's interest includes increasing legislative visibility, achieving third-party reimbursement, and interpreting the nurse's role in preventive care, geriatric care, and consumer education.

MODELS OF MANAGED CARE

A preferred provider organization (PPO) is a type of managed care health plan that uses its provider network to administer care to employers and other groups in a provider network. It has been described as one of the most powerful marketing tools that providers can use. Providers are usually paid on a discounted fee for service. PPOs have decreased costs by creating a network of health care providers who provide services for a specified fee. Characteristics include formation of a panel of providers (hospitals or physicians), negotiated fee schedules that are discounted, a commitment to utilization review methods of quality management techniques, and flexibility in the choice of provider with a financial incentive to use the preferred provider.

A health maintenance organization (HMO) is a managed care health plan that either administers or arranges for health care to be provided to its members usually on a fixed, prepaid capitated monthly fee. These managed care plans have resulted in an increase in services such as home health care and hospice and have reduced the need for more expensive care. Traditional insurance plans have lagged in offering these additional services, but are also adopting many of these services. Approximately one-half of consumers are enrolled in HMO or PPO plans (Levit et al., 1996).

Another model is the point-of-service (POS) model. This is a hybrid of the PPOs, HMOs and traditional indemnity plans. These three health insurance options are integrated to establish a network of providers to meet the company's requirements. The features of the POS model include: POS choice, fee service discounts by providers, utilization management programs, preventive health coverage, provider risk-sharing, and free choice of health care provider. Cost savings in this model are primarily from negotiating lower provider fees and implementing utilization management programs.

Product Line Management

Product line management (PLM) categorizes services or products that have similar functions into multiple strategic business units or product lines. PLM was introduced in 1928 by Procter & Gamble to market their new product, Lava soap™. Several large manufacturing companies adopted this concept to prosper and survive in their competitive environments. The product line manager is responsible for orchestrating the product or service, from marketing, planning, development, implementation, to evaluation.

MacStravic (1986) defines a product in health services as a "set of activities and experiences that are offered and consumed by an identifiable set of people in ways that are different from other sets . . . or a set of products that when planned, managed, or marketed as a group yields some advantage over being treated as isolated individuals" (p. 35). The PLM approach is currently being implemented to market product lines in a variety of hospital settings. Therefore, PLM is a system of planning, organizing directing, and evaluating within a product line, such as cardiovascular laboratory services or emergency services, for the purpose of providing comprehensive, high-quality, and cost-effective care to clients. It is important to emphasize that product lines represent the hospital's business mission, which is referred to as clear, accurate understanding of the goals and services the hospital desires to represent. Simpson and Clayton (1991) stress that only when this business mission and direction are clear can a hospital proceed with defining and selecting product lines for profitability management.

Newbould (1980) differentiates between programs referred to as "stars" and "cash cows." Stars are programs in high-growth fields in which the institution has market-share dominance in terms of relative numbers of staff. These programs are growing rapidly and typically require extensive resources, such as to add health care personnel, expand the facility, and acquire equipment. If these investments are made and the area proves of enduring interest, the star program will become a cash cow and generate cash in excess of expenses in the future. The cash cows are programs in low-growth fields that attract a high share of the market for such programs. Newbould emphasizes that these programs can be used to support high-growth programs or underwrite those with problems.

Marketing competition is directly affecting the health care industry. As McNerny (1980) eloquently states, "For every force, there will be a countervailing force. Progress will be evolutionary, through competition, voluntary efforts, and regulation."

WELLNESS MOVEMENT

Consumers are better informed and more responsible for their own health. The wellness movement is evident. Physical wellness centers are evident throughout the country in hospitals and community and occupational health settings. Women's centers and sports medicine centers are being developed to specifically market products. In the 1970s it was unusual to see a physician or any other health care professional advertising. A quick look at today's Yellow Pages shows that almost all physicians, optometrists, podiatrists, and chiropractors advertise. When you drive down a city street you will see billboards advertising local hospitals and specialty groups. Hospitals and specialty groups are responding to consumer demand as they see the potential profit and public relations possibilities.

Sports Centers

The following is an example of how a local group creates brand loyalty. Each year one of the local sports medicine groups provides physicals to high school students participating in sports for a $20 fee. Physicians from the group perform the physicals. A volunteer physical therapist, from this group, attends each game to assist with injuries, and also attends practice to help students and coaches learn to prevent injuries. Always dressed in shirts, t-shirts, or a jacket with the name of the group prominently displayed, this therapist is a walking advertisement and great public relations for the clinic. Additionally, this clinic purchases a large banner for the sideline and advertises in the programs. All injured students are accompanied to the hospital by this therapist who guides them through the trauma and red tape of the emergency department. If your child is injured and needs rehabilitation services, you will remember that the "Good" clinic has given support to your school. In this situation, "Who are you going to call?"

The sports medicine group has successfully made both parents and children loyal to them by giving of their time and talent to the sports program. They have supported the athletic program and the athletes and parents in turn will support the group.

Women's Health Centers

The competition for health care dollars is reflected in the following scenario. In response to this increased competition, hospitals are creating specialty centers to meet the market demand. Women's health centers are specialty units that are growing in popularity. Usually attached to a hospital, these centers provide total care for women. Women have responded positively to these centers and have indicated that they would be willing to pay a membership fee if necessary. Services offered by these centers include maternity care, diagnostic testing, weight control, nutrition counseling, oncology, psychological counseling, and occasionally plastic surgery (LaFleur & Taylor, 1996).

Many centers advertise on the Internet and list services and affiliated physicians for prospective clients to read at home. A simple search using "women's health centers will provide a list of heart centers for women, diet and exercise centers, obstetric/gynecologic centers, plastic surgery centers, and sports medicine centers. Religious-, university-, hospital-, physician-, and city-affiliated centers are available within the category of women's health centers.

One way the clinics market themselves is by purchasing a mailing list or database. These lists contain names and addresses of people who are identified as users of the services that a women's center could provide. The lists or databases identify the target market.

The World Wide Web has created a revolution in marketing. Hospitals and clinics are using this medium to attract new clients. In our managed care world it is important to make each marketing dollar stretch as far as possible, and the Web offers this opportunity at a low cost to facilities.

SUMMARY

Nurse executives must understand marketing principles and techniques and be able to develop marketing strategies to survive in today's economy. Such strategies should be devised to meet competition and increase nursing's influence in the health care sector within the realm of professional nursing practice.

By using a marketing model, the nurse executive can analyze needs, preferences, and perceptions of potential users of nursing service as well as assess the capabilities of the organization to meet the demand for services. Strategies are determined for each market segment, goals and objectives are formulated, and marketing plans are implemented and evaluated. Marketing is a management discipline and must be recognized by the nurse executive to promote high-quality, client-centered nursing care within the professional practice of nursing administration.

As the health care environment continues to evolve, we must find new ways to market our services (Crow, 1995). Competition for health care dollars ensures that we must reach out for new clients in innovative ways. As nurses we need to recognize the Web as a powerful tool and learn to harness its power to market our services.

STUDY QUESTIONS

1. What are the similarities between marketing management and health care marketing management?
2. Describe the rationale for using the product and marketing concepts in the health care delivery system.
3. Define marketing management's task. Describe the eight different states of demand and give an example of each that is applicable to the health care marketplace.
4. What are the major differences between marketing information and marketing research?
5. Analyze the impact of issues related to price setting, promotion, and competition within nursing.
6. What are the advantages and disadvantages of product line management in the health care arena?
7. What are the advantages and disadvantages of using the Internet for determining what health care services are available?

REFERENCES

Clarke, R., & Shyavitz, L. (1994). Market research: When, why, and how. Organization design. In P. Cooper (Ed.), *Health care marketing: A foundation for managed quality* (3rd ed.). Germantown, MD: Aspen.

Cooper, P. (Ed.). (1994). *Health care marketing: A foundation for managed quality.* (3rd ed.). Germantown, MD: Aspen.

Crow, K. E. (1995). Advertising health care services. *Journal of Health Care Marketing, 15,* 2.

Drucker, P. (1974). *Management tasks, responsibilities, and practices.* New York: Harper & Row.

Flexner, W., & Berkowitz, E. (1979). Marketing research in health services planning: A model. *Public Health Reports, 94*(6), 503–513.

Hillestad, S., & Berkowitz, E. (1991). *Health care marketing plans: From strategy to action* (2nd ed.). Gaithersburg, MD: Aspen.

Ireland, R. (1979). Marketing: A new opportunity for hospital management. In P. Cooper (Ed.). Health care marketing issues and trends. Germantown, MD: Aspen Publications.

Kotler, P. (1994). *Marketing management analysis, planning, implementation, and control.* (8th ed.). Englewood Cliffs, NJ: Prentice-Hall.

Kotler, P., & Scheff, J. (1997). *Standing room only.* Boston: Harvard Business School Press.

LaFleur, E., & Taylor, S. L. (1996). Women's health centers and specialized services. *Journal of Health Care Marketing, 16,* 3.

Levit, K., Lazenby, H., Braden, B., Cowan, C., McDonnell, P., Sivarajan, L., Stiller, J., Won, D., Donham, A., & Steward, M. (1996). National health care expenditures 1995. *Health Care Financing Review, 18*(1), 175–214.

Lovelock, C. (1979). Concepts and strategies for marketers. In P. Cooper (Ed.). *Health care marketing issues and trends.* Germantown, MD: Aspen.

MacStravic, R. (1986). Product-line administration in hospitals. *Health Care Management Review, 11*(35), 35–43.

McNerny, W. (1980). Testimony on S. B. 1968, the Health incentives reform act, to the subcommittee on Health, Committee on Finance, U.S. Senate, March 19, 1980.

Newbould, G. (1980). Product portfolio diagnosis for U.S. universities. *Akron Business and Economic Review,* (2), 44.

Patton, J. (1991). Nurse recruitment: From selling to marketing. *Journal of Nursing Administration, 21*(9), 16–20.

Simpson, R., & Clayton, K. (1991). Automation: The key to successful product-line management. *Nursing Administration Quarterly, 15*(2), 33–38.

Wandelt, M., Pierce, P., & Widdowson, R. (1981). Why nurses leave nursing and what can be done about it. *American Journal of Nursing, 81*(1), 72–77.

PART

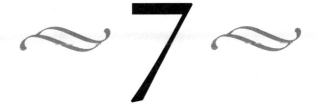

7

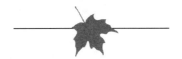

Working in the Year 2000

C H A P T E R

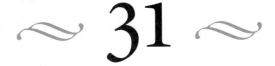

31

Managing a Culturally Diverse Workforce

Karin Polifko-Harris

The most productive vision of diversity employs a full engagement of the human resource potential of the work force. (Malone, 1997, p. 6)

Chapter Highlights

- Key employment trends
- Defining terms of cultural diversity
- Cultural application theories
- Culturally sensitive awareness
- Effective management of a culturally diverse workforce

During the past decade, there has been a growing interest by executives in diversification of our workforce and related implications. Many health care organizations, whether they are located in urban or rural settings, are faced with a similar challenge: how to best "manage" an increasingly culturally diverse workforce. All of us have different expectations based on our backgrounds, and it is often easy to forget that not everyone behaves or reacts to a situation in the same way. Our cultural background affects the manner in which we respond to a conflict situation, to a misunderstood memorandum, and to a nonverbal response. Members of the health care team, and clients and their families, have the right to have their differences and needs respected, accepted, and validated. We may not always understand without asking for clarification. There needs to be an active valuing of individual differences, not automatic assumptions, of what someone's needs may be. The goal of this chapter is to give the reader ideas that may be helpful in working with people of various cultures, races, and ethnicities. Several theories of cultural understanding are presented followed by specific situational issues common to the multicultural organization.

KEY EMPLOYMENT TRENDS

The face of a "typical" American worker is changing, and health care workers are no exception. The changing demographics in our workforce have come about due to two significant influences on American society: a shift from a manufacturing-based economy and globalization of the workplace. It is projected that the labor force will continue to evolve to reflect recent immigration patterns into the United States. According to some forecasters, one of every four new employees into the labor market will be an immigrant by the year 2000 (Smith & Johnson, 1991). Today, almost 25% of the American population is either foreign born or a member of a minority native-born class. Close to 15% of us speak a language other than English in our home or at work, yet almost 97% of people living in the United States can speak English to a degree (Thiederman, 1996). It is anticipated that the influx of white men into the workforce will continue to decline, reaching only about 15% of the total new workers in the next decade (Labich, 1996). We are becoming less homogenous, more female, and older as we progress into the 21st century. It is forecast that the largest growth in the labor market will occur in the Hispanic population, followed by the African American and the Asian labor forces.

Almost 61% of all employable women were in the workforce at the end of the 1990s (Elmuti, 1993), a dramatic change from the "ideal" one wage-earner family of the 1950s. In fact, only 17% of Americans live in a home with the traditional one wage-earner father, a stay-at-home mother, and one or more children (*Virginian Pilot*, May 5, 1998). With nursing being a predominately female profession—it is 94% female—nurse executives have special challenges in women's health and child care needs, because the many health care delivery sites are operational 24 hours a day, 7 days a week.

We are also aging: it is envisioned that within the next 10 years, almost 40% of the workforce will be more than 45 years of age (Labich, 1996). These facts are critically important to keep in mind as we plan for the future of the health care industry—who will our workers be and what needs will they have that potentially may not be met by today's standards? According to *Workforce 2000*, the seminal book that awakened us to diversity issues in the workplace, the health care sector continues to rapidly expand its labor force (Johnston & Packer, 1987). Clearly, our American health care workforce is becoming increasingly more diverse, and as nurse executives, we must become aware of the issues and concerns that arise with diversity if we are to meet the needs of our clients, families, and staff members.

DEFINING TERMS OF CULTURAL DIVERSITY

When defining a culture, one must consider values, norms, beliefs, ethnicity, race, and folkways of a particular group or community. Culture is characterized by a set of people; it is not seen as an individual trait or experience. We are immersed in our culture from birth, learning about spoken words and unspoken traditions from the society in which we are raised. Cultural patterns may be implicit or explicit, arising from the learned experiences of the group who adapt responsively over time, which is primarily unconscious.

Hofstede (1993, p. 89) sees culture as the "collective programming of the mind that distinguishes the members of one group or category of people from another." Leininger (1991) offers that practices in a culture guide actions and decisions in an expected patterned response. Culture is influential over health and illness perceptions (Purnell & Paulanka, 1998; Spector, 1996), and is passed down from generation to generation through time passage. Each culture also has its own symbols with meanings and is dynamic and complex, giving an outsider a perspective on how group members view their environment and their placement within that environment. Culture also refers to a specific group's norms, values, and belief sets that guide the group's behaviors (Kirkpatrick, Katrobos, Sherman, & Hull, 1994).

All members of the societal group share these unique experiences, with defined roles and behavioral expectations. Relationships are also defined from culture to culture; in the Latino culture, the male is considered the "head" of the household and the primary decision-maker, whereas in the Native American culture, the elder female may take a more significant role than male family members. In other societies, the relationships between males and females may appear more equitable, such as in Sweden.

Ethnic Groups

Being "ethnic" is often described as from a certain cultural or societal background. Ethnicity describes the association of belonging to a particular ethnic group, perhaps within a larger community. A sense of affiliation or membership is identified, defining who we are and what we are all about. Many ethnic definitions include descriptors of common geographical origin, race, language (both verbal and nonverbal), feelings, identifications of symbols, traditions and values, religious beliefs, immigration patterns, and distinctiveness, both internally and externally observed (Spector, 1996). Physical characteristics may also identify an ethnic group, whether it is skin color, hair type, facial features, bone structure, or body type.

An ethnic group may also be categorized as a minority group among a majority population. According to the 1990 U.S. Bureau of the Census, by the year 2080, the United States cultural mix will be more than 50% minority ethnic groups: Hispanics, 23.4%; African Americans, 14.7%; Asians and others, 12% (Figure 31.1). Minority groups are becoming the majority group in many areas of the

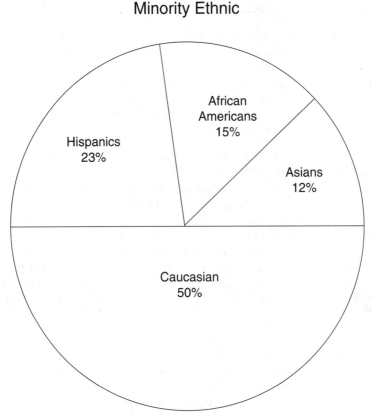

Minority Ethnic

Hispanics
23%

African
Americans
15%

Asians
12%

Caucasian
50%

Figure 31.1 Cultural mix in the United States by the year 2080. Data from 1990 U.S. Bureau of the Census.

United States, such as in the urban cities of Miami, San Antonio, Washington, DC, and Los Angeles.

Cultural Values

Values are often viewed as those internalized attitudes that keep us moral (or immoral), assisting us in making ethical or unethical decisions that only we know as right or wrong (Yukl, 1994). Cultural values are descriptions of a particular group that are accepted, understood, and have designated meanings. For example, how one views the role of a female in a decision-making position outside the home is largely culturally driven. Norms are sometimes interchanged with values, as they are the expected standards within the cultural group, and often provide examples of how a value is to be expressed. These are the visible "rules" that govern human behavior, giving direction to the correct or incorrect manner to act in any given situation.

As you look to interpret a person's behavior, you need to understand that values are a driving force leading to people's decisions. Values are the foundations of one's philosophy and position on many issues, including professional, personal, and social concerns. When the workforce is culturally and ethically diverse, a variety of values may be demonstrated, and occasionally, may be in conflict. It is the astute executive who knows when to intervene, enabling and encouraging differing viewpoints to be expressed and valued.

Diversity, as it relates to management, is a fairly recent label that first began appearing in the literature in the mid-1980s (Gordon, 1992), and became a "hot" topic in human resource management in the early 1990s. Many organizations have diversity awareness training programs in place, encouraging understanding, rather than negating differences among workers.

Diversity addresses those human characteristics different from our own and majority groups to which we belong. The six primary dimensions of diversity include age, gender, ethnicity/culture, physical abilities, race, and sexual/affectional orientation. To effectively manage workforce diversity is to create an organizational climate that accepts each individual employee for what he or she brings to the workplace. Individuality is encouraged, with understanding of differences the goal. It should not be the expectation that employees who are not of the majority culture suppress their culture to work harmoniously, but instead it should be everyone's responsibility to value differences among co-workers. Figure 31.2 illustrates the many ways in which people differ.

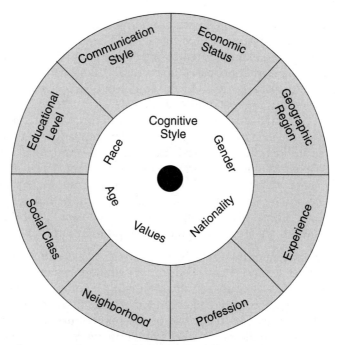

Figure 31.2 Ways in which people differ. From DeLaune, S., & Ladner, P. (1998). *Fundamentals of nursing: Standards of practice.* Albany, NY: Delmar.

CULTURAL APPLICATION THEORIES

When applying cultural theory to one's administrative practice, there are two paths to take. The first is to review the current literature on transcultural nursing theories and conceptual models, which directly address clinical needs individual clients and their families have in a culturally sensitive and competent manner. A second path is to explore cultural theories and models found in the business and management literature that discuss the cultural diversity differences that manifest themselves in the work environment. This section of the chapter will include a brief review of both paths to understanding cultural theory, because nurse executives deal with both issues of direct patient care concerns and interpersonal relationships.

Many nursing courses today include components of cultural awareness in their curricula. The American Association of Colleges of Nursing (AACN) has defined the study of cultural competency and cultural awareness as one of the core knowledge areas expected of a baccalaureate graduate. AACN's 1997 Statement on Diversity and Equality of Opportunity recognizes that diversity is a critical issue for organizations and institutions into the 21st century, stating health care providers overall, and the nursing profession specifically, need to "reflect and value the diversity of the populations and communities they serve."

Transcultural Nursing

Transcultural nursing is concerned with providing care that matches the client's expectations and cultural belief set. Everyone has different perceptions of health, illness and wellness, and expected treatments. Many things influence someone's responses to any given situation, based on cultural beliefs, values, norms, and behaviors approved (or not approved) by the community. A focus of transcultural nursing is to provide an understanding of clients' health care needs who may be from a different cultural background from the health care team members. When providing care to someone of another culture, misunderstandings may arise between the nurse and the client of space, time, communication, food, and community and family expectations, inhibiting the opportunity for the client to reach an optimal health state while in the health care facility. The nurse needs to actively seek clarification of the cultural differences, valuing them within the plan of care. Part of the valuing process is becoming sensitive to our own cultural biases, prejudices, and behaviors and how these may affect our own care and care decisions.

The field of transcultural nursing study began in the 1960s, with Madeleine Leininger as its founder and primary educator. Leininger began the Transcultural Nursing Society in 1974 as a subspecialty of nursing, blending the fields of nursing and anthropology. According to Leininger (1978, p. 8), transcultural nursing is the "comparative study of and analysis of different cultures and subcultures in the world with respect to their caring behavior, nursing care and health-illness values, beliefs and patterns of behavior with the goal of developing a scientific and humanistic body of knowledge to provide culture-specific and culture-universal nursing care practices." Leininger's theoretical model is known as the Sunrise Model (Figure 31.3). Transcultural nursing concepts have incorporated the integral concepts of nursing: person, society, health, and nursing and is extensively reported in the literature (Andrews & Boyle, 1995; Chrisman, 1990; Giger & Davidhizar, 1995). This model has served as the basis for the development of additional models of transcultural nursing and assessment instruments (Block, 1983).

According to Leininger (1978, 1991), several assumptions and precepts are inherent in the practice of transcultural nursing. The first centers around the concept of caring; all cultures have expressions of caring and caring behaviors. A second concept involves that which is defined as "good" care; each culture validates

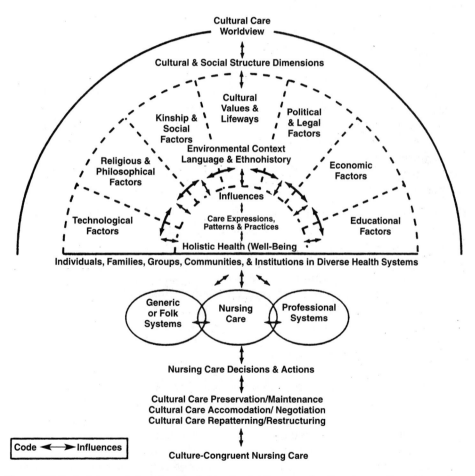

Figure 31.3. Leininger's Sunrise Model to depict theory of cultural care diversity and universality. From Leininger, M. (1991). *Culture care diversity and universality: A theory of nursing* (p. 114). New York: National League for Nursing Press. Reprinted with permission.

what is considered appropriate care, based on any given situation. It is in mutual goal setting and goal attainment that "good" care is evaluated. And lastly, the practice of transcultural nursing is concerned with the awareness of each culture's means of self-identification, in symbols, verbal and nonverbal communications, and shared meanings of health, wellness, and illness.

Transcultural Assessment

Giger and Davidhizar's Transcultural Assessment Model (1995) offers a practical method to completing a cultural assessment and evaluating the meanings of cultural variations. Four concepts are central to understanding Giger and Davidhizar's model, including the notions of culturally diverse nursing care, culturally unique individuals, culturally sensitive environments, and culturally specific illness and wellness behaviors (Giger & Davidhizar, 1995).

When providing culturally specific care, Giger and Davidhizar (1995) assert that six elements need to be considered when completing a cultural assessment. These six concepts are communication, space, social organization, time, environmental control, and biologic variations (Figure 31.4). For example, every culture has specific ideas on nonverbal communications such as touching. Generally, the Japanese consider it disrespectful to look someone directly in the eye or to touch someone, especially in a social context. In contrast, the Hispanic culture is a tactile, but modest, culture. Personal space can be close or expansive, depending on the territorial needs of a person. Social organization includes those enculturated patterns that we learn as members of a society: what are the significant life events of a person, how are they celebrated, and with whom are they shared?

Time is interpreted differently by each culture because there are differences noted between social time, which are those patterns related to societal expectations and actual clock time. Cultural differences are also noted in time orientations of future, present, or past. Likewise, environmental control illustrates the influence an individual has in the surroundings, such as in maintaining health and wellness. Finally, the last concept is that of biologic variations: many ethnic and cultural groups are predisposed to certain diseases, have identifying physical characteristics, and have genetic distinctions.

CULTURALLY SENSITIVE AWARENESS

To be advocates in the changing demographics of the American health care system, nurse executives need to instill in their staffs the need for culturally sensitive awareness for an effective and competent workforce. All individuals are shaped by their cultural, societal, and familial experiences during their lifetime, resulting in expected (and sometimes unexpected) cultural responses. However, it is imperative to not assume that because someone is of a certain cultural heritage that he or she has the characteristic reactions to all given situations.

A challenge for the nurse executive is to foster the staff with processing of new information as they seek to work with others who may be of a culture different

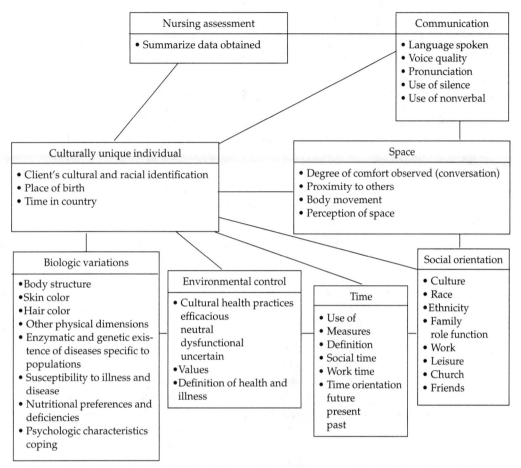

Figure 31.4 Giger and Davidhizar's Transcultural Assessment Model. From Giger, J. N., & Davidhizar, R. E. (1995). *Transcultural nursing: Assessment and intervention* (2nd ed., p. 10). St. Louis: Mosby-Yearbook. Reprinted with permission.

from their own, whether it is a patient, family, co-worker or supervisor. Often we reach a decision based on personal experiences rather than inferring an action based on similar situations and actions.

In the study of culture, there are two significant theoretical viewpoints when analyzing how those culturally determined values, beliefs, and norms are acquired. One viewpoint is the "melting pot theory," which had been popular in the management literature until recently. This acculturation theory asserts the notion that those people raised and living within a culture different from their own should do and learn the host culture's values and norms, acquiring these values and beliefs as their own. Many ethnic groups, especially those living in cultures quite different from their own, may find themselves acquiring certain characteristics as a matter of survival and "fitting in" (LaFrambose, Coleman, & Gerton, 1993).

They may even find themselves living in two cultures simultaneously: one to be seen as "fitting in" with the majority host culture and the other as their ethnic culture.

The opposite theoretical viewpoint is taken by Spector (1996), who has expanded Estes and Zitzow's (1980) Heritage Consistency Model in an attempt to "study the degree to which a person's lifestyle reflects his or her traditional culture, whether European, Asian, African or Hispanic" (p. 68). In this view, it is assumed that ethnic groups keep their traditional values, beliefs, and norms, to be identified as the minority ethnic group within the larger host majority group. This is the current focus of today's diversity awareness training: all people are valued for their differences (Fine, 1996). Employees are no longer expected to conform to the majority ethnic culture in an organization—differences are positive features to be celebrated.

The Heritage Consistency Model distinguishes between those values that are traditionally defined, providing a heritage that is consistent, or the values that contribute to an inconsistent heritage because they are acquired through acculturation. For example, people who live within a "friendly" host culture are more apt to assimilate or acculturate quickly to the values and norms of the host culture. They may even alter their value sets to meet the new value sets in which they live.

Spector (1996) identifies four categories that distinguish the Heritage Consistency Model: socialization, culture, religion, and ethnicity. All categories contain both primary and extended family members. Socialization consists of your name, the place(s) where you are raised, and visits to the primary home. The cultural category contains common language known in the culture and particular folkways and practices. Religion is self-explanatory and includes the historical religious beliefs held by members and formal religious participation. The final category, ethnicity, expands on the symbolic meanings and folkways attached to a distinct heritage, and continues with the socialization of this ethnic group with members of the same ethnicity, identifying as the same entity. Members of an ethnic community also identify closely with similar ethnic groups; all Greek Orthodox members identify with specific religious holiday expectations and preparations regardless where they are living. Being Greek Orthodox is an ethnic identifier by itself.

It is no surprise that most of the research done in the field of cultural diversity as it pertains to management is that of interpersonal and organizational communication (Fine, 1996). Because of the variety of messages each culture has for its communications, many interactions have potential to result in misunderstandings. Further, many employees are judged based on the popular paradigm of white male expectations and responses in an organization. It is beyond the scope of this chapter to discuss the implications of gender and race on communication styles, characteristics, and patterns in the workplace, but it is closely entwined with culture. We are beginning to see more research done in this area, but the majority of the instruments have been developed using the white male's values, offering a rich opportunity for further study and research (Fine, 1993; Limaye, 1994).

A significant theoretical framework developed from Geert Hofstede's work with an intercultural organizational study on values in the late 1970s. Hofstede (1980, 1984) surveyed employees from 39 subsidiaries of the United States-based International Business Machines (IBM) and a Yugoslavian export company that serviced IBM products. He administered a survey to more than 116,000 employees between 1968 and 1972, translating the survey into 29 languages. The goal of the survey was to distinguish the ways in which employees perceived their world, based on cultural expectations. Four dimensions of national cultural variation developed from the data: power distance, individualism, uncertainty-avoidance, and masculinity-femininity. A fifth dimension, Confucian dynamism, was discovered when data were examined from the administration of the Chinese value survey by Michael Bond in 1987. Hofstede later renamed this dimension long-term orientation (Table 31.1).

The first construct, power distance, is the extent to which society accepts inequality both socially and at the workplace. The individualism construct is regarded highly in those cultures where individual achievement is valued over the goals of the group, feeling responsible for only the person and not the family unit or society.

Masculinity has at its opposite end, femininity. Cultures that value masculinity are male-dominated, emphasizing financial matters, achievement, and distinct gender roles. Feminine countries emphasize relationships and caring for others and place importance on life after work. Uncertainty-avoidance measures a culture's risk propensity or how well a culture handles uncertain situations with questionable outcomes. The most recently added construct is long-term orientation, containing the values of thrift, perseverance in activities and observance of the order of hierarchical relationships. Orientation is future oriented.

Hofstede is credited with completing the largest and most significant cross-cultural study applicable to international business theory in the 1980s (Henry, 1989; Hoppe, 1992; Swierczek, 1991). In fact, Hofstede is the most frequently referenced theorist in cultural values in the management literature (Sondergaard, 1994). Through his research, Hofstede determined that although culture influences most of group differences, other characteristics such as gender, age, educational levels, and occupation also significantly contribute to the overall impression of group

Table 31.1 Dimensions of National Cultural Variation

Dimension	Explanation
Power distance	Extent to which society accepts inequality
Individualism	Individual achievement valued over group goals
Uncertainty-avoidance	Measures a culture's ability to handle risk
Masculinity-femininity	District gender roles—male dominance versus caring relationships
Long-term orientation	Values thrift, perseverance, hierarchical relationships—future oriented

differences. Like other theorists, Hofstede believes culture is group rather than individually expressed.

Hofstede's Values Survey Module has been the focus of numerous replication studies. Sondergaard (1994) found that from 1980 to 1993, Hofstede was referenced more than 1,036 times in the literature, and was the focus of 36 book reviews. Numerous researchers have replicated Hofstede's research using populations other than IBM, but to date, there has only been one study applying Hofstede's theory of cross-cultural differences to health care management. Polifko-Harris, in her 1995 study, administered the Values Survey Module to a population of American and Filipino RNs. Unlike most of the research on the Values Survey Module, she found directly contrasting results, especially around the Filipino nurses' results. She concluded that gender, occupation, and time in the host culture affected value orientation considerably more than previously mentioned.

Others have significantly added to the literature on culture's differences in the workplace. Laurent (1983) studied managerial theories in 10 Western countries, surveying more than 800 managers. He found that each person brings to the workplace his or her own values and differences, suggesting that like Hofstede, national culture influences one's understanding and application of management theory. Bass and Burger (1979) surveyed 3,082 managers in 12 countries in an attempt to differentiate the managers' attitudes toward advancement, finding that though there were cultural similarities, other issues such as job satisfaction, motivators, and needs were also influential. Redding and Ng (1982) studied the influence of "keeping face" to Chinese managers in the workplace.

With the continued expansion of our global economy, intercultural research needs to be a focus area, particularly in the field of health care management. Although there is considerable argument for the study of culture's influence on our patient care and management of others, there is a scarcity of information on the "best" directions to take when working with an increasingly diverse health care workforce who is aging, predominately female, and increasingly more diverse in culture, race, and ethnicity (Cejka, 1993; Epting, Glover & Boyd, 1994; Friedman, 1992; Polifko-Harris, 1995). The field of nursing administration will benefit from continued research on the effect of culture on motivation, job satisfaction, conflict management and resolution, communication efforts, preferred leadership styles, and negotiation methods as our health care workforce continues to diversify.

EFFECTIVE MANAGEMENT IN A CULTURALLY DIVERSE WORKFORCE

Nurse executives are challenged to understand the differences in their increasingly diverse employees. Traditional methods of employee management, focusing on the needs of a certain race, gender, or class of people, may no longer be the "best way" of supervision. Each culture has developed its own notion of necessary skills and expectations for effective management. Whether it is communication skills, conflict negotiation techniques, work habits, or leadership ability, people of different cultures have patterned responses and needs based on their indigenous backgrounds. It is the insightful executive's responsibility to be cognizant of those patterned responses and needs. If nurse executives are not aware of how a particular situation may affect their employee, then it is advisable to inquire, rather than assume. All Hispanic workers, though from one cultural background, may not have the same preferences in situational responses. It is inappropriate to band one cultural group together in generalized expectations. People are still individuals and need to be viewed as such.

Studies have shown that the health care industry does not reflect the national trend toward enhanced cultural diversification. Although we may actively seek health care workers who are as diverse as the patient population, Friedman (1992) asserts there is an underrepresentation of minorities among health care professional ranks. According to the National Sample Survey of RNs (1996), 89.7% of the RN population is white (non-Hispanic), 4.2% black (non-Hispanic), 3.4% Asian/Pacific Islander, 1.6% Hispanic, and 0.5% American Indian/Alaskan Native. According to the Association of American Medical Colleges, 12% of the medical students in 1995 were either black, Indian, Mexican American, or Puerto Rican (Moore, 1997). Almost 20% of the practicing physicians today are foreign-born and educated (Wagner, 1991). Compared with the U.S. population during the same census period, 72.3% of the population is white (non-Hispanic), 12.5% is black (non-Hispanic), 3.7% is Asian/Pacific Islander, 10.6% is Hispanic, and 0.9% is American Indian/Alaskan Native.

Health care is a service industry, employing more than 10.5 million workers (Donley, 1995). Moore (1997) reports that in 1996, there were about 5 million hospital workers alone, and of that number, 16.5% were black and 6.7% were Hispanic. The hospital environment offers a variety of positions, ranging from nonskilled to experts in managed systems. With the increasing emphasis on unlicensed assistive personnel, many organizations offer entry-level employment with a large percentage consisting of females and minority members (Wagner, 1991).

Further, the field of health care administration is also lacking in adequate representation with minorities and females; in 1990 minorities accounted for less than 1% of top-level positions, identified as presidents and chief executive officers, as reported by the American College of Healthcare Executives (Friedman, 1992). That trend has not changed at this writing according to the Institute of Diversity in Health Management (Moore, 1997). It is indeed a challenge for all who administer health care organizations today to become aware of the strengths a multicultural workforce brings to the community, and to actively value the differences diversity brings.

Many authors speak of the rationale behind diversity management. Enhanced communication is a desired response to cultural awareness, as both verbal and nonverbal messages are more clearly understood. For example, just holding a meeting or conference with peoples from different countries contains subtle nuances: when should you arrive, who can conduct a negotiation session, is it customary to begin the meeting with "small talk" rather than "getting down to business," who is formally (and informally) in charge of the meeting, are presents exchanged, and if they are, what types of gifts are they and to whom are they given?

Nonverbal gestures also need to be minded when dealing with people of different national cultures. Even a simple "yes" or "no" may have double meaning, depending on the culture of the participants and the situation. Many Asians may nod "yes" when they are actually saying "no"; they are simply acknowledging the other person. The Filipino culture desires harmony and smooth relationships, and to avoid conflict, they may say what they believe the other person wants to hear. Saying "no" may be very difficult for some, especially if they want to please the other person they are working with (Morrison, Conaway, & Borden, 1994).

Just because business is conducted in the United States does not mean that everyone is expected to understand the "American way." It is essential for the nurse executive to understand the subtleties of potential discrimination due to diversity issues of culture, race, gender, age, sexual/affectional orientation, and abilities, and to assist staff in increasing their awareness of their own prejudices and bias. Valuing diversity means appreciating that everyone is different, has strengths to share, and promotes these differences. Diversity is an advantage in the health care environment because it enriches our understanding not only of our co-workers, but of our patients, their families, and the community in which we live. By proactively managing cultural diversity, misunderstandings and conflicts are minimized, and creative problem-solving techniques are applied. Innovative strategies for the organization are encouraged, so critical in today's rapidly changing health care environment. Employees in an organization that values cultural diversity feel empowered not only to suggest change, but to participate in the process itself. Finally, diversity awareness should not be limited to once-a-year programs, or a designated cultural awareness day, but instead be considered part of the health care organization's mission and philosophy on how everyone from the patients to the providers of care are valued. It is not enough to simply acknowledge our differences and similarities—to actually value and respect one another is only human kindness.

SUMMARY

As our health care workforce continues to diversify culturally and ethnically, nurse executives and their employees are asked not only to understand but to place value on the differences between co-workers and clients alike. A population's cultural beliefs, values, and norms all influence behaviors, with the importance placed on understanding the differences and similarities between cultures.

Managing the changing, culturally diverse workforce offers many challenges and opportunities for the nurse executive. It is through awareness of cultural differences that all feel valued and important, with essential knowledge to share.

STUDY QUESTIONS

1. Describe key demographic employment trends in the United States.
2. Define culture, ethnicity, values, norms, and diversity.
3. Discuss cultural theories from nursing and other social sciences.
4. Identify strategies for effectively managing a culturally diverse workforce.
5. Identify potential cultural diversity research topics for the nurse executive to pursue.

REFERENCES

American Association of Colleges of Nursing. (1997). *Statement on diversity and equality of opportunity.* Washington, DC: Author.

Andrews, M. M., & Boyle, J. S. (1995). *Transcultural concepts in nursing care.* Philadelphia: Lippincott.

Bass, B., & Burger, P. (1979). *Assessment of managers.* New York: The Free Press.

Block, B. (1983). Assessment guide for ethnic/cultural variations. In M. S. Orque & B. Block (Eds.), *Ethnic nursing care: A multicultural approach* (pp. 49–75). St. Louis: Mosby.

Cejka, S. (1993). The changing healthcare workforce: A call for managing diversity. *Healthcare Executive, 8*(2), 20–23.

Chrisman, N. J. (1990). Culture shock in the operating room: Cultural analysis in transcultural nursing. *Journal of Transcultural Nursing, 1(2),* 33–39.

De Laune, S., & Ladner, P. (1998). *Fundamentals of Nursing: Standards and practice.* Albany, NY: Delmar.

Donley, R. (1995). Advanced practice nursing after health care reform. *Nursing Economic$, 13*(2), 84–88.

Elmuti, D. (1993, July/August). Managing diversity in the workplace. *Industrial Management,* pp. 19–22.

Epting, L. A., Glover, S. H., & Boyd, S. D. (1994). Managing diversity. *Health Care Supervisor, 12*(4), 73–83.

Estes, G., & Zitzow, D. (1980). Heritage consistency as a consideration in counseling Native Americans. Paper read at the National Indian Education Association Convention, Dallas, TX.

Fine, M. G. (1993). New voices in organizational communication: A feminist commentary and critique. In S. P. Bowen & N. Wyatt (Eds.), *Transforming visions: Feminist critiques in communication studies* (pp. 125–166). Cresskill, NJ: Hampton.

Fine, M. G. (1996). Cultural diversity in the workplace: The state of the field. *The Journal of Business Communication, 33*(4), 485–502.

Friedman, E. (1992, January/February). American's growing diversity: Melting pot or rainbow? *Health Care Forum Journal,* pp. 10–14.

Giger, J. N., & Davidhizar, R. E. (1995). *Transcultural nursing: Assessment and intervention* (2nd ed.). St. Louis: Mosby-Yearbook.

Gordon, G. (1992). This man knows what diversity is. *IABC Communication World, 12,* 8–12, 31.

Henry, N. (1989). *Public administration and public affairs.* Englewood Cliffs, NJ: Prentice Hall.

Hofstede, G. (1980, Summer). Motivation, leadership and organization: Do American theories apply abroad? *Organizational Dynamics,* pp. 42–63.

Hofstede, G. (1984). *Culture's consequences: International differences in work-related values.* Beverly Hill, CA: Sage.

Hofstede, G. (1993). Cultural constraints in management theories. *The Executive, 8*(1), 81–94.

Hoppe, M. H. (1992). *A comparative study of country elites: International differences in work-related values and their implication for management training and development.* Unpublished doctoral dissertation, Chapel Hill, NC.

Johnston, W. B., & Packer, A. H. (1987). *Workforce 2000.* Indianapolis, IN: Hudson Institute.

Kirkpatrick, M. K., Katrobos, S. C., Sherman, C. F., & Hull, A. V. (1994). Health care from a transcultural perspective: A rainbow of diversity. *Perspectives of Patient Care, 8*(2), 3–6.

LaFramose, T., Coleman, L. K., & Gerton, J. (1993). Psychological impact of biculturalism: Evidence and theory. *Psychological Bulletin, 114*(3), 395.

Labich, K. (1996, September 9). Making diversity pay. *Fortune,* pp. 177–180.

Laurent, A. (1983). The cultural diversity of western conceptions of management. *International Studies of Man & Organization, 12*(1), 75–96.

Leininger, M. (1978). *Transcultural nursing: Concepts, theories and practices.* New York: Wiley.

Leininger, M. (1991, April/May). Transcultural nursing: The study and practice field. *Imprint,* pp. 55–66.

Limaye, M. R. (1994). Responding to workforce diversity: Conceptualization and search for paradigms. *Journal of Business and Technical Communications, 8,* 353–372.

Malone, B. L. (1997). Improving organizational cultural competence. In J. A. Dienemann (Ed.), *Cultural diversity in nursing: Issues, strategies and outcomes,* Washington, DC: American Academy of Nursing.

Moore, J. D. (1997, December 15). The unchanging of healthcare. *Modern Healthcare,* pp. 30–34.

Morrison, T., Conaway, W. A., & Borden, G. A. (1994). *Kiss, bow or shake hands.* Holbrook, MA: Adams Media Corporation.

Polifko-Harris, K. (1995). *The influence of national culture on work-related values and job satisfaction between American and Filipino registered nurses.* Unpublished doctoral dissertation, Norfolk, VA.

Purnell, L. D., & Paulanka, B. J. (1998). *Transcultural health care.* Philadelphia: Davis.

Redding, S. G., & Ng, M. (1982). The role of "face" in the organizational perceptions of Chinese managers. *Organizations Studies, 3,* 201–219.

Smith, M. A., & Johnson, S. J. (Eds.). (1991). *Valuing differences in the workplace.* Alexandria, VA: American Society for Training and Development.

Sondergaard, M. (1994). Research note: Hofstede's consequences: A review of reviews, citations and replications. *Organization Studies, 15*(3), 447–456.

Spector, R. (1996). *Cultural diversity in health and illness.* Norwalk, CT: Appleton & Lange.

Swierczek, F. W. (1991). Leadership and culture: Comparing Asian managers. *Leadership and Development Journal, 12*(7), 3–10.

Thiederman, S. (1996, November). Improving communications in a diverse healthcare environment. *Healthcare Financial Management,* pp. 72–75.

Virginian Pilot, May 5, 1998. An older woman's world?

Wagner, M. (1991, September 30). Managing diversity. *Modern Healthcare,* pp. 24–29.

Yukl, G. (1994). *Leadership in organizations* (3rd ed.). Englewood Cliffs, NJ: Prentice Hall.

CHAPTER

32

Assistive Technology

Lillian M. Simms • Mary L. McHugh

Human life, from the miracle of birth to the mystery of death, will be enhanced in countless ways by these technological achievements, by the robot hands performing precise surgical tasks and computers that instantly analyze and comprehend a welter of confusing symptoms. (Clarke, 1986, p. 49)

Chapter Highlights

- Exploring new horizons
- Concept of assistive technology
- Nurses in need of assistive technology
- Assistive technology of relevance to nurse executives
- Personal assistive devices
- Operationalizing receptivity to assistive technology
- The link with quality

Self-care and the use of assistive technologies can be learned and can make a tremendous difference in quality of life of people receiving health care and health care professionals delivering care. The purpose of this chapter is to introduce the nurse executive to the abundance of assistive technology available today that can assist activities of daily living for patients and work for nurses. The chapter is also written to stimulate the development of technology by nurses for nursing.

EXPLORING NEW HORIZONS

Technology is generally recognized to mean knowledge, skills, and equipment (Goodman, Sproull & Associates, 1990). Assistive technology in the 21st century will free health professionals for new tasks as computers free the nurse from routine record-keeping and tireless robots assist both physicians and nurses with various tedious routines. The Planetree Model for health care has set the stage for involvement of patients in diagnosis and self-care (Clarke, 1986; Martin, Hunt, Hughes-Stone, & Conrad, 1990).

The gradual shift to patient-centered care has opened the door to multiple telecommunication technologies that permit nurses and doctors to deliver care via electronic means. Health care has moved far beyond laptops and pen-based computers. Telehealth systems provide two-way simultaneous audio and video capabilities that, in some cases, will fundamentally alter the way nursing care is provided (Warner, 1998). A detailed description of a nursing telehealth business is provided by Warner in Appendix D. In essence, the electronic or video visit will replace many of the physical visits nurses are expected to make to patients. This technology will be especially important in the care of people who live in rural or remote areas.

Telehealth systems (also known as telemedicine systems) involve the transmission of audio, video, vital signs, and data using a client computer terminal and central station connected through a single telephone line (Figure 32.1). Telehealth systems will change the way patients can participate in their own diagnosis and therapy. This is only the beginning, however, because these systems also have the potential for changing the way health professionals interact with each other. It is inevitable that medical applications will migrate to the Internet. Even complicated surgeries have been performed remotely in tests by the Department of Defense.

In a recent Online Industry Standard Magazine, Woody (1999) describes the way doctors will be wired in the future. Ambitious plans are under way to link doctors, health maintenance organizations (HMOs), and insurers on the Web. An online health care company, Healtheon, in California is developing an antidote to the costly paper chase that continues to increase health care costs. Healtheon is developing an online system that will instantly confirm a patient's insurance, make referrals, and submit claims at one Web site. Cost and convenience are not the only factors driving the health care industry online. Patients themselves are savvy about the Internet and are searching the Web for comparative costs and health literature.

These changes in computer technology will affect all health professionals. Nursing will be done differently in the 21st century and nurse executives who cannot expand their thinking will be replaced by other health professionals who perceive that personal health devices can be used by both caregivers and care recipients. Michael Hawley at the 1999 American Organization of Nurse Executives

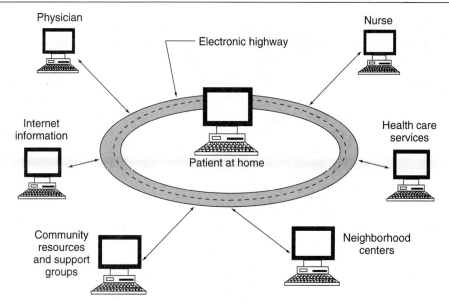

Figure 32.1 Telehealth system

Annual Meeting in Charlotte, NC challenged attendees to think differently. He further challenged the nurse executives to think of computers as "bicycles for the mind." Noting that we are entering a pivotal era, he stated that personal health devices will be as fundamental as the telephone and television. Health care technology will transform aspects of care now considered sacred to nursing (such as pill counting) to sophisticated medical systems that can be effectively and efficiently monitored by patients wearing personal devices. Sophisticated wearable devices will turn health awareness inside out. Biomedical departments are flourishing on college campuses and the expansion of medical studies to include physics, media technology, and life sciences promises even more Star Trek technology.

ASSISTIVE TECHNOLOGY

During the past decade, revolutionary changes have involved every aspect of health care in this country. Extensive basic medical research has yielded an expanding array of diagnostic and monitoring equipment. Life-support systems permit surgeons to remove, repair, or replace components of the body as never before in the history of the human race. The manned space programs have yielded a tremendous amount of knowledge related to physiology and communication systems. Major advancements in robotics and the development of assistive technology are dramatically changing patient education and rehabilitation for self-care. Because nurses are the principle caregivers in various health care delivery settings, it is essential to take a new look at the nature of the work of nursing and propose innovative models for nursing practice that take into account emerging labor-saving assistive technologies as well as rapidly changing health care needs. In essence, nurses must change the way they do their clinical work and how they spend their time in clinical practice. Moving one's thinking about technology as enabling devices for handicapped people to assistive technology that provides labor savings in time and effort is an important leap in thought.

According to Smith (1988), "The evolving technologies and intelligent clinical information systems will enable health care professionals to extend their therapeutic and protective powers beyond the walls of their offices and hospitals. Systems providing continuous medication and patient monitoring will reduce the need to hospitalize patients, perhaps dramatically and may greatly increase the length of life for diabetics and others with chronic diseases. The patients of the 21st century will be connected to their health care providers by webs of telemetry similar to those used in cellular communications; perhaps these communication webs will be coordinated or monitored by computer systems that could trigger responses in advance of crises" (p. 18). Technology will greatly affect the way health care services are organized and delivered in the 21st century. The dichotomy between caring and technology in nursing reflects a fear of technology. Nurses must make technology and humanism function as complementary forces to promote human welfare. Nurses must also be on the forefront of linking assistive technology with patient empowerment and self-care. Nursing could be considered a late entrant into the field of technology-driven services and could offer a highly competitive product in health care delivery.

The Patient Intensity for Nursing Index study, using Division of Nursing definitions, suggests that only one-third of nursing time is spent in direct clinical care (Prescott, Phillips, Ryan, & Thompson, 1971). Other work-sampling studies reported by these authors confirmed this finding. The majority of time (over 50%) is spent in combined indirect care or unit-management activities. Reducing inefficiencies in information flow and charting routines and reassigning aspects of unit management could save approximately 48 minutes per nurse per shift. Based on their review of selected work sampling studies, Prescott et al. (1991) support *(1)* the redesign of work and work groups through restructuring the role of the registered nurse, *(2)* developing assistive nursing personnel, and *(3)* implementing labor-saving assistive technologies.

NURSES IN NEED OF ASSISTIVE TECHNOLOGY

One of the most disabled groups of people may be nurses who are trying to make do with yesterday's curricula. They lack the physics, engineering, and computer science background that would enable them to become intelligent consumers of rapidly changing technology; nor are current faculty in schools of nursing willing to encourage revolutionary changes in curricula. Many nursing faculties believe that as people get older, they do not need technology, they need good supportive nursing care. What could be more supportive than assistive technologies that could keep persons living independently in their own homes?

Many tasks in nursing are so demeaning, dehumanizing, boring, tiring, physically exhausting, and even potentially dangerous that to have a robot perform these tasks would be most useful. Assistance with personal care activities could free the nursing staff to do those things that only humans can do. The automatic washing machine is a robot that has freed American women to perform other activities. Nurses have analogous need for robotics available to them in practice. Many nurses are emotionally unable to deal with introducing robots into nursing care that can conceivably bathe, toilet, feed, and dress people more efficiently and with greater care. Nurses care for a variety of patients who have immobility. Should not there be turning and lifting devices available for those people? Technological support services should be sustained for all disabled citizens and could be available to those seeking prevention of disability, including nurses seeking prevention of back injuries.

Nurses need more of this kind of technology. However, there is much resistance. Convincing nurses of the idea of assistive technology in personal care is difficult even though many devices are already in use. Today, high-technology beds constantly turn and move acutely ill patients. Even 10 years ago, hours of nursing time were consumed in turning and positioning the same kinds of patients. The high-technology beds ultimately cost less and produce better patient outcomes— few decubitus ulcers and a higher degree of comfort for the patient. These devices increase productivity in two ways: *(1)* they save nursing time and *(2)* they decrease costs and improve quality by increasing patient comfort through reducing complications and iatrogenic illness.

Record-keeping, toileting activities, bedmaking, lifting and moving patients, monitoring wanderers and people with tendencies to fall, feeding patients, collecting specimens, and distributing medication are some of the most time-consuming activities in nursing. Several devices are already on the drawing board in a variety of NASA and rehabilitation engineering studies (NASA Spin-off Journals; White, 1998). A portable, noninvasive ultrasonic bladder sensor designed to facilitate independence in toileting could potentially have implications for specimen collection.

The potential for computer-assisted communication is phenomenal. The fact that many hospitals do not have computerized information systems probably accounts for much of the lack of computer knowledge among nurses. Furthermore, faculties in even the best schools of nursing are not fully aware of the potential for computer use in record-keeping, health education, and direct patient care. Before nursing can take full advantage of large databases, computerized care plans, and staffing scheduling systems, the computer must become as much a part of the professional nursing skills as the bandage and stethoscopes of yesteryear.

Computers have remarkable potential to enhance the lives of the aging (Rowe & Kahn, 1998). Books, magazines, and a wide variety of courses could be available on terminals in various health care settings, including nursing homes. The size of print and intensity of brightness could be adjusted to the needs of the viewer. Contrary to increased loneliness, the use of modified computer games in some nursing homes for the frail older people, whose average age is 85, suggests that participants show increased vitality, concentration, and greater interaction. Wandering and propensity for falling frequently require physical or chemical restraints. A variety of restraints such as geri-chairs, beanbag chairs, and tying restraints are commonly used inhumane devices. Surveillance devices could provide wanderers with feedback, which may help them become more oriented in their environment or provide cues that they have entered an unsafe area.

Nurses need new equipment such as levitation devices, people movers, needleless injection equipment, and range of motion exercisers to do their work now and in the future, as described by Arthur C. Clarke (1986) in his science fiction book about life in the 21st century. The significance of the proposed work is that new practice patterns can be designed that will create an environment in which practicing nurses will continue to identify work penetration points at which new technologies and practice patterns can then be tested in practice settings or in newly designed skills labs. It is anticipated that newly designed skills labs could become continuing education centers in which faculty, staff nurses, and even patients and family members could learn how to use new technologies or update practice skills.

Slack (1997) argues that the most neglected resource in health care is the patient. If the Planetree Model predicted by Clarke (1986) for health care in the 21st century is to be fully implemented, surely, it will be the computer as an assistive technology that brings this projection to fruition. Huey (1999) talks about the opportunities for nurses using the World Wide Web. Nurses on the Internet will be able to access research findings and health-related information to an extent unknown in history. Huey (1999) further suggests that health information has become so widely available on the Web that even patients can easily access accurate information about their health problems.

Consumers with computer literacy increasingly expect to play an active role in decisions about their care. They already are entering data for their own clinical records and they will participate actively in various interactive online environments that will mingle home and cloistered clinical settings, thereby closing the gap between prescription and implementation of therapies. Nurses have contributed little to the development of personal assistive devices even though they are closest to personal care. A later section in this chapter provides examples of assistive devices that could dramatically influence independent function in the "smart houses" of tomorrow and the quality of independent living.

ASSISTIVE TECHNOLOGY OF RELEVANCE TO NURSE EXECUTIVES

An abundance of innovations and creative uses of a variety of equipment already exist and more are coming. These innovations have a direct application in the nursing practice domain, because their aim is to increase a patient's independence and thereby decrease the workload of their caretakers. The nursing domains that these innovations may be categorized into are mobility, special senses and communication, maintaining skin integrity, comfort, cognition, elimination, and respiratory areas. Assistive technologies can be conceptualized as personal or nurse assistive as portrayed in Figure 32.2.

In the patient care setting, computers can speed up documentation processes, improve legibility, enhance completeness and accuracy of the medical record, provide clinical decision support, facilitate patient independence, reduce discomfort, and offer facilities reduction of clinical errors. In short, they can improve both productivity and the quality of care delivered at the bedside. Chapter 24 provides detailed information about clinical applications of computers to nursing administration.

Computers can also be used to support information handling in administration. They can make management reports more comprehensive, improve timelines, and permit management to make use of information that was not previously available. In this way, they can help managers make more informed—and therefore more successful—decisions. Computerized management information and decision support systems improve the institution's performance by improving the success rate of management decisions. They can reduce the cost of bad decisions by helping managers simulate the likely results of management decisions—before the decisions are implemented in the organization.

Multiple linked applications can be used to support the computer based patient record. In addition to automating the clinical record of care, other applications such as the patient admission/discharge/transfer (ADT) system, medication and laboratory order entry and results reporting and postdischarge record coding—

Personal Assistive Devices	Nurse Assistive Technologies
Smart houses	Computerized records
Personal computers	Smart cards
Internet access	Telehealth systems
Home security products	Global communication systems
Functional ability systems (respiration, cognition, etc.)	Levitation devices
	Needleless injection equipment
Mobility products	Remote monitoring systems
Telecommunication equipment	People movers
Self-monitoring products	Care assistive products
Emergency alert systems	High-tech beds
	Volumetric IV pumps

Figure 32.2 Assistive technology of relevance to nurse executives.

familiar applications in most hospitals—can be used to form the basis of a management decision support and information system. Unfortunately, the extent to which these processes are fully automated and the integration of the applications are highly variable throughout health care.

PERSONAL ASSISTIVE DEVICES*

When Palmore at Duke University compared trends in surveys conducted by the National Center for Health Statistics, he found less infirmity in 1980 than in 1970 and less disability in 1970 than in 1960. As a group, older people are more fit and in better health today (Belsky, 1988). Many people are physically middle aged in their sixties and the "silver-haired marathon runner has overtaken the image of the passive older person staring into the sunset" (Belsky, 1988, p. 7).

Even older adults with functional impairments resulting from chronic disease and physiologic changes associated with the aging process can be and are more fit if they have been provided information about assistive technology. When impairments are the result of slow gradual changes rather than an acute episode, individuals are rarely aware of assistive devices that might enhance their functional ability. Enhancement of functional abilities both permits independent living and enables older people to participate in meaningful activities. Nurse executives are in a key position to assist the older population by sharing knowledge of available and developing technologies with the potential for enhancing independent function.

Assistive technologies for community-dwelling older adults range from everyday products that are readily available to the general consumer to specialized assistive devices and high-tech solutions such as robotics. Although the use of the word "technology" tends to focus attention on the more complex, it is important also to consider the potential uses of readily available consumer products. Advances in science and industry affect each of us in our daily lives. Technology has, in innumerable ways, enabled us to expend time and energies that would otherwise be spent in self-maintenance or home maintenance tasks on other pursuits. Opening our minds to the potential uses of everyday consumer products as well as products specifically designed for the disabled enlarges the options that can be offered.

Mobility Products

Older people who have difficulty with grasping and twisting motions can operate a lever more easily than a knob. Door knobs can be replaced with levers either by replacing whole mechanisms or by a lever that fits over the existing knob.

*Note: This section has been adapted from a paper presented by L. Simms and S. Fink at the Exploration: Technological Innovations for an Aging Population Conference, Lake Buena Vista, FL, Jan. 31–Feb. 1, 1989 (Simms & Fink, 1989).

Kitchen cabinets are easier to open when knobs are replaced with a c-shaped handle and pull catches replaced with a magnetic latch. Faucets in the kitchen and bathroom that require a grasping twisting motion can be replaced with a lever faucet. A universal turner is available that uses spring-loaded nylon cylinders to grip almost any knob or switch and enables their operation through a lever action. These are particularly useful for stoves, washers, dryers, and other appliances. The small knob-type switch on lamps is particularly troublesome, but a number of alternative adaptations are readily available. The timer can be set to ordinary times of use or a light-sensitive or motion-sensitive device can turn the light on automatically. Lamps also are now available that turn on when the base of the lamp is touched.

Loss of manipulative mobility in the hands may make it impossible for older people to write legibly or may make writing a painful task. The telephone provides one alternative to written communication. This may not be sufficient for people who depend on writing for continued professional activity or as a valued form of communication with distant friends. An electric typewriter with a light touch or a personal computer with word processing software may enable people to meet important goals. If older people cannot manage a standard keyboard, computer adaptations that allow the selection of letters or key words from a menu may be useful. Voice recognition technology can serve people very well under certain circumstances—especially for single-user computers and applications.

Specialized Devices

The number of specialized assistive devices available to older people is staggering. ABLEDATA, a computerized database sponsored by the National Institute for Handicapped Research, lists an extensive number of products. The difficulties lie in maintaining up-to-date information about these products, evaluating their potential usefulness for specific individuals, and funding when the cost exceeds the individual's resources. The American Association for Retired Persons (AARP) and the Western Gerontological Society have published a catalogue of items specifically selected to assist older people to live independently. It is difficult to determine from a catalogue description or picture whether an item is useful. Lending libraries of assistive devices and health fairs that allow for hands-on examination and trial would be useful approaches to educating potential consumers to the usefulness of various devices.

Computer technology has provided a number of options for home monitoring that can increase the security and convenience of older adults. Home-security devices that automatically signal a service or law enforcement agency if there is an intruder may enable people to feel safer. Thermostats are currently available that enable the programming of the desired temperatures for each day of the week with several temperature changes each day. Computerized monitoring-control devices can enable the person to control home heating, lights, other electrical appliances, and even door locks from a control panel that is centrally located or portable. The lifeline system, which is in operation in many communities today, enables the person to call for help by pressing a button on a lightweight transmitter that is designed to be worn. This transmitter is electronically linked to a health care institution 24 hours a day and sends an automatic signal if it is not reset by the person at predetermined intervals.

These devices are merely illustrative. Older people are often extremely creative in finding ways to adapt their own environments to make optimal use of their strengths and to meet personally meaningful goals. Nurse executives can be helpful to older people by keeping staff abreast of new developments in biotechnology and related fields. The creative nurse executive will support the development of new options and resources for maintaining independent function and enhancing the quality of life. Freedom from basic-coping needs can enable older people to reinvest their energies in continuing growth and development and meaningful activities rather than in disease-concentration behavior (Becker & Kaufmann, 1988). The resourceful nurse executive will support the "skunk works" model present in innovative organizations by sponsoring ongoing innovation and invention task forces.

OPERATIONALIZING RECEPTIVITY TO ASSISTIVE TECHNOLOGY

One way to introduce the idea of assistive technology equipment is to introduce an innovation such as the bedside terminal. Another way is to build in self-assessment with the routine health assessment of all clients entering a health care facility. The following self-assessment instrument (Figure 32.3) has been designed to reflect learning needs in the middle and later years. It is important to educate potential users of assistive technology and the addition of self-assessment to current health assessments could encourage a rehabilitation philosophy for living and development over the life span. When basic coping needs are met, the individual is able to move on, meeting needs at a higher level. A person can begin to think beyond physical needs to contributions to society and even transcendence (McClusky, 1974). A minimum of physical adequacy is needed for survival; more than mere adequacy is needed for health and full function.

This self-assessment schedule can also be introduced as part of regular activities in senior centers. Designed for a paper and pencil format, the guide is easily transferred to computer format. Goal setting has been identified as an extremely important part of continued development over the life span and it is possible, in a later stage of our work, that a modified performance plan will be developed for individual measurement of progress. The challenge for nurse executives is to link meaningful assistive technology with self-care and continuing care and the proposed tool could be one way of proceeding. Another way is to link nurses with literature that presents aging and rehabilitation as positive experiences. According to Rowe and Kahn (1998), older Americans are generally healthy and can benefit from a wide range of assistive devices.

HEALTH AND TECHNOLOGY SELF-ASSESSMENT
COPING NEEDS
What are your personal health needs?
What products do you need to assist you in achieving physical well-being? Check all relevant items.

Personal care	___
Mobility	___
Elimination	___
Communication	___
Cognitive function (thinking and remembering)	___
Hearing	___
Vision	___
Other _____	___

What assistive technology do you need to maintain independent living?
What are your strengths?
How can your functional abilities (strengths) be used to balance or offset any
 dysfunctions?
What would you like to learn about physical, mental, and spiritual fitness?
EXPRESSIVE NEEDS
Would you like to learn how to use a computer? Other technology?
Do you wish to take classes that can prepare you for a new career?
What hobbies and personal interests would you like to develop over the next 5 years?
CONTRIBUTIVE NEEDS
Have you ever considered participating in community activities?
What community activities really make you feel fit?
INFLUENCE NEEDS
Have you ever considered sharing your expertise with others?
Do you think it is important to be active in community/societal events?
What assistance do you need that would help you to carry out desired activities?
TRANSCENDENCE/PERSONAL EMPOWERMENT
What are your learning needs that will allow you to achieve your desired state of
 well-being?
What goals do you wish to achieve in your life?

Figure 32.3 Example of a health and technology self-assessment questionnaire.

THE LINK WITH QUALITY IN HEALTH CARE

The use of assistive technology should not be simply for the sake of technology. There must be some positive effect on patients and there must be some impact on outcomes and quality. The definition of quality found in many health care management textbooks is often incomplete. In Chapter 24, outputs are defined not merely as a count of the units of product produced. They are defined as the number of *usable* units of product. Usable means that the produced units are good enough to sell because they meet minimum quality specifications. Units that fail to meet specifications are counted as scrap, not as outputs. Scrap units *lower* productivity because they count as zero units in the formula. Quality is *inherently* part of the measure of productivity in manufacturing. Because of this, the relationship of quality to productivity and profitability in manufacturing is relatively easy to identify and quantify as is the effect of assistive technology on quality of care delivery. Early activation following cerebrovascular accidents and myocardial infarcts has created an unprecedented opportunity to measure the effect of assistive technology (Price & Wilson, 1997).

Quality

The relationships among quality, productivity, and profitability have been more difficult to identify in health care. Traditionally, the health care industry has focused on the "number of units" component of the concept "outputs" while omitting the "quality" component of outputs, simply because service quality has been so difficult to quantify. Even more important, the relationship of quality to profitability has been rather obscure in health care.

In part, the difficulty of linking quality, productivity, and profitability is a function of the extremely poor information handling in the health care system. Patient care information constitutes the *operations* information of health care delivery. Unfortunately, too many nurse executives have viewed clinical information as irrelevant to their work. It is difficult to imagine any other industry trying to operate with so little access to intelligence on their fundamental operations. For example, consider the case of a unit in which many patients experience significant periods of immobility. Immobile patients—such as those typically found in dementia, orthopedic, or neurology/neurosurgical units—are at high risk for decubitus ulcer formation. Their cost of care is high simply due to their inability to feed, bathe, turn, and exercise themselves. If they form decubitus ulcers, their cost of care may increase by as much as 50% to 100%—or even more. High-cost devices such as Flexi-care and other types of motion and air-flow beds, special seating devices, and wheelchairs that electronically lift the patient into a standing position are available for persons who are immobilized below the waist. These devices all cost in the thousands of dollars, but the cost is considered to be a worthwhile investment in the effort to prevent this potentially devastating complication.

A high rate of decubitus formation among a unit's patients might be an indicator of poor care, whereas a low rate might be used as a measure of high-quality care. However, with today's paper clinical records, measuring the rate is almost impossible. The problem is finding the denominator.

To determine the rate of ulcer formation, one must first be able to count the number of patients in the unit. Then one must be able to identify how many of those patients were at risk for decubitus formation. Dividing the latter by the former provides a measure of the proportion of patients served by the unit who are at risk for skin ulcers. Then one must have an actual count of the patients who developed a decubitus. The formula for calculating the rate at which "at risk" patients develop decubitus ulcers is:

$$\frac{\text{Number of patients developing a decubitus}}{\text{Number of patients at risk for decubitus formation}}$$

How can a computerized patient record system help managers determine this ratio? First consider what must be done if the hospital uses a typical paper chart system. The unit manager must develop a special study and determine which nursing diagnoses reflect a patient problem of immobility. Those data cannot be retrieved from old charts in the medical records department because nursing diagnosis is not a key for chart retrieval. So, a prospective study must be done. Then, someone must be given the task of reviewing all patients on a daily basis to identify those with appropriate diagnoses, and someone must examine the patient or the chart (or both if the unit is to be sure the care provider does not miss a small, beginning decubitus ulcer). Finally, the prospective study must be conducted for a sufficient length of time so that a sufficient sample may be obtained.

Productivity

With a well-designed, fully automated patient record system, all diagnoses (nursing, medical, therapy, etc.) should be keys for retrieval. Clinical interventions and patient outcomes, including functional status changes, comorbidities, nosocomial infections, and iatrogenic complications should all be retrieval keys. In fact, most clinical information can be coded for standardized data entry, and all such codes are easily retrievable in a well-designed, relational database management system. Such a system will allow managers to easily and quickly perform studies such as the one described above. Today, performance of more than one or two such studies per year is cost prohibitive. In a fully automated system, the computer itself could be programmed to monitor hundreds of such indicators constantly, and to print an alarm report whenever significant changes in clinical outcomes were detected.

Interventions are services provided to produce some patient outcome. Changes in patient condition, functional status, and the like are results. Managers will still need to track processes of care, and not merely outcomes, because errors in process are likely to produce undesirable outcomes. Generally, when process errors are rare and isolated, they are unlikely to produce deleterious effects on patients. Usually, there is enough redundancy and "fail safe" mechanisms to protect patients against the error of a single person. For example, medication orders are generally checked three or four times before they result in a medication administration. However, when people's performance begins to falter—usually due to a system problem but sometimes due to personal distress—a good process monitoring system will sound alarms before the process deviates too far out of control. These process degradation detection systems can become a key protection for care quality in the highly automated health care delivery system of the future.

Ultimately, quality will be defined by patient outcomes, and in the future, clinical information systems will have to be designed in such a way that managers can use information about clinical results to track the effectiveness of their operations.

Today, the work of developing patient outcome measures has just begun. With hospital stays shortening dramatically, and more care moving into ambulatory care settings, isolated systems that track only short episodic care processes are insufficient to future needs.

As more hospitals, physicians' offices, clinics, home health agencies, nursing homes, rehabilitation hospitals, and other providers form themselves into "cradle to grave" health care organizations, it will become more feasible to have integrated computer systems that span the full period of health care. Patients are discharged from hospitals long before the outcomes of their care are measurable. Without systems that track the patient through the entire care delivery system, managed care decisions will rest on opinion and bias rather than on empirical evidence of effectiveness. Managed care cannot produce quality care for America until sufficient evidence of effectiveness of each and every intervention can be tracked for every patient problem. With today's health care information systems, that is not possible.

Profitability

Managed care profitability depends on restricting utilization of health care services. If increasing numbers of people are enfranchised through universal health care coverage, costs can be contained in only one of two ways. First, health care can be rationed. Explicit decisions about who will live and who will die have to be made. Americans have exhibited a political disinclination to follow that path. The second way to contain costs is to collect and analyze enough data on diagnosis, treatment, and patient outcomes to determine the cost and benefits of virtually every treatment protocol for its appropriate diagnosis. The second approach assumes that at least some standard treatment protocols will be found ineffective under at least some conditions. Most people will not want to endure treatments that are unlikely to produce benefits. Elimination of ineffective care will, for some time, produce significant cost savings. But these savings cannot be realized unless sufficient data are available to make sound judgments about treatment effectiveness. Today's computer systems cannot perform this monitoring function.

In the future, all clinical care should be electronically documented. Paper charts do not facilitate aggregation across time, across settings, and across providers. Nursing will have greater difficulty producing computer systems to track effectiveness of nursing care because unlike medicine, nursing does not have a universally accepted set of words and codes that describe their assessment, intervention, and outcomes data. The American Nurses Association (ANA) has for several years worked in this area, attempting to locate and disseminate the work of nurse researchers in this area. The ANA has recognized the work of researchers such as the North American Nursing Diagnosis Association, Dr. Sue Grobe (Grobe & Hughes, 1993) in Texas (*The Nursing Intervention Lexicon and Taxonomy*), Drs. McCloskey and Bulechek (1992) in Iowa (*The Nursing Intervention Classification*), Dr. Virginia Saba (1992) in Washington, D.C. (*The Home Health Care Classification*), and the Omaha system. However, what is needed is a nationally (or better, internationally) accepted set of terms and codes for describing the work of nursing, just as medicine has the *International Classification of Diseases* for their diagnoses and procedures.

The new customer demands place great challenges before provider organizations. Efficacy of services has not been the focus of profitability. As a result, few mechanisms are in place to identify what service outcomes are, much less to measure them, or to collect, store, analyze, and develop reporting systems for those data. Even worse, the technology necessary to handle the massive amounts of data involved in patient care outcomes reporting is not in place. Manual processing of direct patient care data is still the industry standard. Unfortunately, manual processing is insufficient to meet the changing needs of customers of the health care delivery system. Provider organizations must be able to show what are the end results of treatment on the patients, and how well the organizations' results stand up against national benchmarks. Only computer information systems can provide the data analysis power required to meet customer demands.

Functionally, the definitional change in the concept of *product of health care* changes the old products to throughputs and requires that outcomes of care become the new product. This change is much more complex than it might appear. Outcomes of care are not entirely a result of the care provided. A poor outcome for a single patient may or may not involve care quality problems. A good outcome may be achieved despite poor quality in the care provision process. The meaning of quality in health care will need to be reconsidered as personal assistive technologies play an increasingly more important role in self-care and recovery of functional abilities.

Definitions of Quality in a Changed Health Care Delivery Market

As the concepts, "services" and "patient outcomes" change in health care, the concept of "quality" in health care must also change. "Quality of care" has long been operationally defined as adhering to standards (written or assumed) and identifying what services to provide, how to provide them (performance standards), and specifications for documenting those services. "Quality of care" has actually been a measure of quality of throughputs (process of care). During the late 1990s, corporate purchasers of health care became more involved in defining the product; they also began to demand that providers be able to show the effectiveness of the product. Thus, new measures of quality will have to demonstrate that patient outcomes of care are highly desirable.

Providers will have to be able to use the new outcome measures to market their product. And for many institutions, successful marketing is now a life or death issue. To health care managers who began their careers prior to the 1990s, the health care market has become incredibly competitive. Hospital closures—previously almost unheard of—have become common. Virtually no provider is safe. Even the most protected bastion of hospitals—the university hospital—has had to face competitive stresses. Although a university hospital may not close, it may be sold to another agency if its financial performance is unacceptable to the university's governing board. For the foreseeable future, providers will have to measure outcomes of care, and will have to use this measure of their product—along with competitive pricing—to sell their product to the corporate customer.

Content of the New Measures

The health care delivery paradigm pertaining to quality is rapidly shifting from a focus on measurement of process to a focus on health care outcomes. Therefore, the measures of "quality in health care" most familiar to "quality assurance" nurses—measures of the process of nursing care—will receive less emphasis than newly developed measures of outcomes of care. The new measures will include traditional outcome measures such as cure rates, morbidity, mortality, cesarean rates, and the like. In addition, many surgical procedures are designed to improve functional status. Therefore, providers will need to show that these procedures do what they are intended to do. That is, they will have to follow patients through the rehabilitation process to measure pre- and postprocedure functional status levels.

For example, for the patient who received knee replacement surgery, providers will have to demonstrate that the patient was able to perform more activities of daily living (e.g., walking or working at a job) with less pain (e.g., using less or no pain medication) than before the surgery. In addition, the provider will have to show that its performance for this product was done at a competitive cost and with an acceptable complication rate. This, in turn, means that provider organizations (e.g., hospitals, regional medical centers, etc.) will have to measure the performance of their health professionals, including the nurses. Quality will be a requirement for institutional survival in all care delivery settings. Nurse executives now and in the future will be held accountable for developing and measuring the effectiveness of nurse assistive technologies.

SUMMARY

The literature suggests that emerging assistive technology equipment will dramatically change the way nurses work in all settings. Bold new patterns are needed to liberate nurses and clients; patterns that will allow for the introduction of technology into all redesign activities. As medical technology has increased and reimbursement has changed, health care agencies have minimized the role of the patient. To counteract this trend, several initiatives have been introduced that encourage patients to participate in their care. Among these is the Planetree Model Hospital Project (Martin, Hunt, Hughes-Stone, & Conrad, 1990). The Planetree philosophy emphasizes sharing information about illness and teaches skills regarding self-care and healthy behaviors. Patients receive information not only about their specific diseases and treatments, but also about health-promotion activities and independent living. This model provides a cornerstone for the self-care movement in this country and links well with the current emphasis on assistive technology for personal control of one's life and destiny.

STUDY QUESTIONS

1. Compare and contrast personal and nurse assistive technology.
2. Design a technology for use in nursing. Write an action plan for its implementation.

REFERENCES

Belsky, J. K. (1988). *Making the most of life after fifty.* Baltimore: Johns Hopkins University Press.

Becker, G., & Kaufman, S. (1988). Old age, rehabilitation and research: A review of the issues. *The Gerontologist, 28*(4), 459–468.

Clarke, A. C. (1986). *July 20, 2019 Life in the 21st century.* New York: Macmillan.

Goodman, P. S., Sproull, L. A. & Associates (1990). *Technology and organizations.* San Francisco: Jossey-Bass.

Grobe, S., & Hughes, L. (1993). The conceptual validity of a taxonomy of nursing interventions. *Journal of Advanced Nursing, 18*(12), 1942–1961.

Hawley, M. (1999). *Healthcare technology: The future is now.* Presentation at the 1999 Annual Meeting, American Organization of Nurse Executives. March 18-22, 1999, Charlotte, NC.

Huey, F. L. (1999). Nursing challenges, roles, and opportunities in a world wide web environment. In C. A. F. Andersen (Ed.), *Nursing student to nursing leader.* Albany, NY: Delmar.

Martin, D., Hunt, J. R., Hughes-Stone, M., & Conrad, D. A. (1990). The Planetree model project: An example of the patient as partner. *Hospital & Health Services Administration, 35*(4), 591–601.

McCloskey J., & Bulechek, G. (Eds.). (1992). *Nursing Interventions Classification (NIC): Iowa Intervention Project.* St. Louis: Mosby.

McClusky, H. Y. (1974). Education for aging: The scope of the field and perspectives for the future. In S. M. Grabowski & Mason, W. D. (Eds.), *Education for aging.* Syracuse, NY: ERIC.

NASA Spinoff Journals. Sections on health and medicine. Washington, DC: National Aeronautics and Space Administration.

Prescott, P. A., Phillips, C. Y., Ryan, J. W., & Thompson, K. O. (1991). Changing how nurses spend their time. *IMAGE: Journal of Nursing Scholarship, 23*(1), 23–28.

Price, S. A., & Wilson, L. M. (1997). *Pathophysiology,* (5th ed.). St. Louis: Mosby-Year Book.

Rowe, J. W., & Kahn, R. L. (1998). *Successful aging.* New York: Pantheon.

Saba, V. (1992). The classification of home health care nursing diagnoses and interventions. *Caring Magazine, 11*(3), 50–57.

Slack, W. V. (1997). *Cybermedicine.* San Francisco: Jossey-Bass.

Smith, G. (1988). The evolution of alternative delivery systems: What will be nursing's role? In *Nursing Practice in the 21st Century.* Kansas City, MO: The American Nurses Foundation.

Warner, I. (1998). Telehealth in home care practice. *Journal of Nursing Administration, 28*(6), 3, 16.

White, R. J. (1998). Weightlessness and the human body. *Scientific American, 279*(3), 58–63.

Woody, T. (1999). Doctors get wired. *The Industry Standard. Online Magazine,* March 29, 1999.

CHAPTER

~ 33 ~

Nursing Economics and Politics in a Global Economy

Peter I. Buerhaus

For the health care industry, history will likely record the last decade of the twentieth century as the time when economic discipline slowly, if not painfully, gripped health care delivery organizations and the professionals who make their living providing health care. (Iglehart, 1995)

Chapter Highlights

- Global economics, health care, and nursing
- Changes in the economics of health care and nursing
- Federal and state activities to control health care expenditures
- Adopting traditional market forces in health care
- Political issues facing nursing

When we think about the economics of nursing and health care, it is sometimes difficult to envision examples of how they are influenced by changes in the world economy. This difficulty arises because the effects of global economic changes on health care are usually indirect and stem from complex economic interactions occurring in the broader U.S. economy that often are not well understood or anticipated, even by economists. Therefore, it is useful to begin this chapter by considering some of the ways that the dynamics of an increasingly global economy exert important effects on the health industry and the nursing profession. Following this, changes in the economic environment, resulting from the use of federal and state regulations, and the emergence of economic competition in health care are examined. The chapter concludes by exploring the political effectiveness of nursing and describing areas of political intervention that will make the profession's economic environment less threatening.

GLOBAL ECONOMICS, HEALTH CARE, AND NURSING

In 1981 this country experienced a severe economic recession. At the same time, the value of the U.S. dollar strengthened relative to foreign currencies, which resulted in intensifying competition between domestically manufactured products and foreign imports. Both to survive the recession and to be price competitive with imported goods, American business had to lower the cost of producing its products. When seeking ways to reduce its labor-related costs, business realized not only how expensive employees' health insurance premiums had become but discovered that this was the fastest growing part of labor costs. As a result, the business sector initiated a variety of health care reforms aimed at reducing employees' use of costly inpatient facilities. These reforms included incorporating deductible and copayment provisions in health insurance plans, establishing preadmission screening programs, supporting the development of health maintenance organizations (HMOs) and preferred provider organizations (PPOs), starting health care conditions to monitor the health industry and gather information on providers, offering their own health insurance plans, and pressuring insurers to cover less costly outpatient services and ambulatory surgery. These reforms were so effective that substantial declines in hospital occupancy rates occurred even before the Medicare program's prospective payment system began a few years later and further reduced hospital use (Feldstein, 1986). Had the country not experienced a recession and American firms not found themselves competing with foreign imports in the early 1980s, the business sector might have offset rising health insurance premiums by passing these costs onto consumers in the form of price increases rather than pressuring health insurers and providers to adopt health care reforms.

Although the recession in 1981–1982 slowed the rate of inflation, which had grown significantly during the Carter Administration and eventually reached 10.8% in 1983, unfortunately, the recession also created widespread unemployment. However, rising unemployment had two important effects on the health care system and nursing profession. First, it helped end the national shortage of hospital-employed RNs that had begun in the late 1970s. The shortage ended because, as the spouses of many RNs became unemployed, RNs became the only wage-earner in the family and, consequently, many began to work overtime hours, others switched from part- to full-time employment, and some RNs who were not employed rejoined the labor force. (Increases in real RN wages during this period reinforced the effects of spouse unemployment in stimulating the employment activity of RNs.) Indeed, the overall supply response was so strong that the percentage of employed RNs rose from 76.6% in 1980 to 78.4% in 1984 (Moses, 1986), and full-time equivalent (FTE) RN hospital vacancy rates fell sharply from a national average of 14% in 1979 to 4.4% in 1983 (Buerhaus, 1987).

The second way that high unemployment in the early 1980s affected health care was that, even though the unemployment rate declined after 1983, a significant number of people returning to work, and their dependents, did not regain health insurance (Prospective Payment Assessment Commission, 1991). The plight of these nonaged working Americans and millions of others without health insurance subsequently became a major reason for interest in adopting a national health insurance program. Moreover, this chain of economic interactions—foreign competition, recession, unemployment, growth in the number of uninsured people, pressure to increase access to health care—illustrates the complexity and often paradoxical nature of economic interactions between domestic and global economic events and health care. Consider, for example, if mandating *employer-provided* health insurance is adopted as a way of partially financing expanded access to health care, then labor-related costs will rise and the ability of American business (especially small firms) to compete with foreign companies will be hampered, and business may raise prices (inflation), lay off workers (unemployment), lower wages, or apply greater pressure on providers and insurers to lower health care costs.

Yet another way that the global economy has influenced nursing and the health industry is the policy of the Philippines to export RNs to the United States. Because students are taught to speak English, nursing education programs are similar to those in this country, and because wages in the United States are higher than in the Philippines, it is worthwhile for hospitals facing shortages of RNs to import RNs from the Philippines. Leaving their country to work in the United States also benefits these RNs because part of their earnings are sent to their families living in the Philippines. By increasing the supply of RNs in this country, however, the importation of RNs from the Philippines and other nations puts downward pressure on the wages paid to American-educated RNs. For these reasons the American Hospital Association has sought changes in federal regulations that would extend visas for foreign nurses.

A dramatic example of how global economics influences health care in this country is illustrated by examining the impact of the nation's federal deficit. Despite public calls for smaller government and a balanced federal budget, federal spending under the Reagan and Bush administrations greatly exceeded revenues. Year after year, the excess federal spending was financed in large part by foreign countries (namely, Japan). Had these nations not been in strong economic positions or their government's not willing to lend the United States needed capital, federal spending would probably have been constrained and yearly deficits would not have grown to the point where, now, fully 14% of annual federal spending is used to pay the *interest* on the national debt! The consequence of accumulating huge annual deficits is that essentially all domestic policy decisions, including health care, are made on the basis of how they affect the federal budget deficit.

Consequently, in health care the brunt of federal budgetary policy has been felt by U.S. hospitals who have received Medicare payments less than the cost of providing services for the program's beneficiaries. In 1998, 20% of hospitals have negative Medicare operating margins and their overall financial position has become so vulnerable that managers face extraordinary challenges. Nursing is especially pressured because the costs of labor account for a large portion of hospitals' expenses. Thus, as long as federal budgetary pressures continue, so too will the financial pressure on hospitals and the nursing profession.

Finally, in the early 1990s, the domestic economy was stuck in another recession. Although the economic downturn was not as severe as the recession a decade earlier, the economy recovered more slowly, unemployment stayed above 7%, and corporations were downsizing and laying off workers in large numbers. The resulting fear about becoming unemployed and losing employer-based health insurance made Clinton's national health care reform proposal appealing to many Americans, at least initially. However, once the public began to view the proposal as giving the federal government too large a role in health care and that the quality of care could suffer, support for national health care reform quickly eroded. With the collapse of the Clinton plan, price competition in health care spread so rapidly (discussed later) that the rate of increase in national health care spending fell dramatically in 1994. This sudden economic change made support for any type of national health care reform all but disappear. From the perspective of Congress, the outbreak of true economic competition in health care had accomplished in a very short time what federal regulations were unable to accomplish in 30 years. Support for the role of economic competition has come from the Wall Street financial community that viewed the slowdown in the rate of health spending, which has continued through 1998, as a major if underrecognized reason why price inflation and national unemployment rates have remained at very low levels. The slowdown in the growth of health care spending has also contributed substantially in protecting the U.S. economy from the Asian and world economic downturns, particularly the Japanese recession that has lasted for much of the 1990s.

A final example of the interplay among global and domestic economics and health care occurred in 1997 and 1998 when the economies of many Asian countries (namely Japan, South Korea, Thailand, and Indonesia) experienced severe downturns, marked by rising prices, escalating unemployment, and sagging consumer and investor confidence. Moreover, the sudden demise of the economies of these countries threatened the economic recovery that has been underway in the United States since 1995. However, largely because the rate of increase in U.S. national and per-capita spending on health care spending had been declining since 1993, the effect of the Asian economic crisis on the U.S. economy has not been great. Unlike many other industrial countries, our economy has kept growing (albeit at a slower rate) with sustained low unemployment, little price inflation, and surging consumer confidence.

CHANGES IN THE ECONOMICS OF HEALTH CARE AND NURSING

Beyond these global and domestic economic developments, other changes are occurring that more directly influence the economic environment of health care and nursing. For the most part, these changes are the result of public and private policies aimed at reducing the rate and increase in health care expenditures. The two major strategies that have been used to carry out these policies involve a regulatory approach used by federal and state governments and the adoption of economic competition to guide decisions concerning the production and consumption of personal health care services. Examining these strategies and their effects on the health industry will reveal how the economic environment is changing and provide clues concerning what nursing can expect in the future.

FEDERAL AND STATE ACTIVITIES TO CONTROL HEALTH CARE EXPENDITURES

To understand the federal government's primary motivation for using regulations to control health spending, it is necessary to appreciate the budgetary perspective of the administrations that have occupied the White House since the mid-1980s. They have witnessed federal health expenditures increasing so fast that up until 1997 the annual rate of increase was surpassed only by the annual growth rate of the national debt. Because the administration has responsibility for preparing the federal budget and overseeing federal agencies, it has a political interest to limit spending and reduce the size of budget deficits. But given the political difficulty associated with cutting spending on entitlement programs (namely, social security) or substantially decreasing defense spending, the Reagan, Bush, and Clinton administrations (and Congress) have had little choice but to target health care spending as a primary area for achieving significant budget savings. Despite their publicly voiced disdain of government intervention and regulations, these administrations have consistently directed health agencies, especially the Health Care Financing Administration (HCFA), which administers the Medicare and Medicaid programs, to promulgate regulations aimed at reducing payments to health care providers.

Given the federal government's perspective, it is not surprising that the cost-based retrospective reimbursement system used by Medicare to pay hospitals was replaced by a prospective payment system (PPS) based on diagnosis-related groups (DRGs). Indeed, Medicare's PPS slowed the annual growth rate in Medicare hospital payments to between 4% and 6% in the beginning years of the system and in subsequent years held increases below double-digit levels. But despite these impressive results, Medicare outlays to hospitals were projected to increase as was Medicare's share of total federal spending, which had increased to nearly 12% in 1996. In that same year, the program actually spent more than it received in income and was predicted to be bankrupt in the year 2002 unless changes were made to slow the rate of spending. After the 1996 Presidential election and once partisan rhetoric had subsided, Congress and the Clinton administration worked together to enact comprehensive reform of the Medicare program via the Balanced Budget Act of 1997 (BBA) (P.L. 105-33). Although at the time of this writing this legislation is only beginning to be implemented, the breadth and depth of changes expected to unfold as a consequence of the bill will influence nurses in executive, management, and clinical practice for years to come.

Balanced Budget Act of 1997

Overall, the BBA is expected to reduce Medicare spending by $115 billion between 1998 and 2002 and reduce the rate of Medicare spending from an annual growth rate of roughly 9% to about 6% over this same period (Medicare Payment Advisory Commission, 1998) (MedPAC). These actions are anticipated to forestall bankruptcy of the program until the latter half of the first decade of the new century. The changes to Medicare under the BBA include expansion of Medicare's offerings of health care plans and change in the way plans are paid, extension of the prospective payment system to ambulatory and postacute care organizations and providers, correction of numerous payment policies governing physicians and graduate medical education, availability of new preventive services for beneficiaries, and strengthening of fraud and abuse regulations and provisions.

Expanded Choice of Health Plans for Medicare Beneficiaries

Recognizing changes in the private insurance marketplace, particularly the rapid spread of managed care organizations and increasing enrollment of beneficiaries into HMOs (Figure 33.1), the BBA created the Medicare+Choice program. This program will involve health plans already participating in Medicare's risk-contracting program as well as include PPOs, provider-sponsored organizations, fee-for-service plans, and the medical savings account plans that were created as a demonstration under the BBA. Beneficiaries will receive information that will enable them to compare the benefits and costs among plans in their local market area. Information will also be made available to inform beneficiaries about grievance and appeals processes. In addition, by 2003, beneficiaries will be able to switch or disenroll only during an annual open enrollment period.

Beyond expanding the choice of plans and information about them, the BBA creates a new capitation payment method for the Medicare+Choice plans in which the payment rate for each county is calculated as the highest of a blend of the local and national rate, a minimum payment amount (or floor), or a minimum increase from the previous year's county rate. Moreover, by the year 2000, payments are to be risk-adjusted based on health status. Risk adjusting payments is intended to enable plans that treat sicker beneficiaries to receive higher capitation payments than plans treating healthier beneficiaries, which will reduce the incentives of plans to enroll only healthy patients. The development of an appropriate and equitable risk adjustment methodology has been troublesome for many years, and under the BBA the Secretary of Health and Human Services (HHS) is

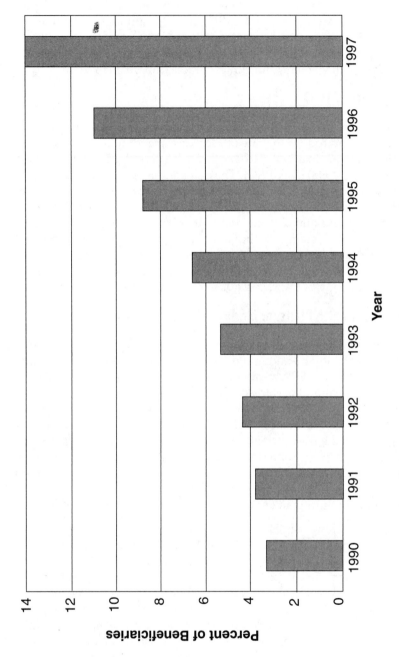

Figure 33.1 Enrollment growth in Medicare risk-contracting plans. Source: Medicare Payment Advisory Commission, March 1998.

responsible for implementing these important and long needed adjustments. Finally, the BBA contains provisions for special populations of beneficiaries, namely the conversion of the Program of All-Inclusive Care for the Elderly (PACE) from a demonstration program to a permanent program (and an option for Medicaid recipients). All of these changes mean that nurses can anticipate continuing growth of Medicare beneficiaries in managed care plans, and as this occurs, pressures to produce and deliver health care services in the most efficient way will increase.

Prospective Payment for Non-Inpatient Providers

The BBA calls for the development or implementation of new PPSs for skilled nursing facilities, hospital outpatient services, home health care agencies, and long-term hospitals and rehabilitation facilities (Table 33.1). These providers have largely been paid on the basis of their costs, which has not provided incentives to produce services efficiently. Consequently, Medicare outlays for nonacute care providers have grown since the late 1980s at a very rapid and unsustainable rate. Based on its success with inpatient PPS, Medicare will try to replicate its experience using PPS in hospitals to accomplish reductions in nonacute care providers' costs, greater efficiency, and simplify payments to providers. However, achieving these objectives will require developing the appropriate unit and level of payment, determining appropriate adjustments for differences in patient mix, and preventing providers from increasing the volume of patient visits. For example, to control for possible increases in outpatient visits, the Secretary of HHS will develop a volume control mechanism, and to prevent providers from receiving too much payment when PPS is implemented, outlays for home health services will be limited to 85% of what would have been paid if the new payment policy were not in place. Although the effects of the new PPS systems are complicated and likely to be onerous for all providers, the full impact of these changes is difficult to predict because the new system will redistribute payments both within and across health care delivery sectors. Further, the new payments to Medicare+ Choice plans will affect nonacute care providers, as will changes to traditional Medicare health plans affect private health plans. Thus, these and other issues (e.g., risk adjustment, benefit levels, data reporting requirements) promise many

Table 33.1 Balanced Budget Act of 1997 Schedule for Developing or Implementing Prospective Payment Systems

Date	Provider Type
July 1998	Skilled nursing facilities
January 1999	Hospital outpatient departments
October 1999	Long-term care hospitals and home health care agencies
October 2000	Rehabilitation facilities

Source: Medicare Payment Advisory Commission, March 1998.

unexpected changes in traditional provider relationships and potentially harmful economic effects. How these changes will affect nurses is also difficult to predict, but it is reasonable to assume that nurses will have fewer resources and will face continued pressures to find new ways to lower the cost and raise the efficiency of producing nursing care not unlike the changes required when DRGs were implemented in inpatient settings.

Payments to Hospitals

The BBA will exert important effects on hospital payments. In fact, PPS payments for all hospitals will be 10.6% lower in 2002 than they would have been under the laws previously enacted. Because PPS payments account for 28% of total hospital revenues (MedPAC, 1998) and 20% of hospitals had negative total margins, the effect of the BBA will be significant and only add to the financial pressures hospitals are already facing.

Payment for Physicians, Graduate Medical Education, and Advanced Practice Nurses

Having implemented many of the payment issues under Medicare's Resource Based Relative Value Scale (RBRVS) methodology used to develop physician fee schedules, the BBA makes additional changes in physician payment. The major change involves phasing in resource-based practice expense values starting in 1999 (it also requires implementation of resource-based malpractice expense values in 2000 but without any phase-in). Under the current method used by Medicare for paying physician fees, only the work component of the payment formula is based on an assessment of resources used to produce services, and practice and malpractice expenses are based on historical charges. By implementing resource-based practice expense values, there is a high likelihood of a redistribution of payments among services and physician specialties whose effects on access to physicians will bear careful monitoring. Also, to control for the possibility that physicians would attempt to increase the volume of patient visits to increase or maintain their personal incomes, the BBA includes special adjustments to constrain total Medicare spending on physician services.

In addition to these changes in physician payments, the BBA directs the MedPAC to study and make recommendations to Congress on a number of payment and other federal policies regarding Medicare's payments to teaching hospitals for indirect and direct costs of graduate medical education. Among the issues to be examined are whether and how payments should be made for training programs in pediatrics, as well as for nursing and other allied health professionals; federal policies regarding international medical graduates; dependence of medical schools on income generated from providing medical services; and methods for promoting an appropriate number, mix, and geographical distribution of physicians and other health professionals. Although the exact changes and their impact are difficult to predict, it is reasonable to anticipate that funding for graduate medical education will be much less generous than previously and, hence, that more teaching hospitals will be turning to advance practice nurses to oversee and provide increasing portions of both inpatient and outpatient care.

Finally, the Primary Care Health Practitioner Incentive Act, part of the BBA, established direct Medicare payment for services provided by nurse practitioners (NPs) and clinical nurse specialist (CNSs) in all practice settings. This legislation is the outcome of years of effort by many nurses in the public policy arena and represents a remarkable achievement given the demographic and financial problems facing the Medicare program. Although this change in Medicare payment policy is being implemented at the time of this writing, NPs, CNSs, and the nursing research community must anticipate that legislators and other interested groups will want to know about the outcomes of this policy change. To be sure, as the changes under BBA are implemented and other actions aimed at restructuring Medicare are undertaken to ensure the program's ability to accommodate the large wave of baby boomers who will enroll in Medicare early in the 21st century, policymakers will examine every aspect of Medicare payment policies, including those affecting NP and CNSs. Questions will be asked about how much Medicare has spent on payments to NPs and CNSs, the benefits obtained, and modifications that may be needed. Some groups may even question whether payments to NPs and CNSs are necessary. Nursing, therefore, should rapidly implement a research agenda aimed at gathering credible data and conducting studies to evaluate the effects of this policy change (Buerhaus, 1998a). If nurses perform studies that show the effects of NPs and CNSs on access to care, total Medicare spending, patient satisfaction, clinical outcomes, innovation, and other effects on the delivery of health care, then nursing will be in a position to shape the policy-related questions that will be asked, as well as influence the outcomes of efforts aimed at changing payment policies.

State Regulatory Initiatives

The rapid increase in state spending on Medicaid that occurred in the latter half of the 1980s and the early 1990s resulted in a steady increase in the number of states mandating enrollment of Medicaid recipients into managed care plans. This led many health policymakers and advocacy groups to fear that quality of care would deteriorate. However, to date there is little evidence that this has occurred; in contrast, many believe that access to primary care and continuity of care have improved for this special population. Today, all but a few states now require recipients to belong to a managed care program, and it is likely that the vast majority of the nearly 35 million Medicaid recipients will be enrolled in an HMO or other form of managed care organization. As more recipients are enrolled in managed care plans, which will be under great financial pressure to take advantage of the least costly and most efficient health care professional to deliver covered services, nurses can anticipate increasing demand for their services.

ADOPTING TRADITIONAL MARKET FORCES IN HEALTH CARE

In addition to federal and state regulations aimed at reducing *payments* to providers, traditional market forces that are based on principles of economic competition emerged in the early 1990s. By introducing incentives to promote efficiency in both the production and consumption of personal health services, economic competition slowed the rate of cost increases and lowered overall spending between 1993 and 1996. However, because competition and regulation are contrasting ways to govern the economic activity of a market, it is somewhat perplexing that the competitive approach emerged at the same time that there was intensifying use of federal price regulations via DRGs (and now RBRVS) and a variety of state level regulations. This contradiction can be explained by recalling the relatively weak form of regulations (with the exception of Nixon's 1971–1974 economic stabilization programs, which affected the entire economy) that were used in the 1970s (e.g., Certificate of Need, Voluntary and State Health Systems Planning, Professional Standards Peer Review, hospital rate setting, etc.). Rather than accomplishing their intended objective of reducing health care expenditures and improving quality, regulatory agencies were so manipulated and controlled by hospitals, insurers, and health professionals (namely physicians) that these groups were able to use the regulatory process to monopolize "their" respective health submarkets. As monopolists, they charged high prices, earned above normal incomes, stifled the development of lower-cost innovations such as HMOs and ambulatory surgery facilities, and prevented competition from other providers. For example, because they would reduce hospital use, hospitals obtained regulatory barriers that slowed the growth of HMOs, and hospitals prevented insurers from covering outpatient surgery because this would have decreased hospital revenues. Physicians have obtained regulatory protection from NPs, nurse midwives, and nurse anesthetists who have sought to expand their practice privileges, gain hospital admitting privileges, or receive fee-for-service payments directly from insurers and the government. Consequently, the output of the health industry was less than optimal, resources were not used efficiently, prices and total expenditures grew rapidly, and too many decisions were made on the basis of how hospitals' and physicians' economic interests were advanced as opposed to satisfying consumers.

During the early 1980s, however, a number of events and economic forces converged such that the emergence of competition could no longer be restrained. Among them were growing doubts about the effectiveness of regulations, several court rulings effectively removing legal issues clouding the application of competition in health care, a growing supply of physicians, an excess number of hospital beds, and pressure by business to control health insurance premium increases and reduce hospital use (Feldstein, 1986). Given these developments and the failure of the 1970s approach to regulating health care, competition in health care began to develop, even though there was a concurrent revitalization of regulatory activity by federal and state governments.

Economic Competition in Health Care

When thinking about competition, it is important to realize that although there may be many hospitals or professionals existing in an area, this does not mean that they compete on the basis of *price.* In economics, competition means price competition, whereas in health care, people usually refer to competition in the sense of nonprice competition, as when hospitals compete for physicians by offering them the latest equipment, modern facilities, etc. Enthoven (1990) explains the true meaning of competition:

> Price competition is present only if alternative suppliers are offering their goods or services to purchasers who really care about price because they are using their own money and must give up something else of value if they choose to pay a higher price. In other words, for there to be price competition, the purchasers must be seeking value for their money. (p. 368)

For competition (in the economic or "true" sense of the word) to exist in health care, suppliers (hospitals, HMOs, among others) must feel economic pressure to compete on price exerted by demanders (employers, unions, consumers, and so forth), or otherwise they will use nonprice competition as a way to increase their market share. Although more competition is developing in health care, most remains nonprice in nature.

Enthoven (1990) and McClure (cited in Iglehart, 1988) believe that competition (price) has been slow to develop in health care because large employers (demanders) have failed to exert appropriate pressures on suppliers. For example, employers do not allow employees to keep any savings that result from choosing a less costly health care plan. This weakens employees' incentive to choose such plans and thereby removes some of the economic pressure on plans to compete on the basis of price. Additionally, many employers do not even offer their employees the opportunity to choose more economical HMO or PPO plans but restrict their choices to expensive fee-for-service providers. Also, employers rarely insist that health care plans provide good information, describing the quality of their services or conveying it in a way that indicators of quality can be compared with other plans. Finally, tax policies give employers an incentive to purchase more costly and comprehensive health care plans, which makes it hard for employers to insist that employees and their unions adopt a cost-conscious approach to selecting health care insurance plans.

In the 1990s the barriers to the development of price competition began to break down, and hospitals and competitive medical plans have faced stronger economic incentives to minimize production costs so that they can price their products and services competitively. Increasingly, formal barriers, such as regulations, or informal ones that rely on traditional ways of doing things, are being removed whenever management believes they are keeping production costs higher than necessary and if their removal will not exert an important negative effect on quality. Employers have lifted restrictions preventing LPNs from giving medications or performing procedures currently done by RNs, or employers have eliminated restrictions preventing nurse aides or nonnurses (e.g., pharmacist technicians) from doing nursing functions. Nurse executives have had to carefully examine their institution's traditional barriers and involve hospital senior management to work with them in cases where they have caused nursing costs to be higher than necessary. To survive in a competitive environment, providers will have to constantly improve their reputations for high-quality patient care, which means that they will truly have to become concerned with satisfying consumers. For nursing to gain, it must visibly demonstrate its unique contribution to increasing consumer satisfaction and anticipate their evolving expectations. Finally, as price competition intensifies in health care, providers will use more promotional initiatives to inform purchasers on the *price* and *quality* of their services and products. Advantages can be obtained if nurse executives are involved in these initiatives so that nurses' contributions to patient outcomes are highlighted and become the means to favorably distinguish the parent organization's reputation (i.e., nonprice competition) from its competitors.

POLITICAL ISSUES FACING NURSING

The extraordinary changes that occurred in health care over the past decade helped national nursing organizations become more effective in representing the interests of the nursing profession. Recognizing that nurses would be excluded from the public policy-making process unless they became more politically sophisticated, national nursing organizations strengthened their lobbying capability, improved the ability to conduct timely policy analysis, expanded information networks, and diminished some of the rivalry existing among them. In the 1980s and early 1990s two nurses in Washington, Sheila Burke, who was Senator Robert Dole's chief of staff (Dole was Senate Majority Leader in the mid-1980s and a presidential candidate in 1996), and Carolyne Davis, who was the administrator of HCFA when DRGs were being implemented, helped nursing's political leaders gain better access to influential political leaders, enrich their networks, and educated countless politicians and federal bureaucracies on the value of nurses' contributions to the health care system. One can argue that today, the nursing profession's political effectiveness at the national level has never been better.

Having a strong influence over national politics in relation to federal health care policy is particularly important as the nursing profession and other health professions confront the inevitable restructuring of the Medicare program. Although the BBA is expected to postpone the financial insolvency of the Medicare program until roughly 2010, the severity of the financial, demographic, and political challenges facing Medicare cannot be overstated (Buerhaus, 1998b). The BBA created a bipartisan Medicare Advisory Commission that over the next 2 years will be examining possible policy changes and strategies to ensure the solvency of the Medicare program. The commission's work will be enormously important in shaping the future of this popular but expensive social program. Thus, there is a huge opportunity for the nursing profession's policy leaders to work with the commission in developing policy options and recommendations. Because the work of the commission is expected to coincide with the presidential election in 2000, there will be the possibility that the new president will take advantage of the traditional honeymoon phase early in the administration to mobilize the American people and Congress to adopt the recommendations of the Medicare Advisory Commission.

Although the BBA and the Medicare commission will be the focus of much public attention, it is important for nurses to keep these developments in perspective relative to the changes that will continue to effect them every work day arising from the private sector's embrace of market competition. In fact, on a daily basis, the pressures and challenges arising from market competition are more likely to affect nurses than are policy developments occurring in Washington. Nurses can anticipate that the focus in the 1990s on eliminating excess hospital capacity through mergers, closings, and consolidation will be replaced by a growing emphasis on the quality of care. In the future, executives, middle managers, and clinicians will come to work each day worried not only about whether they are producing services efficiently and whether they are price competitive, but if they are seen in the marketplace as a high quality provider. As measures of quality of care improve, more information is made available, states enact legislation to protect consumers and ensure high quality, and as it becomes easier to compare plans and providers on the basis of quality and how patients and consumers rate them, it will be essential for an organization's economic survival to have a reputation for high quality. However, nurses need not feel threatened by these developments; rather, the increasing emphasis on quality gives the profession the opportunity, if not the responsibility, to demonstrate the relationship between nursing interventions and the attainment of clinical outcomes and quality that purchasers want and are willing to pay for. Therefore, at the top of nursing's political agenda should be the total dedication of all realms of the profession and by nurses at all levels in organizations to overcome the institutional, professional, and political and policy barriers that retard their ability to fully embrace a quality enhancement agenda. Given the strength of federal and state regulatory actions together with the acceleration of market competition that has been discussed in this chapter, the future well-being of the nursing profession will rest on how well we are able to recognize and deal effectively with these realities that will be unfolding in the 21st century health care system.

SUMMARY

The nursing profession faces significant challenges arising from global economic developments, federal and state regulations, and strengthening price competition among providers of personal health care services. To be sure, it will take a great deal of insight and conviction on the part of nurse executives to direct their nursing departments through such a dynamic economic environment. Their chance of succeeding will be affected by how well nursing's political leaders understand these changing economic conditions and anticipate their political implications.

Because a great number of the challenges that lie ahead can be influenced by political intervention, especially at the state level, it is in the interest of nurse executives to avoid directing all of their energy to solving internal matters but use some of it to develop and implement strategies that promote the political effectiveness of organizations representing professional nurses.

STUDY QUESTIONS

1. Explain in economic terms how nurses function as economic resources.
2. What challenges are arising for the nursing profession from global economic developments and increasing price competition among health care providers?

REFERENCES

Buerhaus, P. I. (1987). Not just another nursing shortage. *Nursing Economic$, 5*(6), 267–279.

Buerhaus, P. (1998a, May/June). Medicare payment for advanced practice nurses. What are the research questions? *Nursing Outlook, 46*(3), 103–108.

Buerhaus P. (1998b). Financial, demographic, and political problems confronting Medicare in the United States. *IMAGE: Journal of Nursing Scholarship, 30*(2), 117–123.

Enthoven, A. C. (1990). Multiple choice health insurance: The lessons and challenges to employers. *Inquiry, 27*(4), 368–373.

Feldstein, P. J. (1986). The changing health care delivery system. *Trustee, 39*(2), 15–17, 21.

Iglehart, J. K. (1988). Competition and the pursuit of quality: A conversation with Walter McClure. *Health Affairs, 7*(1), 79–90.

Iglehart, J. K. (1995). A conversation with Leonard D. Schaeffer, *Health Affairs, 14*(4), 131.

Medicare Payment Advisory Commission (MedPAC). (March 1998). *Report to the Congress: Medicare payment policy. Volume I: Recommendations.* Washington, DC: Author.

Moses, E. (1986). The registered nurse population: Findings from the national sample survey of registered nurses, November 1984. Rockville, MD: Health Resources Services Administration, Bureau of Health Professions, NTIS #HRP-0906938.

Prospective Payment Assessment Commission. (1991). *Medicare and the American health care system. Report to Congress.* Washington, DC: Author.

C H A P T E R

34

Beyond Integrating Practice, Education, and Research: The Next Steps

Lillian M. Simms • Ke-Ping Agnes Yang

Gradually with time, all medical services will move out of the hospital to places of convenience for the patient. The hospital as we know it today—ever larger, more corporate, and more bureaucratic—will disappear. (Slack, 1997, p. 168)

Chapter Highlights
- A historical perspective
- Shift to community
- Nursing-sensitive outcomes
- The genetic revolution
- Globalization of nursing
- The next 100 years

The purpose of this chapter is to chart a course for the future of nursing administration that will be fully integrated by the year 2000. The transition to the 21st century will be marked by a new era of resource discovery. The largest worldwide health care resource will finally be recognized as patients (Slack, 1997). Patients and families will be included in all aspects of care decisions. The shift to community in health care will nurture a world-wide emphasis on nursing-sensitive outcomes and patient-centered care. In addition, globalization of the economy and the genetic revolution mandate a perspective on health care delivery that maximizes the contributions of nursing to quality care. Developing this perspective requires an evolution of insight about management and leadership (Table 34.1).

The application and management of an organization's knowledge resources is perhaps the greatest leadership challenge in modern organizations. The transformation of health care services relies on the development of new service technologies and new models of organization (Gilmartin, 1998). A strong sense of innovation and entrepreneurship leading to the development of improved nursing technologies is a primary component in the evolution of professional nursing administration practice in the 21st century. The best and brightest ideas from nursing practice and education are essential to the development of new products and services. At no time in our history has it been more important for nursing education and practice to collaborate on moving the profession forward, building on the strengths acquired in the various areas of practice.

Nursing practice and education will no longer exist separately. Together, they will blend and build on quality research to bring harmony in the practice setting. Nurse executives hold the key to professional integration and must be the leaders in this effort.

The relationship between nursing practice, education, and research has moved full cycle and is now back on a trajectory of integration with a conceptual framework of "nursing community." The concept of nursing community develops from the highest order of collaboration within nursing, a collaboration such that the separate terminologies of practice and education are no longer meaningful. Within this conception, professional nurses assume key leadership positions and practice clinically, administratively, or both as well as teach. This arrangement negates the guest or visitor faculty role in practice settings and the lack of nursing service involvement in the teaching of students.

Table 34.1 *Evolution of Insight About Management and Leadership*

Power of the few	→	Empowerment for all
Management	→	Leadership
Single managers	→	Self-managed groups
Emphasis on visible	→	Emphasis on invisible
Homogeneity	→	Diversity
Organizational Charts	→	Organizations as energy (chi)
Rational data-based decision-making	→	Combination of intuition and research
Paper-based information systems	→	Global computer-linked networks
Total quality	→	Learning organizations

Nurse executives in practice and education play a unique role in developing this concept and creating the environment in which professional practice can occur and endure. To function in this unique leadership role, nurse executives must have a better understanding of integrated models and collaboration within and beyond nursing as described in Chapters 1 and 4. There must also be a better understanding of the unfortunate separation of nursing education and services over the late 19th and early 20th centuries.

A HISTORICAL PERSPECTIVE

The idea of integration of education and practice has existed since the development of nursing schools in 1873 (Bullough & Bullough, 1969; Gelinas, 1946). Early schools of nursing were hospital based, and nurses were trained through apprenticeship, with little emphasis on formal education. Nearly all schools of nursing were owned and controlled by the hospitals they served. Students were used for service to maintain low costs. Early schools were designed to function in much the same way as religious orders, with the hospital being the training center for educational and practice activities (Goodnow, 1942). There was much confusion as to their purpose: service or education. Differences in the roles of the nursing student and of the graduate nurse were not clearly defined.

By 1923, the need for self-directed, independent schools of nursing was identified. The Goldmark report stressed the need to establish university-based schools of nursing (Goldmark, 1923). The dual role of the hospital school of providing education and service was viewed as detrimental to the needs of patients and students. Furthermore, the training of nurses was considered a serious educational business that required direction by those who were committed to quality nursing education.

Throughout the next four decades, a gradual transition occurred from hospital-based to university- and college-based schools of nursing. Concomitant with this change was a dramatic decrease in faculty involvement in direct service in hospitals. Although the primary purposes of universities are teaching, research, and service, the service component became deemphasized. As faculty moved away from practice, nursing service personnel moved away from education. In the process of developing the strong research focus so important in quality nursing education, many faculty drifted away from problems related to direct care.

In the early 1960s, some nursing leaders began to seriously question the separation and began to devise approaches for reintegrating nursing practice and education. Noted initiatives began at the University of Florida, Case Western Reserve University, University of Rochester, and Rush-Presbyterian-St. Luke's Medical Center (Powers, 1976). Numerous models have developed since that time with research serving as the linking mechanism especially in academic health centers.

These programs have shown great promise, but several persistent difficulties hinder implementation in some settings. Doctorally prepared nurses hesitate to assume leadership roles in practice. Lack of agreement about academic preparation for nurses interferes with professional integrated models. Nationwide, the deficit of nurses prepared for leadership roles interferes with selection of nursing practice patterns appropriate for specific integrated models. Integrated models are not accepted by all nurses, and, indeed, crises are brewing in nursing that demand the most creative thinking by nursing leaders. Visualizing the next steps beyond integration (Figure 34.1) will assist creative thinking.

SHIFT TO COMMUNITY

Increasing unemployment in the acute care sector of health care is causing nurses to rethink their chosen workplace (Corser, 1998). The ambulatory care sector of our nation's health care system is growing 18 times faster than the acute care sector and more changes are predicted. This transformation in acute care settings is having a major impact on organizational commitment among nurses. The group of nurses most affected will be those in current leadership roles. As the concept of leadership changes and becomes integrated at all levels in the system, traditional command and control positions are likely to disappear.

The continued development of staff in a learning environment will be top priority in the health care system of the future. Nurse executives will be expected to design and implement entrepreneurships and intrapreneurships. Telehealth businesses in home care practice (Warner, 1998) will be common and nurses in general will recognize the media as a powerful influence in patient and health education (Ross, 1998). According to Ross, more Americans turn to television for

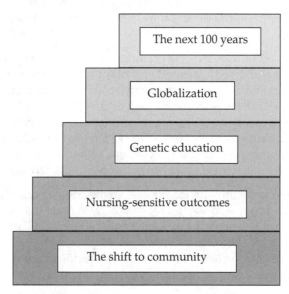

Figure 34.1 The steps beyond integration of practice, education, and research.

medical and other health information, surpassing health professionals for the first time in history. This finding does not include surfing the Internet for health information, an increasingly popular habit among Americans.

Clarke (1986) predicted that these changes would occur and that the shift from inpatient to ambulatory settings will accelerate by the year 2019. People will be increasingly responsible for their own care and insurers will continue to develop benefits that reward good health habits. The winds of change have already blown across the United States and care will continue to move to the community in a variety of outpatient clinics designed for quality and pleasant atmosphere. When possible, people will recover at home or in pleasantly furnished hospital-linked inns/hotels.

NURSING-SENSITIVE OUTCOMES

A nursing-sensitive outcome is the next step in multidisciplinary collaboration and quality care and can serve as the logical link to patient-centered outcomes. The key to nursing sensitive outcomes is patient involvement. Who else can document the nurse's story? In the 21st century, self-care, assistive technology, bloodless surgery, decreased hospital stays, genetic cures, and space travel will forever change how nurse executives view their work and work environment.

The nursing intervention and outcomes classification systems presented in McCloskey and Grace (1997) have a solid place on the bridge to consumer enlightenment. As self-assessment of functional ability becomes standard for all patients, health-related quality of life activities will become as important as drug or gene therapies. By the year 2000, health professionals will be able to monitor clinical outcomes (nursing or medical) much as they monitor financial spreadsheets now. At last we have moved from understanding process to fully appreciating the importance of outcomes.

The role of patients is increasingly at the center of the outcomes debate. Geigle and Jones (1990) argue that patients have remained on the periphery of outcome measurement. They believe this is due to relying almost entirely on objective measures such as mortality and morbidity. Patients are becoming better educated about outcomes and quality issues and have become critical of clinicians' uncertainty about the value of different therapeutic procedures. As patients become better informed, their judgment can augment physicians' judgment (Geigle & Jones, 1990; Slack, 1997). Thus, one of the more crucial developments in the health care field has been the recognition of the importance of the patient's perspective in monitoring quality of health care outcomes.

Ware's (1991) study of the patient's perspective on outcomes of medical care combines traditional clinical measures of disease status with the patient's view of disease and treatment. He concludes that it is impossible to move from efficacy research to effectiveness research unless new instruments to define effectiveness include quality of life, function, and well-being from the patient's perspective.

Patients' experiences with care outcomes are rarely found in existing databases (Ware, 1991). However, research by Flood, Lorence, Ding, McPherson, and Black (1993) on the ability of placebo therapy to alter outcomes suggests that a patient's expectations about therapy can also influence outcomes. In their research on the influence of social-psychological factors on health, they found that positive expectations result in a more optimistic view of improvement after surgery rather than altering reports of outcomes or health.

Outcomes, nonetheless, are sensitive to subjective value judgments and the desirability of one outcome rather than another in any given clinical situation may differ based on the values and preferences of patients. Improved health outcomes can be produced either by lowering expectations or by improving the patient's self-assessment (Slack, 1997). Atchley (1991) addresses the question of whether a strong self-concept can be maintained in the face of normal aging and frailty. Frailty changes the dynamics of quality of life but not necessarily self-concept. Theories about control of destiny in the later years are undeveloped (Atchley, 1991).

Lawton (1991) asserts that indicators of quality must include subjective data. Because individuals' perceptions may differ in their assessment of the quality of their life, the nature of these deviations is itself a matter of interest. Patients and family members are thus the main source of relevant, reliable information as to the patients' capacity to perform an activity and whether they actually do it or not (Lohr, 1993). Lohr argues that patients' reports on interpersonal interactions and the humanistic aspects of care are often included in patient satisfaction measures, although they are attributes more of process than of outcome. However, process and outcomes are directly related.

Patient satisfaction is increasingly considered an outcome in its own right and can be viewed as an objective of care representing the patient's judgment on quality of care. It provides the information on the success of meeting the patient's values and expectations, on which the patient is the ultimate authority. Expressions of satisfaction with certain elements of care can be further considered as an indicator of the art of nursing practice. Patients' subjective perceptions of care thus can certainly be regarded as valid measures on nursing-sensitive outcomes of care.

There are important rationales for believing current health care requires more than medical technology to achieve optimal outcomes. The care versus cure dispute during the past two decades, however, has not identified a clear healing role in contemporary nursing practice (Leftwich, 1993). The medical model has been criticized for the narrow and unsatisfactory view it takes of diagnosis and treatment (Reed & Watson, 1994). Traditionally, nursing care focuses on changing or modifying human behaviors and responses to positively affect quality of life. The role of nursing in acute and chronic illnesses is directed toward preventing illness and disability and promoting health in physical, psychological, and social realms. In addition, nursing care is concerned not only with individuals, but it also recognized that positive outcomes for families and communities are crucial as well.

Nursing research on outcomes focuses most often on the measurement of positive aspects of health, such as status of physiologic, physical, emotional, and functional health, patient satisfaction, and quality of life rather than the negatives of death, disease, and disability to determine effectiveness of care (DeFriese, 1992). Other researchers also have found that reduction of symptoms, improvement in daily functioning, or improvement in a sense of well-being or quality of life are more appropriate than mortality as an outcome. This holistic concept of outcomes directs attention specifically to the patient.

Reed and Watson's (1994) qualitative study of the ways in which nurses assess the mobility of elderly patients indicates that the medical model is occasionally compatible with nurses' values and in certain settings can enhance and support nursing care. In long-term care settings, where cure is clearly not an option for patients, the medical model has little to offer practice in accord with nursing values and may have a negative effect on the development of alternative approaches to care (Reed & Watson, 1994).

THE GENETIC REVOLUTION

The technological explosion of genetic knowledge through the Human Genome Project (Collins & Jenkins, 1997) has created an enormous opportunity for nurses to share leadership for health care in the 21st century. Although health professionals may think that genetic disorders are infrequent, it has become obvious that almost every identified disease has a genetic component. Even trauma may have elements of genetic disposition to accidents. To think of nursing sensitive outcomes without considering human genetics is folly.

According to Collins and Jenkins (1997), genes are the working components of DNA, which carry the instructions for specific products (e.g., proteins) made by the body. When there is a mutation or error in one or many genes, disease may result. The importance of gene identification is that it offers the potential for diagnostic capability to warn people of increased risk. Preventive interventions may be possible as will actual gene therapies in the future. Genetics education will be important for nurses in all types of practice and for health consumers.

Feetham (1997) asserts that the misperceptions of the science and technology innovation continuum as a linear model must be corrected. This model is misleading because it infers that clinical adoption of innovation is the natural outcome of clinical knowledge and practice derived from basic research. There is increasing recognition that clinical questions are often the source of technological innovation. Another misconception is that science (academics) and technology (industry) are separate and distinct paradigms. Science and technology are more intertwined than ever in today's world. Laser technology and magnetic resonance imaging are two examples of cross-over. Education for genetics care for health professionals suggested by Feetham includes:

- Core genetic knowledge base
- Integrated continuum of genetics education
- Didactic and clinically based education programs that ensure genetics relevant knowledge for all populations and across all ages
- Receptive climate to access genetics knowledge
- Research and evaluation base for any program dealing with genetics and primary care

The National Institute of Nursing Research, together with the nursing community, can make a significant contribution to generating research questions that can guide the studies of basic scientists and applied nurse researchers. In the future, treating diseases at the molecular level can build on strong nursing research on children and families, adherence, responses to learning, diagnosis of disease, and coping with acute and chronic illness. In every health care setting, nurses will be involved with the care of patients who have genetic disorders, are members of families with genetic disorders, or undergoing genetic testing or gene therapy. The prevention, diagnosis, and treatment of a variety of health problems is changing significantly in the genetic age (Grady, 1997).

GLOBALIZATION OF NURSING

The globalization of the world economy is also influencing nursing education and practice (Fenton, 1997). There is a tremendous need for students, nurses and faculty to have multicultural experiences. Many of the foreign nursing students who came to American schools for graduate education have now returned to their countries to provide leadership and to provide contact points for developing exchange systems in education and practice. Regional nursing associations around the world are responding to changes in global markets and resultant introduction of new products and services and related occupational hazards and concerns. The global economy has also increased the availability of electronic communication and nurses in less developed countries can now access new health information without traveling great distances at high cost.

Knowledge of health statistics in other countries has made U.S. health professionals aware that the United States no longer ranks at the top for common health data such as infant mortality rates and death rates (Fenton, 1997). It is imperative that we work with other health professionals in other lands to learn about their health promotion and illness prevention practices.

Tlou (1998) suggests that international partnerships can be advantageous in education and service settings. An international partnership is a collaboration in which two or more institutions or departments carry out professional activities aimed at improving and developing more knowledge for nursing education; these partnerships can be teacher and student exchanges, research activities, consultancies, or sabbatical appointments. For a partnership to be successful, both partners must see it as beneficial and the sharing of information, resources, time, and expertise must be mutual. As economies are shrinking, international partnerships in nursing education are growing.

Models of international exchange should go beyond student and faculty educational programs and serious attention needs to be given to clinical exchanges. These could be facilitated by nurse executives much the same way as medical fellowships are arranged. For example, it is not uncommon for foreign physicians to be granted clinical fellowships for clinical study and practice in academic health centers. International health conferences and distance learning programs are bringing health professionals together from all parts of the globe and cross-fertilization of ideas is yielding new and unique therapies and partnerships

According to Possehl (1998), exchange of microbes across global borders requires a universal change in our perspective on health care. A sampling of recent disease outbreaks targets incidents of new viral and bacterial infections in North America, Australia, South/Central America, Asia, Europe, and Africa. Thus cyclospora clusters traveling on fresh fruits and vegetables can be found in California and Washington, DC, far from their original home in Central America. Bubonic plague and cholera have been found in North America, Asia, and Africa and new strains of influenza and pneumonia are transported daily.

THE NEXT 100 YEARS

Regardless of program or degree, Tebbitt (1997) suggests that the job dimensions for the nurse executive over the next 10 years will require a clinical base and knowledge, skill and experience in the following:

- Business acumen
- Strategic and financial planning
- Program development and implementation
- Rapid problem-solving and decision-making
- Teamwork and team building
- Interpersonal and intergroup communication
- Resource allocation
- Negotiation
- Developing employee potential
- Community organizational relations

These activities will require new skills for the 21st century (Figure 34.2) as described throughout this book.

In addition, Joel (1997) asserts that an explosive demand for community services exists today and into the next century. Two distinct markets are forming for patients after an acute illness and for the frail, disabled and chronically ill. A clear picture of reimbursement changes has emerged since the advent of Medicare and Medicaid. Subsequent legislation made home health services a covered benefit. Expansion of the home care market seems to be an irreversible trend that may be

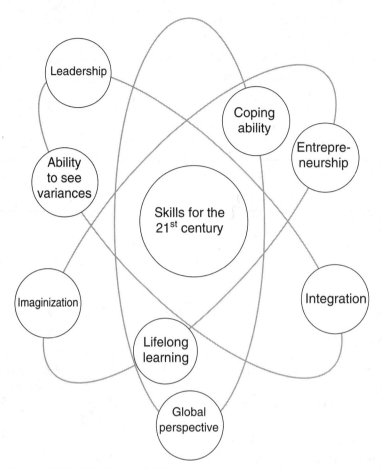

Figure 34.2 Skills for the 21st century.

a response to the declining use of hospitals or other factors such as an increased level of health consciousness.

The shift in the dominant venue for health care, from the hospital to community settings, and the explosion of information on the Internet are creating an unforeseen rise in consumerism and an intelligent recipient of health care who no longer defers to health professionals for personal health decisions. The demand for consumer control of health care decisions will increase with patients and families insisting on quality of life variables to be entered into the health care equation. In the 21st century, physicians will no longer be able to dictate who shall live and who shall die nor will insurance companies. These decisions will be increasingly shared with patient and family members in new professional-client partnerships.

A number of marketplace developments suggest that health care delivery systems will continue to consolidate and the focus on disease and injury prevention will be strengthened (Zelman, 1996). The potential for public-private joint ventures on public health matters will be considerable with jointly sponsored health education projects becoming common.

SUMMARY

Throughout the 1990s and into the 21st century, there will be an increased emphasis on research that has relevance for both nursing practice and education. Faculty members will be increasingly criticized for their lack of practice-based research and their rusty clinical skills. On the other hand, nursing service personnel will be expected to provide sophisticated, cost-effective evidence-based patient care based on research. Research is the primary means of documenting effectiveness and efficiency of nursing education and practice, and nurses in the near future will be expected to provide data to justify nursing's portion of education and health care costs.

This book attempts to reach the heart and soul of the practicing nurse executive. At no time in the history of nursing has there been a better opportunity for the profession to move from adolescence to full maturity. The major studies of the decade carried out by nonnursing groups support the mandate for leadership within nursing. Although leadership must be present in education, research, and clinical practice, it is in administration that leadership is most likely to make the significant difference in bringing the profession to maturity.

This chapter has addressed the major influences on health care in the 21st century: the shift to community and patient-centered care, the genetic revolution, and globalization of the economy. Computerization will continue to impact the entire health care scene and it has been discussed thoroughly in other parts of this book. In closing, the authors look ahead to the next 100 years and give the reader a green light to look forward to a continuously changing health care environment and expanded roles for nurse executives.

STUDY QUESTIONS

1. Review the major themes of this book and design a course that could be Web-based and delivered to schools of nursing in all parts of the world.
2. Search the nursing literature and determine if globalization and the genetic revolution are emerging themes. Write a short article on how these developments will change the way nursing is practiced.
3. Trace the history of nursing-sensitive outcomes and patient-centered care and explain how one affects the other. How do you see the current emphasis on patient-centered care influencing opinions about nursing-sensitive outcomes?
4. Interview four nurses from other countries and find out what common diseases prevail in their homelands and how they are treated.
5. Volunteer to travel with a nurse delegation to another country and visit a variety of health care delivery settings. When you return, write a paper on what you learned during your experience.

6. Trace the disease pattern in your family history and determine if there is a single recurring disease that might possibly be eradicated with genetic therapy.

REFERENCES

Atchley, R. C. (1991). The influence of aging or frailty on perceptions and expressions of the self: Theoretical and methodological issues. In J. E. Birren, J. E. Lubben, J. C. Rowe, & D. E. Deutchman (Eds.), *The concept and measurement of quality of life in the frail elderly,* San Diego: Academic Press.

Bullough, V. L., & Bullough, B. (1969). *The emergence of modern nursing* (2nd ed.). London: Macmillan.

Clarke, A. C. (1986). *Arthur C. Clarke's July 20, 2019, Life in the 21st century.* New York: Macmillan.

Collins, F., & Jenkins, J. (1997). Implications of the human genome project for the nursing profession. In F. R. Lashley (Ed.), *The genetics revolution.* Washington, DC: American Academy of Nursing.

Corser, W. D. (1998). The changing nature of organizational commitment in the acute care environment. *Journal of Nursing Administration, 28*(6), 32–36.

DeFriese, G. H. (1992). Outcomes research: Implications for the effectiveness of nursing practice. In National Institute of Health (Ed.). *Patient outcomes research: Examining the effectiveness of nursing practice.* Washington, DC: Department of Health and Human Services.

Feetham, S. (1997). The genetics revolution: Outcomes and recommendations. In F. R. Lashley (Ed.), *The genetics revolution.* Washington, DC: American Academy of Nursing.

Fenton, M. V. (1997). Development of models of international exchange to upgrade nursing education. In J. C. McCloskey & H. K. Grace (Eds.), *Current issues in nursing* (5th ed.), p. 203–207). St. Louis: Mosby.

Flood, A. B., Lorence, D. P., Ding, J., McPherson, K., & Black, N. A. (1993). The role of expectations in patients' reports of post-operative outcomes and improvement following therapy. *Medical Care, 31*(11), 1043–1056.

Geigle, R., & Jones, S. B. (1990, Spring). Outcomes measurement: A report from the front. *Inquiry, 27,* 7–13.

Gelinas, A. (1946). *Nursing and nursing education.* New York: The Commonwealth Fund, E. L. Hildreth and Co.

Gilmartin, M. J. (1998). The nursing organization and the transformation of health care delivery for the 21st century. *Nursing Administration Quarterly, 22*(2), 70–86.

Goldmark, J. (1923). *Nursing and nursing education in the United States, committee for the study of nursing education.* New York: Macmillan.

Goodnow, M. (1942). *Nursing history.* Philadelphia: Saunders.

Grady, P. A. (1997). The genetic revolution: The role of the National Institute of Nursing Research. In F. R. Lashley (Ed.), *The genetics revolution.* Washington, DC: American Academy of Nursing.

Joel, L. A. (1997). Moving the care site from hospital to home: Whose turf? In J. C. McCloskey & H. K. Grace (Eds.), *Current issues in nursing* (5th ed., pp. 209–215). St. Louis: Mosby.

Lawton, M. P. (1991). A multidimensional view of quality of life in frail elders. In J. E. Birren, J. E. Lubben, J. C. Rowe, & D. E. Deutchman (Eds.), *The concept and measurement of quality of life in the frail elderly,* San Diego: Academic Press.

Leftwich, R. R. (1993). Care and cure as healing processes in nursing. *Nursing Forum, 28*(3), 13–17.

Lohr, K. N. (1993). Outcome measurement: Concepts and questions. *Inquiry, 25,* 37–50.

McCloskey, J. D., & Grace, H. K. (1997). *Current issues in nursing* (5th ed.). St. Louis: Mosby.

Possehl, S. (1998). The long reach of bugs without borders. *Hospitals & Health Networks, 72*(9), 28–40.

Powers, M. J. (1976). The unification model in nursing. *Nursing Outlook, 24*(8), 482–487.

Reed, J., & Watson, D. (1994). The impact of the medical model on nursing practice and assessment. *International Journal of Nursing Studies, 31*(1), 57–66.

Ross, J. (1998). Peabody/FWJ award announced for excellence in health care coverage. *ADVANCES,* Issue 2, p. 3.

Slack, W. V. (1997). *Cybermedicine.* San Francisco: Jossey-Bass.

Tebbitt, B. V. (1997). Nurse executives. In J. C. McCloskey & H. K. Grace (Eds.), *Current issues in nursing* (5th ed., pp. 25–33). St. Louis: Mosby.

Tlou, S. D. (1998). International partnerships in nursing education. *International Nursing Review, 45*(2), 55–57.

Ware, E. J., Jr. (1991). Conceptualizing and measuring generic health outcomes. *Cancer, 67*(suppl), 774–779.

Warner, I. (1998). Telehealth in home care practice. *Journal of Nursing Administration, 28*(6), 3, 16.

Zelman, W. A. (1996). *The changing health care marketplace.* San Francisco: Jossey-Bass.

BIBLIOGRAPHY

Arista II Participants. (1996). *Nursing leadership in the 21st century. Healthy people: Leaders in partnership.* Indianapolis, IN: Center Nursing Sigma Theta Tau International.

Dienemann, J. A. (Ed.). (1997). *Cultural diversity in nursing.* Washington, DC: American Academy of Nursing.

Ditmyer, S., Koepsell, B., Branum, V., Davis, P., and Lush, M. T. (1998). Developing a nursing outcomes measurement tool. *Journal of Nursing Administration, 28*(6), 10–16.

Isaacs, S. L., & Knickman, J. R. (Eds.). (1997). *To Improve Health and Health Care 1997. The Robert Wood Johnson Anthology.* San Francisco: Jossey-Bass.

Lashley, F. R. (Ed.). (1997). *The genetics revolution.* Washington, DC: American Academy of Nursing.

Yang, K-P., Simms, L. M., & Yin, J-C. T. (1998). Nursing-sensitive patient care outcomes in Taiwanese nursing homes. *IMAGE, The Journal of Nursing Scholarship, 30*(3), 290.

APPENDICES

Examples of Community Nursing Businesses as Described by the Nurse Executives Who Started Them

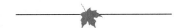

The nursing businesses described in this section can be used by students or practicing nurses to help them become inspired about starting their own professional nursing practices on a fee-for-service basis outside the parameters of traditional employment. As Christine Smith was inspired by her godmother, so we hope will readers, as they experience these new ventures "in print" so aptly described by their authors.

Appendix A: Marcia D. Andersen—Personalized Nursing Corporation, (PNC) and Well-Being Institute (WBI)

Appendix B: Anne F. Darga—Pursuit Health Formulas

Appendix C: Erica Dutton—Wellspring Counseling

Appendix D: Ilene Warner—Insight Telehealth Systems, Inc.

Appendix E: Sandra R. Byers—Parish Nursing: A Health and Wholeness Ministry

Appendix F: Christine M. Smith—Reflections on My Journey to Private Practice as a Small Business

APPENDIX

A

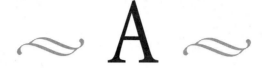

Personalized Nursing Corporation (PNC) and Well-Being Institute (WBI)

By Lillian M. Simms with input from

Marcia D. Andersen, PhD, RN, FAAN, CS; President and Founder

Marcia Andersen may have been born to lead or she developed leadership skills during her nursing studies at the University of Michigan. In any case, she is one of the most successful business women and nurse entrepreneurs in southeastern Michigan with recognition throughout the United States. Marcia has a dream—to set up nursing care delivery systems in many states with her approach to nursing care. Her dream has culminated initially in three nursing companies, the Personalized Nursing Corporation (PNC), proprietary (established in 1983), The Personalized Nursing LIGHT House, nonprofit, (established in 1990), and the Well-Being Institute (WBI), nonprofit, (established in 1994). Gareth Morgan would call her work "imaginization" at its best. These three nursing companies are dedicated to using the Personalized Nursing LIGHT model of care developed by Andersen to address substance abuse and related health issues. Her model of care is a model of the art of nursing care based on the nursing science of Dr. Martha Rogers.

THE LIGHT MODEL

Initially reluctant to start her companies because of her lack of business acumen, she nevertheless went ahead because she wanted to promote her **LIGHT** model of practice. **LIGHT** is an acronym for nurses' duties:

Love the client

Intend to help

Give care gently

Help the client improve well-being

Teach the process.

Then she says patients should Love themselves; Identify a focal concern; Give themselves a goal; Have confidence; and Take action.

The focus of any nursing intervention within this perspective is to assist the client to improve a sense of well-being. The model stresses that the path to optimal health and well-being lies within each person. Clients are taught the LIGHT model as a process to improve their sense of well-being, while remaining free of alcohol and drugs. An improved sense of well-being is associated with an ability to see more options and possibilities when confronted with life's problems.

GETTING STARTED

An RN with a doctorate in nursing, Andersen began Personalized Nursing Corporation in 1983 with a $1,000 tax refund and one employee—herself. Since then she has generated over $16 million in gross revenue and employs over 60 people. Initially headquartered at the Renaissance Center in Detroit, Andersen has moved her companies to Ann Arbor, Michigan, where she continues to oversee her three companies, three affiliated Personalized Nursing LIGHT House Dependency Treatment Centers in Plymouth, Detroit, and Ann Arbor, Michigan; and Well Being Institute's Initiative—a street outreach program on the Cass Corridor in Detroit.

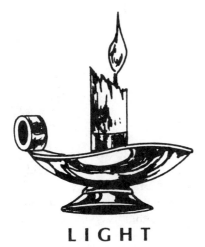

Figure AA.1 Andersen's LIGHT Model Logo. Reprinted with permission of Personalized Nursing Corporation.

NURSING SERVICES

Andersen developed and provides a whole new nursing care delivery system aimed at treating drug addiction. Instead of waiting for government agencies to send addicts to her, Andersen sends her staff out on the streets of Detroit to talk to drug and alcohol abusers and enroll them in her Outreach Early Intervention Program. The outreach program includes counseling, physical and mental health care, transportation to health care appointments, and often, alternative therapies such as body energy work and massage therapy. Those who want to get clean are settled into Andersen's Detroit-area LIGHT House Intensive substance abuse treatment program with a domicile.

Personalized Nursing LIGHT House was opened in 1990 by an experienced team of distinguished nurses, substance abuse counselors, and business administrators. The comprehensive program was developed in response to the needs of clients. These needs were identified by both clients and professional staff during a very successful outreach program in New York, Baltimore, and Detroit, which was funded by the National Institute on Drug Abuse (NIDA). The staff of Personalized Nursing LIGHT consists of PhD, BSN, and MSN nurses, a physician, psychologists, social workers, and recovering and nonrecovering substance abuse counselors. All staff have a deep feeling of respect for the addicted person. Each staff member is dedicated to assisting clients in the recovery process.

Clean, beautiful, and completely furnished apartments are available to clients a place to live while enrolled in the intensive outpatient program. A van shuttles clients from the nearby apartment complexes to the program offices. All major issues that contribute to recovery and relapse prevention are addressed:

- Substance abuse relapse prevention planning (group, individual, and family)
- Substance abuse educational needs
- Legal and financial problems (lawyer on staff)
- Employment/outplacement problems
- Continuing education needs
- Medical and psychiatric nursing needs
- Talent/vocational concerns
- Self-esteem needs
- Family/relationship problems
- General business development education needs

The outpatient program is intensive, with sessions running 3 to 5 hours per day, 5 days per week, up to 70 treatment days. Individual counseling is also provided. Any individual interested in entering the Personalized Nursing LIGHT program must be 18 years of age or older, be willing and committed to participate in treatment, and must have resources to pay for services. Other eligibility restrictions apply regarding medical and psychiatric stability.

OTHER PAYMENT MECHANISMS

Andersen has been highly successful in getting funding from various sources including government grants, contracts, and insurance companies. She seeks funding from other creative ventures to support "scholarship" clients who have no insurance or payer or who have been on the waiting list for over 5 months. She dreams of a $1 million dollar endowment some day to fully support her current and expanded nursing care delivery system.

For more information about these businesses, information may be obtained at Andersen's Web site at www.pnc-wbi.com. Selected publications that describe the results of her efforts to serve hard-to-reach populations are listed below.

Andersen, M. D., & Hockman, E. M. (1997). Well-being and high-risk drug use among active drug users. In M. Madrid (Ed.), *Patterns of Rogerian Knowing* (Chap. 13). New York: National League for Nursing Press.

Andersen, M. D., Hockman, E. M., & Smereck, G. A. D. (1996). Effect of a nursing outreach intervention to drug users in Detroit, Michigan. *Journal of Drug Issues, 26*(3), 619–634.

Andersen, M. D., & Smereck, G. A. D. (1994). Personalized nursing: A science-based model of the art of nursing. In M. Madrid & E. A. M. Barrett (Eds.), *Rogers's scientific art of nursing practice* (pp. 261–283). New York: National League for Nursing Press.

Andersen, M. D., & Smereck, G. A. D. (1994). *The art of nursing: The personalized nursing practice model* (Video). Plymouth, MI: Personalized Nursing Corporation, P.C.

Andersen, M. D., & Smereck, G. A. D. (1994). *The art of nursing: The personalized nursing practice model workbook.* Plymouth, MI: Personalized Nursing Corporation, P.C.

Andersen, M., Smereck, G. A. D., & Braunstein, M. S. (1993). LIGHT model: An effective intervention model to change high-risk behaviors among hard-to-reach urban drug users. *The American Journal of Drug and Alcohol Abuse, 19*(3), 309–325.

Andersen, M. D., & Smereck, G. A. D. (1992, Summer). The consciousness rainbow: An explication of Rogerian field pattern manifestations. *Nursing Science Quarterly, 5*(2), 72–79.

Andersen, M. D., & Braunstein, M. S. (1992). Conceptions of therapy: Personalized nursing LIGHT model with chemically-dependent female offenders. In T. Mieczkowski (Ed.), *Drugs, crime, and social policy: Research, issues, and concerns* (pp. 250–262). Needham Heights, MA: Allyn & Bacon.

Andersen, M. D., & Smereck, G. A. D. (1989, Fall). Personalized nursing LIGHT model. *Nursing Science Quarterly, 2*(3), 120–130.

A P P E N D I X
B

Pursuit Health Formulas

Anne F. Darga, RN, MS, CS-FNP, President

Anne E. Oleszek, RN, BSN, Treasurer

Deborah A. Griffin, RN, MS, Secretary

Prior to January 1996, "entrepreneurship" was an intriguing concept that we hoped to have time to peruse one day. Having vested ourselves in the hospital environment for close to 20 years we were entrenched in the focus and intensity of a hospital system adapting to constant change. We had moved early on from care providers to managing our specialty areas, to directing our specialty service lines, and eventually to developing new business ventures across our organization's continuum. With each transition we accumulated a growing reservoir of experience and knowledge that we applied to our changing work scenarios. With each transition we also accumulated a growing sense of competency, self-confidence, and empowerment that came from successful planning and implementation of patient-centered initiatives. We were used to being leaders, enjoying the status, respect, and power associated with this role.

> You think you understand the situation, but what you don't understand is that the situation just changed.
>
> —*Putnam Investments advertisement*

And change it had! In the context of a usual routine meeting we learned that the organization was again restructuring, that the workforce would be downsized—and that our positions had been eliminated. We were being "economically separated" based on the threatened financial status of our health care system without any relationship to work performance and successful track record. Having positive and outstanding performance account abilities in the past did not influence the nebulous future. The transition to unemployment was numbing and not readily realized. The transformation into a new milieu was not an easy or timely task.

GETTING STARTED

The ensuing months were a period of grief, working through our losses of self-confidence, image, esteem, professionalism, and belongingness. During these months we began to visualize what our future could look like by delving into a world of unknowns that was previously out of our paradigm of a concrete health care system. We began to explore entrepreneurship. Because we each had the luxury of a severance package that cushioned us for a short time, we were able to take some time to search and think about what it was we really wanted to do. In the end it was our past, current, and professional relationships that led us to move toward resolution and action. Some of our initial steps were planned, but we found as many unplanned opportunities and, frankly, stumbled on others as we pushed ourselves toward resolution and action. No longer were we of the mindset of forever, of finding stability within an organization—we began to feel more comfortable with uncertainty and knew we had to develop our own options. Everything old began to look new again.

There was one given for us from the onset of our transition, one we are not sure was ever really overtly discussed. That given was a strong commitment to practice nursing. Our focus as nurses had changed several times over the course of our careers as we took on new and expanded roles. We viewed this current transition as yet another adaptation of our nursing focus, one that presented us with the unique challenge and opportunity of making a contribution to the profession through a completely new avenue while preserving the integrity of our personal lives.

As we made it known throughout our personal and professional networks that we were interested in working as "sole proprietors," work began to emerge for each of us. Professional contacts made during our years as practitioners, administrators, educators, and students in more traditional nursing environment, colleagues who cared about our success, and mentors with whom we had established permanent bonds resurfaced to offer support and opportunities. During these early projects we had each determined to work as a sole proprietor, each developing our own business entity. We would not say that a lot of planning went into this decision because our real focus and concern was on the work. With the freedom to entertain offers we began to individually accept projects and, in several cases, we jointly cooperated on completion of projects. As we left the employment of the inpatient facility, the vice presidents offered multiple consulting opportunities such as developing an organizational response to HCFA's Request for Proposal for Cardiology and Orthopedic Services. These opportunities offered a chance to transition gracefully from the inpatient environment into the world of consulting. However, we struggled with this unfamiliar, new style of working. Questions that needed to be addressed included: How do you price a job? How much information belongs in a contract or letter of agreement to protect your interests? Who does one partner with? The greatest challenge is to write outcome criteria for a specific job that are clear, achievable, commensurate with the pricing, and mutually agreed on with the client.

With respect to the logistics of our business, we have had to reinvent our work environment and processes in a similar fashion to other service industries around the country. The traditional bricks and mortar and systems and structures that dominate corporate America and American health care are not the norm for us. We have had to establish loosely structured mechanisms to manage and accomplish our work commitments. This structure is dynamic by necessity, but it has proven its worth in successful outcomes. Flexible ways of working, constant re-alignment of responsibilities, and fluctuating work teams are now the norm.

Unlike other consulting roles where looking for work in your field consumes 99% of your energy, our work emerged from our past and present professional contacts. With an abundance of potential contracts, we consistently found ourselves relying on each other and teaming with each other to accomplish our commitments. We began to revive a synergy that had begun in our hospital careers and whose foundation was the unique differences we each had to contribute to a project. We found that the sum of our talents was much more potent than working individually. It provided us each with ongoing support and motivation; it balanced our competencies and perspectives; it made work fun and fostered friendship and trust.

FINDING A NICHE

As early successes were realized and the team began to acquire the competencies, tools, and experience needed to compete in the world of health care consulting, we soon noted that finding work was not the issue, we needed to select the right work. We needed to find that niche that would eventually provide some long-term or consecutive contracts. However, we were not ready to totally give up on the assurance of secure income. Through one of the principal's proven track record with a large pharmaceutical company writing clinical overviews for various disease processes as a consultant working through her company, Darga Associates, an opportunity emerged to write a series of cardiac-focused home care training manuals for a large for-profit hospital corporation. This role involved much literature review, design, clinical writing, and outcomes research. The success of this project coupled with the identified need for integrated processes across the continuum of care for cardiac patients prompted the team to develop disease management initiatives. There emerged a confidence among the principals and close associates that fully integrated disease management processes are now and will continue to be the key driver of health care's next paradigm shift. The research and development of this product has been extensive, involving not only the companies' expertise but also the expertise of the multitalented staff at the pharmaceutical company.

DEFINING OUR PRODUCT

Disease management can be defined as a knowledge-based process intended to improve continuously the value of health care delivery for patient populations with chronic diseases from the perspective of those who receive, purchase, provide, supply and evaluate it.

Pursuit Health Formula Inc.'s concept of disease management is an opportunity to take a long-term perspective that optimizes outcomes and health status over the entire life cycle of the disease, decreasing the overall cost of treating patients with congestive heart failure (CHF) while improving clinical outcomes and stakeholder satisfaction. The company has focused on the initiative for CHF in part to build on the strengths of our current clinical and management talent and to augment existing programs and resources the company had previously developed. In addition, our experience and research recognized that most health care organizations were interested and presently involved in improving this area of practice.

THE CHF DISEASE MANAGEMENT INITIATIVE

Pursuit Health Formula's Disease Management Initiative comprises a full-continuum, multidisciplinary approach to coordinating optimizing care for the patient with CHF. The program is based on three core modules: Acute Care, Chronic Care and Comfort Care. Throughout the three modules are woven elements of care coordination, community resource coordination, and disease management. The three modules are interleaved in design, but allow participants to implement in stages or choose to implement only selected modules or components of modules. The program provides practical "how to" manuals that serve as "field reference guides" for a health system's or health plan's Disease Management Program Coordinator, individual intervention implementation plans, as well as instructor training tools to ensure greatest success.

Organizations investigating opportunities in CHF care are provided access to an assessment tool that guides the user in evaluating his current situation and identifying targeted opportunities for improvement. This return on investment (ROI) model estimates overall financial opportunity and assists the user to focus efforts where the greatest improvement may be obtained. With these targets established, the participating organization creates the program infrastructure including selection of program staff, a charter and budget for the endeavor, and a more detailed evaluation of the operations, programs, and effectiveness of the targeted areas. The ROI model allows the user to map a variety of programmatic scenarios, including implementation of only the acute care interventions, implementation of the outpatient interventions, as well as all interventions or specific interventions within one model. Through this iterative process, a health care executive can determine the breadth and depth of the CHF Disease Management Initiative that best serves the organization.

The Clinical Modules: Acute Care, Chronic Care, and Comfort Care

The two organizing principles for the Acute Care Module A are appropriate care and strong coordination. Module A targets best practices for triage, stabilization, diagnosis, treatment, monitoring, education, and discharge planning. Specialized tools are included to facilitate optimum outcomes.

The Chronic Care Module B focuses on aggressive management of the CHF patient the first 90 days following hospital discharge as well as optimizing outpatient management among all care providers. The organizing principles for this module are stabilizing the patient's physical status and empowering the patient to self-manage reducing the use of inpatient services. This initiative includes intensive follow-up during the first 30 days and identification of community support resources, CHF clinic opportunities, and telemanagement components are also included.

Module C, Comfort Care, is concerned with management of care when comfort and palliation become the primary goals. This module provides a process and tools for assessing changes in therapeutic intent. It guides the organization and care team in developing processes, support systems, and tools for facilitating the patient and family in managing end-of-life issues in the home/clinic setting. The organizing principles of this module are optimizing the level of comfort and well-planned choices for care and care settings as the disease progresses to the end-of-life phase.

Meaningful economic, clinical, and quality-of-life outcome measurement and reporting tools are integrated into the platform of care for CHF through the entire continuum of care. Outcome measurement assesses whether changes in behavior, clinical decision-making, and other processes have produced the results set previously by stakeholders-driven goals and against baseline measures. These measures are benchmarked against "best practices" in the field. Emergency room visits, lengths of stay, medication compliance rates, angiotensin-converting enzyme inhibitor utilization rates, use of comfort care protocol, inotropic infusion rates, dietary compliance rates, number of repeat diagnostic studies, and measures of functional ability are just a few potential indices that may be tracked.

Disease management concepts, such as those being developed by Pursuit Health Formulas, are possible in part because of the incredible growth of information technologies. Normative databases and aggregate data files have been collected in repositories across the country and this information is available for analysis. Benchmark performances are based on experience and published literature. Differences between the normative and benchmark performances illustrate the magnitude of opportunities. Pursuit Health Formula's business partners have facilitated access to large databases for information invaluable as we continue to developed our disease management products.

Our experiences with the Disease Management Initiative focused our company not only on CHF, which is becoming a niche for us, but also on the concept of chronic disease management across the spectrum of care. Both offer us the opportunity to practice nursing from a perspective that optimizes the health status and outcomes for patients over the entire life cycle of their disease. This positively affects the larger health system by decreasing the cost of treating patients and provides for the needs of all stakeholders involved in this arena.

OUR CUSTOMERS AND COMPENSATION

Interest in the disease management approach to patient care has emerged from the pharmaceutical industry, health plans and hospital systems, and individual hospitals and practitioners. Members of these entities have approached us to develop proformas and ROI models. Along with our corporate partners, we define the extent of our relationship with the customer in our contractual arrangements. We have made a number of site visits to present the CHF program and assess existing systems and processes. As we prepare proformas, knowing what to charge for our services has been a difficult area for us. There are industry standards for consulting service pricing that we have attempted to use. Because we offer a product that goes well beyond standard consulting relationships, we have had to consider different pricing strategies to include the cost of the product based on the value to individual clients. To determine the resources necessary to complete a project we have begun tracking our hours invested day to day, as time is our most valuable commodity. In addition, we have attended project management training and investigated software programs available as resources.

We have found that the variables involved in pricing strategies are multidimensional. We must consider at one level, the type of entity with whom we contract. At another level we must consider the dynamics of the relationship with our customer. For example, we may be working with a public agency or nonprofit organization with strict grant-driven guidelines for payment for consultation. Also level of consultation (i.e., technical, etc.) is a determinant in pricing strategies—developing an initiative that involves a conceptualization versus a more task orientation such as performing interviews for field study. In addition, when we provide consultation that includes our disease management product, this includes an additional pricing strategy. We have set prices for our product that relate to the relationship we establish with a particular health care entity similar to the relationship established with software application vendors. Often these relationships involve the need for ongoing product development; implementation strategies unique to a particular environment of care may involve communication over an extended period of time. The ROI model assists in determining these specific needs and often drives the initial pricing strategy.

Pricing for us also involves an intuitive process—feel out your client, determine the value of the project to the client, determine their funding source, and determine your personal commitment to the project in terms of time and in terms of opportunities you may be giving up to invest yourself in this project. Is there value added for you and your business? Does the project offer you the prospect of future business? Do you need the experience to enhance the value of your product?

Another approach to establish pricing for our product is to assume a degree of shared risk with the client based on the outcome of the project at various points in implementation. With the disease management platform of care, a strategy is to negotiate a percent of savings at 3, 6, or 12 months into the project. This assumes that specific and measurable data are gathered prior to implementation and change.

STRUCTURING OUR ENVIRONMENT TO SAVE MONEY

We made a conscious decision when we decided to pursue consulting that we wanted a unique and comfortable work environment. Because one of our partners had an empty nest, we were able to use an area in her large home as our base instead of renting expensive office space. This kept our overhead low as well as using outsourcing for printing and design. We were very fortunate in the beginning to have secured several well-paying projects that afforded us the luxury of not having to make a small business loan. We also received some up front monies to develop our key CHF initiative that enabled us to hire writers to assist us with this project. Marketing opportunities were also facilitated through collaboration with a large pharmaceutical company.

As consultants our work has been relatively low tech. Because we choose not to work in a traditional office setting we have embraced laptop technology for its ease of use and mobility. Because of the nature of our consulting the majority of our customers are located throughout the United States and we find that we have had to do some traveling when it is necessary to meet with our customers. In addition to our laptop technologies, we all have Internet access in our homes. We use this global networking technology to work collaboratively when needed. Each principal has fax and printing capabilities. We all share a copy machine at the base office.

THE FUTURE OF PURSUIT HEALTH FORMULA

Despite the success of this business endeavor, we have not put all our eggs in one basket. Other work continues to flow through our company and we struggle to schedule workload to accommodate our need for cash flow and to maintain contacts with clients for work. The combined synergy of the three principals allows the company to diversify its work schedule to accommodate multiple clients. For example, today, Deborah is off to a down-state hospital to complete interviews for an extensive patient and family education project the company took on earlier this spring while Anne, our editor-at-large, is at her cottage on Mackinac Island putting the finishing touches on the CHF Comfort Care Module readying the document for our looming publication date in September. Anne D. is fulfilling her responsibilities as a family nurse practitioner in a collaborative cardiology practice at the Burns Clinic Medical Center managing a full schedule of patients with CHF and postinterventional therapy.

We all agree as professional career nurses that, if you are dedicated to what you love, academically prepared, and have the energy and enthusiasm necessary you can overcome a restructuring and emerge confident and prepared to take on a whole work life. After the initial shock of being the target of a major corporate restructuring, the focus is on channeling energy generated by the experienced change into positive and productive directions. We chose to direct our energies toward aligning immediately with reality of the health care market pushing the organizations that we left to embrace even more radical change with respect to disease management and care delivery. Our opportunity required that we approach working in a whole different way with a new, yet intense, focus. This focus allowed us to continue to have a meaningful impact on health care as advanced practice nurses.

As we sit at our office in Harbor Springs and look out at Little Traverse Bay sipping coffee, returning calls, and working at our virtual and portable work stations we cannot help but think that with all its ups and downs life as independent consultants is indeed rewarding.

A P P E N D I X
C

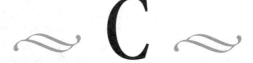

Wellspring Counseling

Erica Dutton, RN, MS, CS, Director

In January 1994, I entered an entirely new area of nursing practice. I became a business owner. I'm a clinical nurse specialist in psychiatric mental health nursing, certified in adult psychiatric-mental health nursing. I specialize in providing therapy to people who are dealing with chronic illness and pain so they can live well and find meaning, satisfaction, and enjoyment in life despite health problems. I own Wellspring Counseling and provide individual, couple, and group therapy as well as teach, consult, and publish a quarterly newsletter on coping with chronic illness called *Living Successfully, Your Resource on Chronic Illness.* I also work with people who are physically healthy, but are in transition or dealing with common life situations such as relationship, personal, or career problems. I've learned a tremendous amount in the past 6 years. Becoming a business owner has changed my perspective on nursing, altered how I view myself, and has re-energized my career.

Previously I worked as a therapist, educator, consultant, clinical nurse manager, and staff nurse, usually for other people. In the frustrating moments of my career, I fantasized about being my own boss, doing things my way without having to jump through hoops. I plotted, planned, and fantasized how wonderful it would feel, how much easier my job would be to do it my way!

I told myself there were practical reasons why I couldn't take the leap to business owner. First of all, I received a decent salary and benefits and seniority. I worked hard to develop respect and credibility in my organization. How could I give that up? How would I manage financially without a regular paycheck? What impact would running my own business have on me and my family. What if I fail?

Most important, I knew next to nothing about running a business. Previously, I'd worked as an independent contractor doing therapy and teaching, but never as my sole career. Those brief forays were just that, brief and temporary. Little did I know that life's circumstances would push me in a new direction.

THE START OF A NEW LIFE

About 15 years ago I was diagnosed with a chronic illness. For the first 8 years, my illness was a minor nuisance, only bothering me if I forgot to take my medications or tired of exercising. But gradually over the past 6 years, the symptoms grew worse and worse until I was forced to take a medical leave. What started as a short respite from work to get well, ended by changing my life.

I fully expected to be off work 6 weeks and then, completely cured, back in the saddle. After 3 months on leave, I was just beginning to feel better. However, I insisted on returning to work. The 12 weeks of the medical leave expired and I knew my job wouldn't be held any longer. Against medical advice, I returned to work part-time. I immediately got much worse and after 6 weeks of a steady downhill course, I left again, knowing I probably wouldn't return. I doubted there would be a place for me in the future.

This was my lowest point. I had tried everything to continue working and failed miserably. My denial about how sick I was evaporated and it terrified me. What was I going to do with the rest of my life? How was I going to pay my bills? What would happen to everything I had worked so hard to build and now had to leave? What would I do in the future? And worst of all, what if I couldn't work. Besides being in physical pain, emotionally I was drained.

Gradually, I dealt with my illness and denial and began to create a new life for myself within the limitations I faced. I began to feel better, physically and emotionally, but I was far from feeling 100%. I made some significant changes in my life. Then, I faced returning to work. My family and doctor urged me not to return to my previous job. Friends encouraged me to think about a private practice again and use what I learned about coping with chronic illness and pain to help others. I hesitated, not sure I was in a position to proceed. I realized a private practice would give me better control over my time, which was important for my health. With much anxiety and planning, I finally started. I opened my private practice, Wellspring Counseling, and began seeing clients.

What I learned on the business side fascinated, intrigued, thrilled, scared, excited, and challenged me. I highly recommend working independently to any nurse who has had visions of running her own show and being her own boss. It's a heady experience.

There's no better time than now to seriously consider working independently. Fewer nurses are being hired at hospitals, there's more demand for your services as the health care industry changes and I'm convinced the public wants to learn what you have to offer.

Now that I've enticed you in, I'll also tell you it's a lot of hard work with many risks and emotional demands. On the positive side, many resources are available to help you succeed.

INITIAL REACTIONS

My previous work experience didn't prepare me for being a business owner. I wasn't even sure I liked the idea of being a "business owner." All I wanted was to do therapy. Business owner sounded foreign and cold to me. I'd worked in hospitals, colleges, clinics, or agencies—as an employee, a health professional. I called myself a nurse, a clinical nurse specialist, a manager, an educator, anything but a business person.

I had a private practice, part-time and full-time for 12+ years, but I didn't view it as a business and I didn't run it as a business. There is a difference! I'd never *owned* a business and knew relatively little in a practical way about what it meant to "go on my own."

Other reactions stirred. Could I make it on my own? Even though I like doing things my way, I would have full and complete responsibility for my decisions, no colleagues to share the responsibility. I could ask other's opinions, but all decisions were mine. What if I made the wrong decisions? How would I deal with being outside an organization, on my own? Who would be my support system? Would I have the long-term perseverance and motivation to keep going.

I had strong reactions to the business language itself especially when I was asked what product or service I was *selling*. I felt more like a used car salesman than a professional nurse. I cared for patients, provided therapy, responded to their needs. I could promote an educational program or clinical service, but was far more uncomfortable promoting myself and my services.

Another word I was uncomfortable with was "profit." I was told over and over "it's okay to make a profit." I was used to providing quality care, not making a profit. Setting realistic fees for my services and calculating a "profit" were difficult. I thought of myself as a health professional who offered services where needed. Unfortunately, Consolidated Gas and the bank who held my mortgage still wanted to be paid in currency, not service. I again had to deal with my reactions and decide what is a fair profit and what is a fair price.

Which led me to another problem. I was used to caring for, teaching, or counseling anyone who came though the door, whether that be the hospital, clinic or agency door. Now the door was my office and I controlled who came through. How was I going to handle people who couldn't afford my services. If I gave it away, I would be out of business in no time and I would become resentful. But the service side of me wanted to give something back to the community. I had to find a way to balance the two and still be successful.

Setting fees, making a profit, pricing services, advertising, and selling myself evoked strong reactions in me. I asked many other health professionals how they dealt with it and after trial and error developed a way that fits for me. I also discovered that my reaction is a common one, especially for people who are in service occupations such as nursing, social work, or psychology. I eventually came to terms with my discomfort and integrated my values, ethics, and standards into what and how I "sell."

GETTING STARTED

How do you get started? What follows are some hard learned lessons. Use what is applicable to your business and discard the rest. Seek many opinions, but remember they are just that, opinions. You have to do what you think is right for you and your business.

First of all, you need **solid nursing skills.** Don't even think about venturing on your own without them. Make sure your level of educational preparation and years of experience are sufficient for what you want to embark on. There is so much to learn in the business world, you don't want the additional stress of lack of skills, knowledge or confidence in your particular area of nursing to distract you. Today's environment is ripe for small business owners but it's very risky. Almost 80% of small businesses fail within the crucial first 3 to 5 years. At the same time, more people than ever are opening their own business, particularly women, so don't let the failure rate stop you. Plan well and go for it!

Learn all you can about starting and running a small business. The Small Business Administration was immensely helpful to me. Because your taxes paid for the Small Business Administration, there are no fees, so take advantage of it. They helped me start my business and continue to provide concrete help and support such as:

- Writing a business plan
- Designing marketing materials
- Developing and implementing a marketing plan
- Pricing services
- Establishing a financial record keeping system
- Dealing with taxes and IRS
- Managing cash flow

They connected me with accountants, legal advisors, and other business people. They also helped me get into a year-long mentoring program. I attended workshops on "Running a Successful Small Business" from a local university and I joined two women's business organizations where I could network with others and continue to learn from them.

This preparation helped me **focus** my business. I had many interests and skills, but I couldn't do it all in one business. There needed to be a coherent focus that the public could easily identify. I had to narrow the range of my interests and skills to one or two related areas.

Ask yourself: What specific skill do I possess? Do I think others would pay for it? What is unique about my business? How does it stand out from my competition?

Describe your business in writing and explain it to others without professional jargon, generalities, or vague promises of well-being and improved health. Be specific and concrete. Try explaining it to a lay person or a 12-year-old child. Do they understand it? If not, keep working on how you explain your business to others.

I was told I needed to explain my business in 30 seconds or less, the **"elevator speech."** That's the time it takes an elevator to travel several floors. Thirty seconds is all the time you have to spark an interest. Longer than that and people get glassy eyed and drift off. It sounds silly but this piece of advice has helped me introduce myself at professional meetings and networking groups, or to potential clients and referral sources. You have 30 seconds to grab people's attention, that's all. Most people are too busy to give more than that. Narrowing and focusing your business to one or two areas will enable you to give a crisp, professional, easy to understand 30 second speech.

Translate skills you've already developed as a nurse to help build your business. One of a nurses's best skills is our natural networking ability. We do it every day as a staff nurse, manager, educator, or administrator. Networking is how nurses get work done. This skill will prove invaluable as you develop your business and is the single most important skill I possess to increase visibility and referrals.

Don't limit yourself to **networking** within the nursing, health care, or medical profession. I found a gold mine of advice and support in real estate, banking, retail, advertising, office services, marketing . . . and in any other field. Nonhealth care people have a unique perspective we don't have. Besides, if your clients are the public, these are your potential clients. If they're not, they may lead you to clients.

In very practical ways, nonhealth care professionals gave me valuable feedback on my marketing materials. For instance, if they couldn't understand my elevator speech or my written materials, I needed to change them. One person thought "chronic illness" meant terminal illness. Another thought I helped people get medical treatment or jobs. If lay people are going to be reading my marketing materials, it needs to be written in language they understand, not "medicalese." My contact with nonhealth care professionals forced me to explain myself to people without health care jargon. It also helped me explain to health professionals who were not familiar with therapy and how therapy could help.

Establish a **referral base.** Develop, nurture and maintain regular contact with your referral sources. Most of my referrals come from physicians, other psychotherapists, physical therapists and massage therapists. But a significant number come from word of mouth via my clients, community groups, and people I have met at Chamber of Commerce meetings, women's business meetings, and even the grocery line.

Don't forget nonprofit organizations and trade organizations as a referral source. I offered my services to the Arthritis Foundation for **visibility** purposes as well as to give something back to the community. In turn, the Arthritis Foundation sent me referrals and offered me opportunities to speak at local and state groups and conferences, which helped expand my visibility. Look for opportunities to become visible in the community. Become known as the expert: offer to speak at agencies, schools, hospitals, and community groups as well as professional groups.

Learn to **advertise** on a shoestring budget, because most likely that's all you'll have in the beginning unless you're independently wealthy or the bank gives you a hefty loan. I had to be extremely careful with how I spent my advertising monies. Other therapists were very helpful in what worked for them and what didn't. Sometimes I advertise, not because it brings in clients but because it keeps me visible in the community. The Small Business Administration told me it takes at least seven repetitions before someone acts on what they read or see. Some of my clients have heard me speak several times or saved articles and press releases from the newspaper for months before they finally called for an appointment.

Learn about your clients. Be able to describe them in detail— age, gender, socio-economic status, location, attitudes, beliefs—everything. The more you know about them, the better you can target your advertising and your services.

Focus not on what services or products you offer, but how your clients can **benefit.** This is a slightly different facet but a powerful tool in advertising. My credentials, the type of services I offer and my skills were less important than the benefits they receive by seeing me. I can help them regain control over their life, find enjoyment and satisfaction, learn to manage pain and fatigue, and create a new life. Benefits capture their attention, not my degrees, years of experience, previous jobs or even the services I provide. These are important and they ask questions about them too, but what captures their attention first is how will it benefit them.

EMOTIONAL DEMANDS

Since I began working on my own, I soon began missing the daily contact with fellow professionals. When I worked at a hospital or clinic, the normal course of my day would bring me in contact with many people. I didn't even have to walk far. Now I was isolated. I had no one readily available, other than my husband, and I couldn't rely on him as my sole support system. Alone, doubts crept in about my decisions. Could I do this alone? What's the best way to handle this? Is this a good idea? I could make any decision I wanted without jumping through hoops now, but sometimes I yearned to be able to talk it over with someone else. And who would that someone else be?

Start early and develop a **support system.** There was so much to do and my energy and stamina were still quite low so it was easy for me to postpone building a new support system. I eventually found I had to schedule weekly contacts with people or I would be alone except for my clients and my husband. Sometimes I met to discuss ideas, brainstorm, or talk about problems or concerns. Other times it was just to relax and talk about the weather or what we did for fun. Nurture and maintain a healthy support system and draw from a variety of businesses for your support system.

Try to maintain some **balance** in your life. Many of today's management guru's talk about having a passion for your work—live, eat, sleep, breathe your work. That's not a passion; it's an obsession. Your new business is exciting, thrilling, time consuming, and demanding and requires hard work. But if you want to succeed in the long run, personally as well as financially, find some balance. Don't become so obsessed with your business that you talk or think about nothing else. If you are single minded to the point of obsession, you can be boring. Don't forget about your friends who have nothing to do with your business. They provide a refreshing and much needed respite.

The stress of starting a new business not only affects you but also affects your **family.** The director of the Small Business Administration asked me how my husband felt about my new venture. He stressed that without the support of my husband, my chances of success were greatly reduced. Family are intimately affected by how your business is doing. When the money doesn't come in, they are affected. When you succeed, they are affected. When you're discouraged or angry about how the business is doing, they are affected. You need to know they will be in your corner offering support and encouragement, not saying "I told you so" or Why don't you do something else."

In every business, at every stage there are **rough times,** particularly in the beginning. Declining cash flow, seasonal changes in business, canceled appointments, lost clients, and gaps in referrals are just a few of the rough times. They test your commitment to your business and your "stick-to-it-tiveness." Rough times are inevitable. No business is smooth sailing. I know, I've had them. I've asked lots of people how they managed theirs. How will you manage them? Sometimes, staying at your desk is the worst thing you can do. Continuing to do what you did yesterday and the day before, plugging away, putting one foot in front of the other can lead to a downward spiral in energy, commitment, and creativity. Get away for awhile—go to a park or indulge in a long leisurely lunch at your favorite restaurant. This will allow you to see things from a new perspective, to refuel and nourish your creative side.

Then take **action.** Determine what is causing the problem and do something about it now! My rough times come when referrals drop off. Most often I've been neglecting marketing, which is one of my weak areas. When I get referrals, I tend to take it easy. Wrong! I need to pay consistent attention to this part of my business, developing new ideas, new angles, and new services.

PERSONAL CHARACTERISTICS FOR SUCCESS

A successful business owner isn't smarter than others and doesn't take more risks. Being lucky isn't necessary either. Personal characteristics for success are initiative, drive, self-motivation, determination, and a willingness to ask for help. These qualities will help you be a success.

There is no one to tell you to get up and go to work today, no one to ask for your monthly report or make assignments for you. On beautiful spring days, you still have to find the motivation to work. *You* have to provide the initiative. Your excitement and need for money will help, but you still need strategies for the stretches of days or weeks when things aren't going well or when the results of your work haven't paid off yet. Balance them with periods of R & R.

One of the wonderful things about having your own business is you make all the decisions. You don't have to ask permission from anyone else. But don't get so full of yourself that you don't ask for help along the way. Asking for and receiving feedback is key to staying in touch with reality. One of my most painful experiences was taking my marketing materials to the director of the small business program at a local university. I worked long and hard on them and was proud of what I accomplished. I knew there was room for improvement, but I was pleased with my efforts so far.

Unfortunately, the director was not pleased at all. He launched into a detailed diatribe of what I did wrong and then invited his secretary and other office staff to witness my humiliation. He regaled them with my shortcomings. He criticized everything—the color of ink, the choice of design, the wording, the tone, the style . . . you name it. I alternated between humiliation and outrage at his insensitivity and crudeness. Frankly, I wanted to choke him. Somehow, I decided I would listen to what he had to say with as much control as I could muster, take what was useful, and tell him to jump in the lake. All the way home, I ranted and raved at him, threatening him with gross bodily harm. If I had a voodoo doll, I would have stuck pins in it!

I must be a masochist, because I attended another workshop led by him a month later. (I already paid for it.) He invited me to be open about my experience when I consulted him. I hesitated, but he invited me to be truthful, so I was. He agreed he was lacking in social skills.

The truth was, I was approaching the brochure the wrong way. His ideas were very helpful and I ended up producing a much better brochure. Most of the time, people aren't so brutal and often they're very helpful. The Director of the Small Business Administration impressed on me, this was my business, my choices, my way. He would give me lots of input, but I make the final decision. This piece of advice helped me avoid throwing out valuable advice given by rude and crude people.

I belong to a women's business owners meeting and every month guest speakers talk about various aspects of developing and running a small business. I take every opportunity to ask for feedback on my ideas. Others are too shy, but I often get good advice from successful people in marketing, computers, advertising, or finance, just by asking. People want to help, particularly other women. Take advantage of new and different ideas, choosing which ones made sense and leaving obnoxious personalities and advice that doesn't fit your business behind.

Last, take care of your own health. As someone who has a chronic illness, I can't afford to ignore this. My body responds very quickly if I ignore it. In some ways that's a blessing. If you don't have any health problems, avoid them in the future by maintaining balance, eating right, sleeping well, exercising, and all the things we know about and sometimes fail to implement in our own lives.

OH, TO DO IT OVER AGAIN!

Hindsight is perfect! If I had it to do over again, I would do many things differently. At the very least, I wish I understood the process of developing a business better. Here are a few lessons I learned.

I underestimated the time it took to make a profit. Most businesses fail because they don't have adequate cash flow to get them through start up, usually considered 3 to 5 years. I felt very discouraged when people didn't rush to my door like I anticipated. I was a good therapist, why didn't they see that!

I grossly underestimated the time and cost to produce my newsletter. Though it was a great marketing tool, it took a lot of time. I priced the newsletter so low it was difficult to raise the price later to cover costs and make a profit.

I underestimated the value of the newsletter. Because the information seemed basic to me, I thought it was basic to others. After I produced a few issues and got some feedback, I realized I was wrong. I couldn't double my subscription rates all at once, even though I needed to. For a long time it was unprofitable. I later asked my family and friends to tell me what they thought it was worth. I was surprised how much they were willing to pay. Most thought I was giving it away and I could almost double my subscription rates. Setting fees is one of the hardest things to do. Even though there are formulas to help you price accurately, I still struggle over this.

Ethical issues are one of the toughest to sort out. My "core business" was therapy, but I received many requests to sell products that others considered a natural extension of my "core business," such as vitamins or supplements. I've been approached by a number of people to sell these products as well as herbs, comfort and support devices, or other products related to chronic illness and pain. People who approach me are ardent believers in their product, often telling me how it helped them personally and could help many other people.

I was tempted to try some of their products. After all, I would love to find a cure. But I felt very uncomfortable selling them to clients. I thought it was a conflict of interest and detracted from my role as a therapist. You may also face similar problems, especially when you are in health care and your stamp of approval enhances a product. Initially I was not firm enough in how I handled this. Later, I decided I was not going to sell any products, period. I was very clear with all requests up front, no hedging. I have solid legal, ethical, and therapeutic reasons and I've never regretted this decision.

THE FUTURE . . .

What does the future hold for me? I hope a growing business including more writing, clinical work, and teaching, especially to health professionals.

I'm glad I pursued my own business. I was thrown into it, out of necessity because I couldn't work at my previous position. I had a chronic illness and the demands and hours were beyond my physical abilities. Starting and running a small business is not easy either. I had to move more slowly because I no longer had almost unlimited energy. It's been very satisfying and professionally challenging. I continue to learn a tremendous amount, not only about the business side, but the clinical side too. My understanding of how people cope with life-changing illnesses and chronic pain have multiplied geometrically. I feel I've found my niche. I can continue to work professionally, take care of my health, control my time, teach, consult, and do therapy.

If you've dreamed of running your own business, now is the time for you to act on it. Get prepared before you quit your job. Talk to people, go to workshops, learn from others, do what you need to increase your chance of success. Then go for it. Good luck!!!

For more information, contact Erica Dutton, RN, MS, CS, Director, Wellspring Counseling.

APPENDIX

D

Insight Telehealth Systems, Inc.

Ilene Warner, RN, C CWCN MA MLSP NHA

Vice-President, Clinical Applications, Insight Telehealth Systems, Inc.

Unlike most of my neighborhood friends, I did not envision myself going into nursing after high school. My father had worked at the CBS-TV station in Philadelphia all my life and I intended to go into communications, seeing myself as a television weather personality. He was quite firm in his opinion that I would likely never succeed in this area and that I should attend nursing school. I eventually went to a diploma nursing program, a bachelor's degree, and three master's degrees. My entire nursing career focused on geriatric patients.

I spent some time in the 1980s as visiting nurse in North Philadelphia. It had occurred to me that as a home care nurse, I spent a great deal of time doing activities that actually took me away from my patients, activities such as driving in traffic jams, finding a safe place to park, and dealing with the weather. Once I finally got into my patient's home, I was not always able to render care on my timeline. I often had to compete with the patient's television to get his or her attention. I also was inundated with paperwork that at times was duplicative. I was sure there must be a better way to be able to carry out my work, spend more time with my patients, and actually improve the way in which health care was delivered.

Twenty years after my father convinced me to become a nurse, I had the opportunity to meet a team of people who were interested in creating a telemedicine system for home health care. The system involved the transmission of audio, video, vital signs, and data, a kind of "mini-television" communication using a client terminal and a clinical station that connected through a single telephone line. Although telemedicine had been around since the 1960s, there had been little effort to use technology to assist home care nurses and patients. I thought the goal should be that technology could be used as a tool to stretch the reach of the nurse.

In essence, the electronic or video visit would replace some of the physical visits the nurse was expected to make to the patient. This would decrease the amount of "windshield" time, but it was also important to actually improve the quality of the nursing visit. This would be accomplished by having a feature on the system, which would remind patients when to take their medications. The system would register when patients took the medications as well as when they did not. For the first time, we could actually deal with issues of noncompliance directly. We could ask patients why medications were not taken and we could address issues such as denial, forgetfulness, cost, side effects, and access.

As a visiting nurse, I frequently made early morning visits to patients, gathered vital sign data, and made assessments regarding their response to medications. What was unknown at the time was the response of the patient to medications, position changes, and other factors throughout the course of the day. What was the effect of antihypertensive agents on the blood pressure after dinner or at bedtime? We had no data, no ability to capture vital signs at off-hours. We had a "slice of life" visit, but little more. Using telehealth, we were actually able to gather patient's vital signs throughout the course of the day. We could teach patients to go to their client station and obtain their own signs. Moreover, we could tailor the medication regime and the dosing times to minimize orthostatic hypotension and other drug-related side effects.

Finally, we could use the comfort that patients have with the television to educate them about their disease processes, signs and symptoms of disease, diet, and medications. Would it improve a patient's ability to retain health-related information if it were delivered using multimedia? Instead of giving a patient a list of foods high in sodium, viewing a clip about foods that are high in sodium may enhance our teaching tools.

My excitement in the field, however, is not always met with open arms. Many are skeptical about delivering health care through these technologies. An old friend, Betsy, who has been doing home care for over 10 years refused my invitation to see the system I helped develop. She was still reeling from being displaced from the hospital and now felt threatened about the possible loss of her job or of control over her situation and was not at all interested in considering telehealth for home care. Others believe it is a good idea, but are waiting for reimbursement from the Health Care Financing Administration, particularly for Medicare patients.

At the present time, my company has received a grant to develop a prototype cardiac disease management system. While we are pursuing sales from home care agencies, social service agencies, and independent disease state management groups, I continue to practice as a wound care consultant for a number of home health care agencies. My career has finally come full circle as my interest in communications has been combined with nursing in the delivery of telehealth services. My only regret is that my father died from cancer just before my company was established. I somehow think that he would have been pleased with the way in which my career has evolved.

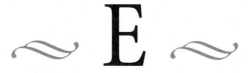

APPENDIX
E

Parish Nursing: A Health and Wholeness Ministry

Sandra R. Byers, Ph.D., RN, CNAA

Parish Nurse and Health and Wholeness Director

PARISH NURSING

Parish nursing is a distinctive and emerging new opportunity for community practice nurses. It requires the planning, organizing, implementation, and evaluation skills similar to beginning a small business. It is a rewarding and challenging service because it has the potential of fulfilling the holistic needs of parishioners *and* of offering the full expertise of the professional nurse. I was unemployed after over 30 years in various health care positions and volunteered to help our pastor and congregation. A new program dealing with health and wholeness was mentioned and my venture began. This is the story of how we planned and developed a health and wholeness ministry and I became the church's first parish nurse and health and wholeness director.

As with any new business, there must be an idea and vision and the energy and desire to make that vision reality. Two individuals aware of the wholistic health needs of the congregation were the catalysts; an RN who is an active church leader and an Interim Associate Pastor. They were intimately in touch with the members and familiar with organized health care, i.e., hospitals, outpatient services, home health, and extended-care facilities. Health promotion and illness prevention efforts are not always emphasized in these settings let alone the body, mind, and soul connection. Because of their enthusiasm, they were able to "sell" the general idea to the pastor. Also, the national church organization was emphasizing health activities as an important area for churches, considering its history and the current state of health care.

STRUCTURE

Following discussions with these individuals, a proposal for a Ministry of Health and Wholeness was developed that included:

- Church philosophy
- Purpose
- Objectives
- Proposed structure
- Evaluation/assessment
- Resources
- Program ideas

This proposal was presented to the church's governing body, the Session, and received approval for an 18-month trial period. Then, members to serve on a Health and Wholeness Committee were appointed and convened, similar to a board. Operating guidelines were developed on:

- General committee operations
- Responsibilities of committee chair, vice chair, and secretary
- Member selection and responsibilities
- Health and wholeness director/parish nurse responsibilities

The Health and Wholeness Ministry is guided by a committee of 12 individuals with diverse health care backgrounds, plus a lawyer and a member with no professional connection to the health care field.

The Health and Wholeness Committee meets 10 times a year and members are asked to serve for 3 years. Initial members were asked to serve varying tenures to develop a strong base. Church members with special interests or expertise are asked to plan activities and many other church members volunteer. A congregational health survey completed in March 1997 provided the assessment needed to identify specific activities and programs desired. A review of over 2 years of clergy visitation cards was made to identify typical congregational problems and needs. The Ministry works in collaboration with other church programs and staff.

MISSION

The Ministry of Health and Wholeness is based on the church's mission statement, "Then the King will say to those at his right hand, come O blessed of my father, inherit the kingdom prepared for you from the foundation of the world: for I was hungry and you gave me drink, I was a stranger and you welcomed me, I was naked and you clothed me. I was sick and you visited me, I was in prison and you came to me" (Matthew 25:34). The objectives are to:

1. Promote the psychological, physical, and spiritual needs of members in all church activities and programs.
2. Deliver all services calling on the enabling grace and presence of God through prayer, scripture reading and Christian caring, and using Jesus' healing ministry as our example.
3. Reach out as Christians to individuals in need of health information, counseling and guidance, support and encouragement.
4. Provide a means for networking within the church and larger community to achieve effective and efficient use of services and expertise.
5. Educate and train volunteers to assist with this Ministry.

As the Ministry developed and grew, three focus areas were identified: education, service and outreach. Members were asked to serve in one of these specific areas. Examples of congregational activities are:

- *Service:* monthly blood pressure screening on Sunday mornings, a Healthy Weight program, a support group for individuals who are or have experienced a loss, a walking group, and a dance group. CPR information sessions were held.
- *Education:* three series of Sunday adult education classes ranging from 5 to 10 weeks each and including a wide range of health promotion topics were conducted; how to help yourself become or stay healthy in body, mind and soul, stress prevention, meditation, communicating with teenagers, values clarification, coping with depression, and "Living Independently as a Senior."

  A special program on "You and Your Medications" was held in conjunction with the Ohio State University College of Pharmacy and the Grant/Riverside Hospital Church Partnership Division to educate members about their medications and questions they should be asking their health care providers to assure that they understand and take all medicines properly.

  A Health and Wholeness Resource Center (Figure AE.1) includes current health and wellness books that underscore personal responsibility for health and ways to achieve personal health goals. Pamphlets on various life situations are available and are popular because of their practical and spiritual guidance.

  A health information bulletin board features different health issues and bimonthly articles are written for the weekly newsletter. These articles emphasize places where health information or services such as immunizations can be obtained or news about a specific health concern, or where the first aid or fire equipment is located in the church.
- *Outreach:* two health fairs were held including one with many basic health screens and mammography screening, a program on Medicare HMOs was co-sponsored with the local senior center and featured a guest speaker from the Ohio Department of Insurance, and Advance Directives, the living will,

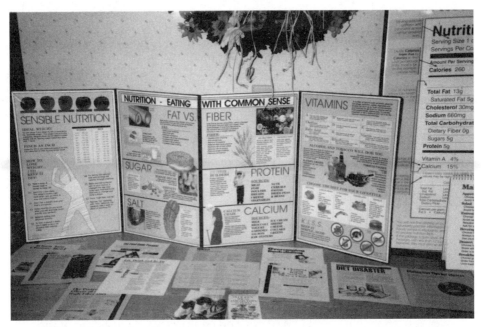

Figure AE.1 Health and wholeness resource center.

durable power of attorney for health care and organ donation, were presented by a panel composed of a lawyer, chaplain, nurse, and physician. A new church Web site includes a distinct Health and Wholeness section with access numbers for health information and local emergency and information telephone numbers.

THE CONGREGATION

The majority of our 1,750 members are white, middle-class, "suburban professionals." There is minimal cultural or economic diversity. The family composition varies; single moms and single dads with children, singles, divorcees, couples of all ages, some with close family connections and others with none. All ages are present and are represented in church functions.

WHAT DOES THE PARISH NURSE DO?

At the start of this new service, the consensus of staff and committee members was the position should be called Health and Wholeness Coordinator and parish nursing was to be a part of the position. It was not to be interpreted or perceived by the congregation as a "hands-on," hospital, or medical model of providing care. After approximately 1 year, the coordinator title was changed to Director. In implementing the various roles and demonstrating its value for the congregation and staff, the position includes many kinds of services, not just coordination.

The Health and Wholeness Director is expected to:

- Work under the accepted theology of the church and the governing body
- Be an experienced licensed professional nurse who has worked in various clinical settings with diverse age populations
- Be committed to helping persons throughout the life cycle meet their total health needs—body, mind, and spirit
- Evaluate and assess health needs of individuals and of the congregation
- Be knowledgeable about community health resources and referral patterns
- Be knowledgeable about the Parish Nursing Standards and strive to maintain those standards.

Terms of Service and Accountability

The Health and Wholeness Director/Parish Nurse volunteers about 20 hours per week and reports to the Pastor. The Director staffs the Health and Wholeness Ministry and carries out additional activities such as home and hospital visits and personal health counseling. Congregation members are the primary clients, but nonmembers are also served as requested. There is no charge for the services. Travel expenses are paid and there is a designated Health and Wholeness budget to cover educational materials, speakers, and equipment as a line item of the church's yearly budget. A budgeted paid part-time staff position is proposed.

Implementation of the Service

The church environment has been perceived as a respected and "safe" place for its members. There are few encumbrances in giving to others and implementing the position and services of a parish nurse using clinical and management skills.

The parish nurse assists individuals to integrate their body, mind, and soul and achieve their highest level of health and well-being. This is accomplished through the nursing process of assessment, diagnosis, outcome identification, planning, implementation, and evaluation.

Assessment in this setting means identifying the parishioners' immediate physical, mental, and spiritual needs that are voiced and desired via conversations, questions and observations. Planning occurs by facilitating the parishioners being in control of their situation and using all their resources to achieve desired results and using other health care providers and services as necessary. Planning is an important task of the committee. Implementing the plan usually means providing resources to accomplish what they cannot do for themselves using family, neighbors, the expanded church family, and community resources. Evaluating results or outcomes is accomplished via direct contact either by telephone or in person. Attendance by the parish nurse in a local forum of parish nurses organized by a local health care system not only assists in evaluating the church's program but provides a mechanism for peer support and evaluation.

APPENDIX
F

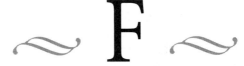

Reflections on My Journey to Private Practice as a Small Business

Christine M. Smith

A Nurse Consultant in Melbourne, Australia

PRELUDE TO THE JOURNEY

For the 8 years prior to my sudden departure from the world of full-time employment I had been a member of a professional organization of nurses in private practice. In that time I had listened to many of their stories and had seen a few decide, after a while, that for one reason or another it was too difficult to continue or that they missed the support and structure of an organization. I had been tinkering with the idea of starting my own business for a number of years and had, several years before, conducted a small consultancy to assist a nurse who had been working part-time in her own business as a clinician.

My vision was to run my nursing practice as a business. I anticipated that there would be a great deal to learn about running a business. I now know that learning would range from understanding where my income would come from, to keeping track of my accounts, to paying the monthly bills, to keeping a roof over my head, and to staying healthy. The enormity of what this could mean may have, but did not, overwhelm me.

For a long time I have thought it important to consider the integration of the four domains of nursing practice into my nursing role. That philosophy has been extended into my business philosophy, making it easier to develop a diverse business plan and to generate the level of income that allows a consultant to survive while the business becomes established. Maybe the issue that keeps many nurses locked into a regular job is knowing where to start and how to take the first step on the journey to private practice. Indeed, starting a business venture is like taking a journey to a new place.

ASSESSING WHAT IS NEEDED FOR THE JOURNEY

I initially assessed three areas in preparation for my journey to a business venture: personal, financial and legal, and professional resources available to me.

Personal Resources

On the evening of departure from the world of traditional employment and my decision to step out on my own, I called my family and broke the news about my former job, and put forward my plans. Everyone supported my plan and some even said that I should have done this sooner. It was more than encouraging to know that I had their support.

I knew my professional integrity was intact and that gave me great confidence to step out the next day. Along with that integrity and confidence I had a wealth of experience in nursing. I had had the opportunity to take part in the planning and implementation of several projects and, therefore, knew what was expected and what level of commitment was required to go out and deliver a service as an independent consultant or contractor. I also had initiative, time, and imagination.

Financial and Legal Resources

On my first day in business I called my accountant/CPA to let him know what I was doing. He provided advice on what I might need to think about and do in the short term from a taxation and financial perspective. He also called several times over the next couple of months to ask how things were going. There are a number of issues to be addressed with one's accountant/CPA, so it is preferable to seek that advice and support at the beginning of the journey rather than waiting until you take a wrong turn and need to spend valuable time back-tracking and getting reoriented. Better still if you already have an accountant who knows you and the financial aspects individual to you. This is especially important in terms of any capital you have to invest in the business, when to file your tax returns, and how to keep track of your professional and personal income and expenditures.

I also called my lawyer and discussed the issues I needed to consider from a legal perspective, e.g., the business structure I needed to establish, when it would be appropriate to do this, and what work might be entailed with the various options. He also advised on how to handle contracts, invoices, and late payments. A separate but important issue is that of insurance for both professional indemnity and public liability.

Your accountant and lawyer are in a way your travel consultant and sherpa on the timing and the processes to follow on your journey. They look after the ever-moving financial, legal and legislative scenery you pass, so that you can concentrate on the journey, i.e., the core of your business. And every so often you need to rendezvous with them and talk about the journey—about new paths to explore, new vistas to contemplate, and the provisions you may need to plan to pick up.

One of the major issues nurses have to come to terms with when setting up businesses is that professional advice comes at a price. Just as you will charge a fee for your nursing service so do other professionals. From a business perspective that expenditure is an investment in your business. You are their client and they are there to provide the best advice for a fee. The more they know of you and the vision for your business, the easier it is for them to assist you to realize your vision.

Professional Resources

On the first day of my business, I also called a few of my close friends to tell them what had happened and what was about to occur. Within 48 hours I had my first consultancy, which was a small but a very positive reinforcement. As part of the redundancy from my previous employment I was given a 3-month outplacement with a large human resource consulting organization. At my first meeting with my outplacement consultant I made it clear that I was not seeking support to find another job. I needed support to set up my own business. I used those 3 months and the resources provided in that organization as a platform to launch my business. My *minder* (business mentor) for those 3 months provided valuable opportunities each week for reflection on how things were going, what other aspects I needed to explore and, importantly, encouragement from an objective perspective.

I knew that I had a good professional network. When I assumed my previous position, I had purposefully joined a couple of professional organizations to get to know some of the nurse leaders in that city. Not long after joining one of these organization I joined one of the working committees and through that membership met many nurses. During that 8 years I devoted much time and energy to the organization. The time and energy were well spent.

SETTING UP THE BASE CAMP (MY HOME OFFICE)

I decided I would initially need to work from home because I was not sufficiently confident nor did I have the cash flow to lease office space. At that time I did not know about business incubators. Business incubators, an important new development in small business, provide new business owners with office space and facilities to use on an "as-needed" basis at reasonable rates until the business is established.

Working at Home

Within my small apartment I allocated specific space to be used as an office. Over several weeks I set up a home office which included: acquiring a computer, printer, and a fax/answering machine. In addition I set up a file of business contacts, a filing system for current clients, an archive system for completed projects and business records, and proformas for stationery such as letters, invoices, and fax cover sheets. Space for records is a continuing problem so at the conclusion of a project I discard everything except the essential information I may need in the future. Over time my home office has grown and I now find I either need to move or find office space close to where I live. More decisions!

Initially I used my own name as the business name. When, sometime later I decided to register a smart new name, I was advised by my business mentor in the small business course that it probably was not a wise action because everyone knew my business by my name and if that disappeared, and was replaced by another, no one would recognize the new name nor connect it with my business.

Other items for day-to-day business should include a diary, mobile or cellular phone or pager, a list of business contacts, a supply of business cards, and other supplies such as pens for a white board or overhead slide, stapler, and paper clips. At the end of the day I empty the briefcase and pack only the items I will need the next day.

Camp Discipline

I knew that working from home would require discipline to focus on the business and not be distracted by interruptions and other interests. When working from home it is very easy to put off doing your work while you catch up on those projects around the house that have been waiting to be done. Then there are the people who call or drop by to have a chat because they know I am at home. The fact that they would not do so if I were in a traditional work environment seems irrelevant to them. The best way I have learned to deal with people who drop by is to say politely but firmly and without apology that I am not able to talk because I am working but that I will call soon to catch up. Most people respect my directness and comply with my request.

DECIDING WHAT TO PACK FOR THE JOURNEY

Over the years of traveling during my career I have learned to travel light. When one goes on a journey there is always some baggage one needs to leave behind. Excess baggage weighs you down and it can also cost money. Although I knew what baggage I needed to leave behind if I was to succeed, I was not so sure what it was I needed to pack. During the first 8 months of my journey I felt I was flying by the seat of my pants. But, I knew that one of the skills I needed to acquire was some plan to help me run the day-to-day operation as well as the longer term aspects of my business.

The Business Plan (Map to the Future for Nurses in Business)

When I first started out on my journey I didn't know that one of the most fundamental and important tools I would need in my private practice bag was a business plan. It is interesting to reflect on all the stories of success and perseverance of nurses' ventures into private practice I have heard over the years. Two aspects strike me as interesting. First, the emphasis on private practice, i.e., nurses who earn income from independent sources and the freedom that gives to nurses to put their philosophy, goals, and vision into practice—freedom from many of the constraints imposed by bureaucratic organizations. The second aspect is the connection between the notion of private practice and what they were trying to create—a viable business which would provide income, security, and a future. I often wonder if some of the early pioneers lasted through the down times and kept their dream alive because they had some plan, i.e., a map to guide them through the wilderness of setting up and managing a business.

One of the most frequently asked questions by nurses who call to talk about private practice is "How do I get started?" Remember it was Alice in Wonderland who asked which way to go. The Cheshire Cat replied that it depended on where she wanted to go, and if she didn't know, then any road would take her there.

Learning About a Business Plan

I decided that to both expedite my goal and to be more sure of the direction I should be taking it would be worthwhile enrolling in a small business course that included the development of a business plan. It was a very busy 8 weeks as I did the course on a full-time basis, juggled some part-time teaching and a 10-day trip to the United States toward the end of the course to attend the Center for Nursing Leadership Program. My colleagues at the Center helped me keep my sense of humor during this hectic time. I wrote much of the plan on long flights, in airports waiting for connecting flights, and late into many nights at the Center. It was an exhilarating experience. I received the 'frequent flyer' award from my fellow students at the graduation of the class.

At the time I was already 8 months into my business and this experience proved helpful especially in terms of conducting the market research and setting out the elements of the projected income and expenditure. I had developed my nursing philosophy statement several years before as a graduate student and this became my customer service statement. At the conclusion of the course I had to do a 40-minute presentation of my plan to a panel of experienced small business owners who had no background in health care. At the presentation I felt very confident, I could answer all their questions, proud that I had accomplished this goal, and reassured that I had a plan for the next 3 years.

The Retirement Plan

In most of the texts we read about preparing a business plan there is rarely any mention of a retirement or postbusiness plan. There is a crucial need to think about a retirement plan if you are serious about running your practice as a small business over the remainder of your career and to fully incorporate a retirement plan into the business plan.

Of course, for most it will be necessary to consult in this field to advise on the development of an investment portfolio based on your unique situation and needs. The aspects to consider include the current level of personal assets, the income needed at retirement, the ability to make regular deposits in a plan when the cash flow is not always steady, and the development of a portfolio of investments to spread the risk over several investment areas. We would all like to think that we could sell our business when we retire. For most nurses in business, it is probably not realistic to rely on the sale of the business to fund retirement.

TALKING AROUND THE CAMP-FIRE

Over the last 2½ years I have enjoyed every venture I have been involved in. Let me tell you a little about my business. I have been in my own practice since November 1995 and have found the experience to be rewarding, challenging, exciting, creative, and perhaps the best time of all my professional life. As a result of preparing my business plan I discerned that there were three core areas of my business: consulting in health service planning, education, and professional development.

Consulting

About 6 weeks into my business venture, I was offered a significant consultancy. I knew that the project would provide the type of experience I could build on over time. This consultancy proved to be a wonderful experience. The project was focused on developing a long-term strategy for the recruitment of nurses to rural practice as a career. It involved meeting and interviewing a number of nursing professionals in key organizations, writing a discussion paper, facilitating a workshop, writing a detailed report, and presenting the key recommendations to the board of the organization that commissioned the consultancy.

At the outset I never dreamed that the report would be so well received that it would be published and launched by a prominent member of the nursing profession. A media release was issued by the organization that commissioned the project and I was interviewed both by the press and several radio stations. Over the last 2 years many of the recommendations have been implemented.

This experience was profound both in establishing my presence as a nurse in private practice and in giving a tremendous boost to my self-esteem and confidence in what I could deliver as a consultant. I have had the opportunity to consult on several projects including reviewing and revising strategic plans, reviewing a nursing education service in a hospital, identifying competencies and assessment criteria for registered nurses practicing in the field of care of the aged, and collaborating on the development of methods to cost clinical pathways. Many of these projects involved the submission of a proposal and a budget. All of them came to me through my professional network.

Education

Sessional teaching has been an interest and part-time activity of mine over several years. As a result of this previous work, I had built up a network of academic contacts. So part of my marketing strategy was to write to contacts and other nurses in academic settings, to express my interest and availability to participate in the delivery of their programs. During the last 2 years I have worked at more than six different universities and have had contact with undergraduate students, RNs in degree articulation programs, nurses studying for an honors degree before proceeding to higher level studies, and nonnurses who are studying health administration. Some of this work has involved marking papers for students undertaking studies by distance education. I learn so much from each of these experiences, in addition to keeping up with the response of nurses and others to the very significant changes occurring in the health care industry.

Professional Development Programs

Today more than ever professionals must keep up to date with changes and be open to new experiences and learning to develop new knowledge and skills for career development. Professional development is one area I enjoy very much. However, in this era of quantum change in organizations there is much competition and it is a continuing challenge to my ingenuity. For several reasons I have found, that at this point, it is best to collaborate with other nurses to develop and deliver professional development programs. Action or experiential learning is the obvious choice when working with professionals, and as a team each member brings different skills to a program and relates differently to participants. Also a team approach provides backup for those occasions when plans fail. As part of the focus on professional development, I have also planned several conferences and provided advice on career development.

Networks—International and Local

Recently I have had the opportunity to act as the agent for two nurses who work internationally. This has been a wonderful experience and allows me to both use and develop my network. Of course the timing of calls and faxes with these colleagues requires working across several time zones and working late hours on some days. I was fortunate to be offered a 2-year contract as the administrative officer with a national nursing organization. This role provided me with the opportunity to learn from new experiences. This work has ensured a steady cash flow during the early days of my business.

Part of my networking activity includes being actively involved in several professional nursing organizations. Professional involvement is a critical way to keep up with what is happening locally and understand issues nurses have to deal with on a day-to-day basis. Conversely, I bring a new dimension to discussions because I am outside the system and can take a different perspective.

There are four discoveries I have made in my business: first, the endless opportunities that exist (in part because of the nature of structural and other changes in the health care system) for nurses to take their knowledge and skill outside their traditional areas of practice; then, second, there is the enormous satisfaction that comes from discovering that other people and organizations value the skills and perspective one brings to a problem situation; third, it is always rewarding to see others learn as a result of one's personal contribution; and I suppose finally and very personally is the fact that one is both contributing to and learning from each assignment and that insight and experience from practice can be used to develop the business.

EXPLORING ALONG THE WAY

When traveling it is always rewarding to take a side tour down a lane or along a road, especially when something tells you to go just a little further and see what awaits around the bend. I've never been hang-gliding but I think I know how it might feel. When one starts out one has a few trial flights to develop a sense for the ways in which the air currents take you up and down and sometimes a bit too close to the mountain and of course landing always calls for more than a little precision.

Several years ago I met and have stayed in close contact with two colleagues in the United States. Over the past few years, I have sought a number of opportunities for each of them to visit Australia to conduct conferences and workshops. But one never knows what the market response will be to the selected topic, the location, or the timing. However, that has not deterred me from continuing to seek opportunities to present new information to the nursing profession from acknowledged leaders in the field. So, though it takes a while to develop the skills of hang-gliding, the challenge is there to ride the currents and see what happens. To date I've not had a crash-landing although it has been close. But experience has taught me to ride the currents and enjoy the up-draft and worry about the down-drafts when they happen. Of course if it looks like it's not a day to fly one cancels the flight. There will be another day!

White Water Rafting (More than Getting your Feet Wet)

And then there is white water rafting. It is not something I have done in real life but I have tried it in my business. We got very wet, laughed a lot, navigated the rapids, survived the day, and learned from the experience. Recently, an experienced and respected nursing colleague and I undertook a small joint venture in 'action learning' and we had an interesting ride. We had planned a workshop in the metropolitan area; another colleague suggested that we also schedule one in a rural location. Competing with yourself is not usually recommended, but on this occasion it was successful. Interestingly, we had more participants at the rural workshop than in the metropolitan group and, of course, each was a different ride. Yes, we traversed the rapids and got very wet but we were not thrown out of the raft. Initially we did not have the registrations we wanted, and my colleague missed the train we were to take on the first day. But the show must go on, so I spent the 2-hour train ride reworking the program, hoping she would arrive by lunch time. When she arrived she was ill with the flu and spent 2 hours in the emergency room. However, when she led the afternoon session, the program proceeded on schedule.

Jay Walking (In Search of Chocolate)

When you are walking along the road there are so many things to see and wonder about. However, at times it takes discipline to resist not stopping to examine each opportunity but just to aimlessly wander along. One will soon find the Cheshire Cat sitting smiling when an opportunity has been passed by and not picked up and examined. You get very tired if you keep walking and don't stop and look and shake every bush you walk past and see what falls out. Sometimes you have to shake that bush more than once and at other times you need to cross the road to shake a bush over there.

But, be careful when something falls out of the bush. Consider what can be achieved with this business opportunity? What are the risks? Does one have the skills? Will it lighten the financial load or could it become a burden? The world of private practice abounds with opportunities for business and we can accommodate almost every one we encounter if we understand the values that guide our practice.

I take an opportunity only if it fits with my business values, and I believe I can carry the project through to completion. This same principle is applied when several projects present at the same time. Time, as we know, has an uncanny way of adjusting many aspects of our lives and so it is with business opportunities. Take the time to cross the road in search of chocolate. Take up the opportunities you feel you can carry and time will work out the logistics. The feeling is like eating great chocolate.

PICKING UP PROVISIONS

As a result of the various work, study, and learning opportunities I have had during my career, my reference point will always be outside the place where I practice. I continue to seek and to draw on new and different experiences to further develop my understanding of my personal and professional world.

Professional Development

During our private practice journey we need to nourish and renew our professional competence as well as our soul. Throughout my career I have considered making time for professional growth and development an absolute necessity and frequently this has meant that I have funded much of my own professional development. This decision has enabled me both to participate and present at conferences in Australia and other countries and has facilitated the development of an extensive network of professional and personal friendships.

Working alone, as most consultants do, can be an isolating experience and can give one a distorted sense of one's competency and expertise. Attention to the development of both the professional and personal self should be considered as an investment in the practice and business. The outlay of time and money, if planned and used wisely, helps to build the platform for the next stage of the development of the business. As a proclaimed expert in a field, one is required to stay on top of new information and skills to continue to be a credible authority in area of expertise.

One has to use common sense and judgment because continuing professional development costs money. Therefore, it behooves the nurse business owner to know what is being offered in the field, who is offering programs, and how attendance at various programs may not only fit into the work schedule but also yield other benefits. Of course, at times difficult decisions may need to be made, e.g., whether to attend a professional development opportunity or to accept the offer for further work and recognition. These decisions need to be made with the knowledge of the opportunity cost, i.e., what may yield the better result in the long run. Of course, another extremely important point must be considered in this area. Networking is an opportunity to find out what is happening in the market place and to sell yourself.

Networking

Networking is the art of acquiring and sharing information and ideas to help in your business and other people in theirs. Networking takes time and commitment but yields results that money alone cannot deliver. After providing a competent and professional service, networking is probably the next most important activity one can undertake in building a practice as a business. Networking puts you in front of people; it puts you in touch not only with people you know, but, perhaps more importantly, also with people you don't know and also with people who know someone you know.

To date all of my work as a consultant, teacher, and agent has come to me from my network. I have not advertised. However, I always carry a supply of business cards and distribute them freely. One never knows when they will be used as a referral point in another network. Now, the skill of networking didn't just happen. Networking has been my hobby and passion for several years. I suppose my business slogan could be described as *bringing people together.* For those who find a crowd of strangers a social challenge, think of the situation as a potential business opportunity and everyone there as potential clients, all of whom want to know you and what you have to offer to help solve problems in their organization. And you have just the service they need.

Reenergizing at Days End

Managing your own business is a full-time, complex, exciting, consuming, and sometimes draining activity. The owner has the responsibility for scanning the environment, identifying new prospects, planning projects, executing and delivering the service, and evaluating the outcome. From the very first day in business I have found it helpful and on most days essential to purposely take the time when I arrive home to sit, relax, and let all that happened that day wash over me, reflecting on what has happened, what went well, what didn't go according to plan and why, and to discern the potential and implications of each. By taking this approach, I sleep well and I don't wake in the middle of the night with a thousand thoughts racing through my mind. I awake feeling rested and prepared for whatever may happen that day. I have also developed a program of walking several mornings each week to keep fit and allow time to think about other aspects of my life and what I want to achieve.

BEYOND THE HORIZON

What lies beyond the horizon of the world of private practice? Many, many opportunities and also some mirages! The challenge is to discern what is a mirage and what is real and importantly to recognize an opportunity before it has passed by and has become a silhouette on the horizon behind you. But what if there are only mirages? Well, you may think the earth is flat and feel that you are going to fall off the edge. It happens to almost everyone who has dared to set out on the journey. What do you do if you keep finding the world is flat? How do you keep walking on?

There are a few things to be conscious of and believe at all times. At the beginning of the journey it is the dream, the vision of the journey, the commitment to running your business and the energy and freedom that can bring to the individual. Then there is the business plan, that map to the future without which one will surely be lost and die in the wilderness. Appreciate your unique perspective of your world, your experience, and what you learn on your journey. Understand that every time one problem is solved another one emerges and that you are passing by and are ready to take up the opportunities and challenges with integrity and all the innovation, energy, and confidence you have within you. I look forward to meeting other business nurses on my continuing journey and comparing notes on our various experiences.

BON VOYAGE!

INDEX